WENNER-GREN CENTER
INTERNATIONAL SYMPOSIUM SERIES

VOLUME 27

SENSORY FUNCTIONS OF THE SKIN IN PRIMATES

With special reference to Man

Already published in this series:

OLFACTION AND TASTE
    Edited by Y. Zotterman, 1963.
LIGHTING PROBLEMS IN HIGHWAY TRAFFIC
    Edited by E. Ingelstam, 1963.
THE STRUCTURE AND METABOLISM OF THE PANCREATIC ISLETS
    Edited by S. E. Brolin, B. Hellman and H. Knutson, 1964.
TOBACCO ALKALOIDS AND RELATED COMPOUNDS
    Edited by U. S. von Euler, 1965.
MECHANISMS OF RELEASE OF BIOGENIC AMINES
    Edited by U. S. von Euler, S. Rosell and B. Uvnäs, 1966.
COMPARATIVE LEUKAEMIA RESEARCH
    Edited by G. Winqvist, 1966.
THE FUNCTIONAL ORGANIZATION OF THE COMPOUND EYE
    Edited by C. G. Bernhard, 1966.
OLFACTION AND TASTE II
    Edited by T. Hayashi, 1967.
MAGNETIC RESONANCE IN BIOLOGICAL SYSTEMS
    Edited by A. Ehrenberg, B. G. Malmström and T. Vanngard, 1967.
STRUCTURE AND FUNCTION OF INHIBITORY NEURONAL MECHANISMS
    Edited by C. von Euler, S. Skoglund and U. Söderberg, 1967.
GROUND WATER PROBLEMS
    Edited by E. Eriksson, Y. Gustafsson and K. Nilsson, 1968.
PHYSIOLOGY AND PATHOPHYSIOLOGY OF PLASMA PROTEIN METABOLISM
    Edited by G. Birke, R. Norberg and L.-O. Plantin, 1969.
THE POSSIBILITIES OF CHARTING MODERN LIFE
    Edited by S. Erixon *and Assisted by* G. Ardwidsson and H. Hvarfner, 1970.
EVALUATION OF NOVEL PROTEIN PRODUCTS
    Edited by A. E. Bender, R. Kihlberg, B. Lofqvist and L. Munck, 1970.
VESTIBULAR FUNCTION ON EARTH AND IN SPACE
    Edited by J. Stahle, 1970.
THE STRUCTURE OF METABOLISM OF THE PANCREATIC ISLETS
    Edited by S. Falkner, B. Hellman, and I. B. Taljedal, 1970.
HUMAN ANTI-HUMAN GAMMAGLOBULINS
    Edited by R. Grubb and G. Samuelsson, 1971.
STRUCTURE AND FUNCTION OF OXIDATION-REDUCTION ENZYMES
    Edited by A. Åkeson and A. Ehrenberg, 1972.
CERVICAL PAIN
    Edited by N. Emmelin and Y. Zotterman, 1972.
ORAL PHYSIOLOGY
    Edited by N. Emmelin and Y. Zotterman, 1972.
CIRCUMPOLAR PROBLEMS: HABITAT, ECONOMY AND SOCIAL RELATIONS IN THE ARCTIC
    Edited by G. Berg *et al.*, 1973.
DYNAMICS OF DEGENERATION AND GROWTH IN NEURONES
    Edited by K. Fuxe, L. Olson and Y. Zotterman, 1974.
THE FUNCTIONAL ANATOMY OF THE SPERMATOZOON
    Edited by B. A. Afzelius, 1974.
BASIC MECHANISMS OF OCULAR MOTILITY AND THEIR CLINICAL IMPLICATIONS
    Edited by G. Lennerstrand, Paul Bach-y-Rita, C. C. Collins, A. Jampolsky, and A. B. Scott, 1975.
ANTIPSYCHOTIC DRUGS: PHARMACODYNAMICS AND PHARMACOKINETICS
    Edited by G. Sedvall, B. Uvnäs, and Y. Zotterman, 1976.
GASTROINTESTINAL EMERGENCIES
    Edited by F.R. Bárány and A. Torsoli, 1976.

SENSORY FUNCTIONS OF THE SKIN IN PRIMATES

With special reference to Man

*Proceedings of the International Symposium
held at
The Wenner-Gren Center, Stockholm,
January 1976*

Edited by
Yngve Zotterman
Wenner-Gren Center, Stockholm

PERGAMON PRESS
OXFORD · NEW YORK · TORONTO · SYDNEY · PARIS · FRANKFURT

U.K.	Pergamon Press Ltd., Headington Hill Hall, Oxford OX3 0BW, England
U.S.A.	Pergamon Press Inc., Maxwell House, Fairview Park, Elmsford, New York 10523, U.S.A.
CANADA	Pergamon of Canada Ltd., P.O. Box 9600, Don Mills M3C 2T9, Ontario, Canada
AUSTRALIA	Pergamon Press (Aust.) Pty. Ltd., 19a Boundary Street, Rushcutters Bay, N.S.W. 2011, Australia
FRANCE	Pergamon Press SARL, 24 rue des Ecoles, 75240 Paris, Cedex 05, France
WEST GERMANY	Pergamon Press GmbH, 6242 Kronberg-Taunus, Pferdstrasse 1, Frankfurt-am-Main, West Germany

Copyright © 1976 Pergamon Press

All Rights Reserved. No part of this publication may be reproduced, stored in a retrieval system or transmitted in any form or by any means: electronic, electrostatic, magnetic tape, mechanical, photocopying, recording or otherwise, without permission in writing from the publishers

First edition 1976

Library of Congress Cataloging in Publication Data

Main entry under title:

Sensory functions of the skin in primates, with special reference to man

(Wenner-Gren Center international symposium series ; v. 27)

1. Skin--Congresses. 2. Sense-organs--Congresses.
I. Zotterman, Yngve. II. Sweden. Statens medicinska forskningsrad. III. Wenner-Gren Center IV. Series.

QP450.S46 1976   599'.8'04182   76-20572

ISBN 0-08-021208-5

In order to make this volume available as economically and rapidly as possible the author's typescript has been reproduced in its original form. This method unfortunately has its typographical limitations but it is hoped that they in no way distract the reader.

International Symposium on
SENSORY FUNCTIONS OF THE SKIN IN PRIMATES
held at Wenner-Gren Center Stockholm January 13-15 1976

*Sponsored by
The Swedish/Medical Research Council,
The Wenner-Gren Center Foundation*

Printed in Great Britain by A. Wheaton & Co. Exeter

CONTENTS

Contributors and Invited Participants. ix

Opening Address. 1
    Y. Zotterman

Natural and Paranatural Stimulation of Sensory Receptors. 3
    A.S. Paintal

Towards a Theory of Sympathetic-Sensory Coupling: 15
The Primary Sensory Neuron as a Feedback Target of
the Sympathetic Terminal.
    M. Santini

The "Receptripse": The Desmosome-Like Lamellar-Axonal 37
Junction Subserving Mechano-Electric Transduction and
Effecting the Sympathetic Actions on the Pacinian Sensor.
    M. Santini

MECHANOCEPTION

Rapidly Adapting Cutaneous Mechanoreceptors (RA): Coding, 45
Variability and Information Transmission.
    H. Dickhaus, M. Sassen and
    M. Zimmermann

Coding of Velocity of Skin Identation in Man and Monkey. 55
A Perceptual-Neurophysiological Correlation.
    O. Franzén and U. Lindblom

Differential Excitation of Dorsal Horn and Substantia 67
Gelatinosa Marginal Neurons by Primary Afferent Units
with Fine (Aδ and C) Fibers.
    T. Kumazawa and E.R. Perl

The Spinocervical Tract: Organization and Neuronal 91
Morphology.
    A.G. Brown

Tactile Thresholds of Normal and Blind Subjects on Stimulation of Finger Pads with Short Mechanical Pulses of Variable Amplitude.
    U. Lindblom and B. Lindström   105

Tactile Intensity Functions in Patients with Sutured Peripheral Nerve.
    O. Franzén and U. Lindblom   113

Somatosensory Potentials from the Exposed Cortex in Monkey and from the Scalp in Man Related to the Sensory Magnitude of Tactual Stimulation.
    O. Franzén   119

Microneurography in Man.
    K.-E. Hagbarth   129

Studies on Cutaneous A and C Fiber Afferents, Skin Nerve Blocks and Perception.
    R.G. Hallin and H.E. Torebjörk   137

A Method for Mechanical Stimulation of Skin Receptors.
    G. Westling, R. Johansson and Å.B. Vallbo   151

Skin Mechanoreceptors in the Human Hand: Receptive Field Characteristics.
    R. Johansson   159

Skin Mechanoreceptors in the Human Hand: An Inference of Some Population Properties.
    R. Johansson and Å.B. Vallbo   171

Skin Mechanoreceptors in the Human Hand: Neural and Psychophysical Thresholds.
    Å.B. Vallbo and R. Johansson   185

Stimulus-Response Functions of Primary Afferents and Psychophysical Intensity Estimation on Mechanical Skin Stimulation in the Human Hand.
    M. Knibestöl and Å.B. Vallbo   201

Mechanoreceptive Unit Activity in Human Skin Nerves Correlated with Touch and Vibratory Sensations.
    T. Järvilehto, H. Hämäläinen and J. Kekoni   215

Differences in Timing of Corticocuneate and Corticogracile Actions.
    J.D. Cole and G. Gordon   231

Cellular Mechanisms in the Parietal Cortex in Alert Monkey.
    J. Hyvärinen   241

THERMOCEPTION

Response of Central Trigeminal Neurons to Cutaneous Thermal Stimulation. 263
    D.A. Poulos and J.T. Molt

Thermosensory Mechanisms in the Spinal Cord of Monkeys. 285
    A. Iggo and R.L. Ramsey

Correlations of Temperature Sensitivity in Man and Monkey. A first Approximation. 305
    D.R. Kenshalo

Correlations of Neural Activity and Thermal Sensation in Man. 331
    H. Hensel

Conduction in the Afferent Thermal Pathways of Man. 355
    H. Fruhstorfer

The Origin and Projections of a Spinal Nociceptive and Thermoreceptive Pathway. 367
    D.L. Trevino

Role of Thermoreceptors in Thermoregulation. 379
    T.H. Benzinger

Temperature Sensations among Other Sensations to the Stimuli of Focused Ultrasound. The Comparison with the Temperature Sensations by Mechanical Stimuli. 399
    E.M. Tsirulnikov and E.E. Shchekanov

NOCICEPTION

The Development in Regenerating Cutaneous Nerves of C Fiber Receptors Responding to Noxious Heating of the Skin. 415
    H. Dickhaus, M. Zimmermann and Y. Zotterman

Pharmacological Modulation of the Discharge of Nociceptive C Fibers. 427
    H.O. Handwerker

The Effects of Anti-Inflammatory Agents on the Responses and the Sensitization of unmyelinated (C) Fiber Polymodal Nociceptors. 441
    J.S. King, P. Gallant, V. Myerson and E.R. Perl

Mechanisms of Muscle Pain: A Comparison with Cutaneous Nociception. 463
    K.-D. Kniffki, S. Mense and R.F. Schmidt

Skin Receptors Supplied by Unmyelinated (C) Fibers in Man. 475
    H.E. Torebjörk and R.G. Hallin

Preliminary Observations on the Pathophysiology of 489
Hyperalgesia in the Causalgic Pain Syndrome.
  G. Wallin, H.E. Torebjörk and
  R.G. Hallin

Single Afferent C Fiber Activity in the Human Nerve during 503
Painful and Non Painful Skin Stimulation with Radiant Heat.
  J. Van Hees

Temperature Sensitivity and Pain Thresholds in Patients 507
with Peripheral Neuropathy.
  H. Fruhstorfer, J.M. Goldberg,
  U. Lindblom and W.G. Schmidt

Modulation of Clinical and Experimental Pain in Man by 521
Electrical Stimulation of Thalamic Periventricular Gray.
  J. Gybels and P. Cosyns

Effects of Multifocal Brain Stimulation on Pain and 531
Somatosensory Functions.
  J. Boethius, U. Lindblom,
  B.A. Meyerson and L. Widén

Activation Patterns Induced in the Dominant Hemisphere by 549
Skin Stimulation.
  D.H. Ingvar, I. Rosén, M. Eriksson
  and D. Elmqvist

Evidence Pertaining to an Endogenous Mechanism of Pain 561
Inhibition in the Central Nervous System.
  J.C. Liebeskind, G.J. Giesler Jr
  and G. Urca

Acupuncturelike Electroanalgesia in TNS-Resistant Chronic 575
Pain.
  M. Eriksson and B. Sjölund

Immunohistochemical Studies on the Distribution of Substance P 583
and Somatostatin in Primary Sensory Neurons.
  T. Hökfelt, J.-O. Kellerth, R. Elde,
  R. Luft, O. Johansson, G. Nilsson,
  B. Pernow and A. Arimura

Concluding Discussion: WHAT ABOUT THE FUTURE? 603

Editor's note

In the interests of making these contributions available as rapidly as possible, no subject index to the volume has been produced.

CONTRIBUTORS AND INVITED PARTICIPANTS

Theodor Benzinger
United States Department of Commerce
National Bureau of Standards
WASHINGTON D C 20234
USA

Jörgen Boivie
Department of Anatomy
Karolinska Institute
S-104 01 STOCKHOLM
Sweden

Ernst Brodin
Department of Pharmacology
Karolinska Institute
S-104 01 STOCKHOLM
Sweden

Alan Brown
Department of Physiology
Royal School of Veterinary Studies
University of Edinburgh
EDINBURGH EH9 1QH
Scotland

Hartmut Dickhaus
Institute of Physiology II
University of Heidelberg
Neuenheimer Feld 326
D-6900 HEIDELBERG
West Germany

Lennart Edwall
Faculty of Odontology
Karolinska Institute
S-111 60 STOCKHOLM
Sweden

Dan Elmqvist
Department of Clinical Neurophysiology
University Hospital
S-221 85 LUND
Sweden

Margareta Eriksson
Department of Clinical Neurophysiology
University Hospital
S-221 85 LUND
Sweden

Curt von Euler
Department of Neurophysiology
Karolinska Institute
S-104 01 STOCKHOLM
Sweden

Åke Flock
Department of Physiology II
Karolinska Institute
S-104 01 STOCKHOLM
Sweden

Ove Franzén
Department of Psychology
University of Uppsala
S-752 20 UPPSALA
Sweden

Heinrich Fruhstorfer
Institute of Physiology
University of Marburg
Deutschhausstrasse 2
D-355 MARBURG/Lahn
West Germany

George Gordon
University Laboratory of Physiology
OXFORD
England

Ragnar Granit
Department of Neurophysiology
Karolinska Institute
S-104 01 STOCKHOLM
Sweden

Jan Gybels
Department of Neurosurgery
A.Z. Sint Rafaël
Kapucijnenvoer 35
B-3000 LEUVEN
Belgium

Karl-Erik Hagbarth
Department of Clinical Neuro-
 physiology
Academic Hospital
S-750 14 UPPSALA
Sweden

Rolf Hallin
Department of Clinical Neuro-
 physiology
Academic Hospital
S-750 14 UPPSALA
Sweden

Hermann Handwerker
Institute of Physiology II
Neuenheimerfeld 326
D-69 HEIDELBERG
West Germany

Johan van Hees
Department of Neurosurgery
A.Z. Sint Rafaël
Kapucijnenvoer 35
B-3000 LEUVEN
Belgium

Göran Hellekant
Department of Physiology
Veterinärhögskolan
S-750 07 UPPSALA
Sweden

Herbert Hensel
Institute of Physiology
University of Marburg
Deutschhausstrasse 2
D-355 MARBURG
West Germany

Martin Holmdahl
Department of Anesthesiology
Academic Hospital
S-750 14 UPPSALA
Sweden

Eddy Holmgren
Department of Physiology
University of Göteborg
S-400 33 GÖTEBORG
Sweden

Juhani Hyvärinen
Institute of Physiology
University of Helsinki
Siltavuorenpenger 20 a
SF-00170 HELSINKI
Finland

Heikki Hämäläinen
Department of Psychology
University of Helsinki
Ritarikatu 5
SF-00170 HELSINKI
Finland

Ainsley Iggo
Department of Physiology
Faculty of Veterinary Medicine
University of Edinburgh
EDINBURGH EH9 1QH
Scotland

David Ingvar
Department of Clinical Neuro-
 physiology
University Hospital
S-221 85 LUND
Sweden

Elzbieta Jankowska
Department of Physiology
University of Göteborg
S-400 33 GÖTEBORG
Sweden

Roland Johansson
Department of Physiology
University of Umeå
S-901 87 UMEÅ
Sweden

Timo Järvilehto
Department of Psychology
University of Helsinki
Ritarikatu 5
SF-00170 HELSINKI
Finland

Contributors and Invited Participants

Jan-Olof Kellerth
Department of Anatomy
Karolinska Institute
S-104 01 STOCKHOLM
Sweden

Dan Kenshalo
Department of Psychology
Florida State University
TALLAHASSEE
Florida 32306
USA

Martin Knibestöl
Department of Physiology
University of Umeå
S-901 87 UMEÅ
Sweden

Klaus Kniffki
Department of Physiology
University of Kiel
Olshausenstrasse 40/60
D-23 KIEL
West Germany

Sven Landgren
Department of Physiology
University of Umeå
S-901 87 UMEÅ
Sweden

John Liebeskind
Department of Psychology, UCLA
LOS ANGELES
California 90024
USA

Olov Lindahl
Department of Orthopedic Surgery
University Hospital
S-581 85 LINKÖPING
Sweden

Ulf Lindblom
Department of Neurology
Huddinge Hospital
S-141 86 HUDDINGE
Sweden

Sivert Lindström
Department of Physiology
University of Göteborg
S-400 33 GÖTEBORG
Sweden

Siegfried Mense
Department of Physiology
University of Kiel
Olshausenstrasse 40/60
D-23 KIEL
West Germany

Björn Meyerson
Department of Neurosurgery
Karolinska Hospital
S-104 01 STOCKHOLM
Sweden

Bengt Nilsson
Department of Clinical Neuro-
  physiology
Södersjukhuset
S- 100 64 STOCKHOLM
Sweden

Göran Nilsson
Department of Pharmacology
Karolinska Institute
S-104 01 STOCKHOLM
Sweden

Akintola Odutola
Department of Physiology
University of Göteborg
S-400 33 GÖTEBORG
Sweden

Leif Olgart
Department of Pharmacology
Karolinska Institute
S-104 01 STOCKHOLM
Sweden

David Ottoson
Department of Physiology II
Karolinska Institute
S-104 01 STOCKHOLM
Sweden

Autar Paintal
Vallabhbhai Patel Chest Institute
University of Delhi
DELHI-110007
India

Edward Perl
University of North Carolina
Department of Physiology
CHAPEL HILL
North Carolina 27514
USA

Dennis Poulos
Albany Medical College
Department of Neurosurgery
ALBANY N Y 12108
USA

Ingmar Rosén
Department of Clinical Neuro-
  physiology
University Hospital
S-221 85 LUND
Sweden

Maurizio Santini
Department of Pharmacology
Via Vanvitelli 32
I-20129 MILANO
Italy

Robert Schmidt
Department of Physiology
University of Kiel
Olshausenstrasse 40/60
D-23 KIEL
West Germany

Bengt Sjölund
Department of Physiology
University of Lund
S-223 62 LUND
Sweden

Erik Torebjörk
Department of Clinical Neuro-
  physiology
Academic Hospital
S-750 14 UPPSALA
Sweden

Daniel Trevino
Department of Physiology
University of North Carolina
CHAPEL HILL
North Carolina 27514
USA

Börje Uvnäs
Department of Pharmacology
Karolinska Institute
S-104 01 STOCKHOLM
Sweden

Åke Vallbo
Department of Physiology
University of Umeå
S-901 87 UMEÅ
Sweden

Gunnar Wallin
Department of Clinical Neuro-
  physiology
Academic Hospital
S-750 14 UPPSALA
Sweden

Göran Westling
Department of Physiology
University of Umeå
S-901 87 UMEÅ
Sweden

Lennart Widén
Department of Clinical Neuro-
  physiology
Karolinska Hospital
S-104 01 STOCKHOLM

Manfred Zimmermann
Institute of Physiology II
University of Heidelberg
Neuenheimer Feld 326
D-6900 HEIDELBERG
West Germany

Yngve Zotterman
Wenner-Gren Center
Sveavägen 166
S-113 46 STOCKHOLM
Sweden

OPENING ADDRESS

Y. ZOTTERMAN

Somebody reminded me the other day that it is 50 years ago that Adrian and I started leading off the action potentials from plantar nerves of the cat in response to mechanical stimulations of the skin. That was at the end of January 1926. We had just finished a bit of work on muscle spindles in the frog. We had recorded from a single afferent fibre to natural stimulation. That was on the 3rd of November 1925 when as old Linnaeus once said we were allowed to look into God's secret chamber of knowledge.

In January 1926 Adrian planned to lead off from the optic nerve of the cat and we tried to split up the optic nerve in fine strands but we never succeeded in recording from any fibres in that nerve. After sacrificing some few cats we gave up and started to work on the plantar nerves of the cat. I remember how I said to Adrian: "What a pity that we did not succeed with the optic nerve." And that he replied: "Oh, never mind, it is better to turn to the skin; if we had succeeded with the optic nerve I might have been stuck to vision for the rest of my life."

Yesterday I rang up Lord Adrian in Trinity College in Cambridge and he was kind enough to send a message via the telephone. I am happy being able to give you his message from a tape record. Here it comes.

"I wish I could have come to this meeting to tell you how lucky we were fifty years ago amplifying potential changes in nerve and muscle fibres and how lucky I was to have some of the apparatus and such collaborators as Yngve Zotterman and later Detlev Bronk. If Bronk had lived I am sure he would have brought me over here today but perhaps we would have spent most of our time talking about Cambridge and Stockholm when we were young. I should certainly have been full of stories about the congress in Stockholm in 1926 when we turned out to the archipelago at midnight in Bertil Josephson's motorboat with my wife Hester, Brita Zotterman, Hugo Theorell and Pierre Gley. But now it is time to go down to the business. All I shall do is to send my love to Brita and Yngve and to wish you all a successful symposium in one of the most agreeable cities in the world".

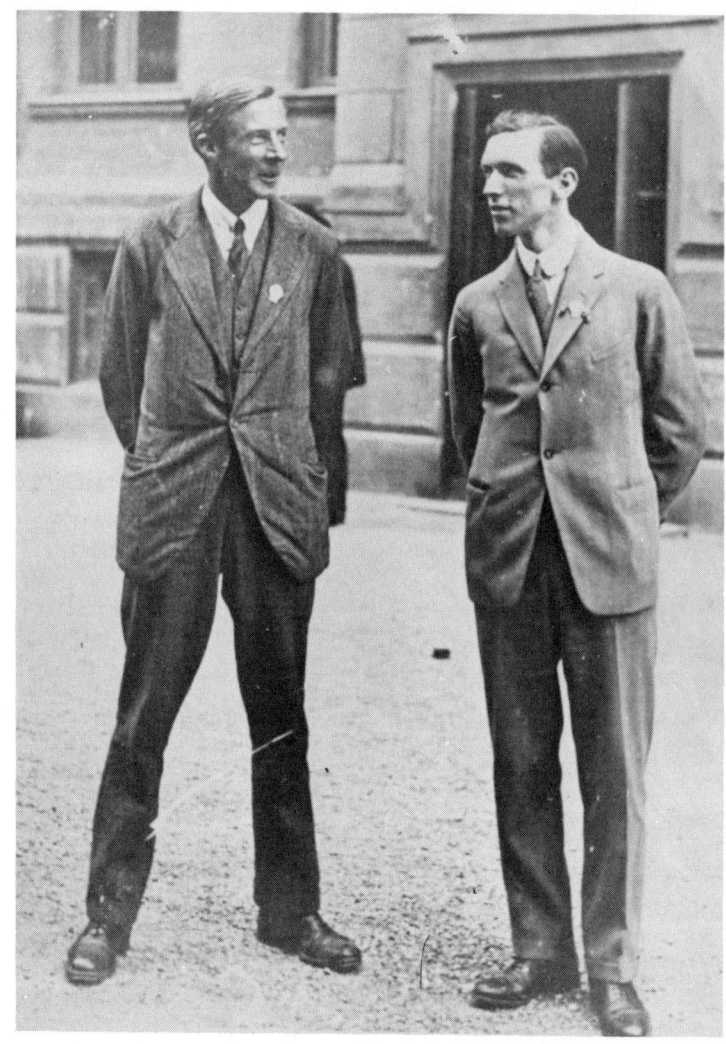

Edgar Douglas Adrian and Yngve Zotterman attending the XIIth International Congress of Physiology in Stockholm 1926.

NATURAL AND PARANATURAL STIMULATION OF SENSORY RECEPTORS

A. S. PAINTAL
Department of Physiology, Vallabhbhai Patel Chest Institute, Delhi University, Delhi-110007

Definitions

Ordinarily, a sensory receptor is stimulated by its natural stimulus ("adequate" stimulus*) *i.e.* that stimulus which by its unique effect on the receptor produces activity that bears a well-defined relation to the natural stimulus. As a result the receptor provides quantitative information about the intensity and rate of change of the natural stimulus (Adrian, 1928). For example, the natural stimulus of pulmonary stretch receptors is change in volume of air in the lungs (Adrian, 1933) and as shown in Fig. 1 the activity of these receptors is linearly related to the volume of lung inflation. Most of these receptors, in spite of the proximity of the heart and pulsatile vessels are not stimulated by movements of the heart and vessels in the thorax and lungs. However, there are some that, under certain conditions relating to lung volume or position of the thoracic viscera, are stimulated by such pulse-synchronous stimuli that occur under ordinary physiological conditions (Adrian, 1933; Whitteridge, 1948; Bianconi & Green, 1959). This results in the appearance of a pulse-synchronous discharge which may come and go at different lung volumes (Fig. 2) and which, quantitatively, bears no relation to intravascular pressures. Such stimuli, which occur physiologically under certain conditions and which play a minor, insignificant or inconstant role when compared to the natural stimulus, may be termed as paranatural stimuli.

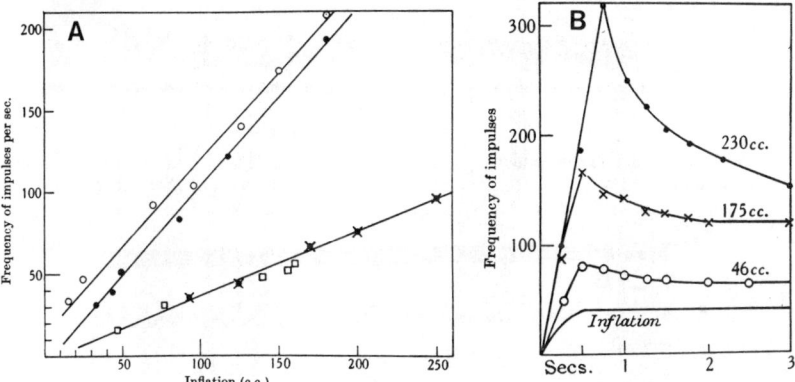

Fig. 1A. *Maximum discharge frequency in single pulmonary stretch fibres with varying inflations of lungs. Spinal cats. The two upper curves are from a small animal and show two series of measurements made within 10 min. The lower curve (also two series) is from a larger animal. (Adrian, 1933).*

Fig. 1B. *Frequency curves from a single fibre to show adaptation and responses varying with the stimulus (volume) (Adrian, 1933).*

Another behaviour of the same kind is to be seen in certain mesenteric Pacinian corpuscles which serve as vibration receptors — their natural stimulus being vibrations at a frequency of 20-1000 Hz (Sato, 1961). In view of their great sensitivity to vibrations (Hunt & McIntyre, 1960a; Hunt, 1961) it is not surprising that some of them are stimulated by transmitted arterial pulsations (Fig. 3). This was first reported by Gammon & Bronk (1935) and later further observations relating to it were made by Gernandt & Zotterman (1946) and Leitner & Perl (1964). The variable nature of the responses and the absence of a well defined relation to the pressure in the vessel (Fig. 4) indicates that the pulsatile stimulus can be regarded as a paranatural stimulus.

---

*The term 'adequate' stimulus was used by Sherrington initially (Sherrington, 1906) but subsequently he along with his collaborators, Creed, Denny-Brown, Eccles & Liddell omitted the term 'adequate' stimulus and preferred to use the term 'natural stimulus' (Creed *et al.*, 1932).

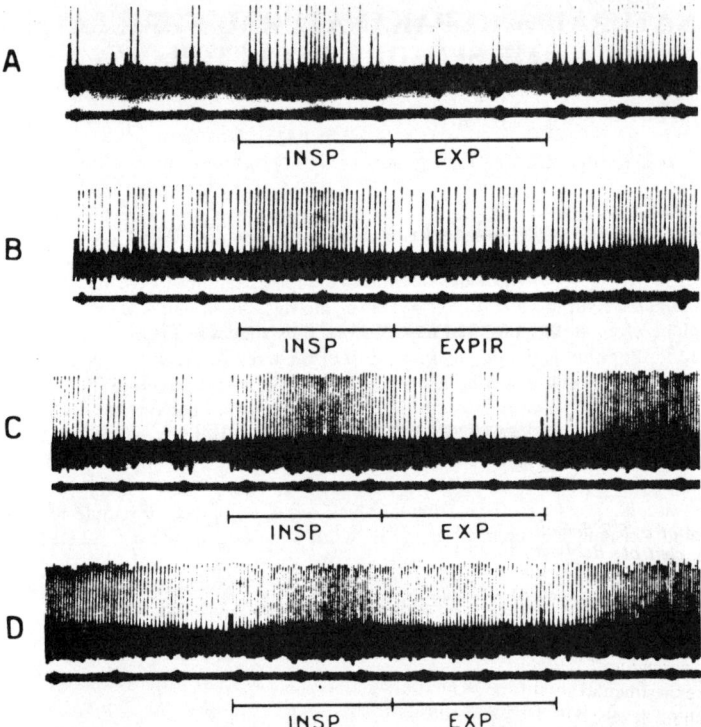

Fig. 2. Activity in a pulmonary fibre showing pulse-synchronous activity (due to paranatural stimulation) that disappears during inspiration. The lower trace in each record is e.c.g.—(From Bianconi & Green, 1959).

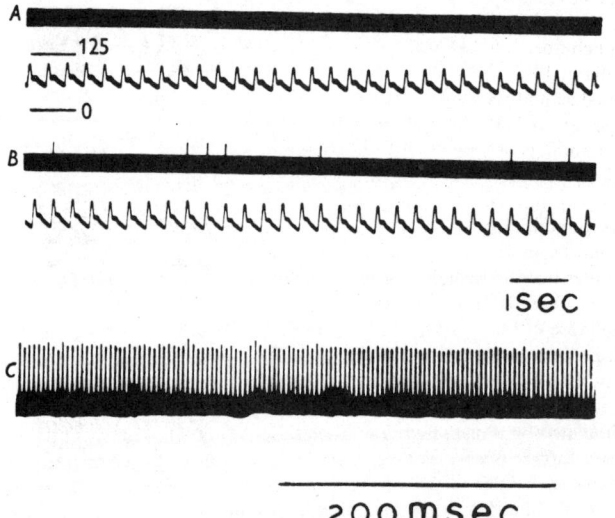

Fig. 3. Response of a T 12 afferent fibre (presumed to arise from a Pacinian corpuscle). A, control; B, after 10 ml of Plasmagel injected intravenously. Note the appearance of impulses with a fixed relation to the pressure pulse during certain cycles only. C, response to sinusoidal vibration at a nominal frequency of 300/sec (From Leitner & Perl, 1964).

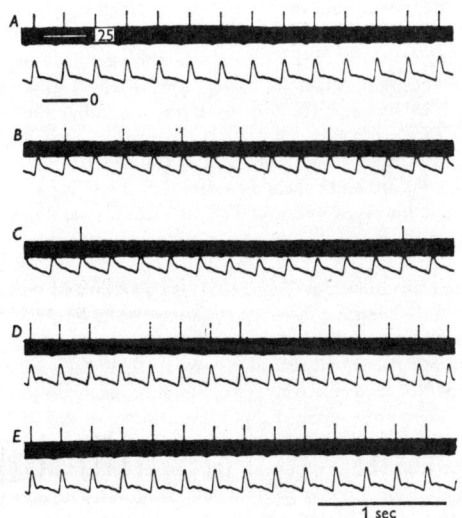

Fig. 4. Discharge of a T 7 dorsal root fibre (*presumed to arise from a Pacinian corpuscle*) *following injection of adrenaline. A, control; B 24 sec; C, 36 sec; D, 50, sec; E, 90 sec after intravenous injection of 10 µg adrenaline. Note there is no relation between activity and blood pressure. This fibre responded to sinusoidal vibration only when it was applied to a localized point in the 7th and 8th intercostal spaces. BP Calibration 0-125 mm Hg. (Leitner & Perl, 1964).*

Prevalence of paranatural stimuli
Under ordinary experimental conditions in anaesthetized animals the natural stimuli of certain types of receptors are below threshold levels but the paranatural stimulus is of sufficient magnitude to activate the endings. Therefore in the absence of knowledge regarding the natural stimulus erroneous conclusions have been arrived at in the past. Examples of such cases are the intestinal Pacinian corpuscles (Gammon & Bronk, 1935) and the Type J pulmonary receptors (Paintal, 1969b). In addition to these there exist several visceral receptors whose natural stimuli we do not know, but whose activity, *on the face of it*, seems to be manifested by paranatural stimulation. Examples of such endings are the epicardial receptors (Coleridge, Coleridge & Kidd, 1964; Sleight & Widdicombe, 1965; Oberg & Thoren, 1972) endings with 'sympathetic' afferent fibres (Brown, 1967; Brown & Malliani, 1971; Malliani *et al.*, 1973; Nishi & Takenaka, 1973; Nishi *et al.*, 1974; Uchida & Murao, 1974); the mediastinal receptors (Adrian, 1933; Widdicombe, 1954). Some of the receptors described recently by Coleridge *et al.* (1973) and Banzett, Coleridge, Coleridge & Kidd (1976) fall into this group. Most of these endings are apparently stimulated by movements in the respiratory and cardiovascular system but their activity bears no defined relation to lung volumes or intravascular or intracardiac pressures.

The Type J receptors (juxta-pulmonary capillary receptors) provide a good example of how misleading the paranatural stimuli can be under ordinary experimental conditions. It is now known that the likely natural stimulus of these endings is pulmonary congestion that occurs during exercise (Paintal, 1969b; 1970) but when they were first encountered they could be obviously stimulated only by chemical substances, notably phenyl-diguanide, and by collapse of the lungs in cats with open chest. They were therefore called deflation receptors (Paintal, 1955). Subsequently Coleridge, Coleridge & Luck (1965) found that they were stimulated by hyper-inflation of the lungs. Both the stimuli used were of an intensity that would occur only under extraordinary physiological circumstances. However because they are silent in the resting cat, there being no congestion, and the effects of brief periods of congestion were not as noteworthy as that of deflation (Paintal, 1955) the role of congestion was overshadowed till, in a subsequent study (Paintal, 1969b), it became obvious that congestion was the likely natural stimulus of these endings.

In the case of pulmonary stretch receptors and the vibration receptors it is easy to distinguish the paranatural stimulus from the natural stimulus because of the variable and inconstant responses produced by the former when compared to the well-defined relation of the response to the natural stimulus *i.e.* lung volume or vibration respectively. However, there are receptors both in the visceral group and the somatosensory group where it has not been established which is the natural stimulus and which is the paranatural stimulus. The difficulty arises when two qualitatively different types of stimuli produce generally comparable effects on a receptor *i.e.* both produce activity that varies with the intensity of the stimulus and are influenced by their rate of change and both occur under physiological conditions. A good example of this is the carotid chemoreceptor which is stimulated by both hypoxia and by hypercapnia (Black, McCloskey & Torrance, 1971; Fitzgerald & Parks, 1971; Fitzgerald, 1976; Lahiri & DeLaney, 1975; 1976). However, unlike the excitatory effect of fall in local P_{O_2}, the effect of increase in CO_2 tensions does not affect the aortic chemoreceptors within the physiological range in a similar way (Paintal & Riley, 1966; Sampson & Hainsworth, 1972; Fitzgerald, 1976). Indeed the effect of CO_2 is variable and inconstant and depends on several factors. Thus if it is assumed that each sensory receptor has only one natural stimulus then one would be justified in assuming that the local P_{O_2} is the natural stimulus and that CO_2 is the paranatural stimulus in aortic chemoreceptors.

The case of the gastric mucosal chemoreceptor (Iggo, 1957) is a particularly difficult one. In this case as shown by Iggo, the endings yield a slowly adapting discharge to *either* acidic or alkaline solutions (not both) applied to the mucosal surface of the stomach. The intensity of the discharge varies with the pH of the solution. However these endings are stimulated equally effectively by stroking the surface of the mucosa — even with cotton wool which can be regarded as a relatively light stimulus when compared to the nature of the gastric contents after a meal. It was therefore suggested that these endings signal the passage or presence of gastric contents and that such a process is facilitated by an appropriate pH of the gastric contents (Paintal, 1973). This conclusion fits in with the recent observations of Harding & Titchin (1975) who found mechanoreceptors in the thoracic oesophagus that were stimulated by acidic solutions and also by 2% NaCl. In both these instances one would be justified in concluding that the natural stimulus for the endings is the mechanical movement or presence of food and fluids and that the pH is a paranatural stimulus. Such endings also appear to be present in the dog's stomach as indicated by the observations of Takeshima (1974).

Paranatural stimuli of cutaneous receptors
Paranatural stimulation is also commonly seen in receptors of the skin. For example certain thermoreceptors are also stimulated by mechanical stimuli that can be assumed to occur under physiological conditions (Witt & Hensel, 1959; Bessou & Perl, 1969; Hensel & Kenshalo, 1969; Burgess & Perl, 1973). Contrariwise there are also mechanoreceptors that are influenced by changes in temperature (Hensel & Zotterman, 1951; Witt & Hensel, 1959; Iggo, 1959; 1960; Hensel *et al,*, 1969; Hunt & McIntyre, 1960 *b*). The slowly adapting mechanoreceptors of the monkey's skin which have a high sensitivity to mechanical stimuli are also stimulated by cooling the skin (Iggo, 1969). This is shown in Fig. 5 from which it is clear that the response to cooling is significant; on warming the skin the receptor is silenced. One could, when comparing its response to mechanical stimuli, conclude that cooling is a paranatural stimulus for this receptor. However, these receptors also have a static sensitivity to temperature which suggests that under constant mechanical stimulation, there is a relation between temperature and the static discharge of the receptor. Under these conditions, in borderline cases, it would not be easy to establish conclusively that cooling the skin is not the natural stimulus.

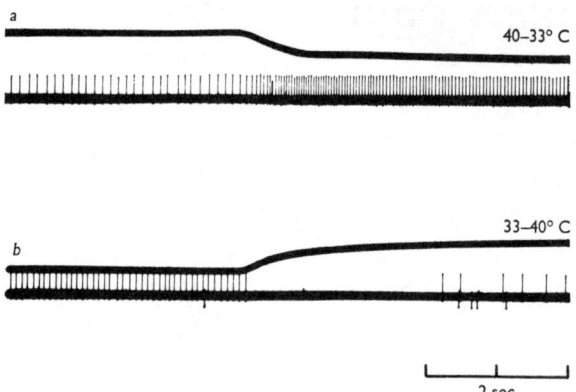

Fig. 5. Responses of a type II slowly adapting mechanoreceptor of monkey. In (a) is shown the steady discharge caused by the pressure of the thermode at 40°C; this is accelerated by the fall to 33°C. When the temperature was held at 33°C the discharge settled down to a new frequency and this was temporarily silenced when the skin temperature was raised to 40°C in (b). (Iggo, 1969).

There is much evidence to support the conclusion that the polymodal receptors of Bessou & Perl (1969) are nociceptive receptors since they are excited by noxious heat, certain chemical irritants, and by strong mechanical stimuli. Bessou & Perl (1969) imply that all these stimuli produce their effects by a common mechanism arising out of tissue damage. This leaves open the question as to what the actual natural stimulus of these receptors is. If one could, by further analysis of the responses produced by the various stimuli, separate the likely natural stimulus from the paranatural stimuli one could then proceed to investigate the mechanisms further. In this connection Bessou & Perl (1969) have suggested that all high threshold receptors of the integument should be regarded as nociceptors. This may not be helpful because a strong mechanical stimulus may be a paranatural stimulus of several types of cutaneous receptors with unknown natural stimuli. Such an approach might therefore impede the search for the natural stimulus, a point that is of particular importance in the case of "unclassified" or "inexcitable" receptors (Bessou & Perl, 1969).

MODE OF ACTION OF NATURAL AND PARANATURAL STIMULI

Natural stimuli
Natural stimuli produce their effects by acting on the sensory meter, of the sensory receptors complex, (Fig. 6), which filters out unsuitable signals. The meter (*e.g.* the corpuscular part of the Pacinian corpuscle) is deformed in magnitude and rate of change of the stimulus. This deformation is transmitted by suitable mechanical coupling to the generator region of the sensory ending (Fig. 6). The generator region is thereby mechanically deformed and this results in the flow of current between the generator region and the regenerative region of the ending where the propagated impulse is produced provided the strength of the generator current attains threshold level. In many instances the sensory meter consists of specialized cells or structures *e.g.* Pacinian corpuscle but in the vast majority of the endings of non-medullated fibres it must consist largely of elements of connective and epithelial tissue in which the endings lie (Paintal, 1971).

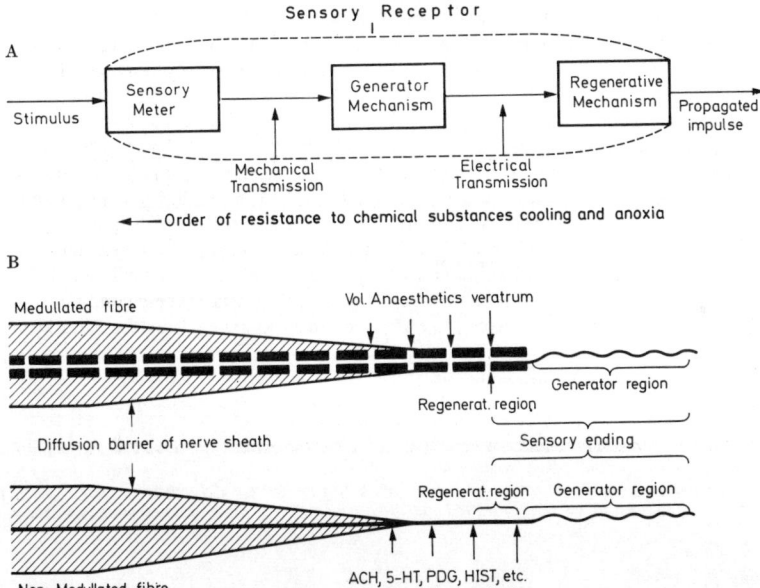

Fig. 6. *A, Mechanisms involved in the excitation of sensory receptors and their relative resistance to chemical substances, cooling and anoxia (Paintal, 1971a). B. Schematic diagram of sensory endings of medullated and non-medullated nerve fibres showing the two parts of an ending and the probable site of action of drugs at the regenerative region, where there is no diffusion barrier. A greater variety of drugs effect the ending of non-medullated fibres because the fibres themselves are more susceptible to these drugs (Paintal, 1964).*

Clear evidence relating to the mechanism of impulse initiation is available only in the case of the frog's muscle spindle (Katz, 1950; Ottoson, 1964; 1965; Ottoson & Shepherd, 1970; 1971) the Pacinian corpuscle (Diamond et al., 1956; 1958a, 1958b; Gray & Diamond, 1957; Gray, 1959; Loewenstein, 1958a 1958b, 1971; Loewenstein & Rathkamp, 1958) and the crayfish stretch receptor (Eyzaguirre & Kuffler, 1955a; 1955b; Edwards &

Ottoson, 1965). It is established that impulse initiation does not depend on a chemical transmitter in the case of the muscle spindle and the Pacinian corpuscle (see Paintal, 1971a for references). Moreover no decisive evidence for the involvement of a transmitter is available in the case of any other sensory receptor including the chemoreceptors (Paintal, 1967; 1969 a; 1971 a; 1971 b). This gave rise to the mechanical hypothesis relating to initiation of impulses at chemoreceptors (1967; 1971 a; 1971 b) and was extended to cover other sensory receptors notably the auditory and vestibular receptors (Paintal, 1971 b). It was pointed out (Paintal, 1971 b) that "Mechanical deformation of the generator region could be the rule even in receptors other than mechanoreceptors, because if the generator membrane is electrically inexcitable (Grundfest, 1965) and there is no chemical transmitter, then we are left with only mechanical transmission e.g. as postulated in the case of arterial chemoreceptors (Paintal, 1967)." It may therefore be presumed that the mechanical hypothesis is also applicable to nociceptive and thermal receptors. In the case of thermal receptors it follows that cold and warmth could cause, by an action on their respective sensory meters, mechanical deformation of the generator region which then leads to the production of the generator potential and the initiation of the propagated nerve impulse.

Transmission at nociceptors

The consideration of mechanical transmission at nociceptors, instead of primary involvement of postulated chemical agents such as histamine 5-HT, bradykinin, acetylcholine, would now seem ripe because of failures to observe any excitatory effects of these substances on endings of non-medullated fibres. In fact some of these substances e.g. histamine desensitize the receptors (see Iggo, 1959; Fjalbrant & Iggo, 1960; Burgess & Perl, 1973). However it is necessary to postulate a special mechanism in the case of nociceptors because both mechanical and thermal stimuli can stimulate the same ending (Bessou & Perl, 1969). Keeping in view observations regarding the temporal relation of pain to the vascular reactions following application of noxious heat it is suggested that the non-neural element (sensory meter) in which the generator region of the sensory receptor complex lies consists of collagenous material and fibro-elastic elements. It is further suggested that it swells on transudation of fluid or blood from the capillaries on application of noxious heat or noxious mechanical stimuli. The suggested scheme is illustrated in Fig. 7. It is similar to the Type J mechanism (Paintal, 1969 b; 1970) for which there is now substantial electron-microscopic evidence (Meyrick & Reid, 1971; Hung et al., 1972).

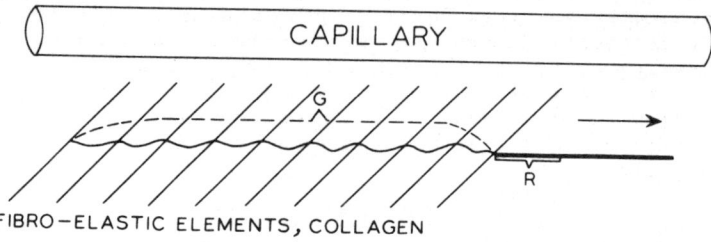

Fig. 7. Schematic diagram showing possible mechanism of initiation of impulses at nociceptors through a mechanical process involving swelling of collagen following leakage of fluid or blood through the capillaries on application of mechanical and thermal nociceptive stimuli. This then leads to mechanical deformation of the generator region, G, thereby causing flow of generator current and the consequent initiation of propagated impulses at the regenerative region, R.

Paranatural stimuli

The mechanism of action of paranatural stimuli can be regarded as being similar to that of the natural stimulus in many cases e.g. pulmonary stretch receptors and Pacinian corpuscles with pulse-synchronous activity. One could assume that the paranatural stimuli have transient components that fall within the filtrable range of stimuli and that they therefore act via the sensory meter (site 2 in Fig. 8). Alternatively, one may speculate that these stimuli perhaps bypass the sensory meter of the ending and act directly on the generator region (site 3, Fig. 8). A good example of how this could happen is provided by the Type J receptors. The available evidence indicates that the Type J receptors are stimulated by increase in interstital volume owing to accumulation of additional fluid which then deforms the ending mechanically (Paintal, 1969 b; 1970). If it is assumed that the swelling of the collagen, in which the endings lie, leads to mechanical deformation of the generator region then it would seem likely that the paranatural stimuli of Type J receptors (deflation and hyperinflation) perhaps act directly on the generator region (site 3, Fig. 8) itself since the collagenous sponge would presumably have a long response time as judged by their response to sudden congestion (Paintal, 1969 b) compared to the much shorter duration of the paranatural stimulus. An even better example of how the sensory meter mechanism could be bypassed is provided by certain arterial chemoreceptors that can be stimulated by mechanical stimuli provided by the natural pulsatile events in the vessels or sudden injection of fluids (Paintal, 1976a). In the case of chemoreceptors the sensory meter is the P_{O_2} sensor. When the local P_{O_2} is reduced during hypoxia, it is believed that this P_{O_2} sensor undergoes mechanical deformation which then leads to the deformation of the generator region (Paintal, 1967; 1973). One would not expect that the mechanical stimuli could cause the appropriate type of deformation in the P_{O_2} sensor. Thus in this case also there is the possibility that the paranatural stimulus bypasses the sensory meter. It should be noted that impulses can be initiated in the absence of the sensory meter (see Loewenstein & Rathkamp, 1958).

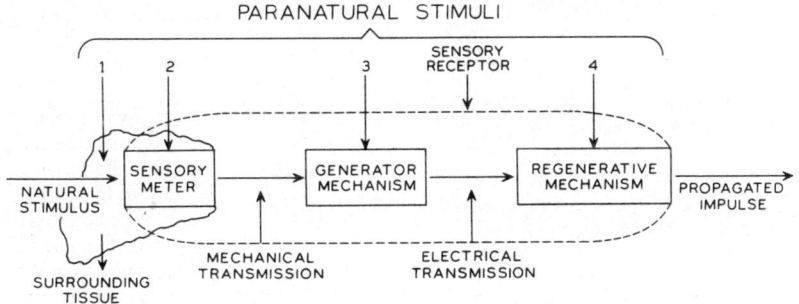

Fig. 8. Possible sites of action of paranatural stimuli at 1, tissue surrounding the sensory meter; 2, sensory meter; 3, generator region and 4, regenerative region of the sensory receptor complex.

Finally, paranatural stimuli of a chemical nature e.g. CO_2 and pH could act on the regenerative region (site 4 in Fig. 8) as has been suggested (Paintal, 1976b) since there is ample evidence to indicate that chemical substances produce their effects by acting on the regenerative region of the sensory receptors (Paintal, 1964; 1971a). If cooling is the paranatural stimulus for the Type I and Type II mechanoreceptors of the monkey described by Iggo (1969) (Fig. 4) one wonders how lowering the temperature produces excitation. Clearly, the effect could not be on the regenerative region because cooling this section would reduce the frequency of discharge by increasing the relative refractory period (see Paintal, 1972; 1973). Moreover cooling tends to reduce the amplitude of the generator potential (Inman & Peruzzi, 1961; Ishiko & Loewenstein, 1961). Therefore the questions are: does cooling deform the generator region mechanically (site 3) or does it deform the sensory meter itself directly (site 2) or by action on the tissue in which the sensory meter lies (site 1)? These are questions that have to be answered by future research.

Differentiation of natural and paranatural stimuli

As already mentioned natural stimuli of receptors give rise to responses that are related to it in a definable manner i.e. the discharge (mean frequency or instantaneous frequency) varies systematically with the magnitude of the stimulus and with its rate of change (dynamic sensitivity). This is not so in the case of paranatural stimuli which generally produce variable and erratic responses depending on experimental conditions. For example the appearance of pulse-synchronous bursts of impulses in pulmonary stretch receptors depends on the level of lung inflation and the position of the lungs. Similarly, the responses of Type J receptors to deflation and hyperinflation (paranatural stimuli) are greatly influenced by the degree of congestion of the lungs (Paintal, 1969b).

Natural stimuli produce the same type of response in endings of the group with different anatomical locations. Thus vibration which is the natural stimulus of the Pacinian corpuscles produces the same type of response in the endings whether they occur in the leg (Hunt & McIntyre, 1960 a; Hunt, 1961) or in the mesentery of the intestines (Sato, 1961). On the other hand the effects of paranatural stimuli vary from location to location. Thus the Pacinian corpuscles of the leg do not have pulse-synchronous activity (Hunt & McIntyre, 1960a) even though as stated by authors, the endings are extremely sensitive to vibrations — indeed almost as sensitive as a siesmograph. It is therefore surprising that these endings are not influenced by the vibrations produced by the arterial pulsations, although they are stimulated indirectly by muscular contraction (paranatural stimulation). On the other hand the Pacinian corpuscles of the intestines are stimulated by such pulsatile changes

(Figs. 3 & 4) (Leitner & Perl, 1964). A similar difference arising out of location exists in the case of arterial chemoreceptors. Here, whereas both the aortic and carotid chemoreceptors are stimulated by a fall in the local P_{O_2}, it is only the latter that is effectively stimulated by a rise in P_{CO_2} (see above). Similarly although the 'warm' receptors of the skin are stimulated by mechanical paranatural stimuli (Bessou & Perl, 1969) those in the nasal region of the cat are very difficult to stimulate by mechanical stimuli; indeed even strong local pressure (3.5 N/cm^2) sufficient to deform the whole nose is ineffective (Hensel & Kenshalo, 1969).

Chemical substances produce their effects by actions on the regenerative region of the sensory receptor complex (Paintal, 1964; 1971a) (Fig. 6) and so since most paranatural stimuli act through the generator mechanism (sites 1-3 in Fig. 8) it is not possible to distinguish between the two types of stimuli by means of chemical substances. For example sensitizing substances sensitize Type J receptors to both natural and paranatural stimuli. However it should be possible to distinguish between the two types of stimuli in cases where the paranatural stimulus acts at the regenerative region. This possibility is currently under investigation.

Conclusions

It is clear that impulses produced by paranatural stimulation have been observed in several visceral and somatic receptors. It is possible for such activity to arise by action at any one of 4 possible sites of action, *i.e.* (1) the tissue surrounding the sensory meter, (2) the sensory meter, (3) the generator region and (4) the regenerative region of the sensory receptor complex (Fig. 8). In resting anaesthetized animals such activity can, in certain cases, yield misleading information about its relative significance. Indeed it would appear that this is the only type of activity that has been recorded so far in certain visceral receptors (the natural stimulus being unknown). As in the case of natural stimulation there is no evidence for the involvement of a chemical transmitter in the process of paranatural stimulation. Observations on the effects of several presumed transmitter agents on endings of non-medullated fibres indicates that no chemical transmitter is likely to be primarily involved in the process of initiation of impulses at nociceptors also. It is therefore proposed that there exists, at nociveptive endings, a system (like that existing at Type J receptors) involving fibro-elastic elements and collagen that is responsible for mechanical transmission of nociceptive mechanical and thermal information to the generator region (Fig. 7). Verification of this scheme by electron microscopic studies is required. This scheme for certain types of nociceptors is based on the assumption that both mechanical and thermal nociceptive stimuli are the natural stimuli that act through a common mechanism.

With this extension of the mechanical hypothesis (Paintal, 1967; 1971a; 1971b; 1972; 1973) for the transmission of neural information at sensory receptors we come to the following conclusion: that in nature there exist three ways of transmission of neural information (1) electrical, along nerve fibres (2) chemical, at synapses and (3) mechanical at sensory receptors. In each case physico-chemical processes are involved.

REFERENCES

Adrian, E.D. (1928). *The Basis of Sensation*. London: Christophers.
Adrian, E.D. (1933). Afferent impulses in the vagus and their effect on respiration. *J. Physiol.* 79, 332-358.
Banzett, R.B., Coleridge, H.M., Coleridge, J.C.G. & Kidd, C. (1976). Multi-terminal afferent fibres from the thoracic viscera in sympathetic rami communicantes of cats and dogs. *J. Physiol.* In press.
Bessou, P. & Perl, E.R. (1969). Response of cutaneous sensory units with unmyelinated fibers to noxious stimuli. *J. Neurophysiol.* 32 1025-1043.
Bianconi, R. and Green, C.J.H. (1959). Cardio-respiratory afferent fibres in the vagus of the cat. *Arch. Sci. Biol.* 43, 454-463.
Black, A.M.S., McCloskey, D.I. & Torrance, R.W. (1971). The responses of carotid body chemoreceptors in the cat to sudden changes of hypercapnic and hypoxic stimuli. *Respiration Physiol.* 13, 36-49.
Brown, A.M. (1967). Excitation of afferent cardiac sympathetic nerve fibres during myocardial ischaemia. *J. Physiol.* 190, 35-53.
Brown, A.M. & Malliani, A. (1971). Spinal sympathetic reflexes initiated by coronary receptors. *J. Physiol.* 212, 685-705.
Burgess, P.R. & Perl, E.R. (1973). Cutaneous mechanoreceptors and nociceptors. In Handbook of Sensory Physiology, Vol. II, *Somatosensory System*, ed. Iggo, A. pp. 29-78. Berlin: Springer-Verlag.
Coleridge, H.M., Coleridge, J.C.G., Dangel, A., Kidd, C., Luck, J.C. & Sleight, P. (1973). Impulses in slowly conducting vagal fibers from afferent endings in veins, atria and arteries of dogs and cats. *Circulation Res.* 33, 87-97.
Coleridge, H.M., Coleridge, J.C.G. & Luck, J.C. (1965). Pulmonary afferent fibres of small diameter stimulated by capsaicin and by hyperinflation of the lungs. *J. Physiol.* 179, 248-262.
Colerdige, H.M., Coleridge, J.C.G. and Kidd, C. (1964). Cardiac receptors in the dog, with particular reference to two types of afferent ending in the ventricular wall. *J. Physiol.* 174, 323-339.
Creed, R.S., Denny-Brown, D., Eccles, J.C., Liddell, E.G.T. & Sherrington, C.S. (1932). *Reflex Activity of the*

Spinal Cord. London: Oxford Univ. Press.
Diamond, J., Gray, J.A.B. & Inman, D.R. (1958a). The depression of the receptor potential in Pacinian corpuscles. *J. Physiol.* 141, 117-131.
Diamond, J., Gray, J.A.B. & Inman, D.R. (1958b). The relation between receptor potentials and the concentration of sodium ions. *J. Physiol.* 142, 382-394.
Diamond, J., Gray, J.A.B. & Sato, M. (1956). The site of initiation of impulses in Pacinian corpuscles. *J. Physiol.* 113, 54-67.
Edwards, C. & Ottoson, D. (1965). The site of impulse initiation in a nerve cell of a crustacean stretch receptor. *J. Physiol.* 143, 138-148.
Eyzaguirre, C. & Kuffler, S.W. (1955a). Processes of excitation in the dendrites and in the soma of single isolated sensory nerve cells of the lobster and crayfish. *J. gen. Physiol.* 39, 87-119.
Eyzaguirre, C. & Kuffler, S.W. (1955b). Further study of soma, dendrite, and axon excitation in single neurons. *J. gen. Physiol.* 39, 121-153.
Fitzgerald, R.S. (1976). Single fiber chemoreceptor responses of carotid and aortic bodies. In *Morphology & Mechanism of CheMoreceptors,* ed. Paintal, A.S. Delhi: Vallabhbhai Patel Chest Institute (In press).
Fitzgerald, R.S. & Parks, D.C. (1971). Effect of hypoxia on carotid chemoreceptor response to carbon dioxide in cats. *Respiration Physiol.* 12, 218-229.
Fjallbrant, N. & Iggo, A. (1961). The effect of histamine, 5-hydroxytryptamine and acetylcholine on cutaneous afferent fibres. *J. Physiol.* 156, 578-590.
Gammon, G.D. & Bronk, D.W. (1935). The discharge of impulses from Pacinian corpuscles in the mesentery and its relation to vascular changes. *Am. J. Physiol.* 114, 77-84.
Gernandt, B. & Zotterman, Y. (1946). Intestinal pain: An electrophysiological investigation on mesenteric nerves. *Acta physiol. scand.* 12, 56-72.
Gray, J.A.B. (1959). Mechanical into electrical energy in certain mechanoreceptors. *Prog. Biophys. biophys. Chem.* 9, 285-324.
Gray, J.A.B. & Diamond, J. (1957). Pharmacological properties of sensory receptors and their relation to those of the autonomic nervous system. *Brit. med. Bull.* 13, 185-188.
Grundfest, H. (1965). Electrophysiology and pharmacology of different components of bioelectric transducers. *Cold Spring Harb. Symp. quant. Biol.* 30, 1-13.
Harding, R. & Titchen, D.A. (1975). Chemosensitive vagal endings in the oesophagus of the cat. *J. Physiol.* 247, 52-53P.
Hensel, H., Iggo, A. & Witt, I. (1960). Quantitative study of sensitive cutaneous thermoreceptors with C afferent fibres. *J. Physiol.* 153, 113-126.
Hensel, H. & Kenshalo, D.R. (1969). Warm receptors in the nasal region of cats. *J. Physiol.* 204, 99-112.
Hensel, H. & Zotterman, Y. (1951). The response of mechanoreceptors to thermal stimulation. *J. Physiol.* 115, 16-24.
Hung, K.S., Hertweck, M.S., Hardy, J.D. & Loosli, C.G. (1972). Innervation of pulmonary alveoli of the mouse lung: An electron microscopic study. *Am. J. Anat.* 135, 477-495.
Hunt, C.G. (1961). On the nature of vibration receptors in the hind limb of the cat. *J. Physiol.* 155, 175-186.
Hunt, C.C. and McIntyre, A.K. (1960a). Characteristics of responses from receptors from the flexer longus digitorum muscle and the adjoining interosseous region of the cat. *J. Physiol.* (Lond.) 153, 74-87.
Hunt, C.C. & McIntyre, A.K. (1960b). Properties of cutnaeous touch receptors in cat. *J. Physiol.* 153, 88-98.
Iggo, A. (1957) Gastric mucosal chemoreceptors with vagal afferent fibres in the cat. *Q. Jl. exp. Physiol.* 42, 389-409.
Iggo, A. (1959). A single unit analysis of cutaneous receptors with C afferent fibres. In Ciba Foundation Study group No. 1, *Pain, & Itch,* pp. 41-56, London, Churchill.
Iggo, A. (1960). Cutaneous mechanoreceptors with afferent C fibres. *J. Physiol.* 152, 337-353.
Iggo, A. (1969). Cutaneous thermoreceptors in primates and sub-primates. *J. Physiol.* 200, 403-430.
Inman, D.R. & Peruzzi, P. (1961). The effects of temperature on the responses of Pacinian corpuscles. *J. Physiol.* 155, 280-301.
Ishiko, N. & Loewenstein, W.R. (1961). Effects of temperature on the generator and action potentials of a sense organ. *J. gen. Physiol.* 45, 105-124.
Katz, B. (1950b). Depolarization of sensory terminals and the initiation of impulses in the muscle spindle. *J. Physiol.* 111, 261-282.
Lahiri, S. & Delaney, R.G. (1975). Stimulus interaction in the responses of carotid body chemoreceptor single afferent fibers. *Respiration Physiol.* 24.
Lahiri, S. & Delaney, R.G. (1976). The nature of response of single chemoreceptor fibers of carotid body to changes in arterial Po_2 & Pco_2-H^+. In *Morphology and Mechanism of Chemoreceptors,* ed. Paintal, A.S., Delhi: Vallabhbhai Patel Chest Institute (In press).
Leitner, J.-M. & Perl, E.R. (1964). Receptors supplied by spinal nerves which respond to cardiovascular changes and adrenaline. *J. Physiol.* (Lond.). 175, 254-274.
Loewenstein, W.R. (1958a). Generator processes of repetitive activity in a Pacinian corpuscle. *J. gen. Physiol.* 41, 825-845.
Loewenstein, W.R. (1958b). Facilitation by previous activity in a Pacinian corpuscle. *J. gen. Physiol.* 41, 847-846.
Lowenstein, W.R. (1971). Mechano-electric transduction in the Pacinian corpuscle. Initiation of sensory impulses in mechanoreceptors. In Handbook of Sensory Physiology, Vol. 1, *Principles of Receptor Physiology,* ed. Lowenstein, W.R. pp. 269-290. Berlin: Springer-Verlag.

Loewenstein, W.R. and Rathkamp, R. (1958). The sites of mechanoelectric conversion in a Pacinian corpuscle. *J. gen. Physiol.* 41, 1245-1265.
Malliani, A. Recordiati, C. & Schwartz, P.J. (1973). Nervous activity of afferent cardiac sympathetic fibres with atrial and ventricular endings. *J. Physiol.* 229, 457-469.
Meyrick, B. & Reid, L. (1971). Nerves in rat intra-acinar alveoli: an electron microscopic study. *Respiration Physiol.* 11, 367-377.
Nishi, K., Sakanashi, M. & Takenaka, F. (1974). Afferent fibres from pulmonary arterial baroreceptors in the left cardiac sympathetic nerve of the cat. *J. Physiol.* 240, 53-66.
Nishi, K. & Takenaka, F. (1973). Chemosensitive afferent fibres in the cardiac sympathetic nerve of the cat. *Brain Res.* 55, 214-218.
Oberg, L. & Thoren, P. (1972). Studies on left ventricular receptors, signalling in non-medullated vagal afferents. *Acta physiol. scand.* 85, 145-163.
Ottoson, D. (1964). The effect of sodium deficiency on the response of the isolated muscles spindle. *J. Physiol.* 171, 109-118.
Ottoson, D. (1965). The effects of temperature on the isolated muscle spindle. *J. Physiol.* 180, 636-648.
Ottoson, D. & Shepherd, G.M. (1970). Steps in impulse generation in the isolated muscle spindle *Acta physiol. scand.* 79, 423-430.
Ottoson, D. & Shepherd, G.M. (1971). Transducer characteristics of the muscle spindle as revealed by its receptor potential. *Acta physiol. scand.* 82, 545-554.
Paintal, A.S. (1955). Impulses in vagal afferent fibres from specific pulmonary deflation receptors. The response of these receptors to phenyl diguanide, potato starch, 5-hydroxytryptamine and nicotine, and their role in respiratory and cardiovascular reflexes. *Q. Jl. exp. Physiol.* 40, 89-111.
Paintal, A.S. (1964). Effects of drugs on vertebrate mechanoreceptors. *Pharmacol Rev.* 16, 341-380.
Paintal, A.S. (1967). Mechanism of stimulation of aortic chemoreceptors by natural stimuli and chemical substances. *J. Physiol.* 189, 63-84.
Paintal, A.S. (1969a). Mechanism of stimulation of type J pulmonary receptors. *J. Physiol.* 203, 511-532.
Paintal, A.S. (1969b). Further evidence that acetylcholine is not a transmitter at chemoreceptors. *J. Physiol.* 204, 94-95P.
Paintal, A.S. (1970). The mechanism of excitation of type J receptors, and the J reflex. In *Breathing*, Ciba Foundation Hering-Breuer Centenary Symposium, ed Porter, R. pp 59-71. London: Churchill.
Paintal, A.S. (1971a). Action of drugs on sensory nerve endings. *A. Rev. Pharmac.* 11, 231-240.
Paintal, A.S. (1971b). The responses of chemoreceptors at reduced temperatures. *J. Physiol.* 217, 1-18.
Paintal, A.S. (1972). Transmission of sensory information at the periphery. *Proc. Australian Physiol. Pharmac. Soc.* 3 (Special number of Regional meeting of IUPS, Sydney) 2-9.
Paintal, A.S. (1973). Vagal sensory receptors and their reflex effects. *Physiol. Rev.* 53, 159-227.
Paintal, A.S. (1976a). Mechanical transmission of sensory information at chemoreceptors. In *Morphology and Mechanisms of Chemoreceptors*, ed. Paintal, A.S.: Delhi, Vallabhbhai Patel Chest Institute.
Paintal, A.S. (1976b). Effects of drugs on chemoreceptors, pulmonary and cardiovascular receptors In International encyclopaedia of Pharmacology and therapeutics, section 38. Ed. Widdicombe, J.G. London : Pergamon Press (In Press).
Paintal, A.S. & Riley. R.L. (1966). Responses of aortic chemoreceptors *J. appl. Physiol.* 21, 503-548.
Sampson, S.R. & Hainsworth, R. (1972). Responses of aortic body chemoreceptors of the cat to physiological stimuli *Am. J. Physiol.* 222, 953-958.
Sato, M. (1961). Response of Pacinian corpuscles to sinusoidal vibration. *J. Physiol.* (Lond.) 159, 391-409.
Sherrington, C.S. (1906) *The integrative action of the nervous system*. New York: Charles Scribner's sons.
Sleight, P. & Widdicombe, J.G. (1965). Action potentials in fibres from receptors in the epicardium and myocardium of the dog's left ventricli *J. Physiol.* (Lond). 181, 235-258.
Takeshima, T. (1974). Functional classification of vagal afferent discharges in the stomach of the dog. In *Vagotomy*, ed. Holle, F. & Andersson, S. pp. 106-108. Berlin: Springer-Verlag.
Uchida, U. & Murao, S. (1974). Afferent sympathetic nerve fibers originating in left atrial wall. *Am. J. Physiol.* 227, 753-758.
Whitteridge, D. (1948) Afferent nerve fibres from the heart and lungs in the cervical vagus. *J. Physiol.* 107, 496-512.
Widdicombe, J.G. (1954). Receptors in the trachea and bronchi of the cat. *J. Physiol.* 123, 71-104.
Witt, I. & Hensel, H. (1959). Afferente Impulse aus Extremitätenhaut der Katz bei thermischer und mechanischer Reizung. *Pflug. rch. ges. Physiol.* 268, 582-596.

Discussion:

Zotterman: I am sure that Professor Paintal's ideas will be vividly discussed. He has, no doubt, challenged us.

Zimmermann: This is a very interesting and challenging unifying concept of the receptor mechanism. Does it apply also to photoreceptors?

Paintal: Yes, I think my hypothesis of mechanical transmission should cover the visual receptors as well. There is a small hyperpolarizarion in the rods and cones when light falls on them. This is not consistent with classical transmission.

Hensel: Dr Paintal, may I ask why you use the terms "natural" and "paranatural" instead of the classical terms "adequate" and "inadequate"? To my opinion, the "natural" stimulus is as natural as the "paranatural" one. An example would be the response of certain cutaneous receptors to mechanical stimulation as well as to cooling. There might be a certain danger of arbitrarily postulating what "natural" and "paranatural" stimulus are. "The method of postulating what we want", said Bertrand Russell, "has many advantages. They are the same as the advantages of theft over honest toil".

Paintal: It is a question of choice, which terms you wish to use. And I think both terms might be all right. It is simply a question of convenience, what one prefers.

Gordon: I know this is a semantic question but not entirely, perhaps. In recent literature the terms "natural" and "adequate" have been used interchangeably. It had always been my impression that Sherrington originally used the word "adequate" in an extremely specific and analytical way. And it can be best recognised in looking back at his work on the scratch reflex which certainly required a mechanical stimulus. But that had to be of an extremely specific form and could not be reproduced in his early work by stimulation of nerves, for example. There are many forms of stimulus which would now be called "natural" but would not produce the scratch reflex. Did you take my point, Dr Paintal? I had not realized that they depend on the use of the word "adequate" later on. But I do think at the time it had a very special meaning.

Paintal: I have gone through this vexing problem about finding a term and I had looked up all the literature on this point. It was only after looking at the literature that I found that this is what had happened. I live in an academic wilderness and I have to go by the published literature. I found the book by Denny Brown, Creed, Liddell and Sherrington 1932. So I thought that perhaps this was the thing to use. I had noticed what Zotterman had said about natural stimulation of the skin earlier. So it does seem to come naturally to talk of natural stimulation the way I have done.

Iggo: The term "adequate stimulus" was, I think, introduced by Marshall Hall in the second half of the nineteenth century and was subsequently taken up by Sherrington. I think it was intended to be the stimulus that called forth the appropriate reflex. It had nothing to do with the electrophysiologist trying to record afferent fibers. It was intended originally as being the stimulus that most effectively in the natural situation evoked a particular reflex response. This, of course, ties in with George Gordon's remarks. Subsequently if people played around with the word that is another matter.

TOWARDS A THEORY OF SYMPATHETIC-SENSORY COUPLING: THE PRIMARY SENSORY NEURON AS A FEEDBACK TARGET OF THE SYMPATHETIC TERMINAL

Primacy of the sympathetic-sensory coupling over the classical sympathetic couplings, and design of supraspinal and segmental controls of primary sensory neurons via sympathetic bias.

M. SANTINI

CNR Center for Cytopharmacology, Institute of Pharmacology, University of Milan, Via Vanvitelli 32, 20129 Milan

> I propose to trace out the history of this involuntary system and show how our conceptions have been modified from time to time, to give our present knowledge, physiological and anatomical, of the different motor neurons of the system, and to give the evidence upon which it is possible to suggest the reason why the motor neurons of the involuntary tissues of the vertebrate have come to occupy their present position.
>
> W.H.Gaskell, The Involuntary Nervous System (1).

The suitability at this time of the ad hoc selection of the quotation from Gaskell will be best exemplified from the mass of results and arguments presented in this paper. For we are now at a turning point and there are new facts which cause one to take the recurrent leap from the past and to postulate that a definite change must now be made in our present ways of looking both at the sympathetic and at the primary sensory neuron.

The new fact is that the two neurons are coupled, forming a morphological and functional structure which I call "the sympathetic-sensory coupling". This is certainly true for primary sensory neurons with Pacinian and muscle spindle endings, but there are good enough pointers indicating that the case can be safely extrapolated to most if not all primary sensory neurons. These facts and their conditioning premises as well as their central and reflex consequences have certainly outgrown the classical frame which gave stability and intellectual guidance in the past. Pushed furthest to their radical consequences, they help to bring about a breakthrough to a new representation not only of the sympathetic and of the primary sensory neuron but also of the CNS.

FACTS

One of the merits of the use of the Falck-Hillarp technique for the cellular localization of the biogenic amines – which has contributed the turning point to the renewal of last years neurobiology – has been the recognition that, in addition to the smooth muscle, the gland and the myocardial cell, the classical sympathetic effectors, there is a new target site for the postganglionic sympathetic fiber. This is the primary sensory neuron, since adrenergic terminal surround Gasserian (2) and spinal ganglion cells (3) and are present in the innermost core region of the Pacinian corpuscle (4, 5), just to quote the examples relative to the physiological and biochemical data to be referred later.

Such an essential preliminary recognition of the presence of the sympathetic within peripheral sensory structures has been further verified and expanded, the ultrastructural picture now illustrating adrenergic terminals closely apposed to the membrane of Gasserian and spinal ganglion cells and of their satellites (6,7), abutting the sensory terminal of the Pacinian corpuscle (8) and also being present within muscle spindles, notably in close proximity of their neuromuscular junction (9) and also closely ap – posed to their sensory ending (unpublished). All of these adrenergic endings, it must be pointed out, are not related at all to blood vessels.

This paper will further summarize the major results of the structural (6,7), biochemical (10,11) and physiological (12,13,14) work which is at the basis of the outlined theory of the sympathetic-sensory coupling and does not pretend to give a review of the field which will be covered later. But what actions these adrenergic endings exert isolately at either site of the primary sensory neuron to which they are in close apposition – i.e., 1) at the sensory ending, 2) at the ganglion cell – and 3) simultaneously at both sites ?

1) Sympathetic and sympathomimetic effects on the Pacinian corpuscle

Under this heading three experimental situations will be presented:
i) of selective stimulation of the sympathetic endings closely apposed to the sensory terminal (5,8) of the in vivo isolated Pacinian corpuscle;
ii) of sympathomimetic stimulation of in vitro Pacinian corpuscles;
iii) of sympathetic stimulation of both the intracorpuscolar ending (5,8) and of those of the pericorpuscolar structures.

The first design is uniquely accomplished by excluding the Pacinian corpus – cle under study from possible spurious effects of sympathetically co-stim – ulated pericorpuscular structures and also by preventing humoral factors from reaching the receptor. The peculiar presence of Pacinian corpuscles in the cat mesentery (15) provides the unique opportunity for accomplishing the above experimental design. In brief the technique consists in recording from the thoracic sympathetic chain the spontaneous high amplitude spikes discharge of an afferent fiber which is provisionally considered to connect with an abdominal Pacinian corpuscle because of the vibration-induced increase of its discharge frequency (16). Scrutiny of the mesentery, mesocolon and pancreas usually proves the assumption to be correct in that from fine testing with a glass rod the several Pacinian corpuscles therein scattered (15) a corpuscle can be singled out which, on being touched, alters the discharge frequency of the recorded intrasympathetic afferent fiber. If the Pacinian corpuscle thus recognized is mesenteric the regional mesenteric arteries are ligated. The mesenteric area is gently fixed to a rigidly mounted 3 cm dia perspex ring which is discontinuous for a few mm so as to allow access to the regional nerve bundle. It is then excluded from the surrounding structures – mesentery and gut – by dividing the mesentery all along the external perimeter of the perspex ring except for the nerve bundle.

Such in vivo isolated Pacinian corpuscle preparation is clearly the Pacinian replica of Hunt's classical experiment on the in vivo isolated tenuissimus spindles (17), connected as it is to the cat exclusively via its nerve supply. Being deprived of any endogenous source of vibrations, it is discharged by vibrations provided by a closely apposed miniature loud speaker. Preganglionic sympathetic stimulation (10V, 25 Hz, 1 msec, 10 sec) – affecting ganglionic neurons of the coeliac or mesenteric ganglia issuing postganglionic sympathetic fibers directed to the Pacinian corpuscle under study – consistently and significantly decreases the afferent output of the Pacinian corpuscle when this is vibrated. The time course of the effect indicates that, with respect to the beginning of sympathetic stimulation, the decreased Pacinian afferent output is instantaneous, reaches its peak (45% decrease) within 30 sec and goes back to the control prestimulation levels within 100 sec. This result, which is also a physiological verification of the morphologically disputed (18) existence of the sympathetic fibers closely apposed to the Pacinian sensor, is clearly at variance with the long latency (90-180 sec) sympathomimetic enhancement of the Pacinian output as obtained by topical application of catecholamines to the in vitro corpuscles (19).

The present in vivo sympathetic inhibitory results are replicated, also as far as time course goes, when perfusing saline solution containing 1 µg/ml of either norepinephrine or epinephrine in mesenteric arteries connected with Pacinian corpuscles in the in vitro isolated mesentery: in an artificial situation which, however, very closely mimics the in vivo experiment where the adrenergic transmitter is released next to the receptripse (20) (experiment ii). Together, then, the full and consistent parallelism of the physiological and pharmacological experiments presented above – indicating a depressant action of both sympathetic stimulation and of catecholamines on the Pacinian output – challenge the never confirm-

ed or disproved, but tacitly accepted (e.g.21) view of an alleged catechol—
aminergic excitatory action on the Pacinian output (19).

As to the mechanism of this sympathetic as well as sympathomimetic
inhibition on the Pacinian afferent output, I believe that the adrenergic
transmitter released on sympathetic stimulation or brought about by per—
fusion to the sensory ending curtails the coupling of the mechano-electric
transducer represented by the "receptripse", the desmosome-like junction
intervening between the membranes of the innermost lamellae and of the
sensory terminal (20). It is worth pointing out that sympathetic endings
have been seen in close proximity of the"receptripses" (20); and serial
work now in progress has to establish to what extent sympathetic endings
and "receptripses" are in general in close proximity.

The third experimental design iii) aims at altering the Pacinian afferent
output with a preganglionic sympathetic (10V, 25 Hz, 1 msec, 10 sec)
simultaneous co-stimulation of the Pacinian corpuscle and of its perire—
ceptor structures in the mesenteric environment from which it is not
separated. The positional changes produced by the simultaneous sympa—
thetically-induced intestinal relaxation and splanchnic vasoconstriction
no doubt may produce effect on the Pacinian corpuscle. These actions
consist in adequate stimulation of the receptor and interfere with the
inhibitory effects 1) of the sympathetic endings closely apposed to the
sensory terminal and 2) of the increased levels of circulating catechol—
amines released on sympathetic stimulation. Thus, whereas in the in vivo
isolated Pacinian corpuscle only inhibitory effects are found, in the
present experimental situation, besides a decreased (34% of the corpuscles
tested) an increased afferent output is encountered in 29% of them. In
addition there occur two mixed discharge patterns, i.e., inhibition
followed by excitation (13%) and excitation followed by inhibition (8%), no
effect at all being present in 16% of the corpuscles tested. In this context
it is worth pointing out that, on the basis of the above results, the increas—
ed mesenteric Pacinian output obtained by close arterial injection of
adrenaline (22) should be ascribable to uncontrolled spurious perireceptor
effects which are unaivodable in the in vivo non-isolated corpuscle.(See
also the Discussion session.)

2) Sympathetic and sympathomimetic effects on spinal ganglion cells.

As already stated, the other site of the primary sensory neuron to be taken
into consideration as a possible candidate of sympathetic actions is the
spinal ganglion cell which is closely apposed, together with its satellites,
by adrenergic endings (3,6,7) whose dopamine and norepinephrine absolute
identification has been afforded by mass fragmentography (11).

Thanks to certain favourable anatomical situations offering an appropriate
separation of the white from the grey ramus, it is possible to selectively
activate by preganglionic stimulation the postganglionic sympathetic supply

to thoracic spinal ganglion cells (3) connected with their physically recognized abdominal Pacinian corpuscles. The latter are not allowed to be
influenced by sympathetic stimulation by dividing the sympathetic chain
immediately caudal to the stimulated sympathetic ganglion, and anyway
cranial to the metameric white ramus containing the Pacinian afferent
fiber recorded from at dorsal root level. Preganglionic sympathetic
stimulation (10V, 15 Hz, 1 msec, 10 sec) results in an initial but not
significant increase of the discharge frequency which is followed within
10 sec by a sudden and dramatic decrease of the spontaneous Pacinian
dorsal root discharge which soon attains zero and quasi-zero plateau
levels for 60 sec. Recovery to prestimulation spike levels occurs some
100 seconds after the onset of sympathetic stimulation.

The above experiment on Pacinian corpuscle dorsal root discharge is
mimicked in the case of an intercostal muscle spindle by slowly injecting
saline solution containing 1 µg/ml of norepinephrine retrogradely in the
intercostal artery which issues a collateral branchlet running to the metameric spinal ganglion under study: within 17 sec from the beginning of the
norepinephrine injection there occurs a full recovery from the inhibitory
effects which consisted in an instantaneous progressive decrease down to
zero levels of the discharge frequency. The short latency of this as well as
of the previous result on the Pacinian dorsal root fiber rule out that anoxia
following vasoconstriction was the precipitating factor of the inhibitory
effect.

In the absence of conclusive intracellular work still in progress from
spinal ganglion cells subjected to appropriate sympathetic stimulation,
to help interpreting these sympathetic effects brought about by the strategic close apposition of the adrenergic endings to the membrane of the
ganglion cells and of their satellites (2,3,6,7), comes to detailed knowledge
of the geometry of the spinal ganglion cell as uniquely revealed by the
Golgi method (7). The latter indicates that the average length of the common
branch is around 120 µ in the kitten. Extrapolating this value to the spiral
coil into which the common branch developes in the adult animal (23) and
whose length cannot be measured with certainty, one gets an approximate
value of not more than 500 µ. The Golgi method reveals also that the common branch is usually thicker than the peripheral which is in turn always
thicker than the central one (7,24).

With this set of Golgi values one can calculate the extension of the electrotonic spread of a steady potential change set up by a sympathetically-induced hyperpolarization (7). The result is that (7), for an unmyelinated
common branch length around 500 µ, more than 1/3 of the voltage change
taking place at the soma should reach the nodal membrane at the T. If the
common branch is myelinated, this should ensure a still tighter voltage
coupling between the perikaryal and the T nodal membranes. Because of
the low safety factor for impuse conduction at the T (25,26), it might well

be possible that a hyperpolarization of a few millivolts is sufficient to prevent the incoming spike from exciting the T node. A larger effect would obviously be achieved if the conductance changes caused by the adrenergic transmitter should occur either along the common branch or, even better, at the T nodal membrane. Further, the possibility of blocking the impulse propagation at the T should also be favoured by the marked asymmetry in the diameters of the three branches (7,24). Due to the very unfavourable partition of the action current of an incoming spike towards the central branch — because of its thinnest diameter — jumping of the excitation from the last node of the peripheral branch to the first node of the central one should possibly be prevented.

3) Net dorsal root effect of the simultaneous sympathetic stimulation of the receptor (Pacinian corpuscle and muscle spindle) and of its related spinal ganglion cell.

In the case of recording from a dorsal root fiber connected to a physically recognized mesenteric Pacinian corpuscle, the experimental design involves thoracic preganglionic sympathetic stimulation activating two sets of sympathetic neurons: those of the coeliac and mesenteric ganglia innervating the mesenteric Pacinian corpuscle and its perireceptor structures, and those of the sympathetic ganglion innervating the metameric spinal ganglion cells. 1 sec of preganglionic sympathetic stimulation (10V, 15 Hz, 1 msec) causes, with a latency of about 10 sec, a progressive decrease of the discharge frequency which eventually drops down to zero level within 25 sec. Full recovery from the sympathetic effect occurs within 50 sec from the onset of sympathetic stimulation. Longer times of sympathetic stimulation bring about, with similar latencies, larger and larger as well as longer and longer effects which exhibit recovery cycles usually occurring within 50-60 sec from cessation of sympathetic stimulation.

Similar results are obtained with simultaneous preganglionic stimulation of intercostal muscle spindle afferents and related spinal ganglion cells.

Without taking into account that endings of postganglionic sympathetic fibers are present in the avascular inner core region (27) where they closely abut the sensory terminal of the Pacinian corpuscle (5,8), are present within muscle spindles (9) and surround spinal ganglion cells (2,3,6,7) — in all cases also not in association with blood vessels — it will be difficult to dismiss the deep-rooted traditional prejudice (reviews in 80, 81, 98): and the reported sympathetic effects of experiments i), ii) and iii) will be attributed to asphyxia at sites of the primary sensory neuron brought about by sympathetic stimulation acting at its sensory terminal and/or at its sensory ganglion cell.

I oppose this view by stressing first of all the heuristic significance of the sympathetic-sensory close apposition of the Pacinian (5,8) and muscle spindle endings (unpublished) and of the sensory ganglion cells (2,3,6,7)

which are not related at all to blood vessels. This indicates that – for
peripheral sensory structures – there are two well separated and distinct
systems of sympathetic terminal distribution, i.e., to target sites of the
primary sensory neuron, sensory endings and ganglion cells, and to
blood vessels. This fact clearly stands for a discrete selective involve –
ment of primary afferent neuron target sites independent from asphyxia.
But against the prejudiced clichéd challenge of asphyxia, more than the
above argument, there stand the relatively short enough latencies of the
sympathetic effects presently encountered – 1 and never more than 15 sec.

This synopsis of the actions of the sympathetic terminals on the sensory
periphery would not be concluded without briefly referring to the effects of
reserpine and monoamino oxidase inhibition on the amino acid levels of
both Gasserian and spinal ganglia (10). Reserpine significantly decreases
the levels of glutamic acid and of alanine–glycine in the cat dorsal root
ganglia and in the Gasserian ganglion; and pargyline, a monoamino oxidase
inhibitor, significantly reduces the levels of glutamic acid, glutamine,
aspartic acid and alanine–glycine in the dorsal root ganglia. Thus a possible
role attributable to the noradrenergic nerve terminals present in the
Gasserian (2,6) and in the spinal ganglia (3,6,7) could be that of interfering
with the ganglion cell production of those amino acids the levels of which
were significantly altered by the above pharmacological treatment. Fur –
ther, by altering the ganglionic production of amino acids which flow down
the dorsal roots to the spinal cord (28,29), the intraganglionic adrenergic
terminals may contribute to the regulation in the spinal cord at either the
metabolic or the "transmitter" level, or of both, of glutamic and aspartic
acid and of glycine, which are candidate synaptic transmitters of the
spinal cord (30).

THEORY

The preceding section was intended as a brief synopsis of the present state
of research on the sympathetic–sensory coupling as morphologically (2-9),
physiologically (7,12-14) and biochemically (10,11) occurring at target
sites of both the sensory ending and related sensory ganglion cells of
primary sensory neurons with Pacinian and muscle spindle endings. Now
a most important need is to extrapolate a heuristic generalization – in the
form of a theory of sympathetic–sensory coupling – as transpires 1) from
numerous records of "vegetative" fibers present in all kinds of periph –
eral sensory structures which for decades have accumulated in the liter –
ature, starting with the pioneering work of Timofeew (31), Dogiel (32),
Perroncito (33), Ruffini (34), Tello (35) and of many others (e.g. 36-40);
2) from numerous studies by the Falck–Hillarp technique and by electron
microscopy demonstrating adrenergic terminals, among other peripheral
sensory structures, in the retina (e.g.41,42), in the cochlea (e.g.43-45)
in the labyrinth (e.g.46), taste buds (e.g.47) carotid sinus (e.g.48-50) and
aortic arch (e.g.51) reflexogenic zones; and finally 3) from several related

and much disputed physiological and pharmacological studies indicating an action of sympathetic and/or of sympathomimetic stimulation on several of the above and on other peripheral sensory structures (e.g. 17, 52-66): just to quote a few significant papers from the many now available on this huge subject matter which urges one to an extensive and detailed critical review.

Heuristically, one may thus envision a fundamental and pervasive character of the sympathetic in all peripheral sensory structures. To visualize a theory of sympathetic-sensory coupling means to bring to mind those results for which it supplies the schematic arrangement. Clearly this is an achievement which lies within our reach, with an act of force of bringing together and comparing general principles of organization and operation of different peripheral sensory structures as imposing by themselves with considerably enhanced force in relation to the object of the theory. And undoubtedly one may without difficulty impart more depth and vigor to these ideas by carrying out special predictive constructions.

The problem is to set up a unified theory of sympathetic-sensory coupling for all the classes of primary sensory neurons. The most important clue to its solution is that there already exists the answer to the cases of primary sensory neurons with Pacinian and with muscle spindle endings. The theory we are looking for must therefore be a generalization of the facts established for them. Much of the present discussion is concerned with expected experimental analogies and with confirmation by planned and controlled experiments.

Indeed, the first and exacting requirement of the theory of the sympathetic-sensory coupling is that all classes of primary sensory neurons are coupled with sympathetic terminals at strategic vulnerable sites like the sensory terminal and its ganglion cell. I cannot resist such a presumption which is widely albeit indirectly supported by the numerous records briefly referred to above even though, as a matter of fact, as far as I know sympathetic-sensory ending close apposition have been thus far revealed only for Pacinian corpuscles (8), muscle spindles (unpublished), carotid sinus baroreceptor endings (50) and for sensory ganglion cells (6,7).

Further, the fact that increased activity in the adrenergic terminals closely apposed to the membrane of a sensory ending alters the output of the latter to a test adequate stimulus (13-15, 17) makes it necessary, to begin with, for the concept of receptor output to be made relative to the state of activity of its sympathetic supply. We soon realize that a given receptor afferent output is not exclusively determined by the adequate stimulus acting on the receptor ending. Rather, it is biased by the relative sympathetic setting of the sensory terminal threshold. Also, it must be considered that, in cases of sympathetic stimulation, adequate stimuli impinging upon the receptor may derive from actions of contiguous structures co-involved in sympathetic stimulation. Thus it look as if the receptor output – in cases of sympathetic stimulation – is the integrated result i) of the adequate stimulus, ii) of the "sympathetic milieu" around the sensory ending, notably at the "receptripse" (20) and iii) of the adequate actions of perireceptor structures impinging upon the sensory ending when sympathetically co-stimulated.

Ultimately, the receptor output may be subjected to a modulating mechanism of incoming sensory impulses at the T bifurcation point of the sensory ganglion cell when part of the adrenergically-induced hyperpolarization of the somatic membrane has flown down the T along the common branch. (7 and see above): the drastic reduction in axon diameter occurring in the central with respect to the peripheral branch (7,24) greatly reduces the safety factor for an incoming spike to pass centrally (25,26); and a few millivolts of a sympathetically-induced hyperpolarization not surprisingly will reduce or even can shut off the spike traffic travelling along the insecure T.

But why are there two target sites of sympathetic inhibitory control on the very same primary sensory neuron and how and when are they brought into action? One could foresee some kind of logistic arrangement of the two sympathetic inhibitory mechanisms somehow as following. In case of excessive receptor output, the CNS would reflexly first react with its sympathetic inhibitory bias to the sensory ending. Should this counterattack by the CNS fail to significantly reduce the receptor output, then the second line of sympathetic counterattack ultimately operating at the T would be reflexly brought into action.

Together, these results provide the picture of the peripheral aspects and of the initial course of events brought about by the working of the sympathetic-sensory coupling which results in sympathetic modulation of the primary sensory codes. Thus it looks as if the primary sensory neurons may represent the target links through which the sympathetic "re-enters" the CNS by conditioning the afferent codes. These arrangements might be utilized to bring about subtle but still decisive ultimate changes: like, for instance, a "sympathetic deafferentation", which might result in central disfacilitation.

This bringing the sympathetic into the forefront of the fast processing by the CNS of afferent codes stresses the need for a clarification of the fundamental functional concepts of both the primary sensory neurons and of the sympathetic nervous system. Certainly the primacy which I accord to the sympathetic-sensory coupling over the classical, terminal, sympathetic couplings – with target organs as the smooth muscle, the myocardium and the gland cell – is a primacy which is based on the very fact of its feedback actions to the CNS.

The centrifugal actions of the CNS on the primary sensory neurons - as expressed down the final common path of the preganglionic sympathetic neurons - are ultimately centripetal by their re-entering the CNS through the integrated impact of sensory information (fig. 1). Thus the classical concept of reflex arc is replaced by the new one of the circular "sympa-thetic-sensory loop" at whose center is the CNS as the target site of its very actions down to primary sensory neurons.

But upon the final common central path of the "sympathetic-sensory loop" - as represented by the preganglionic sympathetic neuron - there operates a multitude of supraspinal and segmental control systems. In particular there exist two pools of preganglionic sympathetic neurons (67): the lateral pool with exclusively polysynaptic connections from the sensory periphery (69) and from all supraspinal systems (70) except for the monosynaptic serotoninergic (71) excitatory (72) projection from the raphe nuclei and for the monosynaptic adrenergic (73) inhibitory (72, 74) projection from the reticular formation (fig. 2); and the medial pool (67) on whose neurons, by contrast, polysynaptic as well as monosynaptic convergence from both supraspinal and dorsal root projections is likely to occur (67). Thus there may be a differential engagement of the medial versus the lateral preganglionic sympathetic neurons in the operation of the sympathetic-sensory loops in view of the different control systems operating upon them.

From the theory of the sympathetic-sensory coupling as a whole there emerge the unexpected roles i) of the preganglionic sympathetic neurons, in so far as they transact the supraspinal and the segmental bias and ultimately set the threshold of the sensory periphery and ii) of the sensory ganglions cells, in that they may exploit their sympathetically-induced hyperpolarizations and the peculiar geometry of their Ts to reduce and even shut off the central passage of peripheral impulses (7). Thus it looks as if the reticular core of the preganglionic sympathetic neurons - by distributing actions to the target sites of its sensory periphery, therein setting the thresholds, and further up filtering the spike traffic at the T-may control the sensory codes adjusting them according to the specific needs of the CNS.

The issue - that there must exist supraspinal control systems of those preganglionic sympathetic neurons with postganglionic sympathetic relations with primary sensory neurons - is particularly crucial in the muscle spindle, which receives a sympathetic supply (9): such systems may act in parallel with supraspinal control systems which lead to a co-activation of α- and γ- motoneurons (α-γ linkage) (75, 76) thus sympathetically modulating the gain of the γ-loop (9). And one has now to realize that preganglionic sympathetic activation may also contribute to the net dorsal root output of muscle spindle afferents when these are looked upon from the view point of the "exclusive" supraspinal activation

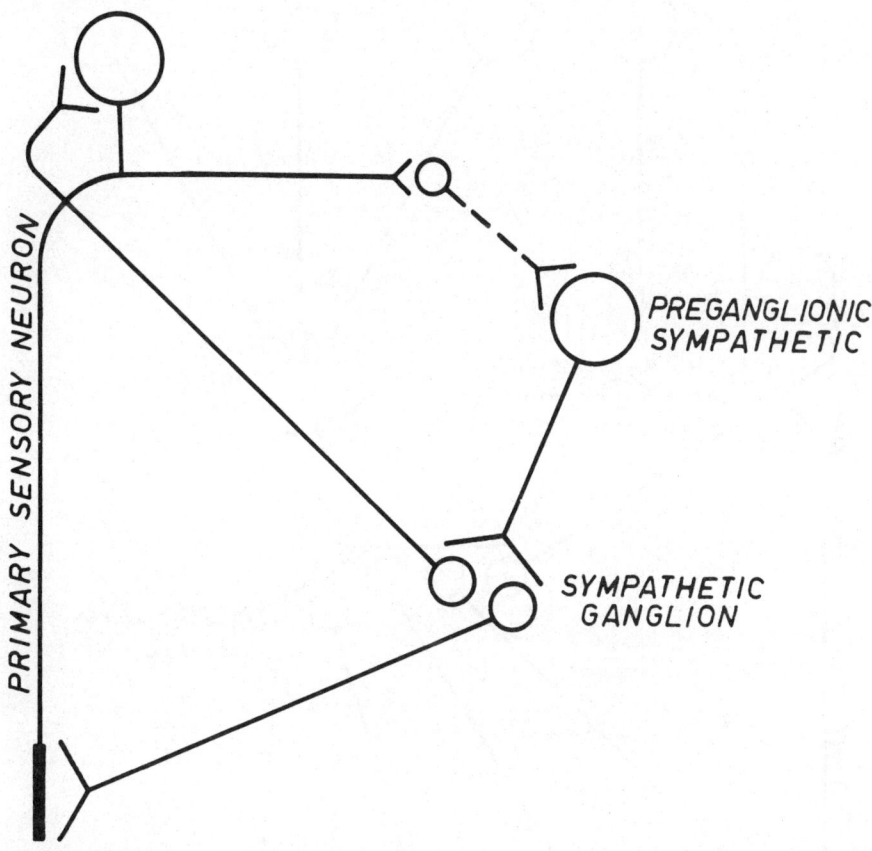

Figure 1. Schematic representation of the sympathetic-sensory loop.

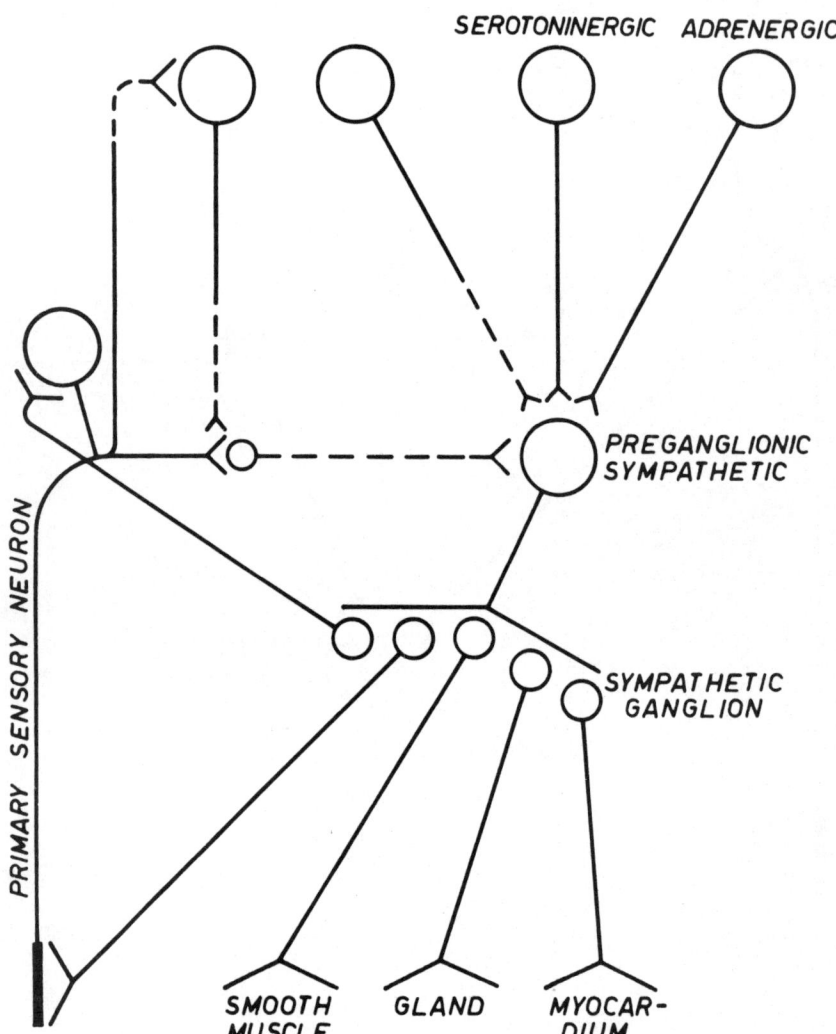

Figure 2. Schematic representation of the sympathetic-sensory loop, of the classical sympathetic couplings and of their supraspinal control systems.

of γ - motoneurons.

This radical theory, besides expounding the heuristic value of a re-interpretation of established facts along its doctrinal guidance, also throws back into perspective old now-disregarded and neglected facts, such as, for instance, those published from Sherrington's laboratory by G. Phillips (77) apropos of the changes in posture and postural reflex actions following sympathectomy in decerebrate cats: all effects which G. Phillips suggested to be due - and rightly so - to an increased excitability in proprioceptive endings in the sympathectomized muscle.

And Peruzzi's group (79) have investigated the issue of the sympathetic actions on the muscle spindle and, more important, of the possible reflex consequences of the sympathetically - altered muscle spindle input to the CNS (78). To start with, they demonstrated that these effects are direct ones since secondary actions due to vascular modifications can be excluded as can be seen from the close parallelism between the effects of in vitro applied catecholamines to isolated tenuissimus spindles and those obtained on the same endings upon sympathetic stimulation in the in vivo experiment. But, most important and thus all the more regrettably neglected or overlooked even by reviewers (81, 82), by exploiting the rhythmical crossed reflex responses of the ankle myotatic unit in chronic spinal cats, Peruzzi's group demonstrated that the proprioceptive or myotatic "after discharge" of the crossed extensor reflex completely disappears within 1.5-2 sec from the beginning of sympathetic stimulation and for about 5 sec in the soleus and is greatly reduced in the gastrocnemius response. They concluded that by keeping the sympathetic stimulation well within the physiological discharge range of 1-16/sec (83) one can definitely interfere with integrated reflex responses by sympathetically altering muscle proprioception.

In view of these results which, it is necessary to re-emphasize, were obtained with stimulation of the postganglionic sympathetic fibers well within the physiological range, with such short latencies as to exclude anoxia due to vascular phenomena, not only should the clichéd challenges (reviewed in 80, 81) and the general discredit about the entire issue fall apart, but an obligatory perspective of sympathetic-sensorimotor integration lies wide open.

The investigation of the connection between the sympathetic and peripheral sensory neurons with Pacinian and muscle spindle endings and the extrapolated theory of the simpathetic-sensory coupling points to new mechanisms which are of considerable theoretical and practical importance having obvious applications to man. Following sympathectomy, unexpected pain patterns, usually in the form of a neuralgia, are "an all too common complaint" (84) -but their incidence varies from 2 to 100% depending upon the criteria of evaluation (85)- and occur in previously pain-free areas later subjected to sympathectomy. Postsympathectomy neuralgia is sudden in onset and usually occurs during the second week after operation. It is severe deep aching and/or burning in quality and its duration is variable from two weeks to 5 months in the untreated cases (85).

The occurrence of this inexplicable neuralgia following sympathectomy may be accounted for by the theory of the sympathetic-sensory coupling. One has to postulate that the sympathetic inhibitory control tonically acting by an electrically silent transudation of the adrenergic transmitter at the target sites of the nociceptor and of its related sensory ganglion cell will still continue to operate following sympathectomy owing to the now passive release of norepinephrine from the degenerating sympathetic ending. But once the last remnants of the adrenergic terminal have disappeared, then 1) an autochthonous activity of the sensory ending and/or of the spinal ganglion cell is released and/or 2) the threshold of the nociceptor is lowered. The development of denervation supersensitivity of the nociceptor and/or of its ganglion cell to circulating catecholamines – mimicking the normal sympathetic inhibitory control over the primary sensory neuron – may account for the disappearance of the postsympathectomy neuralgia.

The sympathectomy "as an experiment in human physiology" which results in unexpected pain patterns in previously pain-free areas is clearly at variance with the sympathectomy which relieves from causalgia (87). By contrast causalgia may thus be looked upon as a pathological case of the sympathetic-sensory coupling of a primary sensory neuron with a nociceptive ending. In my opinion (88) the morbidity would seem to reside not in the sympathetic but in the nociceptor ending because, once "sympathectomized", it reacts to iontophoretically applied norepinephrine as it was used to reacting to increased sympathetic activity prior to sympathectomy, triggering causalgia (87). This clearly points to the possibility of a reversal of response in the nociceptor output as a result of an altered or reversed chemosensitivity of the nociceptive ending to catecholamines. This reversal could derive from a possibly deranged axoplasmic flow along lesioned primary sensory fibers of causalgic patients which might ultimately result in an alteration of the structural and/or functional characteristics, or both, of the receptor ending (88).

It has been stated that "it is possible for central nervous system activities subserving attention, emotion, and memories of prior experience to exert control over the sensory input. There is evidence (89) to suggest that these central influences are mediated through the gate control system" (90).

I would like to hazard my own speculation, namely that in these central activities, such as anxiety, excitement, fighting behaviour and the like, there must be descending control systems operating at the key stations of the various sympathetic-sensory loops represented by the preganglionic sympathetic neurons which are thus pushed into operation i) setting the threshold of various or discrete sensory peripheries and ii) operating the adrenergic gate control at the T bifurcation point of the sensory ganglion cells.

Thus sensory impulses encounter a succession of hazards along the primary sensory neurons i) starting from the sensory ending – subjected as it is to a sympathetic setting of its threshold –, ii) further passing through the insecure T, made even more insecure by sympathetic inhibitory actions which may arrive electrotonically from the perikaryon along the common branch, and iii) finally reaching the central terminal impinged upon by a variety (91) of presynaptic inhibitory actions: the impulses having been again and again subjected to the design of inhibition.

But is there a temporal sequence in the operation of these three inhibitory mechanisms? I would like to propose that the first to enter into operation are the supraspinal excitatory controls of the preganglionic sympathetic neurons which activate the sympathetic bias at the sensory endings first and at the ganglion cell later; and that the last to enter into action are the supraspinal controls – operating the gate control system – which are triggered by the excessive afferent input which escaped the control of the sympathetic bias at the T (fig. 2).

As already stated, there is almost no receptor i) in whose vicinity, contact or interior were not found thin "vegetative" fibers or more recently adrenergic endings by the Falck-Hillarp technique or by electron microscopy and ii) on whose activity was not recurrently tried a sympathetic and/or a sympathomimetic stimulation (see above and to be reviewed). However, the lack of duly exacting appropriate standards, stemming from the unavailability of a general theoretical scheme taking into account all the various facets of this issue, contributed to the confusion which reigns over this uncertain limbo. The intrinsic limited panorama of electron microscopy and the rarely encountered but exacting standards of the Falck-Hillarp technique, to both of which the true "needles" of the unlabeled sympathetic axons "in the haystack" of the receptor are on most occasions destined to escape; the lack of confidence in attributing non-anoxic significance to the experiments of sympathetic stimulation in the absence of well established structural premises: all thse facts have thrown this issue into the realm of discredited and dismissed uncertainties.

No doubt much of the confusion also arises from the lack of a precise scheme considering general laws of sympathetic operation at primary sensory neuron target sites to be adaptively extrapolated to the particular cases of receptor cells storing amines like those of the carotid body (92,93) and possibly also the cochlear (94) and the Merkel cells (95) and of their associated endings of primary sensory neurons. Further, it comes as a surprise that there is a sympathetic control on the sensory ganglion cell – a fact which was ignored even as a possibility in all experiments in volving dorsal root recordings while looking for sympathetic and/or sympathomimetic effects upon sensory receptor discharges. Finally, it has not been sufficiently recognized that a substantial - sometimes even reversing - contribution to the output of a sensory receptor may derive from the "contrapuntal" effects of perireceptor structures co-involved in sympathetic stimulation.

It will be recognized that this explicit assertion to discern relationships, expressible as a simple general theory, between apparently unconnected facts, provides ways out of the confusion and discredit that has arisen around the issue. This present state derives from the retraction of structural views (96) and from the general lack of confidence in the physiological results as well as from the structural and physiological uncertainties and disputes (80, 81, 97, 98); from the general lack of recognition of sympathetic and/or sympathomimetic "spurious" involvement of perireceptor structures in determining the receptor output, from pharmacological misinterpretations (21), from possible species differences in the reactivity of sensory endings to the adrenergic transmitter and finally from apparently contradictory results following sympathectomies, for which the cases of postsympathectomy neuralgia and causalgia discussed earlier are illuminating examples (84, 85, 87, 88).

I still have something essential to add to this sketch concerning the theory of the sympathetic-sensory coupling. Strictly speaking, there are no precise laws concerning the sign - whether excitatory or inhibitory - of the sympathetic actions on primary sensory neurons of different functional classes and of various animal species. In spite of this the theory appears heuristically indispensable if we want to cope with the examples of sympathetic-sensory coupling presently established.

Also, used as we are to consider phenomena occurring in the msec range, it will be difficult to the unprejudiced mind not to receive with skepticism the much longer latencies and duration of effects involved in the operation of the sympathetic-sensory loop couplings. But indeed these nonclassical processes are not the only exceptions to the traditional notions - another example being the long-lasting inhibition (99) - and thus they certainly extend the catalogue of the phenomena which "beg neurophysiology to check and perhaps reconsider classical concepts" (99). There follows from now on the need to use appropriately long enough viewpoints in looking for and evaluating the new phenomena afforded by the theory of the sympathetic-sensory coupling (100).

Thus it looks as if, in addition to the fastest, electrotonic, and to the fast, synaptic, junctional events (101), there are also slower and lasting ones which are peculiar also to the sympathetic-sensory coupling which, in turn, are much faster then the neural trophic actions (102).

The striving towards unification and simplification of the theory as a whole may represent compromises between the old science and the new perspective; which, for this very reason, bears a provisional and incomplete character and is at pains to work out the relations between general concepts and experimental facts more precisely, towards expanding the outlines of the theory with detailing and reinforcing corollaries. There is the emergence in the direction of all primary sensory neurons of a number of problems of sympathetic-sensory couplings whose accurate and extensive elaboration should bring to light a mass of valuable results. And short of resorting of the methodologies involved for the full establishment of the theory, one may prospect that the following lines should be exploited to add details to its basic scheme:

i) ultrastructure of adrenergic terminals - sometime true "needles" to be found "in the haystack" of perpheral sensory structures, and only with some degree of probability only when appropriately labeled - in close apposition to target sites of the primary sensory neurons;

ii) adoption of in vitro and in vivo methodologies to be applied for the unequivocal demonstration of the pure sympathetic effect on the sensory terminal and related sensory ganglion cell - to be clearly differentiated from the total sympathetic effect deriving also from perireceptor influences which obviously may play a substantial and functionally significant role in the receptor output; (there is also to establish how many of the reported cases of enhanced receptor output brought about by sympathetic and/or sympathomimetic stimulation are indeed ascribable to spurious interference of perireceptor structures in turn acting with adequate stimuli on the receptor ending.);

iii) investigation of the circuitries of the various sympathetic-sensory loops and of their segmental (68) and supraspinal control systems acting upon the final common path represented by the preganglionic sympathetic neuron (fig. 2);

iv) investigation of the central consequences of the operation of the various sympathetic-sensory couplings across their successive specific sensory stations.

The theory of the sympathetic-sensory coupling lies wide open to psycho-physiological speculations and experiments. In particular experiments of instrumental conditioning of the type already obtained for classical sympathetic effector organs, indicating learning of visceral and glandular responses (103), may be extended to the primary sensory neuron, the newly recognized target of the sympathetic nervous system.

There is also the emergence of the perspective - for receptors already known to be provided with a centrifugal control system, like the γ-efferents (75), the olivo-cochlear bundle (104) and the like - of an additional efferent control whose functional sign, whether co-operative, antagonistic or modulating the specific gains, must be ascertained.

Also, the large number of examples of sympathomimetic actions on sensory receptors (e.g. 98) adds greatly to the interest which the fact itself commands that there are sympathetic fibres – running to receptors – which are not related to blood vessels; and will help fall into a functional perspective those results otherwise destined to retain an exclusive pharmacological significance. There is also the need for a clarification of the extent of involvement of the primary sensory neuron output when pharmacologically interfering with the sympathetic nervous system.

Further, a number of sympathetic syndromes like causalgia (87), post—sympathectomy pain patterns (84, 85) and the like, together with the various sympathectomies and the sympathetic blocks (86) may provide clues and perspectives of a practical character to the theory and may contribute to the putting of non catalogued and unexplained phenomena into their correct place.

A final remark is addressed to the need for adaptively extrapolating the theory to the specific structural and functional facets of those primary sensory neurons whose receptor cells may or may not be storage sites of monoamines (93, 94, 95).

The whole evolution of our ideas about the sympathetic-sensory coupling and the process of perfecting it reveal a limitation of this wide conceptual system which today still seems to us virtually impossible to overcome. At present the fundamental principles are so satisfactory that the impetus to supplement them can only spring from the strong demands of experi—mental results. Also, with the very little we know today of the sympathetic-sensory coupling, I do not believe that it is justifiable to abstain from formulating this manifesto – however bold may seeem the leap that it forces the present conception to take – whose "raison d'être" was the piercing of the veil of conservation shrouding an as yet unfathomed neuro—biological problem. As noted earlier, there are several points which may rank as prejudiced conservative objections to the theory. And when these challenges have refused to work in spite of their most obstinate efforts, one may gradually get used to the idea of regarding the sympathetic-sensory coupling as a final irreducible basic constituent of nature.

REFERENCES

1. Gaskell, W.H., The Involuntary Nervous System, pp. IX–178, London, (1916).
2. Santini, M., Life Sci. (Oxford) 5, 283 (1966).
3. Owman, Ch. and Santini, M., Acta physiol. scand. 68, 127 (1966).
4. Santini, M., Anat.Rec. 160, 494 (1968).
5. Santini, M., Brain Res. 16, 535 (1969).
6. Santini, M., J.Cell Biol. 55, 226a (1972).
7. Santini, M., Carere Comes, C., Rossi, G. and Abdallah, M., submitted

8. Santini, M., Ibata, Y. and Pappas, G.D., Brain Res. 33, 279 (1971).
9. Santini, M. and Ibata, Y., Brain Res. 33, 289 (1971).
10. Santini, M. and Berl, S., Brain Res. 47, 167 (1972).
11. Santini, M., Cattabeni, F., De Angelis, L. and Raccagni, G., J.Cell Biol. 63, 298a (1974).
12. Santini, M., Benelli, G. and Santini, V., Proceedings of the XXVI International Congress of Physiological Sciences, New Delhi (1974).
13. Santini, M., Benelli, G. and Santini, V., submitted.
14. Santini, M., Benelli, G. and Santini, V., submitted.
15. Santini, M., Anat.Rec. 163, 322 (1969).
16. Hunt, C.C., J.Physiol. (Lond.) 155, 175 (1961).
17. Hunt, C.C., J.Physiol. (Lond.) 151, 332 (1960).
18. Spencer, P.S. and Schaunburg, H.H., J.Neurocytol. 2, 217 (1973).
19. Loewenstein, W.R. and Altamirano-Orrego, R., Nature (Lond.) 178, 1292 (1956).
20. Santini, M., This volume.
21. Schiff, J.D., J.Gen.Physiol. 63, 601 (1974).
22. Leitner, J.M. and Perl, E.R., J.Physiol. (Lond.) 175, 254 (1964).
23. Levi, G., Arch.ital.Anat.Embriol. Suppl.vol.7 (1908).
24. Ha, H., J.Comp.Neur. 140, 227 (1970).
25. Dun, F.T., J.Physiol. (Lond.) 127, 252 (1955).
26. Ito, M. and Saiga, M., Jap.J.Physiol. 9, 33 (1959).
27. Pease, D.C. and Quilliam, T.A., J.biophys.biochem.Cytol. 3, 331 (1957).
28. Duggan, A.W. and Johnston, G.A.R., J.Neurochem. 17, 1205 (1970).
29. Johnson, J.C. and Aprison, M.H., Brain Res. 24, 285 (1970).
30. Graham Jr, L.T., Shank, R.P., Werman, R. and Aprison, M.H., J.Neurochem. 14, 465 (1967).
31. Timofeew, D., Anat.Anz. 11, 44 (1896).
32. Dogiel, A.S., Z.wiss.Zool., 75, 46 (1903).
33. Perroncito, A., Rendic.R.Ist.Lomb.Sci.Lett. 35, 677 (1902).
34. Ruffini, A., Bibliogr.Anat. 11, 267 (1902).
35. Tello, J.F., Trab.Lab.Invest.Biol.Univ.Madrid 22, 295 (1922).
36. Nonidez, J.P., Am.J.Anat. 57, 295 (1922).
37. Sala, G., Anat.Anz. 16, 193 (1899).
38. Jurieva, E.T., Russ.Arch.Anat.Histol.Embryol. 6, 209 (1927)
39. Lawrentiew, B.I. and Lawrenco, V.V. Trab.Lab.Rech.Biol.Univ. Madrid 28, 187 (1933).
40. Palumbi, G., Sci.Med.Ital. 3, 351 (1954).
41. Haggendal, J. and Malmfors, T., Acta physiol.scand. 64, 58 (1965).
42. Ehinger, B., Acta physiol.scand. 67, Suppl.268 (1966).
43. Terayama, Y., Holz, E. and Beck, C. Monatschr. Ohrenheilk. Laringorhinol. 99, 513 (1965).
44. Vinnikov, Y.A., Govyrin, V.A., Leontieva, G.R. and Anichin, V.F., Dokl.Akad.Nauk SSSR 171, 484 (1966).
45. Densert, O. and Flock, Å., Acta Otolaryngol. (Stockholm) 77, 185 (1974).

46. Spoendlin, H. and Lichtensteiger, W., Acta Otolaryngol. (Stockholm) 61, 423 (1967).
47. Gabella, G., J.Neurol.Sci. 9, 237 (1969).
48. Rees, P., J.Physiol. (Lond.) 193, 245 (1967).
49. Reis, D. and Fuxe, K., Am.J.Physiol. 215, 1054 (1968).
50. Knoche, H., Addicks, K. and Schmitt, G., in Schwartzkopff, J. (Ed.) Symposium Mechanoreception, Opladen, p.57 (1974).
51. Khaisman, E.B., Bull.exp.Biol.Med. 78, 109 (1974).
52. Palme, F., Z.ges.exp.Med. 113, 415 (1944).
53. Sampson, S. and Mills, E., Am.J.Physiol. 218, 1650 (1970).
54. Eyzaguirre, C. and Levin, J., J.Physiol. (Lond.) 159, 251 (1961).
55. Mascetti, G.G., Marzi, C.A. and Berlucchi, G., Arch.ital.Biol. 107, 158 (1969).
56. Seymour, J.C. and Tappin, J.W., J.Laryngol. 65, 851 (1951).
57. Beickert, P., Gisselson, L. and Löfström, B., Arch.Klin.Exp.Ohr. Nas.Kehlkopfheilk. 168, 495 (1956).
58. Chernetski, K.E., J.Neurophysiol. 27, 493 (1964).
59. Spray, D., in Santini, M. (Ed.), Golgi Centennial Symposium. Perspectives in Neurobiology p.569, New York City (1975).
60. Niijima, A., J.Physiol. (Lond.) 221, 335 (1972).
61. Edwall, L. and Scott, D.Jr, Acta physiol.scand. 82, 555 (1971).
62. Belmonte, C., Simon, J., Gallego, R. and Baron, M., Brain Res. 43, 25 (1972).
63. Neil, E. and O'Regan, R.J., J.Physiol. (Lond.) 200, 69 P (1969).
64. Aars, H., Acta physiol.scand. 83, 335 (1971).
65. Nilsson, B.Y., Acta physiol.scand. 85, 390 (1972).
66. Rapuzzi, G., Boll.Soc.ital.Biol.Sper. 49, 66 (1973).
67. Santini, M. and Noback, C.R., Brain Res. 26, 399 (1971).
68. Koizumi, K. and Brooks, C.M., Ergebn.Physiol. 67, 1 (1972).
69. Shriver, J.E., Stein, B.M. and Carpenter, M.B., Am.J.Anat. 123, 27 (1968).
70. Nyberg-Hansen, R., Ergebn.Anat. Entwickl-Gesch. 39, 1 (1966).
71. Dahlström, A. and Fuxe, K., Acta physiol.scand. 64, Suppl.247, 2 (1965).
72. De Groat, W.C. and Ryall, R., Exp.Brain Res. 3, 299 (1967)
73. Carlsson, A., Falck, B., Fuxe, K. and Hillarp, N.Å., Acta physiol. scand. 60, 112 (1964).
74. Hongo, T. and Ryall, R., Acta physiol.scand. 68, 96 (1966).
75. Granit, R. Receptors and Sensory Perception, pp. XII-366, New Haven (1955).
76. Grillner, S. Acta physiol.scand., 77,Suppl.327 (1969).
77. Phillips, G., Brain 54, 320 (1931).
78. Peruzzi, P., Staderini, G. and Ambrogi Lorenzini, C., Life Sci. (Oxford) 9 (Part I) 61 (1970).
79. Peruzzi, P. Sperimentale 114, 101 (1964).
80. Matthews, P.B.C., Physiol.Rev. 44, 219 (1964)
81. Matthews, P.B.C., Mammalian Muscle Receptors and their Central

Actions, pp.X-630, London (1972).
82. Hunt, C.C., in Hunt, C.C. (Ed.), Handbook of Sensory Physiology Vol.3/2 p.191 (1974).
83. Mellander, S., Acta physiol.scand. 50, Suppl.176 (1960).
84. Learmonth, J., Lancet 2,505 (1950).
85. Litwin, M.S., Arch.Surg. 84, 591 (1962).
86. Procacci, P., Francini, F., Zoppi, M. and Maresca, M., Pain 1, 167 (1975).
87. Wallin, G., Hallin, R. and Torebjork, E., this volume.
88. Santini, M., Discussant of Wallin, G., Hallin, R. and Torebjork, E., this volume.
89. Hagbarth, K.-E. and Kerr, D.I.B., J.Neurophysiol. 17, 295 (1954).
90. Melzack, R. and Wall, P.D., Science 150, 971 (1965).
91. Schmidt, R.F., Ergebn.Physiol. 63, 20 (1971).
92. Muratori, G., Chiarini, C.N. and Battaglia, G., Riv.Istochim. Norm.Patol. 12, 383 (1966).
93. Biscoe, T.J., Physiol.Rev. 51, 437 (1971).
94. Osborne, M.P. and Thornhill, R.A., Z.Zellf. 127, 347 (1972).
95. Santini, M., unpublished observations
96. Barker, D., in de Reuck, A.V.S. and Knight, J. (Eds.), Myotatic, Kinesthetic and Vestibular Mechanisms, p.3, London (1967).
97. Barker, D. in Hunt, C.C. (Ed.) Handbook of Sensory Physiology vol.3/2, p.1 (1974).
98. Paintal, A.S., Pharm.Rev. 16, 341 (1964).
99. Tauc, L., Physiol.Rev. 47, 521 (1967).
100. Santini, M., Discussant of Nilsson, B.Y. in Iggo, A. and Ilyinski, O.B. (Eds.), Somatosensory and Visceral Receptor Mechanisms, in press (1976).
101. Pappas, G.D. and Purpura, D.P. (Eds.) Structure and Function of Synapses, pp.XI-308, New York City (1972).
102. Guth, L., Physiol.Rev. 48, 645 (1968).
103. Miller, N., Science 163, 434 (1969).
104. Iurato, S., Luciano, L., Pannese, E. and Reale, E., in Santini, M. (Ed.) Golgi Centennial Symposium.Perspectives in Neurobiology p.553, New York City (1975).

THE "RECEPTRIPSE": THE DESMOSOME-LIKE LAMELLAR-AXONAL JUNCTION SUBSERVING MECHANO-ELECTRIC TRANSDUCTION AND EFFECTING THE SYMPATHETIC ACTIONS ON THE PACINIAN SENSOR

M. SANTINI

CNR Center for Cytopharmacology, Institute of Pharmacology, University of Milan, Via Vanvitelli 32, 20129 Milan

Ultrastructural devices for interneuronal transfer of neural messages occurring at either synapses (1) or ephapses (2) have long been recognized (3,4,5). But at the input site of primary sensory neurons with mechano-receptor endings, notably the Pacinian corpuscle, it is not yet known how and where the external non-neural world gains access with its mechanical energy into the peripheral gate of the nervous system.

Electron microscopic scrutiny of the sensory terminal of the Pacinian corpuscle reveals the presence of desmosome-like junctions intervening between the membrane of the innermost lamellae and that of the sensory ending (fig.1). Such junctions are not rare at all and on many occasions several can be seen one next to the other on transverse segments of the membrane of the sensory ending: nine in figure 2 (6).

I believe that this desmosome-like junction – which I call "receptripse" – is the mechano-electric transducer; and this on ultrastructural analogic bases with the other junctional devices, the synapse and the ephapse, which are well known to transduce information between neurons.

So far transduction in Pacinian corpuscles was accounted for by a variation of the ratio longitudinal/transverse diameter of the ellipse of the trans-versely sectioned sensory terminal as brought about by the actions of the innermost lamellae against the sensory ending (7). Hubbard conceived this hypothesis at a time when the only electron microscopic information on the Pacinian corpuscle available to him was the classical paper by Pease and Quilliam (8), which did not disclose the receptripses.

There is no doubt whatsoever that transduction must be the result of a lamellar-axonal interaction. But in order for the innermost lamellae to effect their actions on the sensory ending, there is no other way for them

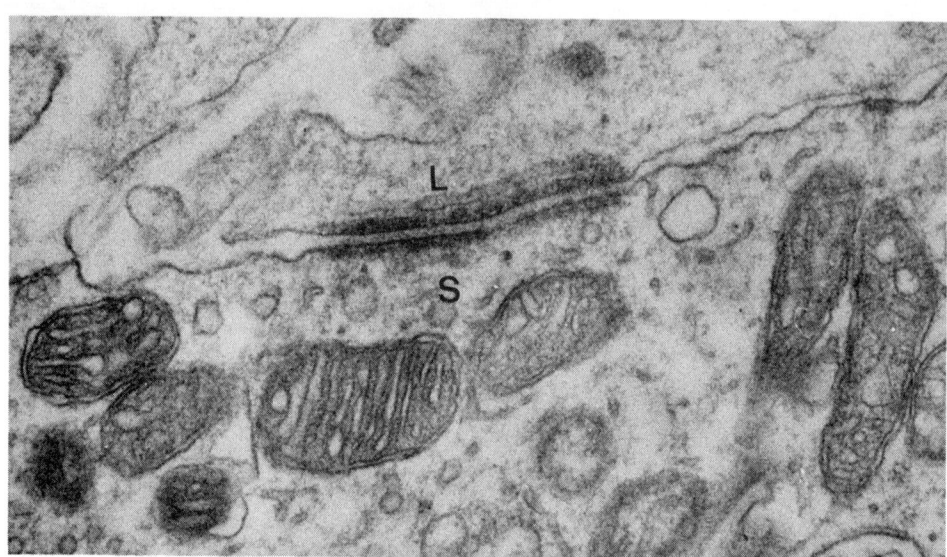

Figure 1. The "receptripse", the desmosome-like lamellar-axonal junction between the membranes of one of the innermost lamellae (L) of the inner core and of the sensory ending (S) of the Pacinian corpuscle. X 80,000

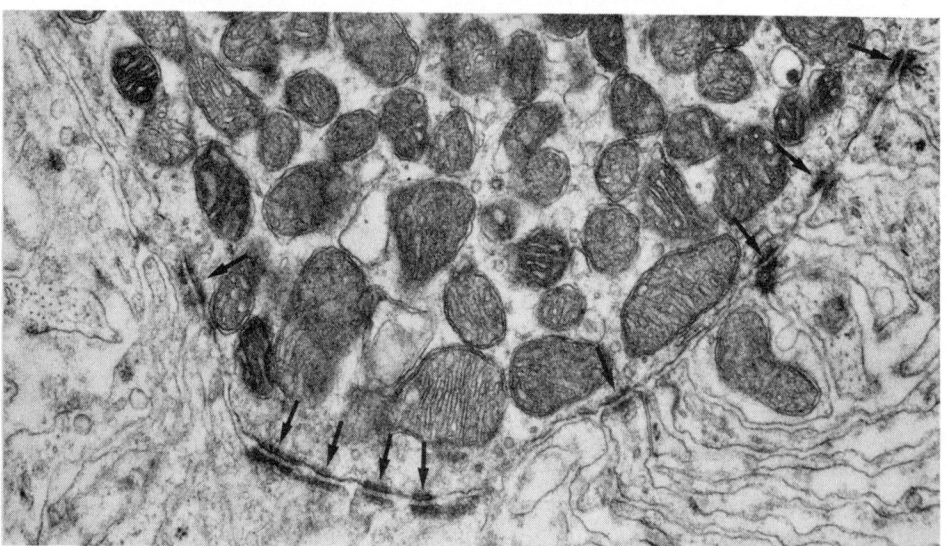

Figure 2. A row of nine "receptripses" (at arrows) along the sensory terminal of the Pacinian corpuscle. X 34,800

but to exploit the natural funnels of which they partake: the receptripses
(9). The receptripses are the obvious terminal focuses through which the
mechanical energy must by all means pass to be conveyed to the sensory
terminal membrane to be transduced in a sum of "miniature excitatory
receptor potentials, m.e.r.p." as they could be called. These m.e.r.p. s
would contribute to the total excitatory receptor potential (ERP) as usually
recorded (10).

Thus, as it seems logical that it is at the receptripse that transduction
occurs, it must be at the receptripse also that the inhibitory action of the
sympathetic stimulation must occur (11). And fig.3 is a strong pro
favouring this view, illustrating as it does a receptripse and two sympa—
thetic axons in its close proximity, as to indicate that the adrenergic
transmitter secreted by the sympathetic fibers will diffuse easily at the
receptripse site there altering its coupling capabilities.

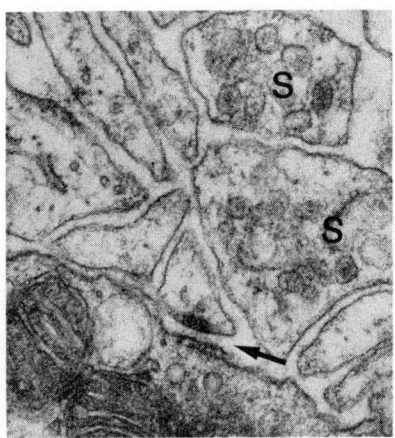

Figure 3. A "receptripse" (at arrow) and two closely located
sympathetic axons (S).   X57,200

Semiserial work of the sensory ending is in progress to asses to what
extent such association of sympathetic terminals to receptripses is the
rule. It should also provide a map as well as the number of receptripses
on either convexity of the sensory ending and this should help to account
realistically for the phenomenon of directional sensitivity which was
interpreted on the basis of the Hubbard model (10).

Now a most important question arises: what is the exact geometry and
topography as well as the functional and biochemical characteristics of the
unidentified cells of the inner core whose terminal lamellae partake with
their feet in the receptripses ? It is in fact just from an appropriate full
knowledge of these cells that we will come to a better grasp of the entire

process of transduction carried out by the receptripse.

To conclude, I would like to propose the term "receptripse" to be extended to the already known examples of junctions occurring between receptor cells and endings of primary sensory neurons.

REFERENCES

1. Foster, M. and Sherrington, C.S., A Textbook of Physiology, Part III: The Central Nervous System, London (1897).
2. Arvanitaki, A., J. Neurophysiol. 5, 89 (1942).
3. Palay, S.L. and Palade, G.E., J. biophys. biochem. Cytol. 1, 69 (1955).
4. De Robertis, E.D.P. and Bennett, H.S., J. biophys. biochem. Cytol. 1, 47 (1955).
5. Bennett, M.V.L., Aljure, E., Nakajima, Y. and Pappas, G.D., Science 141, 262 (1963).
6. Santini, M., Discussant of Iggo, A., in Iggo, A. and Ilyinski, O.B. (Eds.) Somatosensory and Visceral Receptor Mechanisms, in press (1976).
7. Hubbard, S.J., J. Physiol. (Lond.) 141, 198 (1958).
8. Pease, D.C. and Quilliam, T.A., J. biophys. biochem. Cytol. 3, 331 (1957).
9. Santini, M., Discussant of Akoev, G.N., Chelyshev, Yu.A. and Elman, S.I., in Iggo, A. and Ilyinski, O.B. (Eds.), Somatosensory and Visceral Receptor Mechanisms, in press (1976).
10. Ilyinski, O.B., Nature (Lond.) 208, 351 (1965).
11. Santini, M., This volume.

Discussion:

Hagbarth: Are these sympathetic effects upon the mechanoreceptors to be regarded as "natural" or "paranatural"? Or in other words, do the effects occur only in response to the "unnatural" electrical sympathetic stimulation and not to natural sympathetic activation? In microelectrode recordings from human peripheral nerves one can study the afferent responses in individual mechanoreceptive units, muscle spindle afferents or P.C. end organs, and at the same time also record the outflow in efferent sympathetic fibers. And so far we have not seen that maneuvers of different type accompanied by marked changes in the sympathetic outflow in any appreciable way affect the sensitivity of these mechanoreceptors.

Santini: I believe it is important to have disclosed ultrastructural examples of sympathetic-sensory couplings and to have demonstrated that electrical sympathetic stimulation significantly alters the output of primary sensory neurons. I would bet that we may get the same results following a natural sympathetic activation. Also, you will recognize that failures to detect significant changes of mechanoreceptive units such as muscle spindles and Pacinian corpuscles may be due to a too short sympathetic conditioning of the sensory receptors, which is usually just of the order of a few sec in your maneuvers of natural sympathetic activation. On the contrary, to get a significant sympathetic effect on the sole sensory receptor we know now from the experimental results just presented that it is necessary to use a sympathetic conditioning of at least 10 sec. Finally, you will also recognize the unprivileged site of your recording electrode for such kind of experiments using sympathetic conditioning: you cannot say anything of the ultimate sensory input to the CNS since sensory impulses are subjected also to the final sympathetic pre-central control of the sensory ganglion cell and associated T. And from the results presented in the lecture we should also keep very well in mind that in cases of simultaneous sympathetic co-involvement of the receptor ending and of its sensory ganglion cell, only one sec of conditioning sympathetic stimuli will cause a decrease to zero level of the dorsal root discharge; just as if we had a transient, reversible "sympathetic deafferentation" of the CNS, as I would like to call it.

Paintal: How do your results fit in with those of Loewenstein and Altamirano-Orrego published in Nature (London)178, 1292,(1956) who observed increased responses after adrenaline? Also how do they fit in with the observations of Leitner and Perl and Gammon and Bronk? One group observed the opposite of what you found.

Santini: Thank you for giving me the chance to make my point clearer. The results presented in the lecture disprove the never confirmed nor challenged conclusions of Loewenstein and Altamirano-Orrego, Nature (London) 178, 1292 (1956), which however have been tacitly accepted by several authors who have frequently referred to them for twenty years now. Loewenstein and Altamirano-Orrego reported an enhanced output of in vitro isolated Pacinian corpuscles following addition of either epinephrine or norepinephrine to the bath. The latency of the effects obtained was of the order of 90-180 sec and was accounted for by the very slow diffusion speeds of the molecules across the multilamellar layers of the corpuscle to reach the inner core region were the sensory ending is located. Now, in view of the fact that monoamino oxidase activity has been found since then in the sensory ending of the Pacinian corpuscle (Shanthaveerappa, T.R. and Bourne, G.H., Am. J. Anat. 118, 461, 1966), it is probable that the minute amounts of either norepinephrine or epinephrine penetrated as far down as the sensory ending will be easily metabolized by the monoamino oxidase present on the sensory membrane; and that the catabolites may produce the increased Pacinian output. I would like to contrast these results with the pharmacological ones reported in the lecture. The latter consisted in perfusion of either norepinephrine into the Pacinian corpuscles, so as to allow prompt access of the molecules in large enough amount to the sensory ending. And a reversible decreased Pacinian output was consistently obtained. That these pharmacological results were a safe indication of a possible physiological mechanism is demonstrated by the experiments involving appropriate sympathetic stimulation of the in vivo isolated Pacinian corpuscle: the results clearly demonstrate a consistent and significant inhibitory action of the adrenergic transmitter released from the sympathetic axons closely apposed to the sensory ending of the Pacinian corpuscle (Santini, M., Brain Res. 16, 535, 1969) ; (Santini, M., Ibata, Y. and Pappas, G.D. Brain Res. 33, 279, 1971). As to your second question, Leitner and Perl reported an increased Pacinian response following close arterial injection of epinephrine (Leitner, J.M. and Perl, E.R., J. Physiol, London, 175, 254, 1964). In view of the fact that the Pacinian corpuscles thus tested were not isolated from surrounding structures, spurious perireceptor actions were unavoidable. As illustrated in the lecture, the latter may significantly contribute adequate actions on the Pacinian corpuscle which "win" the inhibitory sympathetic actions on the sensory ending, with the final result of increasing the Pacinian output. Such mechanism may account also for the increased receptor output obtained by Leitner and Perl. On the other hand, an inhibitory action of epinephrine on the in vivo non-isolated Pacinian corpuscle was obtained by Gammon and Bronk in their classical experiment (Gammon, G.D. and Bronk, D.W., Am. J. Physiol. 114, 77, 1935). And this result is perfactly in line with the conclusions which were drawn in the lecture from the experiments on the in vivo non-isolated Pacinian corpuscles subjected, with their surrounding structure, to sympathetic stimulation.

Edwall: I could not follow your technique completely but I wonder how can you exclude the possibility that reduction in local blood flow could have caused the reduction in discharge.

Santini: The technique employed on the in vivo isolated Pacinian corpuscles consists 1) in fixing a mesenteric area containing a Pacinian corpuscle under study to a perspex ring which is rigidly mounted, 2) in ligating the major blood vessels contributing to the area and 3) in the division of the area from the surrounding mesentery and gut, except for the small regional nerve twig. Since these small regional nerve bundles consist of just a few fibers and are devoid of vessels, as can be seen from microscopic inspection, there cannot be any reduction in the local blood flow of the Pacinian corpuscle whose sensory ending, anyway, is well known the survive quite well in the isolated situation.

Perl: I feel compelled to comment because our work (Leitner and Perl, 1964) was incorrectly represented in Dr Santini's remarks. In the experiments referred to, small quantities of epinephrine were injected closely into the arterial supply of mesenteric Pacinian corpuscles and measured responses to controlled mechanical stimulation. The corpuscle was mechanically supported on a rigid platform. We observed prolonged (many seconds to minutes) increases in mechanical responsiveness to such injections by artificially increasing the pressure in the arterial supply to the corpuscle. We concluded that the increased responsiveness seen with the epinephrine injections resulted from hydrostatic pressure changes in the corpuscle secondary to vascular rearrangements.

Santini: I did not misquote you at all, I just gave my interpretation of your results. Since I do not see how you can measure the pressure in the arteriolar supply to the corpuscle, as well as hydrostatic pressure changes in the corpuscle secondary to the supposed vascular rearrangements, I must conclude that this is only one possible interpretation just as you did in the discussion of your paper. Rather, I am inclined to think that following close arterial injection of epinephrine one will induce an alteration in the activity of the smooth muscle of pericorpuscular structures such as the vessels and the gut which in turn may impinge upon the receptor with adequate actions "winning" the inhibitory effect of epinephrine on the sensory ending.

MECHANOCEPTION

RAPIDLY ADAPTING CUTANEOUS MECHANORE-
CEPTORS (RA): CODING, VARIABILITY AND
INFORMATION TRANSMISSION

H. DICKHAUS, M. SASSEN and M. ZIMMERMANN

INTRODUCTION

It is well known from psychophysical investigations that moving mechanical stimuli are of particular importance for tactile discrimination (KATZ, 1925). The RA-receptor (RA = rapidly adapting) of the glabrous skin - identified as the Meissner's corpuscle - is one of the movement detectors (LINDBLOM, 1965; JÄNIG, SCHMIDT and ZIMMERMANN, 1968; PUBOLS, PUBOLS and MUNGER, 1971; KNIBES-TÖL, 1973; VALLBO and colleagues, this symposium). Its adequate stimulus has been suggested to be the velocity of skin deformation.

The aims of our investigations were: 1. the quantitative analysis of the coding of the movement velocity by single RA-receptors; 2. the mathematical description of the variability of the afferent discharges; 3. information transmission about the deformation velocity by the receptor and the nerve ending.

METHODS

The experiments were performed on adult cats, anesthetized with pentobarbital sodium (40 mg/kg, further doses if required). The animals were immobilized by gallamine triethiodide (repeated doses of 5 mg/kg, i.v.) and set on artficial respiration. The end-tidal CO_2 was kept at 3%. The left hind foot was embedded with paraffin wax, sole upwards. The posterior tibial nerve and its distal branches, the medial and the lateral plantar nerves, were exposed in two paraffin oil pools. By using watchmaker forceps fine nerve strands were dissected from the posterior tibial nerve, and splitted under microscopic control into single fibres. Single myelinated afferents from RA-receptors were selected for recording. The axonal conduction velocities, determined by electrical stimulation of the plantar nerves, were in the range of Group II (Aβ) fibres.

A moving coil stimulator driven by a function generator and a power amplifier delivered mechanical stimuli with trapezoid waveforms. The excursions of the stimulator probe (1.5 mm in diameter) were controlled by feedback from a displacement transducer (a differential transformer). With this stimulation system deformations of the skin were performed at preselected velocity, amplitude and duration. Examples of the time course of stimulator deflection are shown in Fig. 1. The discharges elicited by these stimuli, the time course of the skin displacement and the trigger pulses were stored on tape for off-line analysis. The interspike intervals were measured on-line with a laboratory computer.

RESULTS

The charactieristic function of the RA-receptor.

The RA-receptors responded only during the rising phase of the trapezoid mechanical stimuli (see records in Fig. 1). With different deformation velocities V generated by changing the rise time at constant amplitude of displacement the receptor responses varied significantly in interspike intervals Δt.

Fig. 1 shows the relation between the velocity of skin deformation V and the averaged interspike intervals $\overline{\Delta t}$. The minimum velocity V_o that generated one interval only, i.e. two spikes, was found in the range from o.1 to 1o mm/sec; the average was V_o = 2.5 mm/sec. The maximum velocity used was 12o mm/sec.

Calculations for the best fit by a mathematical description of data in Fig. 1 yielded a power law of the type

$$\overline{\Delta t} = A \cdot (V-V_o)^p$$

Each of the fibres tested could be fitted by such a relation. The exponents p were in the range between -o.3 and -o.8.

Thus, the average interspike interval $\overline{\Delta t}$ is a monotonic function of stimulus velocity V. The RA-receptor therefore is capable to encode the velocity of skin indentations.

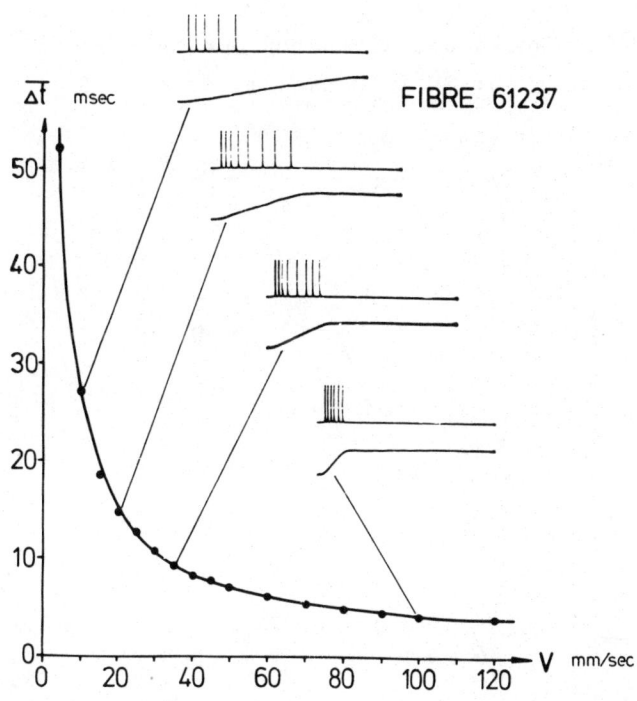

Fig.1. Relationship in a single RA-receptor between the mean discharge interval $\overline{\Delta t}$ and the velocity of the skin displacement V. Each point is the mean of all the time intervals between successive spikes of a discharge averaged from 2o trials.

The stochastic variability of the discharge intervals.

The information content of a spike train depends critically on the degree of fluctuations of the discharges, i.e. the noise. In order to evaluate the amount and the type of fluctuations, the distribution of interspike intervals Δt was determined in some receptors. Up to 12.000 stimuli with identical parameters were delivered at a repetition rate of 5/sec. These measurements revealed that the intervals of any order within the spike train, i.e. the first interval Δt_1, the second Δt_2, etc., usually are distributed symmetrically and can be fitted by a Gaussian distribution function. Since the mean $\overline{\Delta t}$ depends on the velocity V of the skin stimulus (Fig. 1) the question arises what the relationship is between $\overline{\Delta t}$, at various velocities, and the standard deviation SD of the related distribution (VERVEEN and DERKSEN, 1965).

In Fig. 2 the results are given for one RA-receptor of the SD-$\overline{\Delta t}$ relationship: SD increases monotonically with $\overline{\Delta t}$.

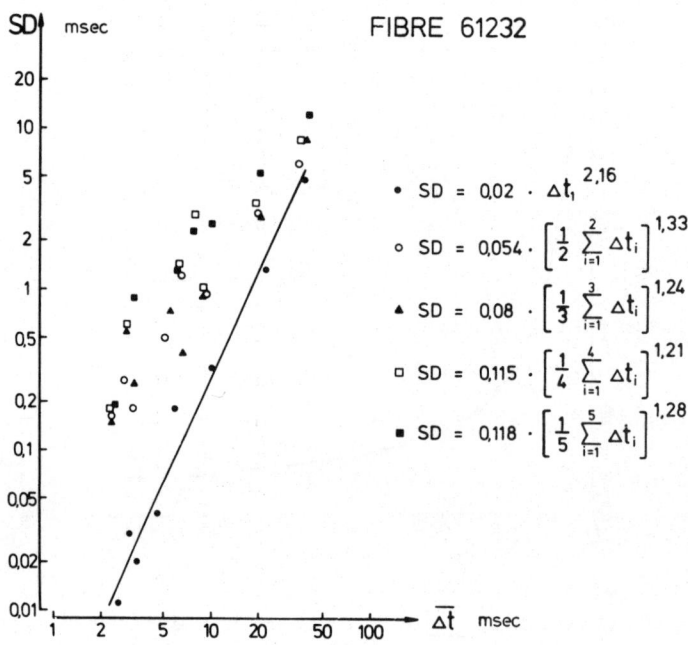

Fig.2. Relationship in a single RA-receptor between the standard deviation SD of the distribution of interspike intervals Δt, and the mean interval $\overline{\Delta t}$. Data refer to the distribution of the first interval Δt_1 only (•), or to the distributions including intervals of increasing order n within each discharge (other symbols, for n=2...5). The formula in the inset are the empirical descriptions of data by power functions; for Δt_1 this power function is plotted. Logarithmic scales of both coordinates.

The points (•) connected by the line represent results obtained when considering Δt_1 exclusively, i.e. the first interval of each discharge. The linear relation in the logarithmic coordinate system indicates a power function, as is fully given in the inset of Fig. 2. The other symbols plot the SD-$\overline{\Delta t}$ relation when intervals of increasing order are taken into account.

The absolute value of SD may be rather small for the first interval Δt_1. The coefficient of variation, calculated as SD/$\overline{\Delta t_1}$, was as low as o.o1, or 1%, at a stimulus velocity of 1oo mm/sec. When higher order intervals were taken into account, the SD was considerably higher; accordingly, the coefficient of variation was greater in these cases(Fig. 2).

Since the power functions relating SD and $\overline{\Delta t}$ (inset of Fig. 2) have exponents greater than 1, the coefficient of variation increases at increasing SD. In the example of Fig. 2 the coefficient of variation grows from 1% to 16% for increasing Δt_1 (•).

To summarize, the relative variability augments with increasing values of Δt, and with discharge intervals of higher order included in the analysis of variability.

Information transmission in RA-receptors

The capability of a receptor to encode a parameter of the adequate stimulus can be expressed in the quantitative measure of information as defined by information theory. Several methods exist to determine the information content of a receptor discharge; they all are derived from the variability of firing (see previous section) that blurs the characteristic function of encoding.

A stright-forward graphic method (ZIMMERMANN, 1975) may give an estimate for the information on stimulus velocity contained in the RA-discharge, as is outlined in Fig. 3. This graph is another way of displaying the characteristic function of the RA-receptor: the stippled band indicates the $\pm$ 3 SD limits of the discharge interval Δt_1, as determined by the procedures of the foregoing paragraph. This approach differs from that used in Fig. 1: There, the charactieristics had been established as a smooth line by averaging many single measurements, as is normally done by receptor physiologists. In contrast, in Fig. 3 the variability of the discharge is displayed, indicating the noise inherent to the receptor processes.

This noise display will yield data on the number of stimulus velocities V that might be discriminated by an ideal observer (i.e. the experimenter) in the receptor discharge: The condition for two V-values to be discernible unambigously in the receptor discharge is that the ranges of uncertainty of the related Δt_1-values do not overlap. Since the ± 3 SD range contains 99.7% of all the Δt_1-responses at either velocity V, the minimum separation practically can be constructed by drawing a horizontal line into the area of variability in Fig. 3; the intersection with the upper and lower 3 SD-limits yields directly the minimum separation of V that can be distinguished in the Δt_1-response of a single RA-receptor.

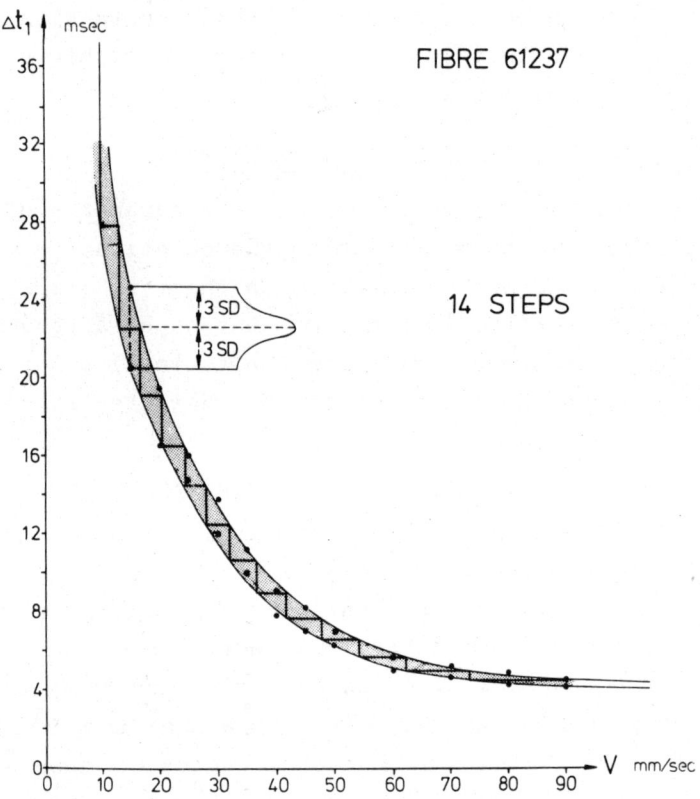

Fig.3. Variability in a single RA-afferent of the first interval Δt_1. The stippled area indicates the ± 3 SD range of Δt_1. The staircase function is fitted into this area; for details of construction see text.

Correspondingly the total number of stimulus velocities V discernible within the total range of the Δt_1-variable will be obtained by drawing a staircase function into the field of uncertainty. In this way, the 14 steps of the experiment in Fig. 3 indicate the maximum number of stimulus velocities V that can be signalled as different by this particular RA-receptor. In terms of information theory the resulting value for the average information T transmitted per stimuls is:

$$T = \log_2 14 = 3.8 \text{ bit/stimulus}$$

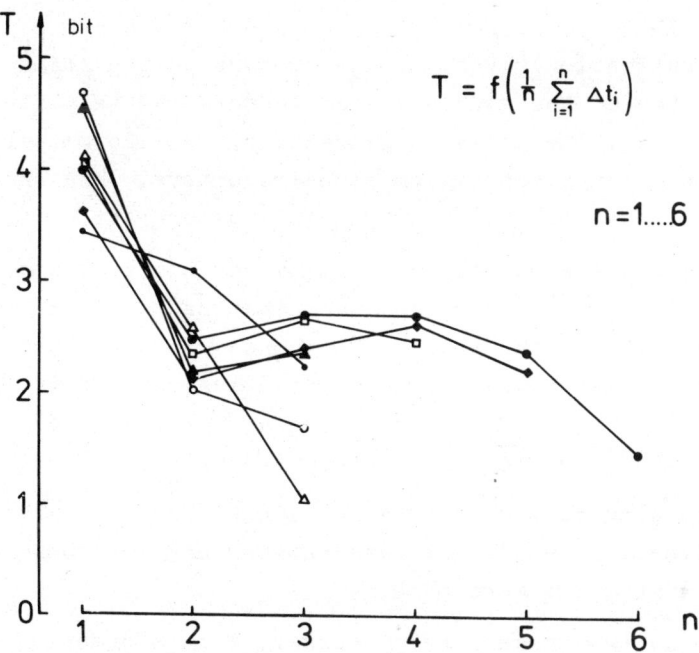

Fig. 4. The transmitted information T calculated for 7 different RA-receptors (different symbols) on the assumption of a pulse interval code. The abscissa indicates the number n of successive interspike intervals of each discharge that have been considered for the calculation of T.

In addition to the above graphic method we performed calculations of the information content of the RA-discharge, by applying two different paradigms that have been used for other systems previously (WERNER and MOUNTCASTLE, 1965; FÄRBER, 1968). These approaches will not be given in detail here. The resulting values for T were practically the same as those obtained by the method of Fig. 3.

The information content T given above was obtained by utilizing Δt_1 only, i.e. the first interval of each response. When the subsequent intervals too were included for the determination of T, smaller values resulted. This is shown in Fig. 4 for 7 receptors. When increasing the number n of intervals considered for the calculations, T decreased from about 4 bit/stimulus at n=1 to 2.3 bit/stimulus at n=5.

Discussion

Our investigation gives further support to the notion that the RA-receptor of the glabrous skin encodes the velocity of skin indentations. The stimulus range of o.1 to 12o mm/sec can be transmitted by a population of RA-receptors, when assuming a pulse interval code as the principle of operation.

Our emphasis was on the reliability and the precision of this velocity detector. We established that particularly the first interval Δt_1 of the receptor response was an accurate measure of the stimulator velocity. The relative variability of Δt_1 was as small as 1%, a value that must be considered as exceptional among the mechanoreceptors investigated for this aspect.

Correspondingly, the information content derived from these small fluctuations of Δt_1 was rather large: values as high as 4.7. bit/stimulus were obtained.

Since only two spikes were necessary for information transmission by this pulse interval code, rather high stimulus repetition rates could be applied (up to 1o/sec); at such high repetition rates our estimates for the maximum rate of information transmission yielded about 3o bit/sec. This is extremely high when comparing with other receptors: for example, about 6 bit/sec have been estimated in SA-receptors under the assumption of a frequency code (WERNER and MOUNTCASTLE, 1965; ZIMMERMANN, unpublished). Thus, the RA-receptor is a precise and fast operating encoder for short moving stimuli.

VALLBO and his colleagues (this symposium) provide evidence that a single impulse in a single RA-fibre might be detected by the human subject. Apart from this significance for threshold of perception it would be challenging to evaluate whether the information content of the first spike bears significance for discrimination in the intensive and time domain, as might be concluded from our work.

REFERENCES

Färber, G. (1968): *Kybernetik* 5, 17-29.

Jänig, W., R.F. Schmidt and M. Zimmermann (1968): *Exp.Brain Res.* 6, 1oo-115.

Katz, D. (1925): Der Aufbau der Tastwelt. J.A. Barth, Leipzig.

Knibestöl, M. (1973): *J.Physiol.(Lond.)* 232, 427-452.

Lindblom, U.F. (1965): *J.Neurophysiol.* 28, 966-985.

Pubols, L.M., B.H. Pubols and B.L. Munger (1971): *Exp.Neurol.* 31, 165-182

Verveen, A.A. and H.E. Derksen (1965): *Kybernetik* 2, 152-16o.

Werner, G. and V.B. Mountcastle (1965): *J.Neurophysiol.* 28, 359-397

Zimmermann, M. (1975): The sensory system seen as a communications network. In: Fundamentals of Neurophysiology. pp. 223-232. Ed. by R.F. Schmidt. Springer Verlag: New York, Heidelberg, Berlin.

This work has been supported by the Deutsche Forschungsgemeinschaft, grant Zi 11o/5.

We wish to thank to Mrs. U. Nothoff for typing the manuscript, to Mrs. J. Peddinghaus for technical assistance, and to Mr. M. Böhm for the electronic engeneering.

Discussion:

Iggo: It was a very fine presentation. I shall take advantage of my privileged position as chairman to ask the first question. In comparison to the hair follicle receptors, these glabrous rapidly adapting receptors show a decreased irregularity or uniformity of interspike interval length as the stimulus continues. Whereas, Brown and I in 1967 described hair follicle receptors where the interspike intervals were much more uniform in length. And I wonder whether, in fact, these receptors of yours may be concerned more with acceleration detection than with velocity detection since they give such inadequate information about continuation of the intervals at different velocities.

Dickhaus: Concerning your second question; all our results are in favour of the RA-receptors being velocity detectors. For example: the tuning curves make reasonable that they do not detect acceleration but velocity. If you plot the amplitude of a sinusoidal stimulus against the stimulus frequency when just one spike is elicited, straight lines with slopes near -1 are obtained in log coordinates. This slope value of the tuning curves indicates that these receptors are sensitive to displacement velocity.

Lindblom: In relation to Professor Iggo's question, I would like to remark on the irregularity of the interval in your discharges. As with the hair follicle receptors, there are the glabrous skin receptors of the monkey which have a fairly regular discharge during the linear indentation. The fact that during the first interval they give the most important information fits well with what might happen during physiological stimuli. Because if the rate is steep the receptor will only have time to discharge two impulses and then there is only one interval which could carry the information. This fits with your analysis, I think.

Dickhaus: Your statements on the first interval; this is exactly my point on the significance of the first interval in daily life. I agree fully with you. Concerning Professor Iggo's and your comments on variability in the hair follicle and the monkey RA-receptors; the papers referred to do not contain detailed analysis of variability, therefore a comparison with our results is not possible - in regard to variability.

Iggo: Perhaps it might be suggested that the central nervous system is interested only in each stimulus, one at a time and not five thousand all averaged.

Dickhaus: To obtain a measure of the variability of interspike intervals it is necessary to apply a high number of identical stimuli. I agree with you that the central nervous system might be not so much interested in this particular experimental situation!

Zimmermann: I would like to give a comment to summarize the new findings on the RA receptors and to emphasize the outstanding significance of these receptors. From the excellent work of Dr Vallbo and co-workers we have learned: 1) That the RA receptors only have a significant small center point distance (1.5 mm at the finger tips) to explain two point discrimination. 2) Single impulses in one afferent RA fiber are detected by the subject. 3) The transmission of these single impulses in single fibers in the CNS is practically free of noise since there is a 1:1 relationship between individual spikes and correct psychophysical detection. This is an extremely outstanding feature of signal transmission in the nervous system. 4) From our work it turned out that the coding of stimulus intensity in the impulse discharge yields values of more than 4 bit per stimulus, and values for the rate of information transmission of 30 bit per sec. Both values are much higher than has been found for all other types of cutaneous receptors. Therefore my conclusion is that the RA receptors are the most important receptors in tactile acuity.

CODING OF VELOCITY OF SKIN INDENTATION IN MAN AND MONKEY A PERCEPTUAL-NEUROPHYSIOLOGICAL CORRELATION

O. FRANZÉN and U. LINDBLOM

*Department of Psychology, University of Uppsala, Uppsala, and
Department of Neurology, Huddinge Hospital, Karolinska Institutet, Stockholm, Sweden*

INTRODUCTION

Information from the sense organs is translated into nervous processes that represent or symbolize events in the external world. It is therefore a question of considerable interest to identify the neural structures whose responses give rise to specific sensations and to determine their operating characteristics by means of behavioral and electrophysiological methods.

This study was undertaken with the purpose of comparing human psychophysical data with the activity in single mechanoreceptive afferents in man and monkey. We will only be concerned with the impulse pattern during dynamic displacement of the glabrous skin of the palm and sole both of which are richly endowed with rapidly adapting intracutaneous receptors (RA) (Cauna, 1956; Montagna, 1960; Winkelmann, 1960) assumed to be associated with the sensation of touch.

METHOD

<u>Subjects</u>. Ten healthy subjects (7 males and 3 females) participated in the experiments. The electrophysiological investigation was performed on only four (2 males and 2 females) of the ten subjects.

Stimulation

a) Linearily rising pulses from a ramp generator was fed to the mechanical stimulator (Brüel & Kjaer type 4810) which was mounted under the arm support of a comfortable chair. The pad of the index or middle finger was stimulated by a 2 mm diameter blunt-ended, plastic probe fixed to the center of the stimulator. Prior to the stimulation the probe was perpendicularly brought in contact with the skin without causing any appreciable indentation as monitored on an oscilloscope with a capacitance meter. The pulse amplitude was constant at 600 microns and the rate of rise was changed between 0.067 and 32 mm/sec. The pulse duration was long in order to avoid interference from the off-phase with the sensation produced by the rising phase.

b) In a second series of experiments where perception and single fiber activity was studied in the same subject under identical stimulation conditions a somewhat different technique of stimulating the skin was used. Half-wave rectified sinusoids from a Wavetek generator (Model 112) energized a vibrator (PYE-ling Model V 47) mounted on a stand that allowed the delivery of pulses to almost any area of the palm of the hand. Probe diameter was as before 2 mm in diameter. The tangent of the pulse ramp was taken as an arbitrary measure of indentation velocity The rates of skin displacement varied between 0.5 and 16 mm/sec spaced logarithmicly. The indentation amplitude was always set to 500 microns.

Measurements of subjective velocity

a) Experiments were performed to examine the subjective appreciation of linearily rising pulses. An equal ratio series of nine velocities in the range of 0.067 and 16 mm/sec were presented at random. The 32 mm/sec ramp always presented before any of the other nine stimuli was assigned the number 100. The subjects had to estimate the velocity of the second ramp in relation to the standard. They also gave verbal reports on what sensations the different stimuli elicited. The observers were given several practise trials before the main experiment. The experimenter asked the subject to pay attention only to the rising phase of the stimulus.

b) Using half-wave pulses for stimulation a different variant of the method of magnitude estimation was employed. A standard velocity of 4 mm/sec was called 10 and the subject's task was to estimate the velocity of other pulses in relation to the standard rate. In the two psychophysical studies the set of stimuli was presented in at least four trials.

Recording of single unit activity

By means of a percutaneous tungsten microelectrode recording technique developed by Hagbarth and Vallbo (Hagbarth and Vallbo, 1967; Vallbo and Hagbarth, 1968) the neural discharge was studied in single mechanoreceptive afferents of the median and ulnar nerves innervating the glabrous skin of awake, healthy human subjects. Recording equipment consisted of a 0.2 mm tungsten electrode with a tip diameter of about 5 microns, a high impedance probe, a preamplifier (Grass P5) with a filter setting of 300 Hz to 10 KHz, an oscilloscope (Tektronix) and a tape recorder (Revox Stereo Model F 36). The recording electrode was manually inserted about 10 cm proximal to the elbow. The receptive fields of the afferent fibers were mapped with a thin handheld glass probe.

RESULTS

The high velocity pulses (16 - 32 mm/sec) produced a sensation of a tap. In the region of a 0.1 mm/sec and below the tactual nature of the sensation was replaced by a vague feeling of rolling pressure. The skin displacement had also to exceed about 100 microns before any sensation at all was reported. The sharply rising threshold can be ascribed to the transition to another receptor of the slowly adapting type. This may account for the very low ratings of subject RT for ramps below 0.1 mm/sec. He may have made some kind of a categorical judgment besides his magnitude estimation.

One observation deserves special notice. When the ramps were systematically varied from high to low in a haphazard fashion the subjects never gave any report of a change in intensity, only of changes in velocity. The subjective magnitude is plotted against indentation velocity in log-log coordinates as shown in Fig 1. All six subjects show a gradual increase in apparent velocity from 0.25 and up to 16 mm/sec. Above this velocity the functions begin to level off.

For the middle range of velocities the estimates fall close to a straight line indicating a simple power function of the form $R = cV^n$ (Stevens, 1957) where R is subjective velocity, c is a multiplicative constant, V is indentation velocity and n is the exponent. The individual exponents and their average (n = 0.51) are presented in Table 1.

TABLE 1.

Subject	Exponent (n)
BB	0.46
AP	0.54
LR	0.43
KP	0.38
RT	0.59
PA	0.63
Mean	0.51

In a previous investigation on the monkey (Lindblom, 1965) single-unit activity was recorded at the level of the 7th lumbar root following linearly rising skin displacements of the monkey sole in order to establish the response properties of intracutaneously located receptors. The range of velocities in the experiment covered almost the same range as the psychophysical study reported above. A typical feature of the discharge pattern is a decreasing interval between the nerve impulses with an increasing displacement velocity. At highest velocities the neural response may be confined to only two impulses which implies that that the coding may depend on a single impulse interval.

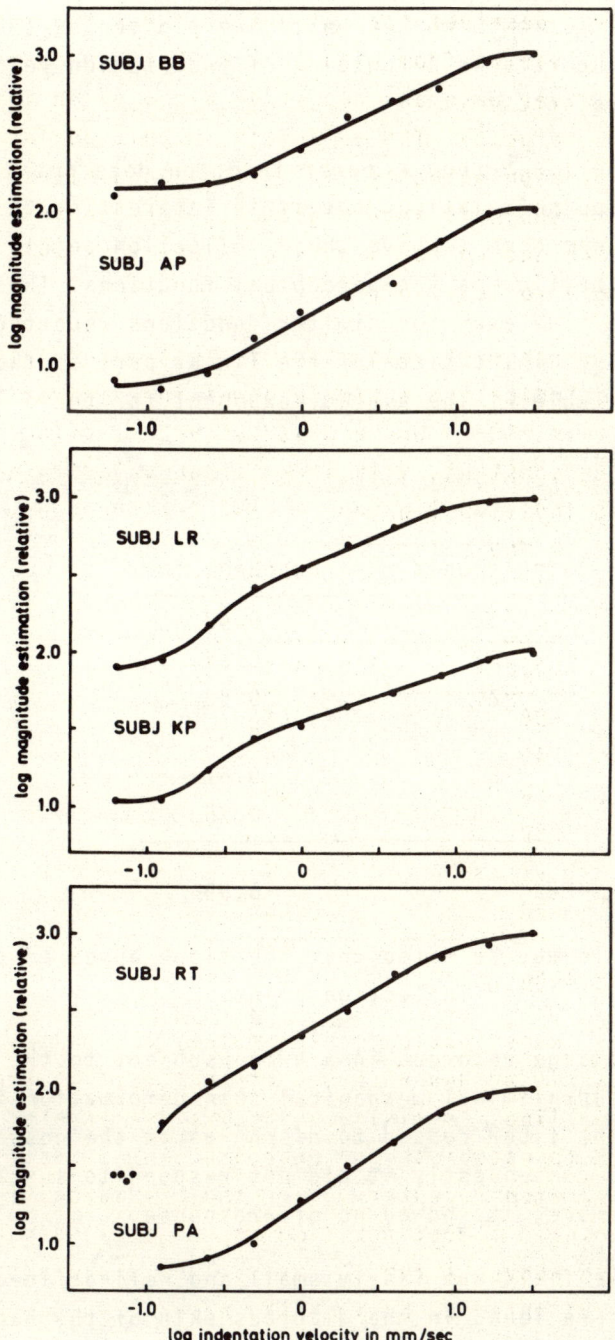

FIG. 1. Magnitude estimations of indentation velocity plotted in log-log coordinates for six subjects.

In Fig. 2 data from 6 monkey units are plotted as the instantaneous firing rate as a function of indentation velocity in log-log coordinates.

Again it is evident that a power function does not describe the stimulus-response relation, but it is interesting to note that these functions seem to have their inflection points at about the same velocities as the perceptual functions. This observation holds true even for similar functions reported by Knibestöl (1973). The slope of the linear part of the functions is found in Table 2. The average exponent for these units was 0.59.

TABLE 2.

Single unit	Exponent (n)
56	0.42
78	0.52
26	0.58
97	0.57
61	0.67
76	0.75
Mean	0.59

In passing, it may be noted that the slope appeared to increase with a raising lower inflection point.

Typical discharge recorded in a human subject to the rising phase of a supraliminal mechanical skin deformation is presented in Fig. 3. The fiber ceased to discharge on the cessation of the movement and consequently it did not respond to sustained pressure. Furthermore, it showed no off-response.

The receptive field was fairly small and well-defined. Seven such units were found in the glabrous skin of the hand. As was pointed out earlier, stimuli of different ramps did not differ noticeably in subjective intensity. It is therefore not considered appropriate to specify the ordinate as impulses per

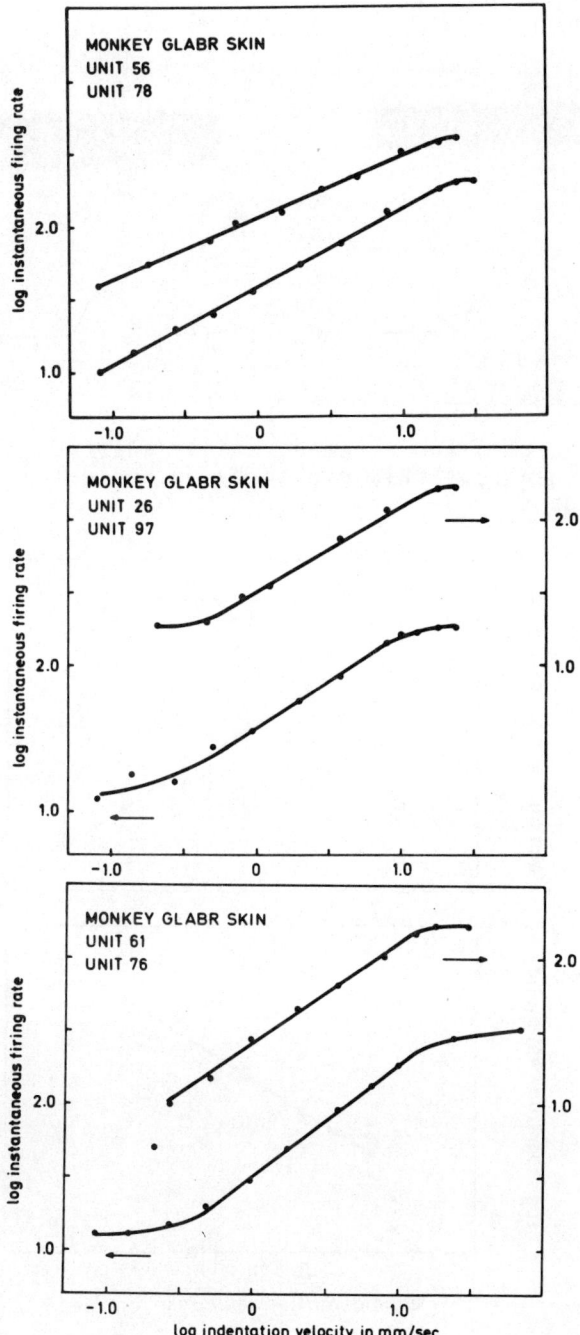

FIG. 2. Stimulus - response relations for six mechanoreceptive fibers ending in the sole of a monkey.

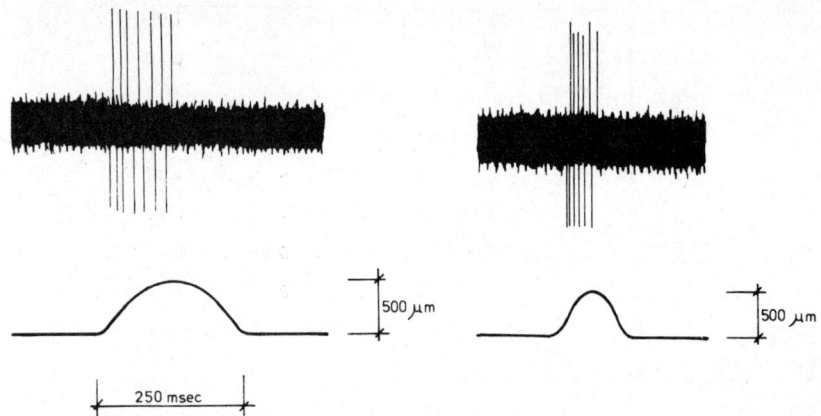

FIG. 3. Discharges from a human rapidly adapting fiber terminating in human glabrous skin evoked by mechanical pulses of different slopes.

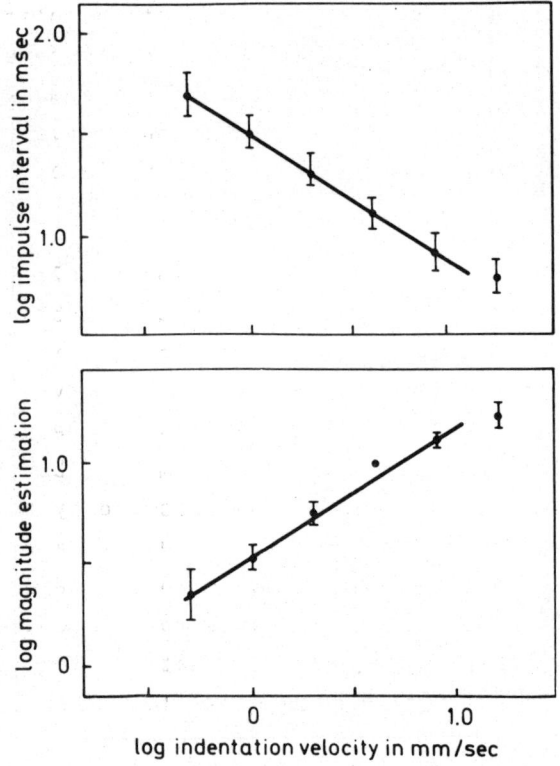

FIG. 4. Spike interval as a function of indentation velocity (upper graph). Magnitude estimations of the same stimuli plotted in log-log coordinates (lower graph).

second (i/s) since this measure is usually related the intensive aspect of a stimulation. The logical way of displaying the neural discharge is in terms of impulse interval (average interval between impulses) as a function of velocity (Fig. 4, upper graph). The data are presented as medians with variability expressed in terms of interquartile ranges. The relation is to a first approximation best described by a power function with an exponent of -0.63 for the neural response. The apparent velocity function grows with indentation velocity raised to a power of 0.61 (Fig. 4, lower graph).

DISCUSSION

The receptor system subjected to quantitative analysis in the present study is specifically sensitive to displacement velocity and ceases to fire upon maintained skin displacement. Plateau discharge was only sporadicly observed in the monkey preparation. Displacement rate sensitivity has also been investigated in the feline hairy skin (Tapper, 1965; Brown and Iggo, 1967; Nilsson, 1969).

With the technique of Hagbarth and Vallbo (1967, 1968) it is possible to intercept the sensory message and by doing so to record the impulse pattern from afferent fibers in man concurrently with the determination of the sensory experience of tactile stimulation. The characteristics of the dynamic discharge were identical for human and primate fibers, a finding that makes interspecies comparisons reported by other authors most meaningful (Talbot et al., 1968). Within a range of 0.5 - 10 mm/sec the majority of fibers seem to discharge with great accuracy. The neural (nerve discharge specified as instantaneous firing rate) and perceptual data are satisfactorily described by a simple power function with exponents less than 1.0 indicating negatively accelerating functions as is commonly found for other sensory systems (Marks, 1974). For instance, the potential of human olfactory receptors follows a power of about 0.5 (Franzén et al., 1970). Nevertheless, it is documented here that the slow increase in nervous activity as well as in subjective velocity at low displacement rates and the levelling off at high rates requires a more complicated mathematical description. It may sometimes be an end in itself to obtain a perfect fit to a straigth line. Instead, genuine departures from a power function may be important anchoring points in the evaluation of the transmission capacity of a sensory system. An attractive model, however, has recently been suggested by Zwislocki (1973).

In the two psychophysical studies a standard ramp of high and medium rate was used. One problem met with the method of magnitude estimation is that the size of the modulus may influence the subject's estimate and therefore the slope of the functions. The difference in exponents between the two present sets of data appears negligibly small although the effect of the standard goes in the expected direction (Stevens, 1956; Hellman and Zwislocki, 1963).

The striking similarity between the single-unit and subjective response implies that the neural information remains invariant as it passes different relay stations on its way to the brain. The successful correlation between perception and single-fiber activity may partly be explained by the fact that we are dealing with the temporal, not the intensive, aspect of the stimulus.

As emphasized in the present investigation the tactile sensation is related to the movement of the skin and to the dynamic characteristics of the mechanical stimulation. Motion is also a fundamental dimension of the visual system (Johansson, 1976) and movement detecting neurons form the substrate for the perceptual quality of motion (Grüsser and Grüsser-Cornehls, 1973). By the same token, velocity of skin indentation produces a primary quality that should be kept apart from that of intensity.

To summarize, the apparent velocity was an inverse function of the interspike interval. The conclusion to be drawn from these parallel studies in man and monkey is that the central structures interprets a decreasing spike interval as an increasing velocity of the deformation of the peripheral tissue. This may constitute the underlying mechanism of the rate component of the sensation of touch.

ACKNOWLEDGMENTS

This work was supported by the Swedish Council for Social Science Research and the Medical Research Council (Project B75-14X-4256-02).

REFERENCES

Brown, A.G. and Iggo, A. 1967. J. Physiol. 193, 707-733.
Cauna, N. 1956. Amer. J. Anat. 99, 315-350.
Franzén, O., Osterhammel, P., Terkildsen, K., and Zilstorff, K. 1970. In: Gustation and Olfaction. (Eds.) Ohloff, G. and Thomas, A.F. Internat. Symposium on Gustation and Olfaction, Geneva, 1970. London and New York: Academic Press. pp. 87-91.
Grüsser, O.-J., and Grüsser-Cornehls, U. 1973. In: Handbook of Sensory Physiology. (Eds.) Autrum, H., Jung, R., Loewenstein, W.R., McKay, D.M. and Teuber, H.-L. Heidelberg, Berlin and New York: Springer Verlag. pp. 334-429.
Hagbarth, K.-E. and Vallbo, Å.B. 1967. Acta Physiol. Scand. 69, 121-122.
Hellman, R.P. and Zwislocki, J. 1963. J. Acoustic. Soc. Amer. 35, 856-865.
Johansson, G. In: Handbook of Sensory Physiology. In preparation.
Knibestöl, M. 1973. J. Physiol. 232, 427-452.
Lindblom, U.J. 1965. J. Neurophysiol. 28, 966-985.
Marks, L.E. 1974. Sensory Processes. London and New York: Academic Press.
Montagna: W. 1960. Cutaneous Innervation. Oxford, London and New York: Pergamon Press.
Nilsson, B.Y. 1969. Acta Physiol. Scand. 77, 396-416.
Stevens, S.S. 1956. Amer. J. Psychol. 69, 1-25.
Stevens, S.S. 1957. Psychol. Review 64, 153-181.
Talbot, H.W., Darian-Smith, I., Kornhuber, H.H., and Mountcastle, V.B. 1968. J. Neurophysiol. 31, 301-334.
Tapper, D.N. 1965. Exp. Neurol. 13, 364-385.
Vallbo, Å.B. and Hagbarth, K.-E. 1968. Exp. Neurol. 21, 270-285.
Winkelmann, R.K. 1960. Nerve endings in Normal and Pathologic Skin. Springfield Ill.: Thomas.
Zwislocki, J.J. 1973. Kybernetik 12, 169-183.

DIFFERENTIAL EXCITATION OF DORSAL HORN AND SUBSTANTIA GELATINOSA MARGINAL NEURONS BY PRIMARY AFFERENT UNITS WITH FINE (Aδ AND C) FIBERS

T. KUMAZAWA* and E. R. PERL

Department of Physiology, University of North Carolina Chapel Hill, North Carolina, 27514 U.S.A.

The classical neuroanatomy of the late nineteenth century led to the first suggestions of a difference in the entry of large and small diameter dorsal root fibers into the spinal cord (Lissauer, 1886; Bechterew, 1887). Subsequently Ranson (1914, 1915) described a division of each dorsal root into a medial portion composed of large diameter, thickly-myelinated fibers and a lateral part containing only thinly myelinated and unmyelinated fibers; he argued that fibers of the medial division passed through the entry zone into the dorsal columns while the lateral bundle ran directly into the neuropil of the dorsal horn and/ or formed part of the tract of Lissauer. A difference in the termination and projection of the large diameter and small diameter fibers would provide a reason for their separation on joining the central nervous system and could reflect different functions for the two groups. Considerable evidence for a relation between afferent fiber diameter and function comes from a variety of sources including experiments in which peripheral nerves were either stimulated or blocked in order to distinguish the contributions from various fiber components. Such studies have consistently indicated that small diameter fibers have a critical place in cutaneous temperature appreciation and pain sense (Lewis, Pickering, Rothschild, 1931; Bishop, Heinbecker & O'Leary, 1932, 1933, 1934; Zotterman, 1933, 1936; Clark, Hughes & Glasser, 1935; Collins, Nulsen & Randt, 1960).

The way fine diameter afferent fibers enter the cord and their part in sensation takes on significance for their linkage to central neurons when considered in the light of Kuru's (1949) findings in human chordotomy patients of a close parallel between the distribution of dorsal horn marginal zone neurons (Waldeyer cells) showing retrograde degeneration and the regional loss of pain and temperature. A somewhat different

*Present address: Department of Physiology, Nagoya University School of Medicine, 65 Tsuruma-Cho, Showa-Ku, Nagoya, Japan.

conclusion was reached by Pearson (1952) from observations on Golgi impregnations; in agreement with Ramon y Cajal (1909) he argued that many fine afferent fibers have an initial bifurcation immediately under Lissauer's tract, with a branch passing into the marginal zone while other branches enter the substantia gelatinosa. In contrast, the thicker, more heavily myelinated fibers appeared to pass through the gelatinous region without signs of termination. The known relationships of activity in fine afferent fibers to pain sensation and these observations on their introspinal termination led Pearson (1952) to propose that the substantia gelatinosa was important for the transmission of information leading to pain.

These lines of reasoning and the underlying evidence are partially circumstantial, and consequently they have not been widely accepted. A more direct tie between the spinal termination of fine afferent fibers and their functional characteristics has been provided by experiments in which slowly conducting fibers (Aδ and/or C) were found to provide most or all of the excitatory drive to neurons of the dorsal horn's marginal zone (Rexed's lamina I) in the cat (Christensen and Perl, 1970). A similar set of experiments in monkey described herein provides additional information on the excitatory projection of afferent units with fine fibers.

<u>Afferent</u> <u>Input</u>. Excitation can be taken as an appropriate measure for determining peripheral sensory projections if it is presumed that primary afferent fibers initiate most, if not all, of their central action by excitation of second order cells. To be meaningful, studies on the central actions of sensory elements must be based upon reasonably complete knowledge of characteristics of primary (first order) sensory units and the use of an experimental design capable of distinguishing possible contributions from each type.

Much work has been done on primary afferent neurons and their responsiveness, but the technical difficulties of studying single elements with slowly conducting fibers has blocked the availability of a reasonably comprehensive picture until relatively recently. Table 1, listing some receptive characteristics of cutaneous receptors with afferent fibers conducting

TABLE I

PRIMATE CUTANEOUS RECEPTORS WITH AFFERENT FIBERS CONDUCTING UNDER 30 M/SEC

	Gentle Mechanical			Thermal		Tissue Damaging			
	Static	Moving (velocity)	Stretch	Cooling	Warming	Mechanical	Heat	Cold	Chemical
MYELINATED									
High-threshold Mechanoreceptor	-	-	-	-	-	++++	none or delayed	-	-
D Hair	+	+++ @ 2*	+ → ++	- → ++	-	+++ (transient)	-	-	-
Cooling	-	-	-	+++	inhibited	+	++	-	?
Heat-Mechanical Nociceptor	-	-	-	-	-	++++	++++	?	?
UNMYELINATED (C)									
Polymodal Nociceptor	+|	+|	-	** -	** -	+++ → ++++	+++ → ++++	+	++
C Mechano-receptor	+	+++ @ 1*	+ → ++	++	-	+++ (transient)	-	-	-
Warming	-	-	-	inhibited	+++	+ → ++	- → ++	-	?
High-threshold Mechanoreceptor	-	-	-	-	-	++++	-	? → ++	?

This listing applies to hairy skin of limbs (particularly proximal regions). Regional differences exist with the proportion of these types varying and others present. Sensory units classified as having C fibers in this table may have thinly myelinated fibers in other areas or species. Magnitude indicated by + signs is relative to maximal responses evoked in that type of element. * refers to most effective velocity of a moving contact graded 1 to 4 ["1" is equal to or below 1 mm/sec and "2" equals about 6 mm/sec. Many mechanoreceptors with fibers conducting over 30 m/sec are best excited by stimuli rated at 3 (30 mm/sec) or 4 (over 60 mm/sec) on this scale.] ** applies only before skin has been roughly handled to stimulated with noxious heat. - indicates no response, ± indicates variable small response to no response, → indicates range where variability exists. Gentle mechanical is defined as static or moving contact with minimal deformation, such as produced by a soft artist's brush. The "thermal" stimuli referred to above are changes from neutral levels (31° to 36° C) of 1° to 5° C.

under 30 m/sec (Aδ and C population) in the primate, is derived from several sources as well as personal experience (Iggo and Brown, 1967; Burgess and Perl, 1967, 1973; Iggo, 1968; Perl, 1968; Bessou and Perl, 1969; Bessou, Burgess, Perl and Taylor, 1971; Hensel, 1973; Kumazawa and Perl, 1976). This tabulation makes several points, including the fact that neither the conduction velocity nor the response to any particular form of natural stimulus, is sufficient by itself to differentiate between types of first order afferent units. For example, a cooling receptor with a slowly conducting myelinated afferent fiber will respond very vigorously to innocuous cooling of the skin, but may also give a considerable response in the transient phase of noxious heating (Dodt and Zotterman, 1936; Long, 1975). Moreover, the cooling receptors can be excited by strong mechanical stimulation, particularly if the stimulating object is below skin temperature. Thus, a response to noxious heat or noxious mechanical stimulation can be anticipated for neurons which receive an excitatory input from cooling receptors, and therefore does not necessarily define an input from nociceptors.

Additional comment also needs to be made on the projection of certain mechanoreceptors. Mechanoreceptors make up a large fraction of the sensory units with unmyelinated fibers in the cat (Bessou, Burgess, Perl and Taylor, 1970); however, in man, equivalent kinds of units have not been observed when C fiber sensory elements have been recorded percutaneously (Van Hees and Gybels, 1973; Törebjork, 1974). In monkey, as in cat, some C fiber sensory units show a maximal discharge to a very slowly moving object lightly contacting the skin; they are found in the innervation of the proximal limb regions in the rhesus monkey, although they appear to be less numerous than in equivalent nerves of the cat (Kumazawa and Perl, 1976). Therefore, as can be deduced from Table I, a spinal cord neuron in the monkey showing (1) a maximal response to a very light, slowly moving mechanical contact with the skin, (2) a moderate response to a sudden drop in skin temperature, (3) no response to skin heating, and (4) an evoked response to afferent volleys only when there are components conducting at C velocity, can be presumed to receive a major excitatory input from C mechanoreceptors. In this set of circumstances an important excitation from cooling thermoreceptors or "D hair" receptors appears unlikely because the cooling response is less than that produced by weak mechanical stimulation, and there is no response to afferent volleys limited to myelinated fibers.

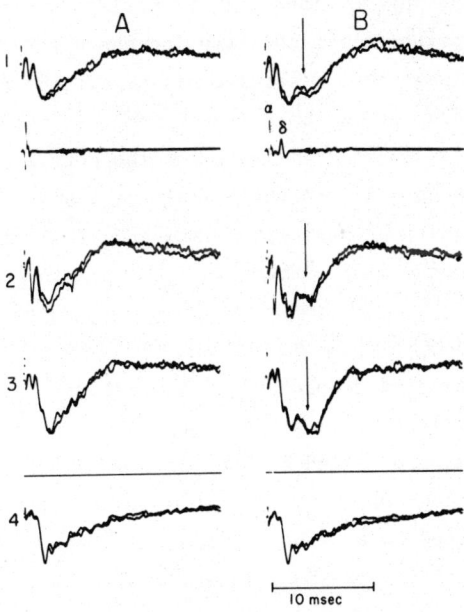

Fig. 1. Relation of responses recorded from the cat spinal cord to the composition of the evoking afferent volley. The upper traces in row 1 are recordings from a microelectrode on the surface of the root entrance zone and in rows 2, 3, 4 at progressively deeper locations within the dorsal horn. Row 3 was recorded at the marginal zone-- substantia gelatinosa interface and Row 4 (amplifier gain reduced to 40% of upper rows) at the level of lamina IV. Column A shows responses evoked by volleys in Aαβ fibers only; column B shows responses to volleys in Aα and Aδ fibers. The compound potentials for the volleys are illustrated by the lower traces of row 1. (from Christensen and Perl, 1970).

Dorsal Cord Potentials. In the earlier work on cat (Christensen and Perl, 1970), the search for evoked responses was selective. Intact dorsal roots or cutaneous nerves were stimulated at intensities chosen to produce one set of volleys in the most rapidly-conducting myelinated fibers of a bundle, and another set which also contained activity in slowly-conducting fibers. Using nerve volleys of different composition as a tool to differentiate responses in cat uncovered the fact that slowly-conducting myelinated fibers (Aδ) initiate a particular component of the dorsal cord potential which often increased relative to other parts of the evoked wave as a recording microelectrode was advanced into the spinal cord. The Aδ component of the cord potential reaches a maximum in the most superficial layers of the dorsal horn gray matter. Deeper, the response to afferent volleys alters dramatically; it becomes larger in amplitude with an earlier maximum and it is unchanged by addition of slowly-conducting elements. These points are illustrated by Fig. 1.

Reliable identification of recording locations is a crucial part in analyzing the projection of primary sensory units. For this purpose recording electrodes were filled with an aniline dye for iontophoretic deposition at each locus of interest. Dye marks made at sites where the potential initiated by Aδ fibers reaches maximal size suggested a close correlation to the marginal zone (Rexed's lamina I). The transition to the response seen more deeply in the dorsal horn was similarly determined to occur at about the dorsal edge of the nucleus proprius (Rexed's lamina IV), a level at which relatively large cells of the dorsal horn are evident. Postsynaptic unitary activity evoked by Aδ afferent fibers occurred at locations where the slow wave component indicated by the arrows in Fig. 1B was prominent. Fig. 2 illustrates the way in which unitary recordings from the cat dorsal horn were compared to the compound action potential of dorsal root fibers to establish that a postsynaptic discharge was related to the slowly-conducting myelinated fibers. While no attempt was made to systematically search for discharges from spinal neurons excited by Aα fibers, they were rarely seen at recording positions superficial to the dorsolateral order of the nucleus proprius (Rexed's lamina III-IV). With stimulus intensities sufficient to excite unmyelinated fibers, a delayed negative wave of variable amplitude appeared at a latency consistent with a C fiber input. The distribution of the C fiber evoked potential coincided in part with that of the deflection of the earlier wave initiated by the Aδ fibers.

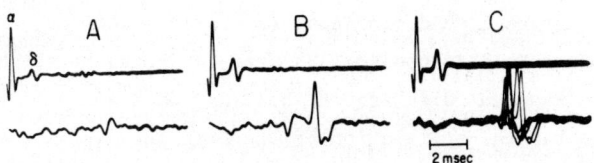

Fig. 2. Response of a unit in the marginal zone of cat dorsal horn to volleys of differing composition. Upper trace of each pair shows the compound dorsal root potential. Lower traces are potentials recorded with a microelectrode inserted into the spinal cord. The large diphasic impulse was first evoked during progressive increase in volley constituents at the level shown in B (40-50% of Aδ deflection). Five superimposed traces for responses to volleys containing all myelinated fiber components (Aα & Aδ) are shown in C (from Christensen and Perl, 1970).

Some units excited by the Aδ fibers did not respond differently when C fibers were recruited to the volleys; when tested with natural stimuli they were excited only when the skin was subjected to intense mechanical manipulation (the case for the unit shown in Fig. 2). In cat, in contrast to monkey, interpretation was simplified by the knowledge that small-diameter, myelinated cutaneous fibers distributed to hairy skin are associated almost exclusively with two types of receptors: high threshold mechanoreceptors, a form of nociceptor, and "D" hair follicle receptors (Burgess and Perl, 1967). Therefore the spinal elements responding to volleys containing slowly-conducting myelinated fibers and only to intense mechanical stimulation of the skin were judged to have an excitatory input from a single class of primary sensory unit, the myelinated-fiber mechanical nociceptor.

A number of units in the cat experiments responded to volleys with a latency and a relation to active fibers which suggested suprathreshold excitation by both Aδ and C fibers. Some of these were excited by intense mechanical stimuli and noxious heat but not to any form of innocuous stimulation of the skin and were presumed to receive strong excitatory inputs from both the high threshold mechanoreceptors with

Aδ fibers and C fiber polymodal nociceptors. Still another group of unitary discharges 1) had prominent spontaneous activity, 2) gave vigorous responses to skin cooling, 3) were inhibited by slight warming, 4) exhibited a transient discharge to heating above 45°C, 5) were activated by mechanical stimulation of the skin only when it was intense, and 6) discharged to afferent volleys only if C components were active. This set of characteristics was inferred to be consistent with excitatory input dominated by C fiber cooling receptors. In cat these three classes of units were recorded from loci distributed around the rim of the dorsal horn, with no evident systematic difference corresponding to functional characteristics. Originally it was believed that all were obtained from the large neurons of lamina I with variability in the location of recording sites attributable to the considerable variation in the location of marginal neurons (some marginal type

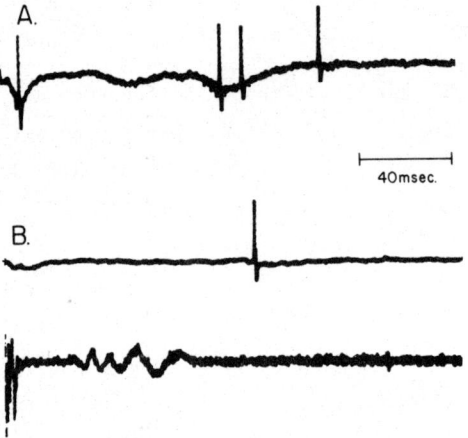

Fig. 3. Unitary responses evoked by maximal dorsal root volleys in superficially located parts of the monkey coccygeal dorsal horn. A: response showing a single impulse occurring at the time of the wave related to Aδ input and three impulses in relation to the later part of the negative wave evoked by C fiber input. The recording location was in the substantia gelatinosa. B: upper trace illustrates the single impulse which appeared only when C fiber components were present in the compound dorsal root potential (lower trace) (from Kumazawa and Perl, 1976b).

neurons are separated from the main body of the dorsal horn by bundles
of fibers, while cells of similar size and appearance are scattered
more deeply among the predominantly smaller elements of the substantia
gelatinosa).

Observations on primate suggest an extension of the concept that receptor-specific projection occurs from primary sensory units with fine fibers
to include neurons of the substantia gelatinosa as well as to those
of the marginal zone. The experimental design was similar to that
employed for the unanesthetized, acutely-spinal cat (Christensen and
Perl, 1970), except that monkeys were anesthetized by chloralose or
pentobarbital. All studies were made in lower sacral or coccygeal
segments. The dorsal spinal cord potential in monkey exhibited components
which were related to the composition of dorsal root volleys in the
fashion described for the cat, and unitary discharges excited only
by more slowly conducting myelinated components also were regularly
seen. A number of units were observed which responded once to myelinated
fiber input, and when C fiber activity was present, a second time
after the arrival of the unmyelinated afferent volley (Fig. 3A).
Moreover, the frequency of recordings from elements, apparently receiving
effective excitatory inputs only from the unmyelinated fibers (Fig.
3B) was relatively high. (The apparent increase of the latter from
the cat experience may have resulted from a change in the experimental
protocol, since in many of the cat experiments testing with C fiber
volleys was not systematic.) As explained above, further qualification
of the nature of the afferent projection is not as simple in the monkey
as in the cat. Table 1 shows that the cutaneous receptor population
with small diameter myelinated fibers consists of at least four receptive
types; at the same time, receptors with unmyelinated fibers also represent
a diverse population. What could have been an impossible situation
was simplified by an apparent selectivity in the afferent projection
to most elements encountered.

Some spinal cord neurons in the monkey which received a major excitatory
input from the small myelinated fibers, had little (or no) background
activity and were excited by intense mechanical stimulation of the
skin. They did not respond either to any form of gentle mechanical

stimulation or cutaneous temperature changes, including noxious heat. As in the cat, it was concluded that this group received their dominant excitatory input from the myelinated fiber, high-threshold mechanoreceptors.

A second class of dorsal horn unit in the monkey also responded to volleys when slowly-conducting myelinated fibers were present, generally did not have a demonstrable excitatory input from C fibers, and exhibited a conspicuous background discharge. The ongoing activity promptly ceased upon warming the receptive field and increased proportionally to the degree of innocuous cooling. Such elements were not excited by any innocuous mechanical stimuli, showed weak reactions to intense mechanical stimulation but often gave a considerable response when heating was carried to noxious levels. Their constellation of characteristics appeared consistent with an excitatory input from the cooling type of cutaneous receptor but did not eliminate the possibility of a weak excitatory convergence from other receptor types such as the high threshold mechanoreceptors. (One unit with persistent background discharge was inhibited by cooling and excited by warming; the effect of C fiber activity in volleys on its discharge was equivocal.)

The largest number of identified units responded consistently to afferent volleys in relation to C fiber activity but most (20 of 21) also gave an earlier response attributable to the $A\delta$ fibers and were not driven by innocuous cooling or gentle mechanical brushing. Firm pressure to skin usually evoked some impulses from elements of this group; however, vigorous responses followed only upon skin-damaging mechanical stimulation (forceful jabbing with a needle, or pinching with a toothed forceps) or cutaneous heating over $45°$ C. Typically, in the absence of prior noxious stimulation of the skin, cooling in the range from $35°$ to $20°$ C was without effect. This set of properties suggested that a major excitatory input came from polymodal nociceptors with C afferent fibers. A projection from either high threshold mechanoreceptors or from heat-mechanical nociceptors with myelinated fibers appeared to be present in addition for those elements which responded to the $A\delta$ volleys.

A fourth group of unitary elements shared the common characteristic

of a vigorous response to innocuous mechanical stimulation. The majority
(7 of 11) in the category responded consistently to afferent volleys
only when they contained active C fibers; the others were excited
by volleys with Aδ components (3 of 4 gave a second delayed response
when C fibers were added to a volley). They were most effectively
driven by a slowly moving mechanical contact with the skin. Other
features included a response to stretch of the skin outside of the
receptive field defined by light contact, a behavior which probably
contributed to the recruitment sometimes observed as the stimulus
progressively increased from contact through firm pressure. In addition,
sudden cooling of the skin initiated a variable increase in activity
which differed from the thermoreceptive elements described above in
that larger temperature swings were necessary and the thermally induced
response was always less than that produced by gentle moving contact.

Recording Location. The marginal zone of the dorsal horn is well-
defined in the monkey; the large neuronal perikarya composing it are

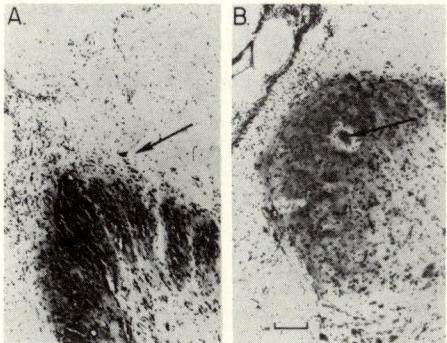

Fig. 4. Histological sections illustrating dye
marks at recording locations for two of the elements
studied in the monkey. The arrows indicate the
point of maximum dye concentration. A: at dorsal
column-dorsal horn junction near to a large pericornual
cell. B: large dye mark in the deeper part of
the substantia gelatinosa. Calibration-100μ (from
Kumazawa and Perl, 1976b).

more numerous than those of the equivalent regions in the cat. As
a consequence, in the monkey it was easier to distinguish between
recording loci (marked by dye deposition) which were related to the
marginal zone and those which were within the substantia gelatinosa
(equivalent to Rexed's lamina II). A well-defined mark was recovered
in the histological material for 51 recordings of unitary discharges
meeting the criteria for a selective activation by Aδ and/or C afferent
fibers and for which some useful characterization was available on
the pattern of effective cutaneous stimuli. The data on another 30
unitary recordings were consistent with the description which follows;
however, some important information for them was lacking (either an
adequate spectrum of stimuli had not been tried or the identification
of the recording site was equivocal).

A number of the marked recording locations were within the distribution
of the large pericornual cells making up the marginal zone. An example
is illustrated in Fig. 4A; large cells such as the one appearing immediately left of the arrow, apparently separated from the main body of
the dorsal horn grey matter, are relatively common both in primate
and cat (Bok, 1926; Christensen and Perl, 1970). Other recording
positions were unequivocally within the substantia gelatinosa (as
defined by Szentagothai and Rethelyi, 1973). A typical instance is
shown in Fig. 4B. To make comparisons possible, Fig. 5 illustrates
the 51 recording sites plotted on a standardized cross-sectional diagram
of the coccygeal spinal cord with care taken to maintain the relative
position to the grey-white matter boundaries, the distinctive cell
population of the substantia gelatinosa and the larger cells of nucleus
proprius. These positions were plotted from the histological material
without knowledge of the afferent characteristics. When this material
is grouped according to information on the afferent excitation, a
notable correlation appears. Units excited by myelinated primary
fibers conducting under 30 m/sec, but without evidence for an important
input from C afferent units, were recorded from locations in or immediately
adjacent to the marginal zone (Fig. 6A and B). Looked at in another
way, this analysis indicates that spinal elements with a major excitatory
input from the Aδ high threshold mechanoreceptors (Fig. 6A) and specific,
low-threshold thermoreceptors (Fig. 6B) cluster in the marginal layer.

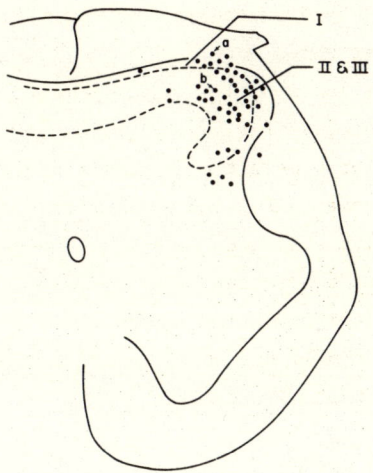

Fig. 5. Plot of recording loci in monkey for units excited only when Aδ and/or C fiber primary afferent elements were active. Each dot represents a histologically determined dye mark location positioned on a standardized diagram of a coccygeal segment according to measured distances from white matter-dorsal horn junction and the exterior of the spinal cord. All recovered marks are plotted. a: location for Fig. 4A; b: location for Fig. 4B. (from Kumazawa and Perl, 1976b).

It should be noted that one unit of the category with thermoreceptive characteristics was excited by warming, implying a C fiber projection; its recording site was also located on the inner limits of the marginal zone (Fig. 6B2).

Recording loci for units with a prominent or major excitatory input from the C fiber population of receptors tended to be more deeply located. The trend for a deeper location was well-marked for elements whose excitation was attributable in part or whole to the C fiber polymodal nociceptors (Fig. 6C). Therefore, even though some recordings from the units with a C fiber excitatory input were obtained from

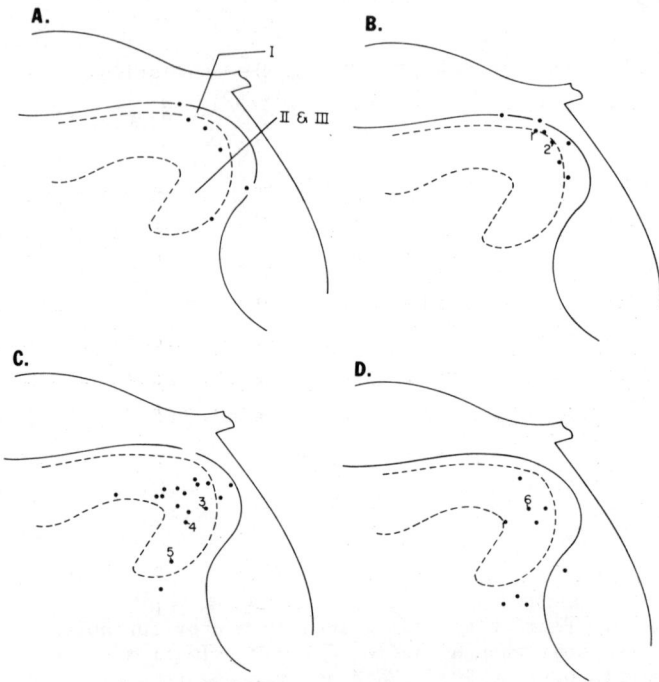

Fig. 6. Plot of recording loci according to most effective kinds of cutaneous stimulation. A: units excited only by intense mechanical stimulation, responded to volleys containing Aδ activity; but showed no evidence of C fiber input. B: units excited by innocuous cooling type except #2 which increased discharge on warming. All responded only to the Aδ component of single volleys except one which gave a second discharge when C activity was also present. C: units which responded to strong mechanical stimuli and noxious heat and were excited by C fiber components in dorsal root volleys. Most units also responded to the Aδ component of afferent volleys. D: units excited by innocuous low-velocity mechanical stimulation skin stretch. The five shown in the substantia gelatinosa responded to afferent volleys only when C fiber components were present (from Kumazawa and Perl, 1976b).

regions defined as the marginal zone, the modal distribution of these recording sites was shifted more deeply to center on the substantia gelatinosa.

Units excited by the kind of innocuous mechanical stimulation which implied an input from the C fiber mechanoreceptors had a less concentrated distribution, as illustrated in Fig. 6D. None were clearly in the marginal zone while a number were in the small cell layer of the substantia gelatinosa (equivalent to Rexed's lamina II). Four units evidencing an input from the Aδ and from C afferent fibers, whose responses were consistent with excitation by D hair receptors and C mechanoreceptors, were located in the lateral part of the neck of the dorsal horn. One mark for the latter type of unit was associated with a cluster of cells often seen separated from the remainder of the dorsal horn by a substantial band of fibers.

DISCUSSION

These results and analyses, taken together, provide evidence that the superficial layers of the dorsal horn--in particular, the marginal zone and the substantia gelatinosa Rolandi--contain neurons whose major excitatory input is derived from somatosensory receptors with thinly myelinated and C afferent fibers. It must be emphasized that experimental evidence supporting this conclusion was obtained by a particular experimental arrangement which focused attention exclusively upon activity specifically related to an excitatory input from slowly-conducting afferent fibers. Neither the studies on monkey nor the earlier work on cat (Christensen and Perl, 1970) have attempted to explore fully the spectrum of characteristics for neuronal elements making up the marginal zone and the substantia gelatinosa. For this reason, the negative aspect of these observations, the absence of units receiving a major excitatory input from the large diameter, rapidly-conducting myelinated fibers or a convergent input from both rapidly-conducting and slowly-conducting fibers must be viewed with this limitation in mind. Nevertheless, the apparent paucity of postsynaptic unitary activity excited by afferent volleys confined to Aαβ myelinated fibers in the most dorsolateral parts of the spinal grey matter cannot be ignored.

The elements from which recordings were obtained under the conditions of the present experiments showed a considerable specificity in terms of afferent projection; most received an important excitatory convergence from only one or a coherent class of peripheral sensory units. In particular, the data obtained from an anesthetized primate are consistent with the conclusion by Christensen and Perl (1970) that the posterior horn marginal zone (lamina I) is partially or exclusively a sensory nucleus receiving specific nociceptive or thermoreceptive afferent input. In addition, the primate experiments add an important facet in suggesting a differential distribution of primary afferent input between neurons of the marginal zone and those located more deeply in the substantia gelatinosa. One interpretation of these differences is that the marginal zone represents an area concerned with afferent input from primary sensory units with slowly-conducting myelinated fibers, while C afferent units project in some special excitatory fashion to certain neurons of the substantia layer. Some of the latter also receive an input from the thin myelinated fibers. These interpretations are predicated on the assumption that most or all of our extracellular recordings of unitary discharge derived from activity in the soma-dendritic part of neurons. This assumption appears reasonable because of the typical sequence seen for a unitary recording (Christensen and Perl, 1970) and the probability that the extracellular current generated by a cell would be greater where the surface membrane area was largest.

The distribution of recording loci itself mitigates the assumption on the origin of the recorded activity. Neurons of the marginal layer have a principal distribution of processes in the longitudinal or sagittal axis, an orientation also typical for many cells of the substantia gelatinosa (Ramon y Cajal, 1909; Earle, 1952; Pearson, 1952: Szentagothai, 1965; Scheibel and Scheibel, 1967). Considering the largely dorsal-ventral microelectrode penetrations used in the two studies, it is unlikely that the noted differential distribution of electrical activity stemmed from cells with somata in other regions such as those of deeper layers. For example, neurons of the dorsolateral rim of the nucleus proprius with dendrites extending into the substantia gelatinosa (Rethelyi and Szentagothai, 1973) could produce impulses in their dendritic trees, but the deeper-lying proximal dendrites and/or soma should also generate readily-recordable, extracellular impulsive potentials. The fact is that penetration of the microelectrode in the ventromedial direction usually caused loss of the unitary recording before the characteristic change in the field potential related to the edge of the nucleus proprius was seen. There is no direct evidence on the source of the potentials recorded from the substantia gelatinosa. For reasons given elsewhere, it seems unlikely that the very small cells of this layer are good possibilities (Christensen and Perl, 1970), particularly since such recordings were rare in penetrations through the region. More probable candidates would appear to be the less common, larger cells of this region which more closely resemble neurons of the marginal zone in size (Pearson, 1952). It appears to be likely that an important functional significance underlies the differential distribution of recording loci for elements principally excited by the small diameter myelinated dorsal root fibers and those receiving a large or major input from the C afferent fibers.

The earlier morphological analyses (Ranson, 1914; Pearson, 1952; Szentagothai, 1964; Scheibel & Scheibel, 1968; Rethelyi & Szentagothai, 1969) and the present correlation of morphological, locational and functional properties taken together provide insight into the functional significance of the substantia gelatinosa. They suggest to us that a principal function of the substantia gelatinosa is to act as a receiving and distribution region for the unmyelinated primary afferent input. Even if this were its entire functional role, then the required organization could be expected to show a substantial complexity. Afferent information to the spinal cord coming from unmyelinated fibers has importance for thermal changes affecting the skin, noxious stimulation of the skin and probably deeper tissues, as well as innocuous mechanical events involving the skin. The possibility of sensory terminals from C fibers in association with blood vessels and viscera raises still further intricacies. The sensory impulses with so diverse an origin must be appropriately distributed and interacted with other sensory inputs to account for many reactions including the initiation and modulation of perception and of reflexes with both somatic and visceral distribution. The idea that the cells of the substantia gelatinosa and the marginal zone receive their input from the small diameter

afferent fibers directly, i.e., monosynaptically, is implicit in this
proposal for functional organization. Physiological studies cannot
provide adequate evidence on this point since the latency for the
first arrival of activity over the more slowly-conducting afferent
fibers is difficult to predict accurately, and the range of conduction
velocities involved has too great a variation to allow useful deductions
on relations between the arrival of activity and the time of a postsynaptic
activation. Some direct evidence on this point has come from morphological
studies which, on the grounds of degenerating synaptic complexes,
conclude that fine calipered dorsal root fibers do terminate directly
on cells of the marginal zone and the substantia gelatinosa (Ralston,
1965; Rethelyi and Szentgothai, 1969).

The proposal that the substantia gelatinosa represents a receiving
zone for unmyelinated afferent fibers is not new. Ranson (1914) suggested
this possibility in his classical studies on the unmyelinated fibers
of the dorsal roots and Lissauer's tract. On the basis of Golgi work,
Pearson (1952) and Earle (1952) also described termination of very
fine primary afferent fibers in the substantia gelatinosa and from
this, argued that the substantia gelatinosa has an important part
in pain perception. The latter, of course, would fit with our description
of neurons within the substantia gelatinosa which apparently are effectively
excited largely by polymodal nociceptors.

SUMMARY

1. In both cat and monkey, recordings of activity evoked by a specified
afferent input showed that neurons of the spinal dorsal horn marginal
zone and substantia gelatinosa were selectively excited by small diameter
dorsal root fibers.

2. In both species, the important excitatory projection to individual
units was most commonly limited to a single or coherent class of sensory
receptors. Spinal elements with specific nociceptive, with thermoreceptive
and with low-velocity mechanoreceptive properties were found.

3. In the monkey, units powerfully excited by primary units with
fine myelinated (Aδ) fibers were recorded from positions centered
in the marginal zone. In contrast, units receiving a powerful excitatory
projection from unmyelinated (C) fiber primary afferent units were

recorded from more deeply placed loci within the substantia gelatinosa.
4. On the basis of these observations and the existing morphological evidence of a fine afferent fiber projection to the same regions it was proposed that in the primate a) the substantia gelatinosa in part acts as a receiving and integrative nucleus for sensory information arriving over primary sensory units with unmyelinated fibers and b) the posteromarginal zone in part serves as a receiving and projecting nucleus for afferent information principally stemming from the myelinated fiber nociceptors and thermoreceptors.

REFERENCES

1. Bechterew, W. (1887). Le cerveau de l'homme dans ses rapports et connexions intimes. Arch. slaves de biol. 3, 293-321, 4, 1-30.

2. Bessou, P., Burgess, P.R., Perl, E.P., and Taylor, D.D. (1971). Dynamic properties of mechanoreceptors with unmyelinated (C) fibers. J. Neurophysiol. 34, 1, 116-131.

3. Bessou, P. and Perl, E.R. (1969). Response of cutaneous sensory units with unmyelinated fibers to noxious stimuli. J. Neurophysiol. 32, 6 1025-1043.

4. Bok, S.T. (1926). Das Ruckenmark. Hdb. d. mikr. Anat. d. Menschen. vol. 4, pp. 478-578, ed. von Molhendorff. Berlin: Springer.

5. Brown, A.G. and Iggo, A. (1967). A quantitative study of cutaneous receptors and afferent fibres in the cat and rabbit. J. Physiol. 193, 707-733.

6. Burgess, P.R. and Perl, E.R. (1973). Cutaneous mechanoreceptors and nociceptors. Handbook of Sensory Physiology. vol. II, pp. 29-78, ed. Iggo, A. Berlin: Springer-Verlag.

7. Burgess, P.R. and Perl, E.R. (1967). Myelinated afferent fibres responding specifically to noxious stimulation of the skin. J. Physiol. 190, 541-562.

8. Cajal, Ramon y S. (1909). Histologie du Systeme Nerveux de L'Homme et Des Vertebres. Paris: Maloine.

9. Christensen, B.N. and Perl, E.R. (1970). Spinal neurons specifically excited by noxious or thermal stimuli: marginal zone of the dorsal horn. J. Neurophysiol. 33, 293-307.

10. Clark, D., Hughes, J. and Gasser, H.S. (1935). Afferent function in the group of nerve fibers of slowest conduction velocity. Am. J. Physiol. 114, 69-76.

11. Collins, W. F., Nulsen, F. E., and Randt, C. T. (1960). Relation of peripheral nerve fiber size and sensation in man. Arch. Neurol. 3, 47-51.

12. Dodt, E. and Zotterman, Y. (1952). The discharge of specific cold fibres at high temperatures (The paradoxical cold). Acta physiol. scand. 26, 358-365.

13. Earle, K. M. (1952). The tract of Lissauer and its possible relation to the pain pathway. J. Comp. Neurol. 96, 93-109.

14. Hees, J. van and Gybels, J. M. (1973). L'activité unitaire des fibres C en registrée dans un nerf cutané chez l'homme et sa relation avec la douleur. Acta Neurol. Belg. 73, 39-43.

15. Heinbecker, P., Bishop, G. H. and O'Leary, J. (1932). Allocation of function to specific fiber types in peripheral nerves. Proc. of the Society for Experimental Biology and Medicine 30, 304-305.

16. Heinbecker, P., Bishop, G. H. and O'Leary, J. (1933). Pain and touch fibers in peripheral nerves. Arch. Neurol. Psychiat. 29, 771-789.

17. Heinbecker, P., Bishop, G. H. and O'Leary, J. (1934). Analysis of sensation in terms of the nerve impulse. Arch. Neurol. Psychiat. 31, 34-53.

18. Hensel, H. (1973). Cutaneous thermoreceptors. Handbook of Sensory Physiology. Vol. II, pp. 79-110, ed. Iggo, A., Berlin: Springer-Verlag.

19. Iggo, A. (1969). Cutaneous thermoreceptors in primates and sub-primates. J. Physiol. 200, 403-430.

20. Kumazawa, T. and Perl, E. R. (1976). Primate cutaneous sensory units with unmyelinated C afferent fibers. (Submitted).

21. Kumazawa, T. and Perl, E. R. (1976b). Specific excitation of neurons of the spinal cord dorsal horn marginal zone and substantia gelatinosa by cutaneous sensory units with $A\delta$ and C fibers in the monkey. (Submitted).

22. Kuru, M. (1949). Sensory Paths in the Spinal Cord and Brain Stem of Man. Resumé, pp. 675-713. Tokyo: Sogensya.

23. Lewis, T., Pickering, G. W. and Rothschild, P. (1931). Centripetal paralysis arising out of arrested bloodflow to the limb, including notes on a form of tingling. Heart 16, 1-32.

24. Lissauer, H. (1886). Beitrag zum Faserverlauf im Hinterhorn des Menschlichen Rüchenmarks und zum Verhalten desseben bei Tabes dorsalis. Arch. f. Psychiat. 17, 377-438.

25. Long, R. R. (1973). Cold fiber heat sensitivity: dependency of "paradoxical" discharge on body temperature. Brain Res. 63, 389-392.

26. Perl, E. R. (1968). Myelinated afferent fibres innervating the primate skin and their response to noxious stimuli. J. Physiol. 197, 593-615.

27. Pearson, A. A. (1952). Role of gelatinous substance of spinal cord in conduction of pain. Arch. Neurol. Psychiat. 68, 515-529.

28. Ralston, H. J. III (1966). Dorsal root projections to dorsal horn of cat spinal cord. Anat. Rec. 159, 406.

29. Ranson, S. W. (1913). The course within the spinal cord of the non-medullated fibers of the dorsal roots: A study of Lissauer's tract in the cat. J. Comp. Neurol. 23, 259-281.

30. Ranson, S. W. (1914). The tract of Lissauer and the substantia gelatinosa rolandi. Am. J. Anat. 16, 97-126.

31. Ranson, S. W. and von Hess, C. L. (1915). The conduction within the spinal cord of the afferent impulses producing pain and the vasomotor reflexes. Am. J. Physiol. 38, 128-152.

32. Rethelyi, M. and Szentagothai, J. (1969). The large synaptic complexes of the substantia gelatinosa. Exp. Brain Res. 7, 258-274.

33. Rethelyi, M. and Szentagothai, J. (1973). Distribution and connections of afferent fibres in the spinal cord. Handbook of Sensory Physiology, Vol. II, ed. Iggo, A., pp. 208-252. Berlin: Springer-Verlag.

34. Scheibel, M. E. and Scheibel, A. B. (1968). Terminal axonal patterns in cat spinal cord. II. The dorsal horn. Brain Res. 9, 32-58.

35. Szentagothai, J. (1964). Neuronal and synaptic arrangement in the substantia gelatinosa rolandi. J. Comp. Neurol. 122, 219.

36. Törebjork, E. (1974). Single unit activity in afferent and sympathetic C fibres recorded from intact human skin nerves. Acta Univ. Upsal 211, 1-23.

37. Zotterman, Y. (1933). Studies in the peripheral nervous mechanism of pain. Acta Med. Scand. 80, 1-64.

38. Zotterman, Y. (1936). Specific action potentials in the lingual nerve of cat. Skandinav. Archiv. 75, 105-119.

ACKNOWLEDGEMENT

The work on primate was supported by a grant NS10321 from the National Institute of Neurological and Communication Disorders and Stroke of the United States Public Health Service. Computer, electronic, and histological facilities were provided by NINCDS, USPHS grant NS-11132.

Discussion:

Gordon: May I ask a little about identification of cells? I noticed that in your first diagram showing the set-up of your experiment, that you had a pair of stimulating electrodes sitting on the dorsal-lateral cord at about cervical four. Were you able to establish which groups of these cells projected into ascending systems and if so, how far and where they went?

Perl: The electrode that was at the cervical spinal cord was to be used for testing of antidromic projections. We used, actually, several types, I am sorry to say, not a constant kind. The majority of the experiments were done with a needle electrode placed into the lateral columns of the spinal cord at a position where we could record evoked activity from stimulation of the dorsal root. A number of our experiments were done with ball electrodes placed on the surface of the spinal cord. We were not very satisfied and are still not satisfied with our antidromic stimulating arrangements because it was easy to show that movements of the electrode could influence whether or not we could excite the unit antidromically. All we can say is that we did have positive results from a certain group of units and there was a consistent characteristic, namely that they were located in the marginal zone. This may have something to do with the way the axon projects from this region or with the size of the axon. That is, only one of our projecting neurons had a fiber whose conduction velocity was under five meters per second.

Gordon: It was specifically the question of antidromic identification that I was talking about. Which one of them, if any were you able to identify?

Perl: Let me summarize by saying that we tested about twenty units in the monkey for antidromic activation. Those that we proved were antidromically excited by the kind of response they gave to the stimulation of the cervical cord are marked by triangles (in Fig 5, Kumazawa, Perl, Burgess & Whitehorn, J. Comp. Neurol. $\underline{162}$: 1-12, 1975). This is the quality of our data. We did not test every unit that we recorded from, because in many experiments we did not have an adequate antidromic stimulating electrode. Those where we thought there was a reasonable possibility of exciting with our cervical cord electrode are plotted here.

Gordon: And you did not go on into the thalamus?

Perl: No, we did not.

Zotterman: In 1951 Dodt and I found in the lingual nerve of the cat a great number of A-delta fibers responding specifically to warming. Did you find

A-delta fibers responding to warming the skin?

Perl: I waffled a little bit on that, Sir. What I did say was that we had one unit recorded in the spinal cord which was at the edge of the marginal zone which responded as if it had a specific input from warming receptors. That particular element probably responded to both C-fibers and to delta units in afferent volleys. In our experience in the monkey in this particular region, the warming units tend to have unmyelinated fibers.

Boivie: Please look at Dr Perl's last slide again. (See fig. 5, Kumazawa Perl, Burgess & Whitehorn, J. Comp. Neurol. 162: 1-12, 1975). In our lab in Stockholm and in Dr Trevino's lab in Chapel Hill it has been demonstrated that those cells with the triangles (cells with that location) project both to the intralaminal region of the thalamus and to the ventroposterial region. This has been shown by injecting horse radish peroxidase (HRP) into either the intralaminal or the ventroposterial region of the thalamus of the monkey. We do not know if one cell projects to both areas or if they are two different cells.

Perl: Prior to the HRP experiments Trevino, Coulter and Willis (1974) have shown that one can antidromically excite spinal cells from various loci in the thalamus some of which are located along this rim region. I do not want to give the impression that some of the cells which we could not antidromically drive are not projecting cells. We do not know that. All we know is that projecting cells exist out in this rim region.

Zimmermann: I have a comment concerning the type and size of neurons involved in your 1970 paper with Christensen (in the cat). All these neurons having AS input had been found in the marginal layer of the dorsal horn. This finding was compatible with your suggestion that the cells recorded from these were the large Waldeyer cells. In your contribution today you report locations of such cells all over the substantia gelatinosa, which is said to contain only very small neurons. Do you claim to have recorded from such small cells?

Perl: Let me make two comments. Professor Zimmermann has quite correctly focused on something. If he looks carefully at the paper with Christensen, he will see that units which responded to heat, in fact, were also plotted in a distribution similar to Fig. 6 C. Our conclusion was that we were recording from the Waldeyer cells because a large cell always was close to our marked recording site. We cannot say that in the present analysis. However, it is wrong to think that there are only small cells in the substantia gelatinosa. A number of Golgi studies, including recent ones by Gobal at the N.I.H. and by Rethely of Budapest show that there are a substantial number of rather large cells in the substantia gelatinosa interposed among the very small cells. It is conceivable that our recordings were made from these larger cells.

THE SPINOCERVICAL TRACT: ORGANIZATION AND NEURONAL MORPHOLOGY

A. G. BROWN*

Department of Physiology, Royal (Dick) School of Veterinary Studies, University of Edinburgh, Edinburgh EH9 1QH, Scotland

The spinocervical tract (SCT) is the spinal part of the spinocervical-lemniscal system described by Morin in 1955 [1]. It is particularly well-developed in carnivores but is also present in primate species (Bryan, Coulter and Willis [2]). Physiological studies of the SCT have been reviewed recently by Brown [3] and Boivie and Perl [4].

The present report is an account of experiments designed to determine, 1. how SCT cells are arranged in the lumbosacral spinal cord, 2. the morphology of their somata and dendritic trees, and 3. whether or not their axons have collateral branches. All experiments were performed on cats, either anaesthetized with chloralose (70 mg.kg^{-1}) or decerebrate and paralyzed with gallamine triethiodide. SCT neurones were always identified electro-:physiologically by antidromic activation from the dorsolateral funiculus at the third cervical segment and absence of such activation from the first cervical segment or reduction of antidromic conduction velocity of at least 1/3 between the first and third cervical segments.

THE LOCATION AND DISTRIBUTION OF SCT NEURONES

Neurones which give rise to SCT axons are thought to lie in the dorsal horn

---

*Experiments reported in this article were performed in collaboration with Drs. C.R. House, P.K. Rose and P.J. Snow. The work was supported by a grant from the British Medical Research Council.

of the spinal cord between about 1.0 and 2.0 mm from the cord dorsum (Hongo, Jankowska and Lundberg [5]; Bryan, Trevino, Coulter and Willis [6]) which would place them in Rexed's [7] laminae III, IV and V. It had been noted by Hongo et al. [5], however, that SCT neurones were often well separated from one another. Since we were determining the dimensions of the dendritic trees of SCT neurones (see below) it seemed worthwhile to determine the location and distribution of all SCT neurones in parts of the spinal cord of individual cats. Accordingly 2 experiments were performed in which SCT cells were recorded extracellularly. In one experiment 77 micro-:electrode tracks were made at the intersections of a 250 μm grid in the seventh lumbar segment, each track being taken to a depth of 3000 μm from the cord dorsum. In the other experiment a longitudinal row of 36 electrode tracks was made, 1.0 mm from the midline, to a depth of 3000 μm and also with inter-track spacing of 250 μm. The 250 μm spacing was chosen in these experiments because previous experience had shown that it was always possible to record extracellularly from SCT neurones at distance of up to 150 μm from the cell soma.

The results of the first (grid) experiment are shown in Fig. 1. Fifty-three SCT neurones were recorded from a 2.5 mm rostro-caudal length of cord in the seventh lumbar segment. The neurones formed a band across the dorsal horn (Fig. 1A) all except one at depths between 1000 and 2200 μm from the cord dorsum. Most (85%) were within a 500 μm band centred on Rexed's lamina IV with more cells laterally than medially. The medio-lateral distribution, as well as the rostro-caudal distribution, of SCT neurones is shown in Fig. 1B which also includes an indication of the average medio-lateral and rostro-caudal extents of SCT neurone dendritic trees determined by Procion dye injection (see below). In the second experiment the electrode tracks passed through the lateral 1/3 of the dorsal horn and a similar density of SCT neurones was encountered as in the lateral parts of the grid in the first experiment (about 1.3 cells in a track). In the 8.5 mm length of cord examined 45 SCT cells were recorded in 35 tracks. Statistical examination of the numbers of cells in individual tracks and in adjacent pairs of tracks indicated a strong probability that the distribution of cells was random (Poissonian) in the sagittal plane (x^2 test, P=0.9-0.95 and 0.05-0.1 respectively).

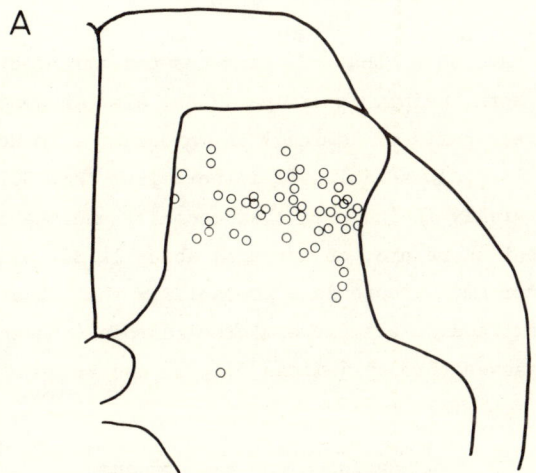
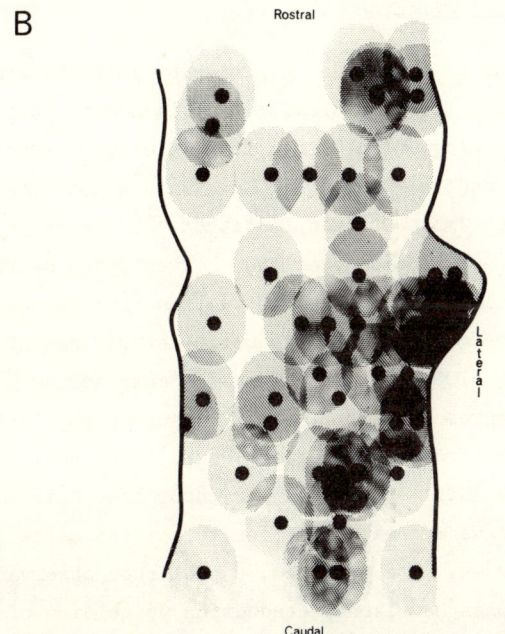

FIG. 1. The distribution of SCT neurones in the lumbar dorsal horn. A. The positions of 53 SCT neurones record‑
:ed extracellularly from a 2.5 mm length of L7 cord shown on a transverse section of the cord. The positions were determined from histological reconstructions.
B. The positions, in the horizontal plane, of 52 SCT neurones. The stippled region around each location in‑
:dicates the average extent of SCT dendritic trees as determined by Procion dye injection. The one very deep neurone has been omitted.

These experiments have shown that SCT neurones are arranged in a sheet across the dorsal horn, mainly in lamina IV but also in ventral parts of lamina III and dorsal parts of lamina V in agreement with Hongo et al. [5] and Bryan et al. [6]. In addition it is now clear that SCT neurones are more plentiful laterally in the cord than medially and the density of cell packing is such that there are, on average, about 14 SCT neurones below each mm^2 of cord dorsum. There is a probability that about one SCT neurone will be recorded extracellularly as a microelectrode (chosen for isolation of single units) passes through laminae III, IV and V.

THE MORPHOLOGY OF SCT NEURONES

Somata and dendritic trees

Intracellular staining of individual neurones by iontophoresis of Procion dyes, introduced by Stretton and Kravitz [8], is a most powerful technique for studying the morphology of neurones from which electrophysiological recordings have been made. We [9, 10] have used a modification of the technique developed by Jankowska and Lindström [11] to stain SCT neurones with Procion Yellow (and Procion Scarlet). Twenty-two neurones were sufficiently well-filled to allow reconstruction from serial sections and they included neurones across the whole medio-lateral extent of the dorsal horn and at depths of 1100 to 2400 μm from the cord dorsum. In these respects they were representative of the SCT neurone population. In their conduction velocities (from upper cervical cord), however, they were not representative of the SCT. Extracellular recordings have shown that about 30% of SCT neurones have axonal conduction velocities below 30 $m.s^{-1}$ (Bryan et al. [6], Brown, Rose and Snow, unpublished observations). The Procion stained neurones had axonal conduction velocities of 24-79 $m.s^{-1}$ but all except one were within the range 42-79 $m.s^{-1}$. Attempts to impale SCT neurones with axons conducting at less than 40 $m.s^{-1}$ were nearly always unsuccessful. This suggests that these neurones had smaller somata than those with axons conducting at faster than 40 $m.s^{-1}$. Within the stained sample, however, there was no correlation between the axonal conduction velocities and the volumes of SCT cell somata measured planimetrically from photographs of serial sections.

Although SCT neurones are restricted to a sheet running across the dorsal horn they do not constitute a morphologically homogeneous population. Projections of the reconstructed neurones, in the transverse plane, are shown in Fig. 2, where it can be seen that the dendritic trees vary greatly in the frequency of branching of dendrites and in the morphology of the projections of the trees. For ease of description the neurones have been classified into six categories, although these divisions may be arbitrary and the dendritic trees really form a morphological continuum. The six types are, 1) <u>radially symmetrical</u> with dendrites extending for about equal distances from the soma in all directions including the rostral and the caudal ones, 2) <u>semicircular</u> with dendrites extending dorsally, medially and laterally in the transverse plane but not to any extent ventrally, 3) <u>large elliptical</u> with elliptical dendritic trees in which the major axis exceeds 500 μm, 4) <u>bi-lobed</u> with dendrites in two lobes, one each side of the soma, 5) <u>triangular</u> with almost all dendrites projecting dorsally from the soma and which have conical dendritic trees when the rostro-caudal plane is also considered, 6) <u>small elliptical</u> with the major axis less than 400 μm in length.

There was some separation of the different categories of SCT neurones within the dorsal horn. Bi-lobed neurones were found only in the medial third of the horn and small elliptical neurones only in the lateral half. Radially symmetrical, semicircular and large elliptical types were found in the central parts but not in the medial or lateral parts of the horn. Triangular neurones were found across the medial two thirds of the dorsal horn.

Because of the topographical organization of the dorsal horn, see Bryan et al. [6], there were some correlations between the morphology of the den:dritic trees and the cutaneous receptive fields of some neurones. Thus small elliptical neurones always had large receptive fields including parts of the thigh or hip and were the only SCT neurones found in the lateral third of the horn. Bi-lobed neurones had small receptive fields on the toes and were located in the medial third of the dorsal horn. Cells with receptive fields on the toes, however, were not exclusively represented by bi-lobed neurones nor were they restricted to the medial

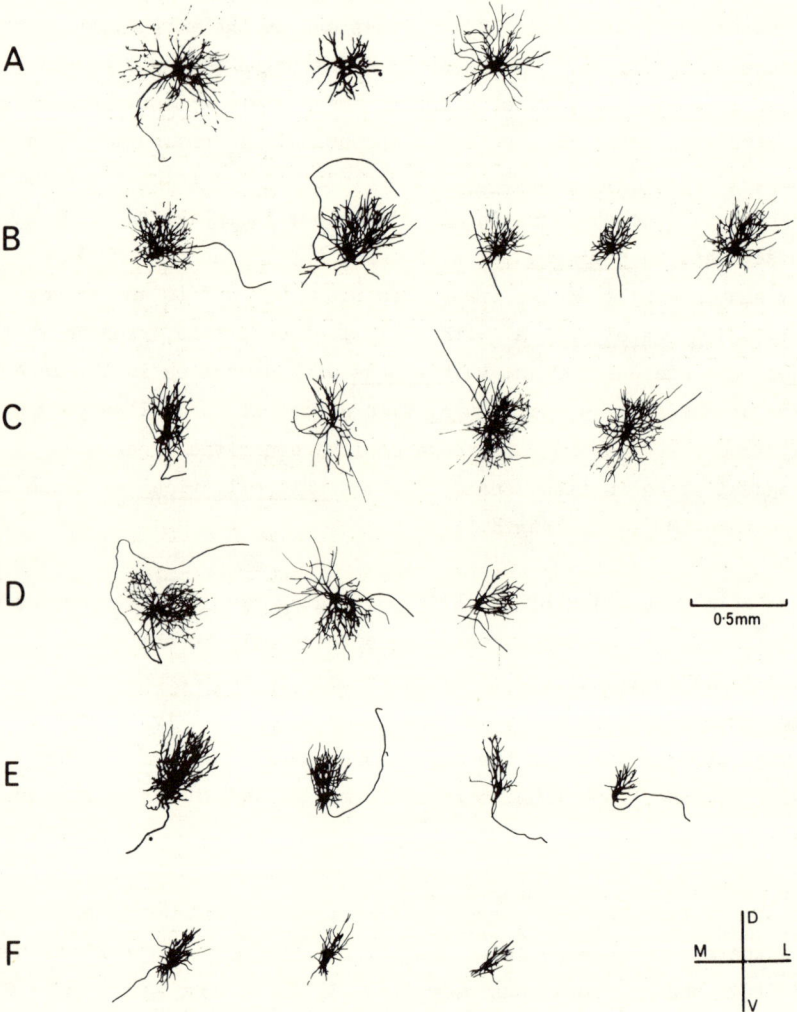

FIG. 2. Projections, in the transverse plane, of 22 SCT neurones reconstructed from serial sections after stain:ing with Procion dyes. The dendritic trees are divided into 6 categories A) radially symmetrical, B) semicircu:lar, C) large elliptical, D) bi-lobed, E) triangular, F) small elliptical.

third of the horn. Furthermore, within the sample of 22 reconstructed SCT neurones there were no clear correlations between dendritic tree morphology and the excitatory input to the neurones (hair movement, skin pressure, strong pinch).

These experiments have demonstrated some of the cells which give rise to the SCT. Scheibel and Scheibel [12] have suggested that lamina IV neurones with conical (our triangular type) dendritic trees are SCT cells and Réthelyi and Szentagothai [13] suggest that 'antenna type' neurones are the cells of origin of the SCT. The present results have shown that the SCT arises from these types of cells but in addition from several other types as well. Jankowska [14] has illustrated 4 neurones stained with Procion yellow which gave rise to SCT axons and which are similar to types that we have seen.

When the extents of the dendritic trees of SCT neurones are considered together with the density of the cells (see above) it is clear that SCT cell dendrites form a rich arborization in laminae III, IV and V. Examination of our original material reveals that there is relatively little extension of the dendrites into lamina II or into lamina VI. Furthermore, within laminae III-V there appears to be few or no spaces in the SCT dendritic arbor and also, except laterally, relatively little overlap between the dendritic trees of individual cells. This leads to the conclusion that the SCT forms a very effective filter for the incoming information from the skin.

Axons and axon collaterals of SCT neurones

Procion dyes are not very successful in staining the axons and axon collaterals of neurones (see Kater and Nicholson [15]). In the sample of 22 SCT neurones stained with this technique the maximum length of axon stained was 1.9 mm. Although nearly all neurones had a few hundred μm of axon stained only one showed any trace of an axon collateral. Similar results have been obtained by Jankowska, Rastad and Zangger (quoted by Jankowska [14]) who only found evidence of an axon collateral in one SCT neurone from a number they stained with Procion yellow. According to classical (Ramon Y Cajal [16]) and more recent (Scheibel and Scheibel [12]) anatomical studies, however, neurones in the dorsal horn have axons which give rise to a number of collateral branches before they enter the ipsilateral dorsolateral funiculus and ascend the spinal cord.

Whether or not the axons of ascending sensory systems give off collaterals near their cells of origin or during their ascent has important functional implications. In order to examine for this possibility it was necessary to develop a suitable staining technique that would allow electro- :physiological recording from an identified neurone followed by the injection of that neurone with a substance that could be visualized subsequently and which would pass into the axon and any axon collaterals that were present. We (Snow, Rose and Brown[17]) have developed such a technique which utilizes microelectrodes filled with a horseradish peroxidase solution which can be injected into a neurone by intracellular iontophoresis. The technique will stain the initial 1.5 cm of axon and its collateral branches together with the soma and dendrites of a neurone. We have applied the technique to cells of the SCT and so far have stained 19 neurones.

<u>The main axon of SCT neurones.</u> Two-dimensional projections of reconstruct- :ions of SCT neurones are shown in Figs. 3 and 4, from transverse and sagittal sections of the spinal cord. The initial parts of the main axons may also be seen in some of the neurones illustrated in Fig. 2 from Procion yellow injected material.

The axon usually arose from the soma but occasionally from a basal dendrite. Immediately after its origin the axon pursued a tortuous path through the grey matter of the dorsal horn, sometimes forming complex loops (Fig. 4). Ultimately the axon reached the most medial and superficial part of the ipsilateral dorsolateral funiculus where it usually made an abrupt turn and then ran in an almost straight line as it ascended the spinal cord. The initial few hundred μm of the main axon were often thinner than the following part and also were often not very well stained. This made reconstruction difficult (Fig. 3B). All main axons ascended the cord in the most super- :ficial part of the ipsilateral dorsolateral funiculus where they have been demonstrated in electrophysiological experiments (Lundberg and Oscarsson[18];

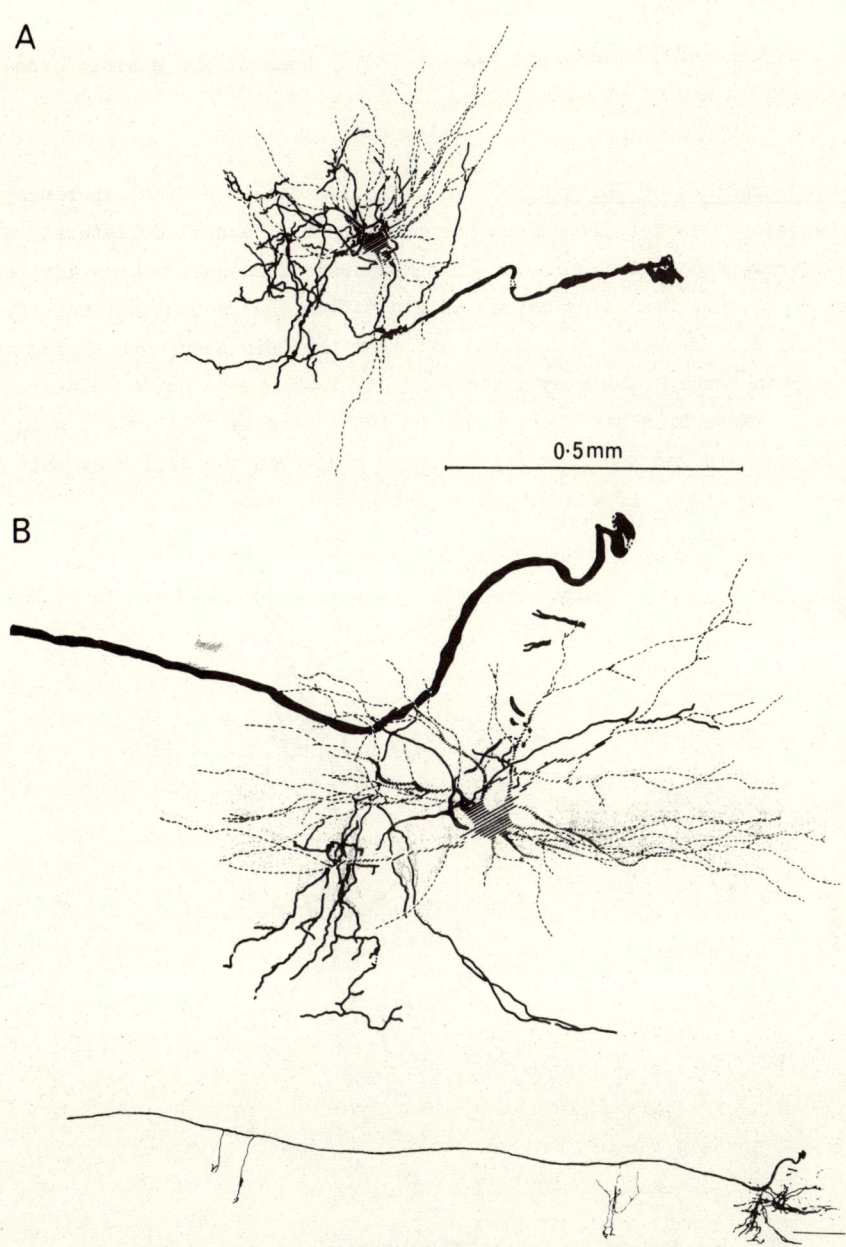

FIG. 3. Projections of SCT neurones reconstructed from serial sections after staining with horseradish peroxi:dase. A. Reconstructed in the transverse plane. B. Reconstructed in the sagittal plane. The axon and its collaterals are shown by solid lines, the soma and dendrites by broken lines.

Taub and Bishop [19]; Brown and Franz [20]). None of the stained axons ascended the cord in any other region.

Collateral branches of SCT axons. The Procion dye injection experiments described above did not prepare us for the extent of axonal collateral branching revealed by the horseradish peroxidase technique. Some idea of the extent of this branching may be obtained from the reconstructions of Figs. 3 and 4. Branches were given off from the main axon both during its tortuous path through the grey matter and as it ascended the dorsolateral funiculus. More branches arose close to the cell body than as the axon ascended the cord and the furthest distance away from the cell body that a collateral was given off was 5.5 mm in the present material.

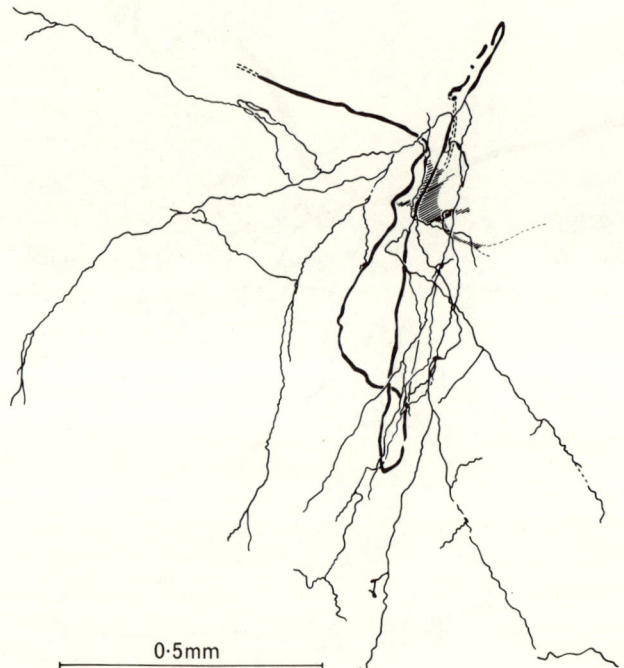

FIG. 4. Projection of a SCT neurone reconstructed from serial sagittal sections. The soma is shown but the dendrites have been omitted. Note the tortuous path of the main axon near the soma and the branching pattern of the collaterals.

Collateral branches nearly always arose from the main axon at a right angle to it and collaterals themselves often branched in this way. This is particularly well seen in Fig. 4 which is a reconstructed SCT neurone in which the soma is shown but the dendrites have been left out for clarity. Collaterals often ran for several hundred μm before branching further. Most collaterals subdivided some 5-8 times before breaking up into their final arborization. The finest branches were at the limit of the light microscope and were less than 0.5 μm in diameter. Ultimately the finest branches often gave rise to two types of expansions which were probably synatic endings; these were, serial swellings similar to the 'climbing' or 'crossing-over' type of synaptic arrangement and disc-like or ring-like expansions some 2.5-4.0 μm in diameter.

In general most of the terminal axonal arborizations of SCT neurones were found close to the position of the parent cell body and dendrites. That is, most terminals were in Rexed's laminae III, IV and V in that part of the dorsal horn (medial, central or lateral) near the soma and dendrites. Occasional collaterals penetrated more ventrally into lamina VI but none have been seen ventral to the level of the central canal and are therefore unlikely to reach motoneuronal dendrites in any number. Also, occasional collaterals ascended into lamina II and in one instance to the dorsal grey-white border and therefore into lamina I.

It is not known which dorsal horn neurones receive an input from the SCT. We have no evidence from our horseradish peroxidase material or from electro-physiological experiments that SCT neurones themselves receive such an input. We have some evidence that dorsal horn neurones without long ascending axons receive this input, since we have been able to stain such a neurone with Procion yellow and demonstrate (at the light microscope level) SCT horseradish peroxidase stained axonal terminals ending upon it (see Snow et al. [17]). Since the axonal terminals are generally within about 500 μm of the parent cell body then, because of the topographical organization of the dorsal horn, the neurones which receive these SCT inputs should also receive other inputs from the same or closely adjacent receptive fields. The present results have shown that the SCT must now be considered, not only as part of an ascending somatosensory system but also as having actions at the segmental level.

SUMMARY AND CONCLUSIONS

By using a combination of electrophysiological and intracellular dye inject-
:tion methods it has been possible to determine the anatomical organization
and density of SCT neurones in the lumbosacral cord of the cat and to
describe the morphology of these neurones. SCT cell bodies are arranged
in a sheet across the dorsal horn, centred on lamina IV but including
ventral parts of lamina III and dorsal parts of lamina V. There are about
14 neurones under each square mm of dorsal cord surface, with more neurones
laterally than medially. The dendritic trees of SCT neurones vary from
cell to cell and do not form a morphologically homogeneous group. Six
main types of dendritic tree have been identified in the present work.
The dendrites of SCT neurones also form a sheet across the dorsal horn
mainly located in laminae III, IV and V and with relatively little overlap
between dendritic trees of individual neurones. SCT axons give rise to a
number of collateral branches which ramify and terminate mainly within 500
μm of the parent cell body, also in laminae III, IV and V.

REFERENCES

1. Morin, F., Amer. J. Physiol. 183, 245 (1955).
2. Bryan, R.N., Coulter, J.D. and Willis, W.D., Expl. Neurol. 42, 574 (1974).
3. Brown, A.G., In Handbook of Sensory Physiology II Somatosensory System (A. Iggo, ed.), Springer-Verlag: Berlin-Heidelberg-New York, p.315 (1973).
4. Boivie, J.J.G. and Perl, E.R., In MTP International Review of Science, Physiology I, Vol. 3 Neurophysiology (C.C. Hunt, ed.), p.303 (1975).
5. Hongo, T., Jankowska, E., and Lundberg, A., J. Physiol. 199, 569 (1968).
6. Bryan, R.N., Trevino, D.L., Coulter, J.D. and Willis, W.D., Expl. Brain Res. 17, 177 (1973).
7. Rexed, B., J. Comp. Neurol. 100, 297 (1954).
8. Stretton, A.O.W. and Kravitz, E.A., Science, 162, 132 (1968).
9. Brown, A.G., House, C.R. and Hume, R.B., J. Physiol. 244, 10P (1975).
10. Brown, A.G., House, C.R., Rose, P.K. and Snow, P.J., J. Physiol. 249, 65P (1975).
11. Jankowska, E. and Lindström, S., J. Physiol. 226, 805 (1972).
12. Scheibel, M. and Scheibel, A.B., Brain Research, 9, 32 (1968).
13. Réthelyi, M. and Szentagothai, J., In Handbook of Sensory Physiology, II Somatosensory System (A. Iggo, ed.), Springer-Verlag; Berlin-Heidelberg-New York, p.207 (1973).

14. Jankowska, E., In *Golgi Centennial Symposium* (M. Santini, ed.), Raven Press; New York, p.235 (1975).
15. Kater, S.B. and Nicholson, C., *Intracellular Staining in Neurobiology*, Springer-Verlag; Berlin-Heidelberg-New York (1973).
16. Ramon Y Cajal, S., *Histologie du système nerveux de l'homme et des vertébrés*, Vol. I, Maloine; Paris (1902).
17. Snow, P.J., Rose, P.K. and Brown, A.G., *Science*, in the press (1976).

Discussion:

Jankowska: Have you found early axon-collaterals in all SCT cells stained with horse radish peroxidase, so that all of them could mediate some spinal reflexes in addition to acting as ascending tract cells? Were these early axon-collaterals more abundant at the same or at a more rostral spinal level?

Brown: Yes, and all spinocervical tract. We have seen only one example where the collateral moved quarterly. All those have been in the rostro side of the cell or at the same level and most of them close. This may have been a problem with the method, of course.

Odutola: First, have you studied the properties of the afferent inputs to these cells? Secondly, in view of the localization of cells projecting to the Dorsal Column Nuclei Complex (DCN) through the dorsolateral funiculus (DLF) in the same geographical position as your SCT cells (Rustioni and Dekker, 1974), have you considered the possibility that these SCT cells may also project to the DCN?

Reference: Rustioni A. and Dekker, J.J. (1974): Non-primary afferents to the dorsal column nuclei of cat: Distribution pattern and cells of origin. Anat. Rec. 178, 454 - 455.

Brown: To your first question, we have gathered as much physiological information as possible on each of these neurons which means that we have recorded axon-serially, determined the division, size, receptive field and whether they are excited by only A-fibers or by A- and C-fibers and so on. We had hoped that we could make some correlations between the physiology and morphology. But with the few exceptions I mentioned, at the moment there does not appear to by any obvious correlation. As for your second question, yes, of course, we have considered the problem of the input to the dorsal column nuclei to the DLF. The vast majority of our neurons are not excited from the first cervical segment, which would suggest that either they terminate before that level or they enter the dorsal column right before that level. It is a very difficult problem. In our experiments we always cut the dorsal columns at C-4 so if these options are going to enter they must do so between C-3 and C-1. We have no evidence on this one at all. But it is a real possibility, of course.

TACTILE THRESHOLDS OF NORMAL AND BLIND SUBJECTS ON STIMULATION OF FINGER PADS WITH SHORT MECHANICAL PULSES OF VARIABLE AMPLITUDE

U. LINDBLOM and B. LINDSTRÖM

Department of Neurology, Huddinge Hospital, 141 86 Huddinge and
Department of Medical Biophysics, Karolinska Institute, 104 01 Stockholm (Sweden)

A technique for rapid determination of the threshold for passive touch, and for studying tactile intensity functions, has recently been developed in which half cycle sinusoidal mechanical pulses are used for stimulation (Lindblom 1974). In the present investigation this technique was applied to a larger material to establish the normal inter- and intraindividual variability and to compare the thresholds of various fingers of the dominant and non-dominant hands. Threshold determinations were also made on a series of blind subjects in which special attention was payed to the thresholds of the fingers used for Braille reading.

METHODS

The normal material consisted of 22 indoor working healthy people, 11 of each sex, between 18 and 54 years of age (average 37 years). The blind subjects, 5 of each sex, were from 18 to 41 years of age (average 29 years). They had all been blind from birth or early childhood but were otherwise healthy. They were all Braille readers, In a pilot study, the results of which will be presented first, four normal and three blind subjects took part.

For stimulation with single short mechanical pulses half sinusoids of 100 Hz were used with the technique described earlier (Lindblom 1974). The pulses were applied perpendicularly to the skin of the finger pads via small blunt-ended probes. A minimum indentation of the order of 5 μm was used to assess contact between the probe and the skin prior to stimulation. Control measurements showed that a preset displacement of this small magnitude was without influence on the threshold value. The stimulus displacements were displayed and measured on a storage oscilloscope. On increasing or decreasing the amplitude of the stimulus pulse in small steps, recording was made of the lowest amplitude which was felt on at least 3 or 4 consecutive stimulations, i.e. the "yes response", and the highest amplitude which was never felt, i.e. the "no response". The difference between the yes and no responses was called the threshold gap and the average was taken as the threshold. The stimulation and reporting procedure was easily understood by all subjects which were well attentive and not fatigued. The measurements on one occasion were completed within one hour.

Measurements were made on all fingers of both hands in random order. The normal subjects were examined twice with an interval of at least one week and the blind subjects only once. All subjects were right-handed. The measurements were analysed by standard methods for analysis of variance. For the normal subjects there were five classifications, sexes, subjects, sides, fingers and occasions, four of which were crossed, and sexes and sides nested. For the blind subjects there were four classifications, sexes, subjects, sides and fingers, three of which were crossed.

RESULTS

Mechanical stimuli of the type used in this study are typically felt as a tap at the point of stimulation. They are usually but not always precisely located. On stimulation with threshold strength, the sensation produced by successive stimuli varies somewhat and is either a clear "yes" or a vague uncertain sensation which some subjects want to report as a "maybe" response. This occurs in the "threshold gap", i.e. at stimulus strenghths between the yes and no values, and especially during the descending series. The threshold response may thus be a graded one rather than an all or none phenomenon. On supra-threshold stimulation the sensation is characterized by an intensity continuum as will be reported in a subsequent paper (Franzén & Lindblom, this volume).

The stimulation method was designed for clinical application with the hope that it might be a sensitive measure of nerve lesions, even subclinical ones. The first series of measurements (Lindblom 1974) had shown that the threshold was of the order of 5-10 μm on the finger tips of normal subjects, but a greater sample had to be investigated to define the interindividual variation and the upper normal limits. It was convenient also to collect, in the same investigation, data for various fingers, from the thumb to the little finger, and from both hands to compare the sensitivity of the dominant and non-dominant sides. Since the method was aimed to be applied repeatedly in the same patient to achieve a profile of the course of a particular disease, it was important to show if the sensitivity for this kind of stimulus was altered by experience which would constitute a source of error on repeated testing. The subjects were therefore measured twice with an interval of at least one week, and Braille reading blind subjects were included because of their long training of the tactile sense, especially in the fingers which they had been using for reading. If such training, especially Braille reading, influenced the sensitivity to passive touch, the lower thresholds would be expected.

The results of a pilot study performed on 3 blind subjects are presented in Fig. 1 B-D. Fig. 1 A shows, for comparison, the thresholds for various points of the glabrous skin of the hand of normal seeing people. The figures are the average values of 4 healthy laboratory workers, which were all about 40 years old. It is seen that the finger tips are about equally sensitive. Proximally the thresholds

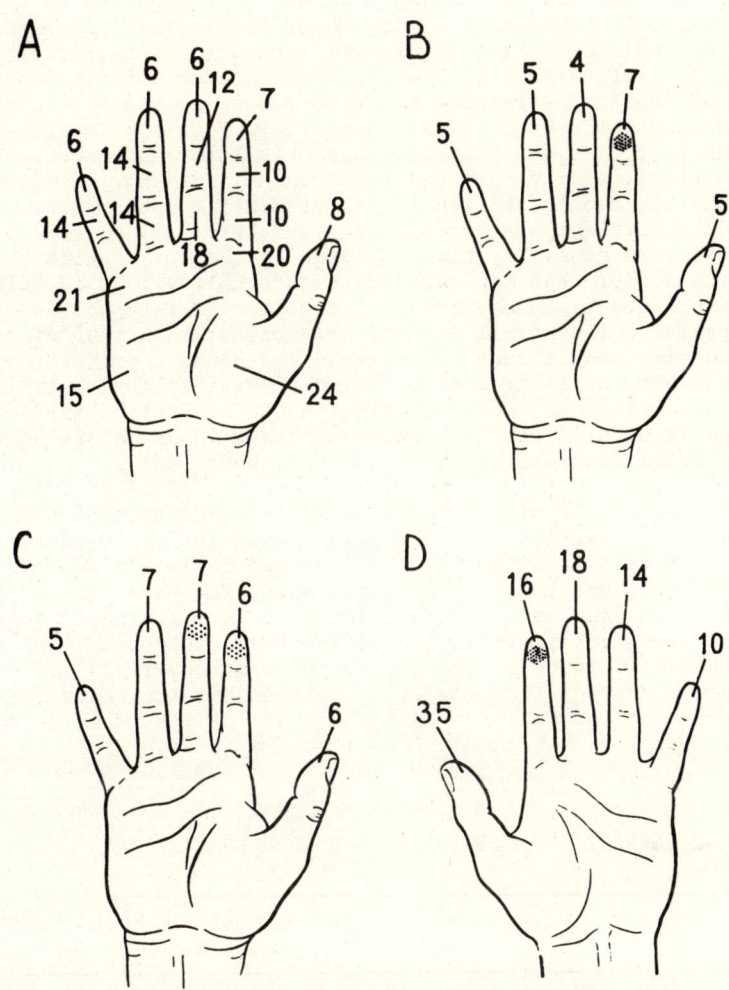

FIG. 1. Tactile thresholds in terms of amplitude of skin displacements in µm on stimulation with short mechanical pulses. A, average values of four healthy seeing subjects; B, from a 22 year old male blind subject who was a good Braille reader; C, from a 17 year old male blind who was a poor Braille reader; D, from a 54 year old male blind teacher. Fingers used for Braille reading are indicated by dots.

are about 2-4 times higher which most probably reflects the fact that the receptor density is lower than on the finger tips.

Fig. 1 B shows the finger tip thresholds of a male blind subject who was a skilled Braille reader. Most values were found to be in the low normal range. The threshold of the index finger which he used for reading was not lower, rather higher, than the thresholds of the other fingers. The values in Fig. 1 C are from another blind subject who inspite of ambitious training was a poor Braille reader. As can be seen his thresholds were of the same order. Fig. 1 D is from a middle-aged Braille reader who primarily used his left hand because he had lost his right index finger and thumb in an accident. He was an early blind, who had been a skilled and eager Braille reader during his whole adult life and was working as a teacher. Yet, as appears, the thresholds were generally higher including that of the index finger which he used for reading. The higher threshold values in this case may be explained by an age-related reduction of receptor density. His skin appeared quite normal and was not thicker than that of other indoor working people such as those of the control material of this study. Further, apart from being blind he was healthy, which should be mentioned since an increase of the touch perception threshold can be a sign of subclinical neuropathy as has been demonstrated for diabetic blind subjects (Heinrichs & Moorhouse 1969).

The statistical analysis of the data from the samples of seeing and blind subjects revealed that the greatest variation in threshold was between different individuals. The standard deviation was 22% for the seeing subjects and 16% for the blind ones. The mean values for sexes, sides, fingers (numbered I-V from thumb to little finger) and occasions are given in Table I. For the blind subjects there was no significant difference between males and females, right and left hand or between different fingers. This implies that the index fingers which were used for Braille reading did not differ from the other fingers.

TABLE I. TACTILE THRESHOLDS (MEAN VALUES IN μm)

		Normal subjects	Blind subjects
Sex	Males	7.01	4.99
	Females	6.44	4.73
Sides	Right	6.99	4.81
	Left	6.46	4.90
Fingers	I	7.22	4.94
	II	6.40	4.94
	III	6.56	4.62
	IV	6.58	4.58
	V	6.86	5.21
Occasions	1	6.98	
	2	6.46	

For the seeing subjects there was no significant difference between males and females, but between right and left there was a small difference which was significant on the one per cent level. The variation between the fingers was not significant. The thresholds obtained on two different occasions did not differ significantly.

Table II shows the total means of the thresholds as well as of the "yes" and "no" values and the threshold gap. It appears that the values of the blind subjects were on average about 30% lower than those of the normal subjects. The threshold gap was 34% of the threshold for both normal and blind subjects.

TABLE II. TOTAL MEANS (IN μm)

	Normal subjects	Blind subjects
Threshold	6.72	4.86
"Yes"-value	7.87	5.68
"No"-value	5.58	4.04
Threshold gap	2.29	1.64

DISCUSSION

It is probably a common thinking that the index and 3rd finger are more "sensitive" than the rest of the fingers, and many blind persons believe that their "reading fingers" are more sensitive than the others. The present results show that there is no difference as far as the threshold of passive touch is concerned. Any difference between fingers which might exist must refer to suprathreshold intensity functions or the power of spatial or temporal resolution.

Among the blind subjects the absolute threshold values were lower and the variation less than in the seeing group which may indicate a generally higher sensitivity. However, the difference was not greater than could be explained by e.g. less manual work and a thinner outer skin among the blinds. Another explanation may lie in the circumstance that the blind subjects were in the average 8 years younger although the individual scores did not indicate an age regression. One exception from this was the middle-aged blind (Fig. 1 D), the values of whom were not included in the statistically treated sample since he was missing two fingers, and a further investigation of the age factor is well motivated. An age variation of the tactile threshold has been reported for children (Ghent 1961). Heinrichs and Moorhouse (1969) did not find any difference of the threshold for light touch, vibration or two-point discrimination between healthy normal and blind which were of equal age.

The threshold was the same on the two sides in the blind group but in the seeing group there was a small but significant difference so that the threshold was lower on the non-dominant side. A similar difference has been reported earlier (Semmes et al 1960) and may not be related to differences in skin thickness (Weinstein & Sersen 1961).

In a previous paper (Lindblom 1974) it was concluded that the threshold sensation on stimulation with short mechanical pulses was mediated by Pacinian corpuscles since these receptors were the only ones whose discharge threshold was known to be low enough to explain a perceptual threshold of the order of 5 µm. This conclusion must now be revised since it has been found that the rapidly adapting (RA) receptors of the glabrous skin of the human hand actually may have a threshold of this low value for the discharge of one afferent impulse (Vallbo & Johansson, this volume). The fact that the RA and not the Pacinian afferents may be responsible for the threshold sensation fits better with the finding that the perceptual threshold remains low at low velocities of skin indentation (Lindblom 1974), even at velocities lower than the "critical slope" of the Pacinian afferents (Lindblom & Lund 1966). Perceptually, the threshold rises below an indentation velocity of about 0.15 mm/sec which corresponds well with the critical slope values of the RA receptors (Lindblom 1965). To which extent the highly sensitive Pacinian afferents, which easily will be excited by rapid displacements, may contribute to the threshold or suprathreshold subjective response needs further study, e.g. with differential anaesthesia.

SUMMARY

The threshold for perception of tactile stimuli was measured in terms of skin indentation amplitude. In a sample of healthy indoor working people it was 6.72 µm ± 22% (SD). There was no significant variation between fingers, sexes or occasions but the threshold of the non-dominant side was on average 0.53 µm less than that of the dominant side which was a statistically significant difference. In a sample of blind subjects the threshold was 4.86 ± 16% (SD), i.e. about 30% lower. There was no difference between fingers, including those which were used for Braille reading, sides or sexes. The lower values of the blind were not greater than can be explained by differences in skin thickness and age. The results do not indicate that training increases tactile sensitivity measured as the threshold for passive touch.

REFERENCES

Franzén, O. & Lindblom, U.: Tactile intensity functions in patients with sutured peripheral nerve. This volume.

Ghent, L.: Developmental changes in tactual thresholds on dominant and nondominant sides. J. Comp. Physiol. Psychol. 1961, 54, 670-673.

Heinrichs, R.W. & Moorhourse, J.A.: Touch-perception thresholds in blind diabetic subjects in relation to the reading of Braille type. N. Eng. J. Med. 1969, 280, 72-75.

Lindblom, U.: Properties of touch receptors in distal glabrous skin of the monkey. J. Neurophysiol. 1965, 28, 966-985.

Lindblom, U.: Touch perception threshold in human glabrous skin in terms of displacement amplitude on stimulation with single mechanical pulses. Brain Res. 1974, 82, 205-210.

Lindblom, U. & Lund, L.: The discharge from vibration-sensitive receptors in the monkey foot. Exp. Neurol. 1966, 15, 401-417.

Semmes, J., Weinstein, S., Ghent, L. & Teuber, H.L.: Somatosensory changes after penetrating brain wounds in man. Cambridge, Harvard University Press, 1960.

Vallbo, Å.B. & Johansson, R.: Skin mechanoreceptors in the human hand: Neural and psychophysical thresholds. This volume.

Weinstein, S. & Sersen, E.A.: Tactual sensitivity as a function of handedness and laterality. J. Comp. physiol. Psychol. 1961, 54, 663-667.

ACKNOWLEDGEMENTS: This study was supported by the Swedish Medical Research Council (B75-14X-4256-02).

Discussion:

Vallbo: I would like to give a couple of comments in relation to the report by Lindblom and Lindström. One of the conclusions presented in this report was that the PC-units account for the detection of threshold touch stimuli. The argument was that all the other types of mechanoreceptors in the human glabrous skin have been found to have higher thresholds than the perceptive thresholds found by Lindblom and Lindström, whereas it is known that, in the monkey, the PC-units have very low thresholds. I am sorry to say that we have found that the RA-receptors in the human hand, in fact, have equally low thresholds as the PC-units, as will be reported this afternoon. On the other hand, I think that it is important to point out that the threshold of a mechanosensitive unit might be highly dependent upon the exact method of stimulation. For instance, it seems likely that the thresholds of the PC-units are highly dependent upon preindentation and we have observations which indicate that preindentation might lower the threshold of the PC-units by as much as a factor of ten. Also it seems likely that preindentation favors the excitation of a fairly large number of PC-units. The effects could be due to a more effective energy transfer of the skin when preindentation is used.

My second comment is related to the connection suggested between absolute threshold and Braille performance. Don't you think that Braille reading required above all a high spatial discrimination rather than high sensitivity to small indentations in the threshold range which after all are much smaller than the indentations produced by the Braille pattern? Also it seems slightly far-fetched to relate the activity of the PC-units which were assumed to be the detectors of weak stimuli to Braille reading as these units, and the system as a whole, presumably have a rather low spatial discrimination capacity.

Lindblom: I will answer the second question first. I don't think it matters if the threshold is five microns or ten microns for a Braille reader, because the elevation of the text pads on the Braille sheet is four hundred microns. You get a superficial stimulation when you move the finger over. The other question was whether the PC receptors would be good for spatial discrimination. I would say no. In the first place, they are easily picked up with a very small deformation even from distant sources. But perhaps, those which lie very close to the stimulation point may have the property of spatial discrimination just at threshold stimulation. As soon as you increase above threshold you will excite a rather wide population in the whole pad, for instance. I would say that spatial discrimination mainly has to rely upon the intra-cutaneous receptors RA and the dynamic range of SA receptors.

Zimmermann: I would expect that larger differences exist in blind and normal subjects when testing the spatial (two-point) discrimination and the intensity discrimination of moving stimuli rather that absolute thresholds in microns. Have you done measurements of this type?

Lindblom: No, we have intended to do measurements of intensity discrimination with this method. As far as two-point discrimination is concerned, Heinrix and Moorehouse found absolutely no difference between blind and normal subjects of the same age.

TACTILE INTENSITY FUNCTIONS IN PATIENTS WITH SUTURED PERIPHERAL NERVE

O. FRANZÉN and U. LINDBLOM

*Department of Psychology, University of Uppsala, Uppsala, and
Department of Neurology, Huddinge Hospital, Karolinska Institutet, Stockholm, Sweden*

INTRODUCTION

Previous investigations on vibrotaction (Franzén, 1969) and vision (Franzén & Berkley, 1975) have demonstrated that growth rate of subjective magnitude functions is inversely related to sensitivity or detection threshold. These findings are consistent with the classical equal-loudness contours of Kingsbury (1927) and Fletcher and Munson (1933) that have been confirmed in a subsequent scaling experiment (Schneider et al., 1972).

Since patients with peripheral nerve injuries have elevated thresholds and impaired discrimination, it would be expected that their imperfect perception would somehow be reflected in their tactile intensity functions.

Conventional methods for the examination of tactual sensibility, such as stroke of cotton-wool or pin-pricking do not satisfy strict requirements as to adequate quantification and reproducibility.

The aim of the present study is to determine threshold amplitude on the finger pad of patients with unilateral median-nerve lesions using mechanical pulses and to measure the sensory magnitude of the same stimuli at supraliminal levels by means of a direct scaling procedure. The sensibility of the patient's injured hand was compared with that of his normal hand. The method employed might be useful in the follow-up of the recovery and rehabilitation process.

METHOD

Subjects

Four male patients at the age of 19 to 22 who had sustained median-nerve injury at the wrist of their right arm took part in the experiments. They had their nerves sutured by a surgeon four to eight years prior to the present investigation.

Stimulation

The distal pad of the index or middle finger of the patient's right and left hand was perpendicularly stimulated by a piston of 2 mm diameter mounted on a Brüel and Kjaer vibrator (type 4810). The probe protruded through a small hole in a flat wooden plate which supported the hand. Half-wave sinusoids of 10 msec duration from a Wavetek generator (Model 112) actuated the minishaker. The piston was brought in contact with the skin without causing any measurable deformation of the skin. The displacement of the rod was measured with a capacitance meter and displayed on an oscilloscope.

The range of intensities is shown by the data points in fig. 1. The lowest intensity was set at two to three times the threshold amplitude. With the exception of the lowest intensities for the normal hand the pulses were rapid enough not to interfere with the velocity component of touch (Franzén & Lindblom, 1976).

Procedures for measuring detection threshold and subjective intensity

Detection threshold was determined by a stair-case method. In the scaling experiment the subject was presented a standard stimulus in the middle of the range that was arbitrarily called 10. The subject's task was to rate all other stimuli presented to him in relation to the prescribed modulus. All levels were presented four times in irregular order. This procedure was repeated twice on the right and left hand. In order to construct a common scale of tactile intensity the subject estimated in per cent the magnitude of a stimulus applied to the affected hand relativt to a signal presented to the normal hand. The subject alternated between his two hands.

RESULTS

The stimulation was sensed as a distinct tap on the skin that increased in subjective magnitude with increasing intensity. On the affected side the sensation was different. The stimuli were felt "like pulses through the finger". The subjects reported a "distortion of sensation". In one case the experience was also referred to a finger adjacent to the digit actually stimulated.

The results of the threshold measurements are shown in table 1.

Patient	Normal hand		Injured hand	
	Threshold in microns	Exponent	Threshold in microns	Exponent
BC	8	0.86	56	1.51
KB	10	0.68	42	1.13
SL	6	0.64	75	1.28
TL	6	0.78	8	0.79

TABLE 1. Tactile thresholds and exponents of the psychophysical power function on mechanical stimulation of the finger pad of the normal and injured hand.

The threshold for the patient's left hand (unaffected) is within the normal range (Lindblom, 1974). For the injured side the threshold is much higher except for patient TL who had recovered almost completely.

The numerical estimates (geometric means) plotted against displacement in log-log coordinates conform to a straight line. Thus, a power function of the form $R = cA^n$ (Stevens, 1957) where R is the subjective response, A is displacement amplitude, c is a constant of proportionality and n is the exponent, describes to a fair approximation the relation between sensory magnitude and stimulus intensity (Fig. 1).

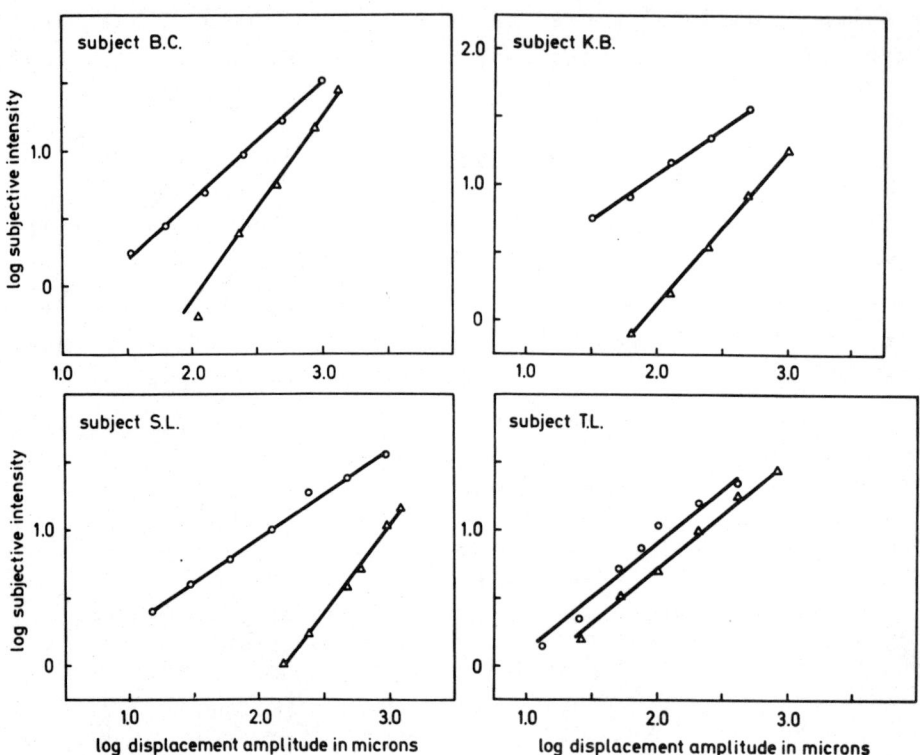

FIG. 1. Subjective intensity plotted against displacement amplitude in log-log coordinates.

However, the right hand curve of patient KB displayed a slight flattening at low levels. The deviation from linearity in the log-log plot was eliminated by subtracting a constant of 0.45 from the response variable. This constant could not be related to any report of paresthesia as would be expected. The individual exponents are listed in table 1. The abnormal hand produced obviously a much higher detection threshold and a steeper slope of the intensity curve than the opposite intact hand. Interestingly, patient TL whose left and right hand thresholds were almost the same had also intensity functions with nearly identical exponents.

DISCUSSION

On examining patients whose afferents have partly been destroyed, different response characteristics may be encountered. A peripheral nerve lesion raises evidently the detection threshold and induces also a power transformation on the psychophysical function.

We find it unlikely that the abnormally high threshold is caused by a general loss of low-threshold dynamic receptors such as pacinian and Meissner's corpuscles (Lindblom, 1965; Lindblom and Lund, 1966, Talbot et al., 1968; Franzén, 1969; Franzén and Lindblom, 1976). An increased threshold would rather be interpreted as a sign - and very reasonably so - of a reduced receptor density which would require larger displacement amplitudes in order to elicit a threshold sensation. The log-log slope of the straight line is greater for the abnormal hand than for the intact hand. Once the threshold is attained, sensory experience grows more rapidly than on the normal side, i.e., the recruitment of units occurs faster on the affected side. This phenomenon is suggestive of similar recruitment functions for hearing losses (Miskolczy-Fodor, 1960). Analogous observations were made by Békésy (1960) who matched a vibratory stimulus on a less densely innervated locus with a corresponding stimulus on an area of higher density of neural elements. Differences in sensibility are determined by differences in peripheral innervation. Furthermore, with larger stimulus probes more distant receptor populations will be activated which may result in even lower thresholds for the normal hand than those of the present study (Franzén and Offenloch, 1969). The exponents of their power functions tended also on the average to be somewhat less steep than those shown in Fig. 1. The growth rate of sensory magnitude seems to be inversely related to the sensitivity and the number of neural units excited.

As instantaneous firing frequency in e.g., rapidly adapting receptors (Franzén and Lindblom, 1976) is not expected to change much in response to such a fast tactile pulse as employed in this investigation, the discharge in these units could not effectively serve as an intensity cue. The magnitude of the tactual sensation will mainly depend upon recruitment of new units progressively brought into action with increasing amplitude of skin indentation. Our results may not either be consonant with any "single-unit doctrine" stating that the detection threshold is set by the threshold discharge in a single fiber.

ACKNOWLEDGMENTS

This work was supported by the Swedish Council for Social Science Research and the Medical Research Council (Project B75-14X-4256-02)

REFERENCES

Békésy,G. 1960. Experiments in Hearing. New York: McGraw-Hill
Fletcher, H. & Munson, W.A. 1933. J. Acoust. Soc. Am. 5, 82-108.
Franzén, O. 1969. Scand. J. Psychol. 10, 289-297.
Franzén, O. & Berkley, M. 1975. Vision Res. 15, 655-660.
Franzén, O. & Lindblom, U. 1976. Coding of velocity of skin indentation in man and monkey. This volume.
Franzén, O. & Offenloch, K. 1969. Exp. Brain Res. 8, 1-18.
Kingsbury, B.A. 1927. Phys. Rev. 29, 588-600.
Lindblom, U. 1965. J. Neurophysiol. 28, 966-985.
Lindblom, U. 1974. Brain Research 82, 205-210.
Lindblom, U. & Lund, L. 1966. Experimental Neurology, 15, 401-417.
Miskolczy-Fodor, F. 1960. J. Acoust. Soc. Am. 32, 486-492.
Schneider, B., Wright, A.A., Edelheit, W., Hock, P. & Humphrey, C. 1972. J. Acoust. Soc. Am. 51, 1951-1959.
Stevens, S.S. 1957. Psychol. Rev. 64, 153-215.
Talbot, W.H., Darian-Smith, I., Kornhuber, H.H. & Mountcastle, V.B. 1968. J. Neurophysiol. 31, 301-334.

Discussion:

Zimmermann: After experimental nerve lesions in cats, Burgess et al, (1973, J. Neurophysiology) have found regeneration of all types of mechanoreceptors in the hairy skin but at reduced numbers. If you apply this finding to your present results, your suggestion of increased stimulus intensity in nerve injured areas to increase recruitment is well supported.

Franzén: Lindblom and I missed one kind of control experiment. We should have studied the vibratory threshold in these patients. If the PC receptors had been regenerated we should obtain the U-shaped threshold curve.

SOMATOSENSORY POTENTIALS FROM THE EXPOSED CORTEX IN MONKEY AND FROM THE SCALP IN MAN RELATED TO THE SENSORY MAGNITUDE OF TACTUAL STIMULATION

O.FRANZÉN
Department of Psychology, University of Uppsala, Uppsala, Sweden

INTRODUCTION

Under natural conditions the skin is subjected to different changes in indentation velocity and amplitude. Franzén and Lindblom (1976) have investigated the velocity component of tactile sensation by recording the discharge in primate and human single fibers. They concluded that there were great similarities in the response pattern between the two species and that the resolving capacity of the central mechanism as evaluated with a psychophysical method was set by the receptor organ. The limitations besetting each method makes it important to study the sensory functions by psychological as well as by neurophysiological experiments. This line of research has been pursued on the somatosensory system with great success by e.g., Mountcastle et al. (1972) and LaMotte and Mountcastle (1973).

The objective of the present study is to record gross signal-averaged potentials from the exposed cortex in monkeys evoked by a brief skin deformation of varying amplitude and to compare these results with psychophysical and primary cortical responses in man obtained under identical conditions.

METHOD

Material

Three adult rhesus monkeys were used in the experiment. They were anesthetized with intraperitoneal sodium pentobarbital (30 mg/kg). The head of the animal was attached to a stereotaxic holder. The pial surface was exposed and covered with mineral oil. Body temperature was maintained between 36.5 and 37.5°C.

Stimulation

The apparatus for delivering the tactile pulses is given in full detail in an earlier report (Franzén & Offenloch, 1969). The 1 cm^2 plastic probe was applied to the distal pad of the middle finger of the monkey's right hand. The stimuli were delivered at a rate of one pulse per second. Displacement amplitude was varied in seven steps between 25 - 280 microns as seen in Fig. 2.

Recording of evoked cortical surface potentials

An Ag - AgCl electrode mounted on a micromanipulator was used. The reference electrode was clipped to the remains of the parietal muscle. The exposed pial cortical surface of somatosensory area I was explored by moving the electrode in successive steps while tactually stimulating the monkey's finger in order to obtain a response of minimum latency, maximum amplitude and appropriate waveform, i.e., an initial positive phase followed by a small-amplitude, long-duration negative phase. The EEG was amplified by Grass amplifiers with filter settings of 0.3 to 500 Hz and stored on FM magnetic tape. All evoked potentials were sampled from a homogeneous and noise-free EEG as best it could be monitored on an oscilloscope. An averaging trial consisted of 64 stimulus presentations per intensity level. One channel of a Nicolet 1070 computer accumulated and processed the 64 sweeps.

RESULTS

As is well-established, the configuration of the primary response changes with the recording position. With the criteria mentioned above a typical signal-averaged cortical potential monopolarly recorded from the contralateral surface of somatosensory area I is shown in Fig. 1. It was recorded over a very restricted field.

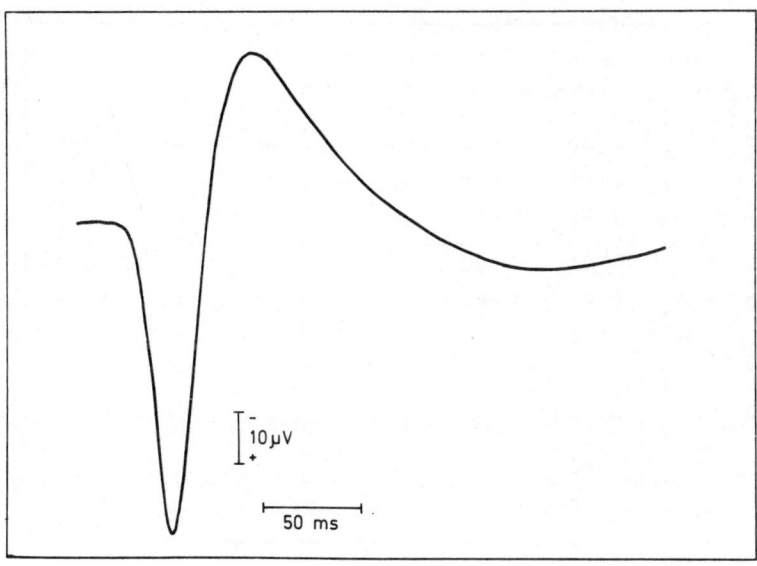

FIG. 1. Potential recorded from the left exposed somatosensory area I on tactile stimulation of the middle finger of the monkey's right hand.

Its location agrees with the first systematic studies of the somatic afferent representation in the cerebral cortex (Woolsey, Marshall, and Bard, 1942) and subsequent investigations by Woolsey (1947,1960,1963). These observations have been refined in single-unit experiments by e.g., Towe and Amassian (1958), Powell and Mountcastle (1959) and Werner and Whitsel (1968).

The onset latency from the application of a tactile pulse of 40 microns was about 25 msec (see Fig. 1). The peak-to-peak amplitude (maximal positive and negative deflection) was measured and plotted against indentation amplitude in log-log coordinates (Fig. 2). Each point represents the geometric mean of six observations. The best fit of the line was calculated with the method of least squares. The slope of the line is 0.53 which is the exponent of a power function of the form $R = cS^n$ where R is the response, S is the stimulus and n is the exponent characteristic of the function. The exponent for the individual

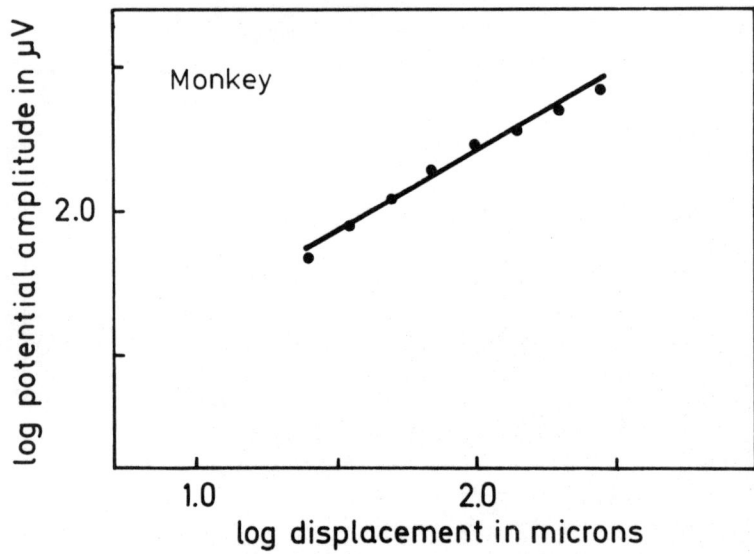

FIG. 2. Potential amplitude plotted against displacement in log-log coordinates.

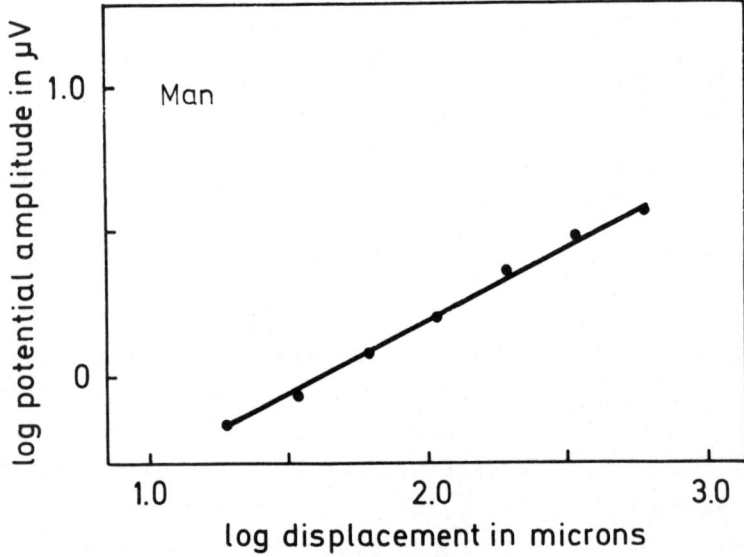

FIG: 3. Amplitude of human cortical responses plotted against displacement in log-log coordinates.

curves ranged between 0.40 and 0.65. In Fig. 3 the peak-to-peak values of human primary cortical potentials are plotted versus stimulus strength (replotted from Franzén and Offenloch, 1969). The exponent of this function is very close to 0.50. Finally, a function from a scaling experiment (unpublished group data for the same, well-practised subjects as in Fig.3) is displayed in Fig. 4

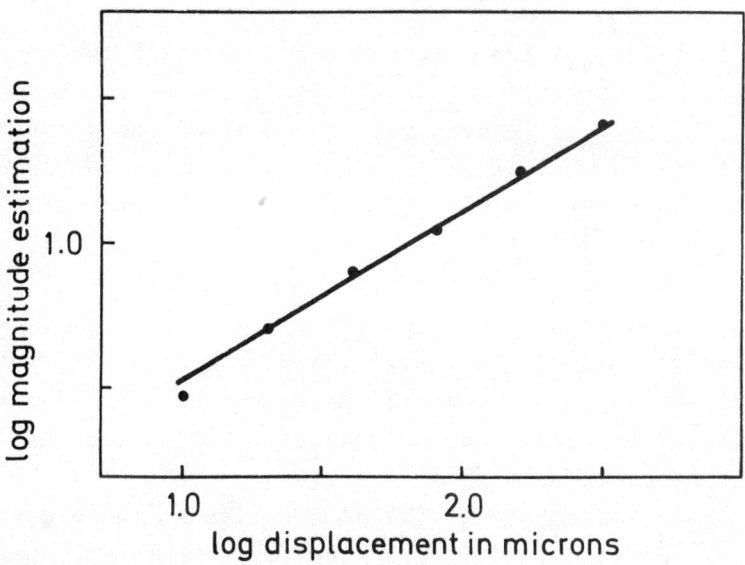

FIG. 4. Plot of log magnitude estimation versus log displacement.

In order to minimize any response bias a variation of magnitude estimation was applied in which no standard stimulus was introduced. No restrictions were placed on the subject who was free free to select numbers appropriate for the stimuli presented. Again, the data conform to a power function with a slope value of 0.58. There is evidently a good accordance between the different studies in primates and humans.

DISCUSSION

A prominent feature of the system(s) under study is the remarkable and powerful synaptic security of the central linkages in the presence of an anesthetic agent as sodium pentobarbital (Rose and Mountcastle, 1959). The neurones of the somatosensory area I reproduces faithfully the mechanical stimulation and a power function was adequately descriptive of the input-output relation. The mean value of the exponent ($n \approx 0.50$) was nearly the same for primates and humans despite the fact that the monkeys were anesthetized. This circumstance raises the somewhat disconcerting but challenging question whether the dorsal column activity leads to perception. Maybe the discharge in the dorsal columns triggers processes that control the analysis of the neural messages travelling over other routes (Wall, 1970). Now, it could be argued the human somatic cortical potentials recorded in awake state exhibit a more complex waveform (see Franzén and Offenloch, 1969, p. 5) than the responses from the animal preparation. It may be so that other components than those selected by Franzén and Offenloch (1969) are directly involved in the conscious experience of the signal. These late waves may be a reflection of the elaboration and the organization of neuronal activity in different central structures. However, Franzén and Offenloch did choose a response index (largest positive and negative deflection from the baseline) that had the best correlation with the sensory scales. It appears rather strange that components of the cortical waveform that show no or very remote relation to perception would play a more important role in the subjective appreciation of the stimulus than those components that really do so. We may therefore conclude that a precise neural replica of the stimulus in the parietal lobe is a necessary but not sufficient condition for our sensory experience. This conclusion may be supported by the observations of Penfield and Rasmussen (1950) who stimulated electrically the sensory hand area of postcentral gyrus during the course of operations. They also asked the patient for his reactions to the stimulation. The patient had a sensation of tingling or numbness in his hand but it was never experienced as though anything was touching the skin. The sensations were never interpreted as induced by events in the external world.

The double-positive early waveform characteristic of a human primary response (see Franzén and Offenloch, 1969, p. 5) was only occasionally observed in this animal experiment and that of Andersson, Norrsell, and Norrsell (1972). In a recent paper Stowell (1972) favored the opinion of Franzén and Offenloch (1969) that the fast double positive was the specific electric sign of the arrival in sensory cortex of information from mechanoreceptive afferents. The different results may among other things be related to the size of the active recording electrode. In the monkey experiment the cortical potentials were recorded with a knobshaped electrode with a diameter of 1.5 mm whereas in the human study the disc electrode had a diameter of 8 mm.

From the evidence so far available it is difficult to bring out clearly whether the double positivity is of peripheral or central origin. After a transection of the dorsal columns in monkeys leaving other tracts intact the latency of cortical potentials evoked by peripheral stimulation increased as the over-all amplitude decreased (Andersson, Norrsell, and Norrsell, 1972).

We may take a speculative leap by proposing that the first positive peak represents information transmitted over the dorsal column pathway and the second positive peak information relayed over the spinothalamic and/or Morin's pathway (1955).

ACKNOWLEDGMENTS

This work was supported by the Swedish Council for Social Science Research.

REFERENCES

Andersson, S.A.,. Norrsell, K., and Norrsell, U. 1972. J. Physiol. 225, 589-597.
Franzén, O. and Lindblom, U. 1976. Coding of velocity of skin indentation in man and monkey. This volume.
Franzén, O. and Offenloch, K. 1969. Exp. Brain Res. 8, 1-18.
Morin, F.1955. Am. J. Physiol. 183, 245-252.
LaMotte, R.H. and Mountcastle, V.B. 1975. J. Neurophysiol. 38 No. 3, 539-559.
Mountcastle, V.B., LaMotte. R.H., and Carli, G. 1972. J. Neurophysiol. 35, 122-136.
Penfield, W. and Rasmussen, T. 1950. The cerebral cortex of man. New York: MacMillan.
Powell, T.P.S.,and Mountcastle, 1959. Bull. Johns Hopkins Hosp. 105, 133-162.
Rose, J.E. and Mountcastle, V.B. 1959. In: Neurophysiol. Vol.1. (Eds.) Field, J., Magoun, H.W., and Hall, V.E. Baltimore: Williams & Wilkins. Pp. 387-429.
Stowell, H.1972. Internat. J. Psychobiol. 2, 305-320.
Towe, A.L. and Amassian, V.E. 1958. J. Neurophysiol. 21, 292-311.
Wall, P.D. 1970. IEEE Transactions on Man-Machine Systems MMS-11, 39-44.
Werner, G. and Whitsel, B.L. 1968. J. Neurophysiol.31, 586-869.
Woolsey, C.N., Marshall, W.H., and Bard, P. 1942. Bull. Johns Hopkins Hosp. 70, 339-441.
Woolsey, C.N. 1947. Fedn Proc. 6, 437-441.
Woolsey, C.N. 1960. In: Structure and Function of the Cerebral Cortex (Eds) Tower, D.B. and Shadé, J.P. Amsterdam: Elsevier.
Woolsey, C.N. 1963. Internat. J. Neurol. 4, No 1, 13-20.

Discussion:

Hensel: Franzén's argumentation seems not convincing. Stevens' dictum that the sensory magnitude is proportional to the magnitude of the stimulus raised to a power is based on the assumption that the internal structure of the estimated magnitude scale is, in fact, a ratio scale. This assumption has yet to be proved. The only way of doing this is to investigate the subjective magnitude scale per se and not by comparing sensation with other parameters, such as stimuli, modalities, neuroelectric responses etc.

Franzén: I am certainly aware of the fact that the opinion is far from unanimo as to the validity of scales of sensation obtained by means of direct scaling methods. However, a mathematical consequence of Stevens' dictum that equal stimulus ratios produce equal response ratios is a power function, i.e. the sensory magnitude is proportional to the magnitude of the stimulus raised to a power. For instance, estimations of 2-to-1 ratios in loudness of a 1 000 Hz tone correspond approximately to 10-to-1 ratios in sound intensity. This finding is consistent with a power function with an exponent of 0.30 if the stimulus variable is specified in terms of energy. Moreover, the growth of loudness of a 100 Hz tone is more rapid as can be easily understood from inspection of the equal loudness contours of Fletcher and Munson (1933). Analogous results have been presented for vibration (Franzén, 1969).

With respect to Fechner's equation, it is based on two false assumptions, namely that differens limen (DL) is subjectively equal along an intensive continuum and that DL can be used as a differential in calculus.

A significant contribution to the theory of measurement is an article by Luce (1959) where he reduces the possible relations between independent and dependent variables to an attractively small set. If the two variables are measured on ratio scales, are independent and continuous functions, the only possible relationship is a power function. If the dependent variable is an interval scale a power function or a logarithmic function may be obtained. The cross-modality matching functions give support to the assumption that the direct methods yield ratio scales because if two continua are governed by power functions, then, if a crossmodality match is performed, the exponent of the matching function is simply the ratio of the exponents of the individual magnitude functions. On the other hand, if they are logarithmic, then the exponent of the matching function is nothing but the ratio of two arbitrary constants (Luce and Galanter, 1963). An analogous problem arises when meaningful comparisons between perceptual and neuroelectric responses are called for with respect to growth rate of different intensity functions as is the case in the present study.

Finally, it should be pointed out that the power-law relation is considered as a first-order approximation. Systematic deviations from a simple power function have been observed many times, especially at low intensity levels. Genuine departures were also noted by Franzén and Lindblom (1976) in their study on coding of velocity of skin indentation (This volume). Maybe, the direct scaling methods developed by Stevens will be of greater importance for sensory psychology than the law.

References:

Fletcher, H. and Munson, W.A. (1933). Loudness, its definition, measurement and calculation. J. Acoust. Soc. Amer., 5, 82-108.

Franzén, O. (1969). The dependence of vibrotactile threshold and magnitude functions on stimulation frequency and signal level. Scand. J. Psychol. 10, 289-298.

Luce, R.D. and Galanter, E. (1963). Psychophysical scaling. In Handbook of Mathematical Psychology (Edited by Luce, R.D., Bush, R.R. and Galanter, E.), Vol. 1, pp. 245-307. John Wiley, New York.

Luce, R.D. (1959). On the possible psychophysical laws. Psychol. Rev. 66, 81-95.

Stevens, S.S. (1957). On the psychophysical law. Psychol. Rev. 64, 153-181.

Zotterman: In our experiments on human taste nerves we found that independently of whether our data fitted Steven's power law or a Fechnerian function, there was a very close correlation between the perceptual data and the electrical response recorded from the nerve. (Borg, Diamant and Zotterman, J. Physiol. 1967).

MICRONEUROGRAPHY IN MAN

K - E HAGBARTH

Department of Clinical Neurophysiology, Academic Hospital, Uppsala, Sweden

The following five papers and also some reports to be presented later during this meeting deal with microneurography in man. Tungsten microelectrodes are percutaneously inserted into human peripheral nerves where recordings can be obtained from different types of afferent nerve fibres with various receptive functions. This recording technique in man has now been in use for 10 years, and it is gradually being adopted by an increasing number of basic- and clinical neurophysiologists in various countries.

My intention is not to present any new data. I rather want to give some comments and initiate a discussion about the general value and applicability of this recording method, possible ways of improving the technique and ethical aspects of doing studies of this type in man.

Value and applicability.
Microneurography in man can provide information of both basic-physiological and patho-physiological interest. Whether it will ever be used as a diagnostic tool in routine clinical work remain to be seen.
Basic-physiological studies. The reports on microneurography, published so far, can be divided into three main groups: recordings from skin afferents, recordings from muscle afferents and recordings from postganglionic efferent sympathetic nerve fibres in the peripheral nerves.

Single unit recordings from skin nerve afferents indicate that, both with respect to glabrous and non-glabrous skin, the human being is equipped with receptors rather similar to those previously described for other mammals. Thus the various main types of fast- and slowly adapting A-fibre mechanoreceptive units, known from previous animal work, have been identified also in man. Also for sensory units within the C-fibre conduction range receptive properties have been encountered that agree with findings in cats and monkeys: many of them are high threshold polymodal nociceptors, but also C-fibre warm receptors can be identified, as will be shown in succeeding reports during this meeting. In microelectrode recordings in cooperative human subjects it is possible to get direct information of how the impulse messages in the primary afferents correlate to the sensory experiences of given stimuli. Many of the succeeding reports deal with psychophysical studies of this type involving tactile, nociceptive and thermal sensory functions.

The advantage of using cooperative human subjects is also apparent in studies dealing with muscle receptor functions and the fusimotor control of muscle spindles in normal voluntary movements. Awake animals can certainly be conditioned to do purposive movements of different types but it is difficult to do single unit recordings from peripheral nerves at the same time to see how the spindle endings in the working muscles behave. Many studies of this type have now been done in man with the microneurographic technique, and no doubt these studies have contributed a great deal to our knowledge of how the fusimotor system normally operates.

In microelectrode recordings from human peripheral nerves it is also possible to identify discharges in postganglionic sympathetic nerve fibres and thus to study the neural sympathetic outflow in skin and muscle nerves, as well during resting conditions as during various manoeuvres engaging different vaso- or sudomotor control mechanisms. Here again, the awake human subject gives us excellent opportunities to see how these control systems operate under normal conditions in intact organisms, undisturbed by anaesthetic drugs.

Patho-physiological studies. For all the three research fields mentioned above it is easy to see that the microneurographic technique also has clinical applicability, not primarily as a diagnostic tool but as a technique to be used in pathophysiological investigations. The questions that can be raised are numerous. For instance, how do the receptive properties of cutaneous end-organs change in different types of dermatological diseases accompanied by itching? The itching relief by scratching - is that due to peripheral or central mechanisms or both? What can microneurography tell about A- and C-fibre receptive characteristics in pain-syndromes following peripheral nerve lesions, or about the mechanisms involved in the pain relief by sympathectomy or electrical nerve stimulation in such cases? Some of these problems have been dealt with in a study that will be presented later during this meeting. It would also be interesting to know to what extent the sensory disturbances in peripheral neuropathies of different types are due to impaired receptor functions rather than to impaired impulse transmission in the axons.

With recordings from muscle spindle afferents it is possible to investigate pathophysiological mechanisms involved in spasticity and rigidity, and a number of microneurographic studies have already been devoted to the problem of fusimotor system involvment in these pathological states. Finally we have the groups of patients with various types of disturbances in vasomotor regulatory functions and where it is of interest to make direct recordings of the sympathetic neural outflow in skin and muscle nerves. Are there any abnormalities to be seen in the resting sympathetic activity or the sympathetic responses to various manoeuvres in patients with essential hypertension, Raynaud's disease, migraine etc? Some reports on microneurographic findings in patients with essential hypertension have been published and further investigations in this field are in progress.

What I have said illustrates, I hope, that with microelectrode recordings from human peripheral nerves it is possible to study various sensory and motor functions with a precision similar to that achieved in animal experiments. And as Sherrington said to Penfield "it must be wonderful to have an experimental animal who could speak to you and tell you what he felt". This is certainly true when psychophysical methods are used for correlation with sensory processes, especially in studies of pain. We must not forget however that the subjects' reports are not always reliable and different words may be used by different subjects to describe the same sensation. Still if an intelligent and cooperative subject tells that a stimulus is painful, this is a more reliable indicator of subjective pain than are avoidance reactions and autonomic responses to nociceptive stimuli in experimental animals.

Technique.
All of us doing this type of microelectrode recordings in man know that the procedure is often quite tedious. It may take hours to hit the nerve and to get the electrode tip through the perineural sheath and into an adequate intrafascicular recording position. Quite often the electrode slips out of the nerve bundle and then it may be surprisingly difficult to find it again. These difficulties are probably related to the fact that the nerve fascicles within a nerve trunk are separated by fairly large spaces of loose connective tissue and the electrode may pass within these spaces right through the nerve without penetrating the dense and high-impedance collagen sheaths of individual fascicles. After impalement of a fascicle it is possible to record afferent multiunit responses to mechanical stimuli within the fascicular innervation zone, but it is also possible to adjust the electrode position so that more selective recordings from individual nerve fibres are obtained. Single unit recordings are much more easily obtained from fast conducting A-fibres than from fibres within the A-delta or C-fibre conduction range. The shape and polarity of the A-fibre single unit potentials indicate that they derive from fibres

which have been impaled or damaged by the electrode tip. C-fibre activity, afferent and- or sympathetic, may be quite clearly seen in certain intrafascicular regions but not in others, probably due to the fact that the Schwann's cells containing these fibres are not evenly distributed.

A question that may be raised for discussion is whether there is such a thing as "the ideal electrode" for these recordings. I think it is more likely that we will learn to use differently shaped electrodes with different impedance depending upon what type of nerve fibres we want to record from. It is certainly true that an electrode with a fairly long bare tip and low impedance is to be preferred if one wants to obtain multi- rather than single unit recordings, but what I am suggesting is that one day it may be possible to make "A-fibre electrodes" and "C-fibre electrodes". Or is it just a coincidence in Uppsala that those interested in doing A-fibre recordings have such an amazing ability to get hold of "C-fibre electrodes" and vice versa? In fact we all use disposable electrodes with a shaft diameter of 200 u, a relatively short taper and a tip diameter of 1-5 u, the length of the bare tip varying between 10-50 u. We have made attempts with platinum coating of the tips to reduce noise but without much success. The platinum was too easily scraped off and besides, the electrodes became too expensive to be disposable. And we do prefer the disposable type because of the infection risks.

What can be done to facilitate these searching procedures, to obtain more stable recording positions and better signal to noise ratios? I suppose we have all tried different modifications of the electrodes and different ways of handling them, different amplifiers, different stimulating techniques to find the nerve more quickly etc. To my knowledge however, no major advances in the recording technique have been made during these 10 years. We have all acquired more experience and better skill and for that reason the quality of the recordings tends to improve. It is important, however that we don't give up in our efforts to refine the method.

Perhaps, it will be possible with computer techniques to get single unit data out of recordings which we today can not analyze because of low signal to noise ratios. For analysis of C-fibres recordings the compressed-time display of successive responses to electrical skin shocks, that will soon be described by Hallin, implies a definite step forward in the single unit analysis technique. However, it should not be forgotten that multi-unit recordings can also give valuable information. In correlative studies of neural and perceptual events a single unit recording never tells the whole story since even weak localized stimuli tend to excite a large number of receptive units. Since single unit recordings probably imply that the fibre investigated has been damaged by the electrode tip, it is even possible that the impulses recorded do not pass the recording site. In pathophysiological studies it may also be difficult to get a large enough unit material to tell whether a certain receptor population behaves in an abnormal fashion. Here mass recordings give often a valuable compliment to the single unit data.

Ethics.
The question of ethics in "experiments" on human subjects has been raised on numerous occasions, and we must certainly consider these problems when we do our microelectrode recordings. A common principle that applies to both animal and human studies has to do with the avoidance of suffering and pain. I suppose most of us consider it ethical, however, to make observations on nociceptive stimuli in man, providing the studies are made with the consent of the subject and providing they may contribute to a better understanding of pain or pain treatment.

There are also ethical considerations especially pertinent to studies on human subjects. Any procedure which involves risks with respect to the health and welfare of the subject must be

avoided, and in all instances a physician with full medical
qualifications should be responsible for the studies, even
though collegues in the theme without such qualifications may
certainly do major contributions. These considerations agree
with the principles put forward by Jasper at the Paris Symposium on "Neurophysiology studied in man", 1971.

In many papers dealing with microneurography in man the authors
report that they have noted no enduring signs of neuropathy
as a consequence of nerve impalement. To my knowledge there
is so far not a single case reported with symptoms of a lasting
nerve lesions as a result of the experiments. It is well-known
however that a few days following microneurography from a skin
nerve fascicle the subject may experience sensory paraesthesias
within the fascicular innervation zone, paraesthesias which
are enhanced by local pressure on the nerve at the recording
site. These symptoms usually subside within a week, and in
Uppsala we have only had a few cases where the paraesthesias
have remained for as long as a month. We believe these symptoms
are due to local neural oedema with increased intrafascicular
pressure. It is important that the subject before the experiment is told that this may occur and that, on the whole, he is
well informed about the experimental procedure and the purpose
of it all. In studies on patients, all procedures employed
should strictly speaking make a significant contribution to
diagnosis or treatment. However, with the patient's consent
and with full explanation it is usually considered ethical
to do studies which have no chance of benefitting the particular patient concerned but which may contribute to the understanding of a disease process.

In many medical centers there are now committees which are
supposed to judge about the ethics of various research projects involving human subjects. Such committees in Sweden
have had no objections against microneurography carried out
according to the above principles, but I have heard about similar committees abroad which have been more hesitant. When

Vallbo and I started we did during the first two years all recordings on ourselves before we asked other subjects to volunteer. And today we feel confident that even though there must be some risks involved, infections for instance if proper sterilization is not performed, microneurography can be regarded as a non-harmful method. Still I would be hesitant to apply the method on certain patients with severe neuropathies where there in some muscle nerves may be only a few functioning motor axons left. In patients with severe spasticity in certain muscle groups, on the other hand, one may consider the possibility of using the microelectrode to make selective thermal lesions in the nerve to relieve the hypertonus. But this is a different story which has nothing to do with the topic of the present symposium.

Discussion:

Vallbo: In his review report, Microneurography in man, Professor Hagbarth indicated a difficulty in relating neural activity to psychophysical responses of individual tests in recordings from human nerves. He pointed out that the impulses of a single nerve fiber recorded from, might be blocked at the recording site due to injury by the impaling electrode. As it is relevant for the communications which will be presented later, I am happy to have this opportunity to mention that I have done a separate study of this particular problem. It turned out that it is possible to predict impulse block with a high probability in A-fibers from the impulse shape and the changes of the impulse shape during the recording. The study is in the course of publication . (Prediction of propagation block on the basis of impulse shape in single unit recordings from human nerves, Acta Physiol. Scand. 1976).

STUDIES ON CUTANEOUS A AND C FIBRE AFFERENTS, SKIN NERVE BLOCKS AND PERCEPTION

R. G. HALLIN and H. E. TOREBJÖRK

Department of Clinical Neurophysiology, University Hospital, Uppsala, Sweden

Introduction.
Previous investigators of cutaneous sensibility have utilized local anaesthetics (7, 14, 15, 19) or nerve compression produced by a sphygmomanometer cuff (14, 15, 18, 19) for differential blocking of nerve fibres of variable diameters when studying perceptual events in man. In other approaches perception has been directly correlated with evoked neural activity (2, 12) but the number of such studies has been limited possibly because of the technical difficulties involved in recording activity from fibres of thin diameter in man.

Recently it was shown that both multiunit activity (8, 10) and single unit impulses (9, 22, 25) from the entire spectrum of nerve fibres, including C fibres, can be recorded with microelectrodes inserted into intact human skin nerves. In a number of studies to be summarized this technique was used to elucidate the role in perception of afferent A and C fibres. Experiments were also made to evaluate the reliability of cutaneous nerve blocks for use in clinical experiments aimed at investigating pathophysiological mechanisms in patients with chronic pain syndromes (30).

Electrically induced A and C fibre activity correlated with perception.
Afferent A and C fibre activity was elicited by electrical shocks (0.5-50/s) delivered through small needles in the skin and recorded from fascicles of the median, radial, saphenous or peroneal nerves. For analysis of the electrically induced nerve responses a computer of average transients was used.

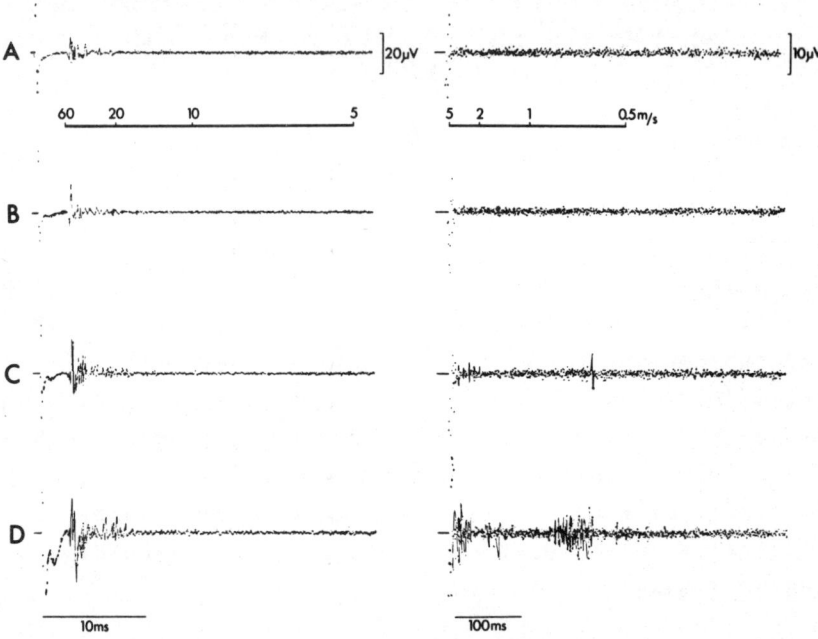

Fig. 1. Radial nerve responses induced by electrical shocks delivered at 1/s to the receptive field on the dorsum of the hand 15 cm from the recording site. Electronic averaging of 200 successive sweeps. To emphasize deflections in the records individual dots in the computer display have been joined by lines in Figs. 1, 2, 4 and 6.
A. On stimulation under the threshold for perception of the stimulus a small short latency A response was induced.
B. The A fibre response was more pronounced to electrical shocks just perceived by the subject.
C. When the stimulus was felt as a pricking sensation both A delta and some C fibre deflections were identified in the neurogram.
D. On painful stimulation additional components were recruited especially in the A delta and C responses.

In fascicles supplying hairy skin a prominent spontaneous activity was sometimes recorded but not felt by the subjects, confirming previous observations on nerve activity led off from fascicles innervating hairy skin (12, 28). In such situations a short latency A fibre response could be recorded at a stimulus intensity below the threshold for perception with stimulus frequencies up to 10/s (Fig. 1A). Spontaneous afferent neural activity was not prominent in fascicles supplying glabrous skin. Electrical stimulation in the finger pulps at intensities below the threshold for perception failed to elicit any neural response.

Electrical stimuli at the threshold for perception were felt as light repetitive touch or tapping and regularly induced a short latency A fibre response in recordings from both glabrous and non-glabrous skin nerve fascicles (Fig. 1B). With increasing stimulus strength perceived as stronger tapping or throbbing several A fibre components were recruited, and at a stimulus strong enough to produce pain, A delta and C fibre activity could also be identified in the fascicular response (Fig. 1C-D). However, in some cases when exploring fascicles supplying hairy skin a few C fibre components were even elicited at low non-painful stimulus intensities near the threshold for perception (11, 23).

Correlation between the evoked neural activity and the perceptions reported by the subjects suggested that tactile sensations were dependent upon activity in thick myelinated fibres. A delta and C fibre activity was considered important for the experience of pain.

With intense low frequency stimulation (0.5/s) the dominating experience was a prolonged pain with each stimulus. The averaged nerve response consisted of prominent series of A and C fibre deflections (Fig. 1D, 2A). On raising the stimulus frequency to 5/s the subjects initially felt an augmented severe burning pain, which diminished markedly over the following seconds of stimulation. The decrease in painful sensation was accompanied by a reduction of the averaged C fibre response (Fig. 2B), whereas the A fibre response remained essentially uninfluenced by such a moderate increase in stimulus frequency.

High stimulus frequencies of 50-100 Hz have been used in trials aimed at inducing local electrical analgesia in patients with chronic pain syndromes (29). With similar skin stimuli

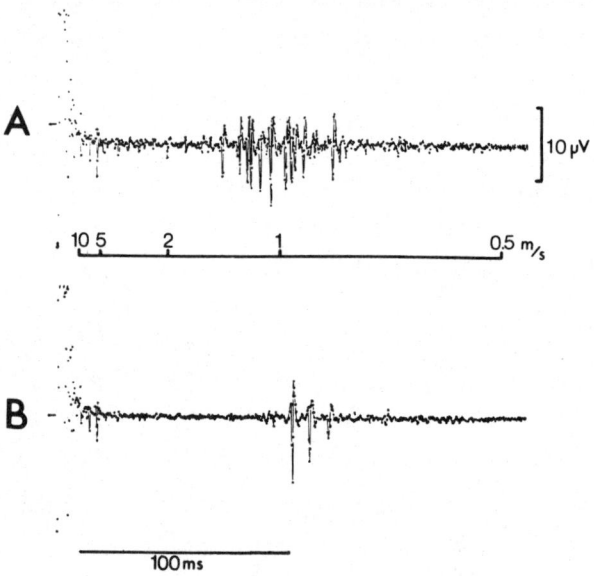

Fig. 2. Changes in the averaged C response following variations in stimulus frequency. Corresponding A response is not shown. Conduction distance 10.5 cm. Each computer record is based upon the averaging of 100 successive nerve responses.
A. On painful stimulation at a frequency of 0.5/s a pronounced C response was recorded.
B. When raising the stimulus frequency to 5/s the C response was reduced and the latencies of its components increased (24).

blockings occur in individual A delta and C fibre elements as signs of decreased excitability, the critical frequency for excitation failure being higher for A delta fibres than for C fibres (Fig. 3A-B). Thick myelinated fibres are less influenced by increases in stimulation frequency up to 50/s. The results of these studies are in accordance with those of other workers showing that conduction block in thin myelinated fibres can be achieved by both direct (17) and percutaneous (20) high frequency electrical stimulation of a whole nerve. These data suggest that, besides central mechanisms, peripheral neural events may contribute to the beneficial effects of local electrical stimulation.

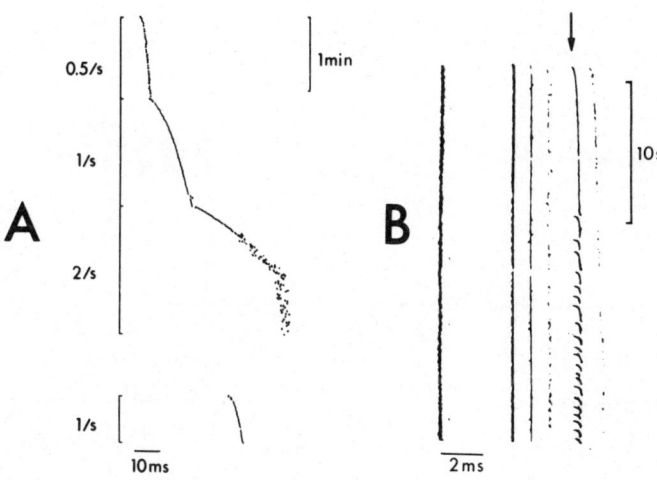

Fig. 3. Latency changes and blockings of afferent A fibre elements and one C unit triggered by electrical skin shocks of variable frequency. The nerve spikes time-locked to the stimulation were dot-converted and successive responses displayed under each other as the oscilloscope sweep moved downwards. Different experiments are shown in A and B.
A. Responses of a C unit recorded from the saphenous nerve 23 cm from the stimulating site near the medial malleolus. The unitary responses appeared with a latency of 260-265 msec when stimulating at 0.5/s. The first 250 msec after the stimulus artefact are omitted. With small increases in stimulus frequency the unit latency increased considerably and at 2/s latency irregularities and blockings appeared.
B. Responses in A fibres in a radial nerve fascicle when the stimulus frequency was set to 50/s. Distance of conduction 10.5 cm. Stimulus artefact to the extreme left. Arrow indicates an A delta unit with a conduction velocity of about 17 m/s. Initially this unit was excited by each shock, but after some 10 seconds an increasing number of blockings appeared (26).

Perceptual events accompanying changes of the nerve response during lidocaine blocks.

Previous investigations on differential nerve blocks with local anaesthetics have shown that small axons are generally more susceptible to block than are larger axons (6, 7). Similar blocking experiments with lidocaine, 0.25%, were performed on the radial nerve at the wrist (24). Changes in the activity of different fibre groups were monitored and concurrently correlated with alterations in the perception of the applied

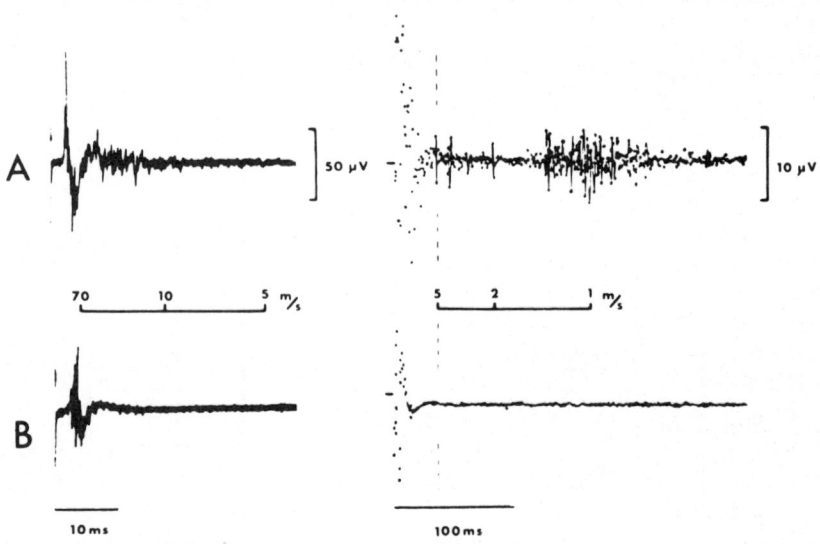

Fig. 4. Cutaneous nerve block with lidocaine, 0.25%. Radial nerve recording at the wrist. Conduction distance 16 cm. Strong electrical shocks were applied at 0.5/s to the receptive skin field (refers to Figs. 4 and 6). In Figs. 4 and 6 the vertical interrupted line to the right delimits the extension of the response shown to the left on displaying the induced activity with long time base. In this figure the left row shows part of the A fibre response (5 superimposed responses) and to the right the late A and C fibre activity is visualized (average of 50 successive responses).
A. In the control situation both A and C fibre activity was recorded.
B. Soon after injection of lidocaine between the stimulating and recording sites the C fibre activity and most of the A delta response was abolished whereas some large A fibres still were conducting (24).

physiological or electrical stimuli.

Typically the perceptual events to be described started proximally, just distal to the injection site and then spread peripherally as the block progressed involving larger skin areas within the innervation zone of the radial nerve on the dorsum of the hand. Before blocking, intense shocks evoked a prolonged painful sensation. On such occasions an extended multifibre response deriving from both A and C fibres was regularly recorded (Fig. 4A). Soon after injection of the anaesthetic between the stimulating and recording sites there was an impairment of warmth discrimination and a reduced appreciation of the prolonged painful component of the skin shocks. Cold discrimination was also rapidly affected, as was the perception of pricking pain. The intrafascicular neurogram showed a decreased A fibre response and abolition of the C fibre potentials (Fig. 4B). In a few experiments the subjects acknowledged a pricking or sharp sensation when C activity was blocked. Light touch continued to be felt as a tactile sensation when mainly large myelinated fibres were conducting.

In these trials there were difficulties in determining when A delta activity and C waves of the averaged response disappeared and reappeared in the course of the rapidly changing nerve block. Therefore the neural events were studied in detail in unitary recordings on some occasion (Fig. 5). Using a compact time presentation of electrically induced nerve activity described previously (26) the responses in both A and C fibres were monitored. Soon after injection of the anaesthetic (Fig. 5, upper arrow), and at about the same time, both A and C fibre elements exhibited transient latency increases. Subsequently when more anaesthetic was injected (Fig. 5, lower arrow) conduction in many of the fibres was blocked (Fig. 5A-B, bottom). Of particular interest was the finding that some thick myelinated fibres and A delta fibres were blocked at about the same time as the C fibres.

Our results accord with those of Franz and Perry (1974) showing that small diameter axons generally are more susceptible to lidocaine than are larger axons, even if some large and small myelinated fibres block almost simultaneously with the non-myelinated fibres. The outcome of the experiments were also consistent with other studies on perception using lidocaine nerve blocks (7, 16, 19, 31).

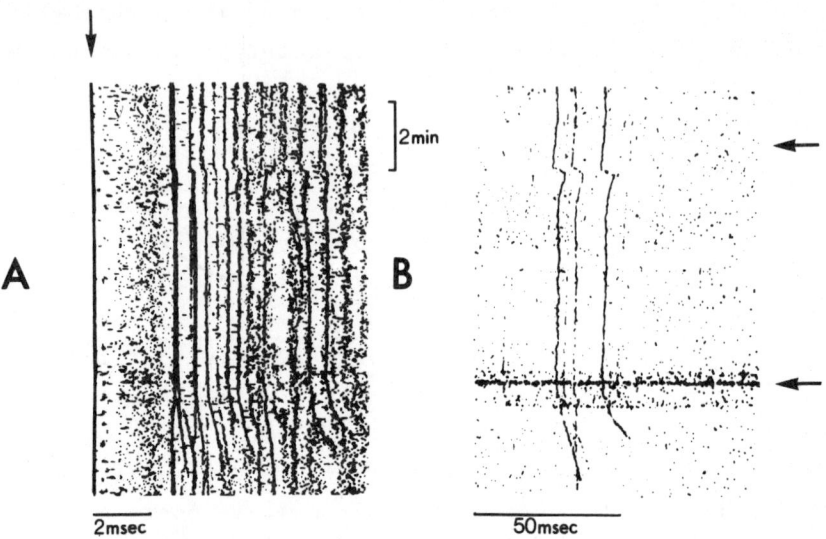

Fig. 5. Detailed demonstration of the neural events occurring in A and C fibres during lidocaine blocks. Conduction distance 15 cm. Stimulus artefacts marked by vertical arrow. Lidocaine injections indicated by horizontal arrows.
A. Responses in A fibre components with conduction velocities ranging 60 to about 15 m/s. Soon after injection of lidocaine, 0.25% (upper arrow) the A fibre components exhibited transient latency increases indicating slowing of conduction. Following next injection of lidocaine (lower arrow) many of the A fibre components blocked but some still remained in the response.
B. Simultaneously with the events occurring in the A fibre response transient latency increases and blockings also appeared in three C fibre elements (conduction velocities 0.8-0.7 m/s) in association with the lidocaine injections.

Preferential nerve blocks with pressure and accompanying changes in perception.

The compression block experiments were performed on the radial nerve at the wrist by applying an inelastic band tightly to the nerve between the stimulating and recording sites (24).

Typically the perceptual changes started at the periphery and then spread centripetally engaging larger areas within the cutaneous region supplied by the radial nerve distal to the compression. The first sensations to be affected were percep-

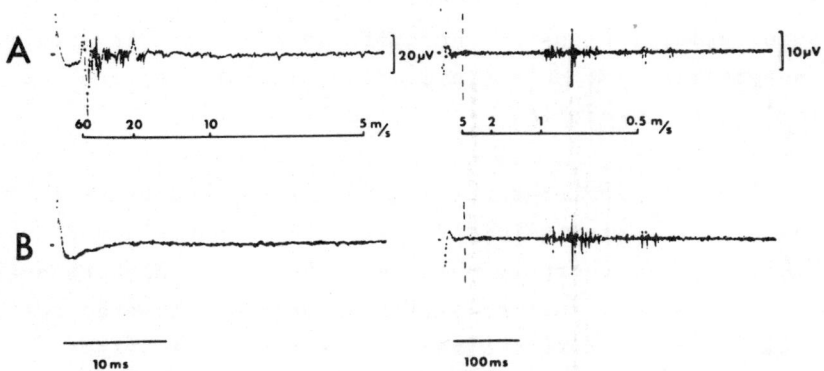

Fig. 6. Preferential blocking of myelinated fibres. The same recording site as for Fig. 5. Averaged nerve activity based upon 50 successive responses are shown.
A. Control.
B. When the pressure had been exerted for more than 40 minutes the averaged response was composed of C fibre deflections only (24).

tions of tactile and vibratory stimuli, and this was accompanied by a temporal dispersion and a progressive amplitude reduction of the short latency A fibre response. With progressive abolition of activity also in thin A fibres the perception of cold and fast pricking pain gradually disappeared. The A fibre activity was usually abolished after nerve compression for 40-60 minutes (Fig. 6B). At this stage no apparent reduction of the C fibre response was observed, but after prolonged pressure for about 2 hours an amplitude reduction and latency increase in the C fibre response could also be detected. When only C fibres were conducting differentiation between rough and smooth surfaces of emery cloth was rendered impossible and the tickling sensation of hairs being moved, mimicking the movements of an insect, had disappeared. However, the subjects retained the ability to perceive warmth, heat and delayed pain. This accords with our recent findings that human skin receptors supplied by afferent C fibres can be excited by warmth, heat and painful, noxious stimuli (21, 25, 27).

Of particular interest was the observation that sticking a

needle into the skin was perceived as delayed pain but of a more uncomfortable, unpleasant character than before. Several subjects reported that an extreme cold stimulus produced a paradoxical "heat" sensation.

Upon release of the pressure early A fibre components in the neurogram reappeared within the first 30 seconds and cutaneous sensibility was generally restored within some minutes even if on a few occasions full sensibility had not recovered until several hours had passed after the experimental session.

The general results of the experiments are in good agreement with those of other studies suggesting that high sensitivity fibres for touch fall within the A beta-gamma group whereas pain and temperature fibres in human skin nerves fall within the A delta and C groups (1-5, 7, 13-16, 24, 32, 33).

The pressure block was more selective than the lidocaine block, leaving the C fibres conducting at a stage when impulse conduction was blocked in the A fibres. Pressure blocks have therefore been used in experiments aimed at elucidating the relative role of afferent A and C fibres for the perception of hyperalgesia in the causalgic pain syndrome (30).

Conclusions.
The outcome of the studies confirms the belief that touch sensibility in hairy skin is dependent upon intact transmission in thick myelinated fibres, cold and pricking pain on thin myelinated A delta fibres, and warmth, heat and delayed pain on C fibres. Additional support was lent to the notion, that, besides central mechanisms, peripheral neural events may be involved in the pain-relieving effects of transcutaneous electrical stimulation. Pressure blocks of cutaneous nerves are to be preferred to lidocaine blocks in pathophysiological studies when the role of afferent C fibre activity for pain is to be evaluated in chronic pain syndromes.

References.

1. Clark, D., Hughes, J., and Gasser, H.S. Amer. J. Physiol., 114, 69-76, (1935).
2. Collins, W.F., Nulsen, F.E., and Randt, C.T. Arch. Neurol., 3, 381-385, (1960).
3. Collins, W.F., Nulsen, F.E., and Shealy, C.N. Pain, Boston, (1966).
4. Dyck, P.J., and Lambert, E.H. Arch. Neurol., 20, 490-507, (1969).
5. Dyck, P.J., Lambert, E.H., and Nichols, P.C. Handbook of E.E.G. clin. Neurophysiol., 9, 83-118, (1972).
6. Franz, D.N., and Perry, R.S. J. Physiol., 236, 193-210, (1974).
7. Gasser, H.S., and Erlanger, J. Amer. J. Physiol., 88, 581-591, (1929).
8. Hallin, R.G., and Torebjörk, H.E. Acta Soc. Med. Upsal., 75, 77-80, (1970a).
9. Hallin, R.G., and Torebjörk, H.E. Acta Soc. Med. Upsal., 75, 277-281, (1970b).
10. Hallin, R.G., and Torebjörk, H.E. Exp. Brain Res. 16, 309-320, (1973).
11. Hallin, R.G. and Torebjörk, H.E. Advances in Neurology, Vol. 4, Raven Press, New York, (1974).
12. Hensel, H., and Boman, K.K.A. J. Neurophysiol., 23, 564-578, (1960).
13. Heinbecker, P., Bishop, G.H., and O'Leary, J. Arch. Neurol. Psychiat., (Chic), 29, 771-789, (1933).
14. Landau, W., and Bishop, G.H. Arch. Neurol. Psychiat., (Chic), 69, 490-504, (1953).
15. Lewis, T., and Pochin, E.E. Clin. Sci., 3, 67-76, (1937).
16. Mackenzie, R.A., Burke, D., Skuse, N.F., and Lethlean, A.K. J. Neurol. Neurosurg. Psychiat., 38, 865-873, (1975).
17. Nyquist, K.J., and Ignelzi, R.J. Personal communication.
18. Sinclair, D.C., and Glasgow, E.F. Brain, 83, 668-676, (1960).
19. Sinclair, D.C., and Hinshaw, J.R. Brain, 73, 480-498, (1950).
20. Taub, A., and Campbell, J.N. Advances in Neurology Vol. 4, Raven Press, New York, (1974).
21. Torebjörk, H.E. Acta physiol. scand., 92, 374-390, (1974).
22. Torebjörk, H.E., and Hallin, R.G. Acta Soc. Med. Upsal., 75, 81-84, (1970).
23. Torebjörk, H.E., and Hallin, R.G. Cervical Pain, Pergamon Press, New York, (1972).
24. Torebjörk, H.E., and Hallin, R.G. Exp. Brain Res., 16, 321-332, (1973).
25. Torebjörk, H.E., and Hallin, R.G. Brain Res., 67, 387-403, (1974).
26. Torebjörk, H.E., and Hallin, R.G. J. Neurol. Neurosurg. Psychiat., 37, 653-664, (1974).
27. Torebjörk, H.E., and Hallin, R.G. This volume.
28. Vallbo, Å.B., and Hagbarth, K-E. Exp. Neurol., 21, 270-289, (1968).
29. Wall, P.D., and Sweet, W.H. Science, 155, 108-109, (1967).
30. Wallin, B.G., Torebjörk, H.E., and Hallin, R.G. This volume.

31. Zenz, M., Fruhstorfer, H., Nolte, H., and Hensel, H. Pflügers Arch. ges. Physiol., suppl. 339, R. 86, (1973).
32. Zotterman, Y. Acta med. scand., 80, 185-242, (1933).
33. Zotterman, Y. J. Physiol. (Lond)., 95, 1-28, (1939).

Supported by Swedish Medical Research Council Grant No. B76-14X-02881-07B, Jörgen Schaumanns fond för dermatologisk forskning, Finsenstiftelsen, Tore Nilssons fond för medicinsk forskning and AB Förenade Liv, Stockholm.

Discussion:

Gordon: (to Hallin) I wondered if you had any evidence to show whether the uncomfortable pain experienced during A fiber block can be attributed even in part, to increased discharge of single unmyelinated fibers or whether it must be regarded as a central release phenomenon.

Hallin: In those experiments when we have recorded C fiber impulses after all A fiber activity has been abolished, we have not seen any signs of increased firing in afferent C units responding to natural skin stimuli.

Zimmermann: You speculated that blocking of A delta and C fibers after repetitive electrical stimulation may contribute to pain relief by electrical stimulation of nerves transcutaneously in patients with chronic pain syndromes. The difficulty raised by this hypothesis is that you must produce strong pain by the repetitive stimulation in order to have a few seconds of conduction block and hence of pain relief. Since much of the electroanalgesia is produced by stimuli which are subthreshold for nociceptive afferents, I believe that the predominant factors in electro- and hypalgesia is central inhibition.

Hallin: I only wanted to draw attention to a peripheral mechanism that might contribute to the pain relief experienced by some of these patients during peripheral electrical stimulation. I did not say that this mechanism is the all-important factor. It is a fact that both A delta and C fiber endings when stimulated in the skin exhibit decreased excitability during repetitive high-frequency stimulation. There is also evidence from other workers who have stimulated percutaneously on a whole nerve, that thin myelinated fibers during these conditions exhibit similar excibility changes. I am now referring to for instance, Taub. I do not exclude the great importance of central mechanisms in this context.

Paintal: I would like to address a question to both Dr Hallin and Dr Iggo. Is it not true that as shown by Young and Iggo there is some dispersion of the delta compound action potential after application of a local anaesthetic and this gives a misleading impression about fiber block. Have you Dr Hallin considered this point while correlating the changes in the electroneurogram with the change in sensation.

Hallin: I agree that temporal dispersion of impulses contributing to the averaged nerve response may give a misleading impression about fiber block during local anaesthesia. To overcome this difficulty individual units in the electrically induced responses were followed during the block using the dot-display technique. Some thick fibers blocked at about the same time as A delta fibers and C fibers. Thus even with this display technique it was difficult to attribute certain sensations to activity in a particular fiber group during lidocaine blocks.

Iggo: It is true that there can be difficulties in the interpretation of the compound action potentials during the nerve blocks. But nevertheless, I think your results in man fit quite well with single unit afferent recordings in animals because you find that the loss of cold sensation accompanies block of impulse transmission in thin myelinated fibers and most of the cold afferent fibers in monkeys seem to be slow A delta fibers. There's preservation of the sensation of warmth, and most of the information suggests that warm function in monkeys is mediated by non-myelinated fibers. These fit together quite well in spite of the problem that is raised by Dr Paintal that the technique may not reveal the correct blocking point. There's a second question that I would like to direct to Dr Hagbarth. You did raise the matter of the advantage of being able to use the human subject to report when he was able to experience the pain and suggested that this might be a more satisfactory method than when you did the animal experiment and had to use other criteria for testing. Have you had the opportunity to make in the human subjects a comparison between the report of the subject and some of these other criteria in the same subject. Have you recorded the reported sensation as well as looked for these other autonomic changes, perhaps?

Hagbarth: No we have not made any comparative studies of the subjective experience of pain and the reflexes induced by noxious stimuli.

A METHOD FOR MECHANICAL STIMULATION OF SKIN RECEPTORS

G. WESTLING, R. JOHANSSON and Å. B. VALLBO
Department of Physiology, University of Umeå, S-901 87 Umeå, Sweden

There have been a number of methods for stimulation of skin mechanoreceptors ever since von Frey introduced his hair in 1896. For many years different mechanical arrangements were used to apply a controlled force or indentation. In the fifties electronically controlled stimulators opened up new possibilities. Electromechanical devices, i.e. moving coils or piezoelectrical crystals, were used to generate skin indentations. The moving coil is relatively slow, load-sensitive and has considerable non-linearity and hysteresis, whereas the crystal is fast, but has a small amplitude range. To improve the performance of the former, a position servo controlled system was introduced.(Werner and Mountcastle 1965, Chubbuck 1966). The system included an amplifier, an electromechanical moving coil stimulator, a mechanoelectrical position transducer and a negative feedback loop. In this type of system it was also possible to compute, although with limited accuracy, the external force acting upon the mechanical system by measuring the electronically generated force and the effective displacement (Chubbuck 1966). Nowadays fast force transducers permit true force controlled servo system, although there are some problems with thermal stability (Byrne 1975).Our system is a further development of the basic position servo principle.

THE POSITION TRANSDUCER

The most essential component in a system of this type is not the electro-mechanical device but the mechano-electrical position transducer as it acts as a reference upon which the accuracy of the whole system is dependent. Thus, the transducer must be selected with great care. The main problem with position transducers is nonlinearity which gives rise to a deviation from the preset stimulus although the position signal looks perfect. In the most commonly used types of transducers, such as differential transformers and capacitive bridges, residuals of the carrier frequency after filtering reduce the dynamic range. Further, input-output phase shift and limited frequency response may dramatically reduce the negative feedback performance and possibilities. For these reasons the differential transformer and the capacitive bridge were rejected and an optical position transducer was developed. Its light source is a lens suited neon bulb which in turn is driven by a constant current generator. The light transmission is modulated by a flag connected to the stimulus probe, before the beam reaches a photodiode, working in energy transformation mode. The photodiode current is converted to a voltage before passing through a carefully selected filter. The linearity of the position transducer, and thus the linearity of the whole stimulator, is $\pm 0.2\%$. The total noise is normally distributed with a standard deviation corresponding to 0.05 μm, as shown in Fig.1. With this transducer the servo system has an amplitude range from 0.1 μm to 8 mm.

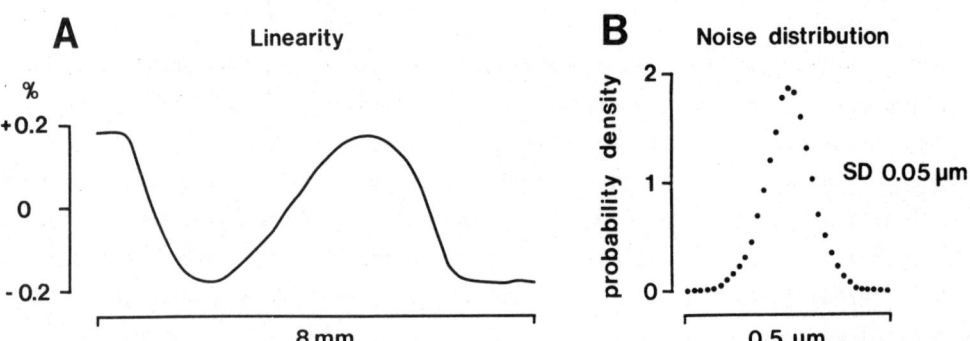

Fig.1. Characteristics of the optical position transducer.
A. The linearity in per cent of total range.
B. The normally distributed noise with a standard deviation corresponding to 0.05 μm.

THE POSITION SERVO

When a position servo is used, the moving coil does not need to be attached with stiff springs, as in commercially available vibrators. On the contrary, stiff springs would just take a lot of power reducing the stimulator efficiency as soon as the moving coil deviates from the midposition. For this reason a loadspeaker was modified by removing the acoustic membrane, leaving only the soft, moving coil centering membrane, which provided some damping to the system properties. For the above reasons, it is possible to have a very effective negative feedback, giving the stimulator a frequency response from DC to 600 Hz as illustrated in Fig.24, and a stiffness of 80,000 N/m. The movable mass is 10.5 grams and the maximal force 30 N giving a maximal acceleration of 3,000 m/sec^2, over the whole amplitude range of 8 mm. These data are several times better compared to what has been described before. The stimulator may be driven by any external signal generator, and it has its own generator, giving square, trapezoid or triangular waveforms. This is realized in an analouge integrator with independent up-and-down integration times and slopes. The slopes can be varied between 0.1 m/sec and 3,000 mm/sec. Fig.2B shows the mechanical step response of 5 mm when applying leading edge slopes from 10 mm/sec to 300 mm/sec. The controls of the slopes and amplitudes are completely independent.

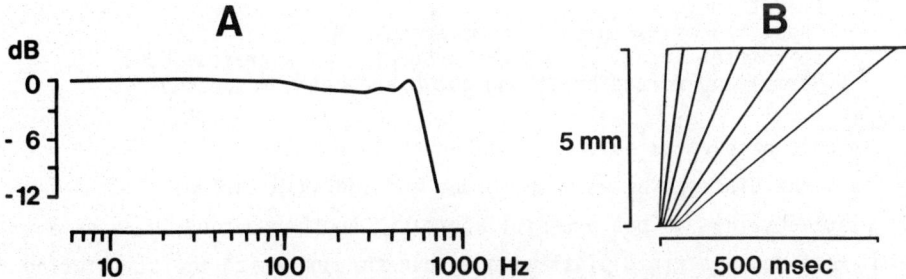

Fig.2. Characteristics of the position servo.
A. The mechanical frequency response.
B. The mechanical step response with slopes of 300, 100, 50, 30, 20, 15 and 10 mm/sec.

SKIN MOVEMENT COMPENSATION

Thus, some problems in generating a very precisely controlled deviation have been solved. However, there remains an important question: What is the effective skin indentation?

This question is very pertinent in the stimulus range below approximately 1 mm where body movements may seriously interact with the stimulator probe movements. Even if the fixation of a limb is very good, there are still variations in the volume caused by breathing and pulsations, which give rise to movements of the skin surface. These complications are illustrated in Fig.3 showing skin movements in the glabrous skin of a human hand which was firmly fixed to a special adhesive clay. The skin surface movements in the upper trace are very well correlated to breathing as measured with a spirometer, as well as to ECG. Normal breathing is shown above and forced breathing below. It may be seen that the skin movements amounted to 10 μm to 100 μm.

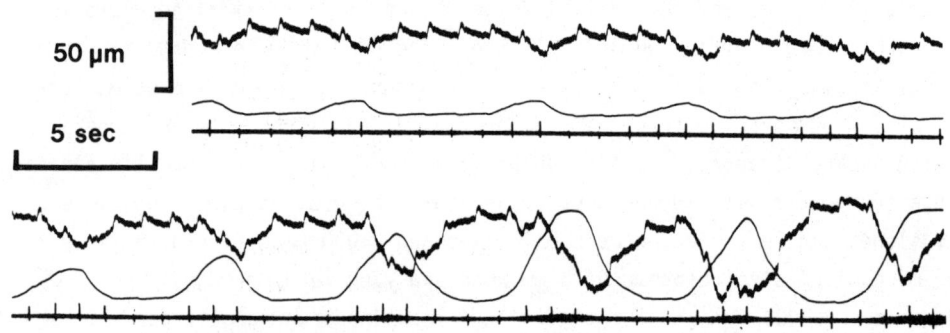

Fig.3. Skin surface movements caused by breathing and pulsations.
Upper traces: skin surface movements. Middle traces: spirometer signal from a thoracograf. Lower traces: ECG. Normal and forced breathing above and below respectively.

How could this problem be solved? A way which in principle seems simple would be to check the distance between the probe and the skin through a microscope but in practice, this is not a useful approach. Another method is to have the limb resting on a rigid plate with a hole through which the stimulating probe comes up (Verrillo 1963). We rejected this method as it might introduce lateral effects which may be particularly relevant in psychophysical studies. In addition, only a small fraction of the total glabrous skin area of the human hand may be reached with this method. Another solution is to use pre-indentation, but this method has its place only in the study of rapidly adapting receptors. Further, the skin movements described above will complicate the analysis. Still another method is demonstrated in Fig.4. The effective skin indentation is indicated as the distance from the point when the stimulating probe makes electrical contact with the skin to the moment when the probe motion stops (Lindblom 1958). This method has been further developed at our laboratory.

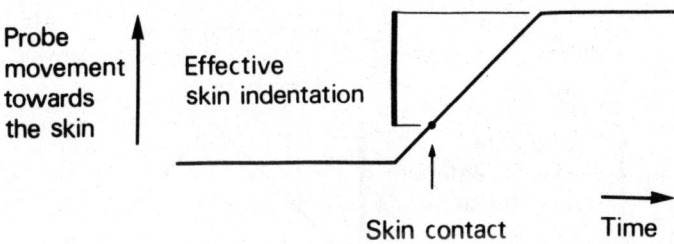

Fig.4. The principle for measuring the effective skin indentation with an electrical contact pulse. The effective skin indentation is indicated as the distance from the point at which the stimulator probe makes electrical contact with the skin to the stop of the probe motion.

In order to have a high accuracy in determining the moment of skin contact, we measure the skin conductance and its time derivate with a small current. This current is fed supracutaneously and it is limited to 80 n amps in order to safely avoid electrical stimulation of cutaneous endings. A skin contact pulse is generated when the skin conductance exceeds $11 \cdot 10^{-11}$ mho. However, if the skin is very dry, this level is reached very slowly, and some skin indentation might be required to attain this level. In order to eliminate this uncertainty we have set the condition that the time derivate of the skin conductance must exceed $9 \cdot 10^{-4}$ mho/sec for the skin contact pulse to appear. If this is not the case, we moisture the skin with a solution of 10% glycerin in water which is allowed to dry into the skin. The skin contact device is floating and battery powered to minimize artefacts in the nerve recording. We have used this method during the last four years in amplitude estimation studies, in which fairly high stimulus amplitudes were employed (Knibestöl 1973, Knibestöl 1975, Knibestöl and Vallbo 1976). One disadvantage is, however, that you cannot preset an amplitude, but only measure it after the stimulation has been delivered. This complicates threshold studies in which the stimulus amplitides are only a small fraction of the skin movements as described above.

THE STIMULATION METHOD

In order to come by these difficulties a new control method has been developed which is demonstrated in Fig.5.

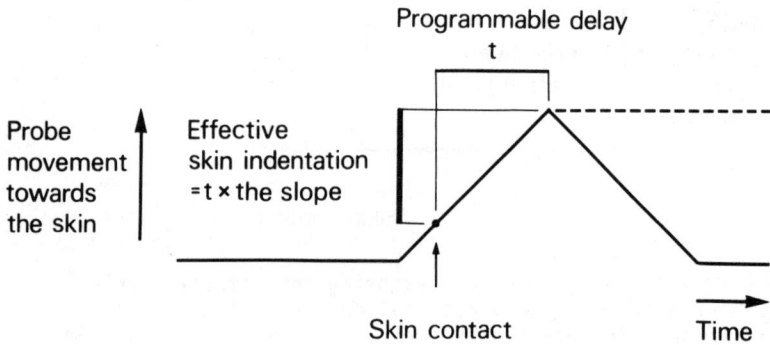

Fig.5. The principle of the stimulation method. The position of the stimulus probe at the moment it makes electrical contact with the skin acts as a reference for a preset indentation amplitude.

The earlier described up-integration starts the probe movement towards the skin at a certain speed. When the probe makes electrical contact with the skin a programmable counter starts. After a preset time it stops the up-integration or turns it into down-integration. The effective skin indentation is equal to the preset delay period times the slope. Thus, the position of the stimulus probe at the moment when it makes electrical contact with the skin, acts as a reference from which a preset amplitude of indentation starts. This method has been used during the last two years in threshold and receptive field studies (Johansson 1976a, Johansson 1976b, Vallbo and Johansson 1976, Johansson and Vallbo 1976). Fig.6 demonstrates the total accuracy of the system. The two curves show the distribution of the deviation from two preset amplitudes of 3 μm and 500 μm, when a triangular indentation was used with a slope of 4 mm/sec. All errors of the stimulation devices as well as skin movements caused by breathing and pulsations were taken into account.

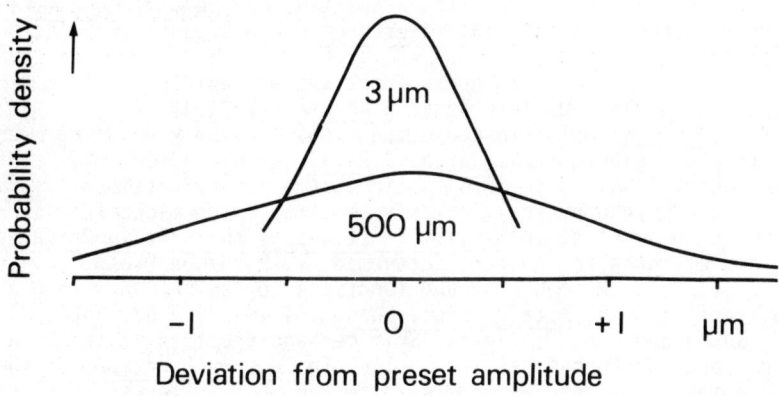

Fig.6. The total accuracy of the system. The two curves show the distribution of the deviation from preset amplitudes of 3 µm and 500 µm, when a triangular indentation was used with a slope of 4 mm/sec. All errors of the stimulation devices as well as skin movements caused by breathing and pulsations were taken into account.

Thus, in summary the stimulator has the following advantages. It has a large amplitude range and a high accuracy. It is presettable and it compensates for inevitable skin movements.

This investigation was supported by grants from the Swedish Medical Research Council, project no. 04X-3548, and by Gunvor och Josef Anêrs Stiftelse.

REFERENCES

Byrne, J. (1975). A feedback controlled stimulator that delivers controlled displacements of forces to cutaneous mechanoreceptors. Trans.Biomed.Engng. 1, 66-69.

Chubbuck, J.G. (1966). Small motion biological stimulator. APL.Tech.Digest. 5, 18-23.

Frey, M. von. (1896). Untersuchungen über die Sinnesfunctionen der menschlichen Haut:Druckempfindung och Schmerz. Abhandl.sächs.Ges.Wiss math-phys. 23, 175-266.

Johansson, R. (1976a). Receptive field sensitivity profile of mechanosensitive units innervating the glabrous skin of the human hand. Brain Res.106. In press.

Johansson, R. (1976b). Skin mechanoreceptors in the human hand: Receptive field characteristics. In Sensory Functions of the Skin in Primates,with special reference to Man. Ed. Zotterman,Y. Pergamon Press.

Johansson, R. and Vallbo, A.B. (1976). Skin mechanoreceptors in the human hand. An inference of some population properties. In Sensory Functions of the skin in Primates, with special reference to Man. Ed. Zotterman, Y. Pergamon Press.

Knibestöl, M. (1973). Stimulus-response functions of rapidly adapting mechanoreceptors in human glabrous skin area. J.Physiol. 232, 427-452.

Knibestöl, M. (1975). Stimulus-response functions of slowly adapting mechanoreceptors in human glabrous skin area. J.Physiol. 245, 63-80.

Knibestöl, M. and Vallbo, A.B. (1976). Stimulus-response functions of primary afferents and psychophysical intensity estimation on mechanical skin stimulation in human hand. In Sensory Functions of the skin in Primates, with special reference to Man. Ed. Zotterman, Y. Pergamon Press.

Lindblom, U. (1958). Excitability and functional organization within a peripheral tactile unit. Acta Physiol. Scand. 44, suppl. 153, 1-84.

Vallbo, A.B. and Johansson, R. (1976). Skin mechanoreceptors in the human hand: Neural and psychophysical thresholds. In Sensory Functions of the skin in Primates, with special reference to Man. Ed. Zotterman, Y. Pergamon Press.

Verrillo, R.T. (1963). Effect of contactor area on vibrotactile threshold. J.Acoust: Soc.Amer. 35, 1962-1966.

Werner, G. and Mountcastle, V.B. (1965). Neural activity in mechanoreceptive cutaneous afferents stimulus-response relations. Weber functions and information transmissions. J. Neurophysiol. 28, 359-397.

Discussion:

Lindblom: Was the small layer of moisture you put on the skin a source of error to any appreciable amount because the moment of contact will not be with the actual skin but with the moist layer on the skin, the glycerin solution. My second question was how could you calibrate such small movements as .5 microns in that reading?

Westling: Dr Lindblom has put two questions: one regarding the moisturing procedure and the other one was how it is possible to measure such small distances.

1. As I mentioned, the solution of 10% glycerin in water is allowed to dry into the skin, and thus there is no supracutaneous layer which might reduce the preset amplitude. This moisturing procedure is used to reduce the skin resistance to below the skin contact triggering level of 9000 Mohm, but it also acts as a mechanical standardisation procedure.

2. It is possible to measure such small distances either with a laser or with measuring blocks, manufactured by Johansson, Eskilstuna, Sweden, with an accuracy of 0.1 µm, but I measured the total accuracy by using statistical methods e.g. averaging.

SKIN MECHANORECEPTORS IN THE HUMAN HAND: RECEPTIVE FIELD CHARACTERISTICS

R. JOHANSSON

Department of Physiology, University of Umeå, S-901 87 Umeå, Sweden

It has been shown by using the percutaneous microelectrode technique developed by Vallbo and Hagbarth (1968) that there are four types of large diameter mechanosensitive units innervating the human hand glabrous skin: two types of rapidly adapting units, the RA and the PC units, and two types of slowly adapting units, the SA I and the SA II units. The RA and SA I units have been found to have small, well defined receptive fields, whereas the PC and SA II units are sensitive to remote stimuli: mechanical transistents and skin stretch respectively (Knibestöl and Vallbo 1970, Knibestöl 1973, Knibestöl 1975). These 4 types of mechanosensitive units have striking similarities with 4 well-defined types which have been described in subhuman mammals (for references see Burgess and Perl 1973).

In order to specify quantitatively how events at the human hand glabrous skin surface set up patterns of activity within the population of afferent units, it is necessary to know the characteristics of the unitary receptive fields in some detail. Some preliminary results will be reported in the present communication on the sensitivity profile of the unitary receptive field when the skin was stimulated with indentations of various amplitudes.

Preliminary observations regarding the skin stretch sensitivity of the
SA II units will also be reported.

The subjects were healthy adults. Single unit impulses were recorded from
the median nerve with the method of Vallbo and Hagbarth (1968). Well controlled skin indentations were delivered with the stimulator described by
Westling et al.(1976). Triangular indentations with a slope of 4 mm/sec
were employed except for the PC units for which the velocity was 8 and
16 mm/sec. The tip of the stimulus probe was 400 μm in diameter and its
contacting surface was rounded to a hemisphere. The receptive fields of
single sensory units were mapped. Stimuli of constant displacement amplitude were delivered, while the position of the probe tip in the plane
corresponding to the appropriate skin surface was traced with an X-Y-plotter. Neuronal responses were indicated by dots on the X-Y-plotter
paper at the appropriate positions, and an iso-sensitive field bondary
was outlined from the dot pattern. This procedure was repeated with several indentation amplitudes and thus a sensitivity profile was obtained.

THE RA RECEPTIVE FIELD

The receptive fields of the RA units were characterized by several zones
of maximal sensitivity distributed over an approximately circular or oval
area covering 5-9 epidermal ridges. A map of an RA receptive field is shown
in Fig. 1A. The closed lines are iso-sensitive lines referring to different
threshold amplitudes. The thinner lines mark the grooves between the papillary ridges. The inner most closed lines indicate the zones of maximal
sensitivity. The mean number of such zones for five receptive fields was
14.7 with a range of 12-17. An asymmetric location of the individual zone
on the papillary ridge was frequently seen. This is consistent with the
notion that the end-organs of the RA units are the Meissner corpuscles
(Jänig 1970, Munger 1971) which mostly are located on either side of the
intermediate epidermal ridge (e.g. Miller, Ralston and Kashara 1958). The
diagram in Fig. 1B shows a section through the receptive field with regard
to the threshold variations along the straight horizontal line in the map
in Fig. 1A. The two ordinates give the threshold amplitude in multiples of
the lowest threshold of the unit as well as in actual threshold amplitudes
in μm. Considering the shape of the curve, it may be seen that the inden-

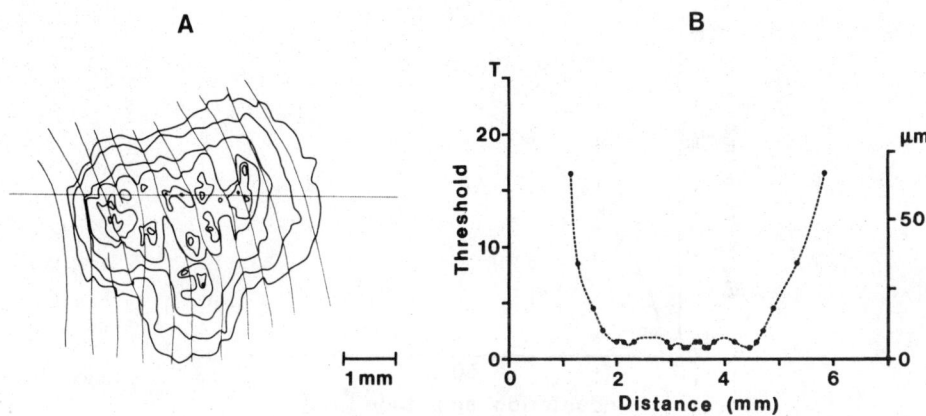

FIG. 1. Receptive field characteristics of an RA mechanosensitive unit. A: Receptive field sensitivity map. The closed lines are iso-sensitive lines referring to the following threshold amplitudes: 66 µm, 34 µm, 18 µm, 10 µm, 6 µm, 4 µm. The thin lines mark the grooves between the papillary ridges. B: Section through the receptive field with regard to the threshold variations along the straight line as shown in A. The left ordinate gives the relative indentation amplitude as multiples of the lowest threshold (T), whereas the right ordinate gives the absolute threshold amplitudes (µm). The abscissa is a distance scale with an arbitary origin.

tation threshold was quite constant among the zones of maximal sensitivity whereas it rose very steeply to the periphery of the receptive field. This finding indicates a close uniformity of the end-organs innervated by the same afferent fibre with respect to the indentation threshold. It is obvious from the map in Fig. 1A that the size of the receptive field of a unit increases with the indentation amplitude. The relation between these two variables could be reasonably well described with a hyperbola. The diagram in Fig. 2 which refers to the RA unit in Fig. 1, shows the hyperbola fitted to the experimental data. The function approached linearity when the indentation amplitude was increased. Linearity in this respect indicates that the stimulus was attenuated in proportion to the reciprocal of the square of the distance from the probe tip. The relation between the indentation amplitude and the field size is of obvious interest for calculations of the population response to skin indentations as a function of indentation

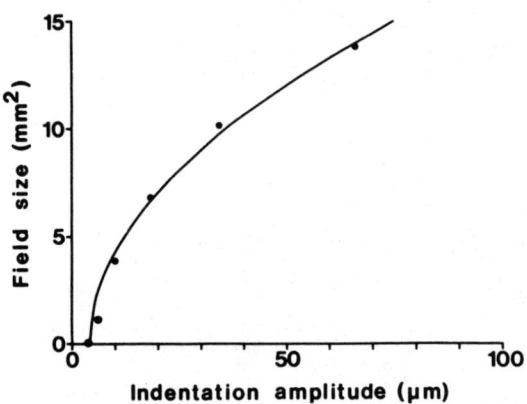

FIG. 2. The receptive field size (ordinate) of an RA unit as a function of the indentation amplitude (abscissa). The curve is a hyperbola fitted to the experimental data indicated by dots. Same unit as in Fig. 1.

amplitude. The relation demonstrated in Fig. 2 indicates that, for an arbitrary RA unit, the field size at any indentation amplitude may be predicted if only information is available concerning the lowest indentation threshold and the field size at a known multiple of the lowest threshold.

THE SA I RECEPTIVE FIELD

Striking similarities were found between the SA I units and the RA units. As illustrated by the sample unit of Fig. 3, the individual SA I units showed several zones of maximal sensitivity, but not as many as the RA units. The mean number of such a zones for five units was 5.4 with a range of 4-7. Sensitivity variations among the zones of maximal sensitivity of a single unit were very small. A hyperbola could adequately describe the relation between the indentation amplitude and the field size as for the RA units.

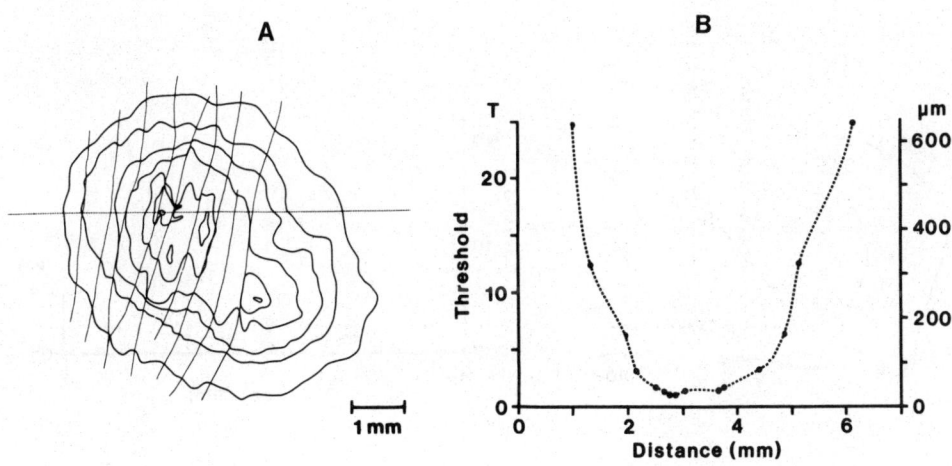

FIG. 3. Receptive field characteristics of an SA I mechanosensitive unit. A and B as in Fig. 1. The iso-sensitive lines refer to the following threshold amplitudes: 642 μm, 322 μm, 162 μm, 82 μm, 42 μm, 34 μm, 26 μm.

THE PC RECEPTIVE FIELD

In contrast to the units described above, the PC units had only one zone of maximal sensitivity. An example is shown in Fig. 4 where it may be seen in the diagram to the right, that the indentation threshold rose very gently from the single zone of maximal sensitivity. In order to facilitate a comparison, the scale of the left ordinate which is divided into multiples of the lowest indentation threshold, is the same as in the receptive field sections of Fig. 1 and 3.

THE SA II RECEPTIVE FIELD

In Fig. 5 is shown a typical map of a SA II receptive field which, as for the PC units, had a single zone of maximal sensitivity and a gentle threshold rise from this zone.

Analysis of the SA II units with regard to their sensitivity to skin stretch and mechanical stimulation of the nails revealed interesting differences

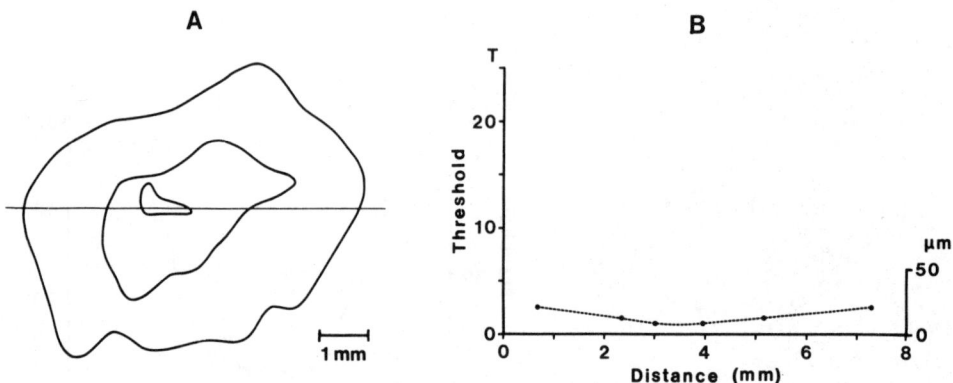

FIG. 4. Receptive field characteristics of a PC mechano-sensitive unit. A and B as in Fig. 1. The iso-sensitive lines refer to the following threshold amplitudes: 20 μm, 12 μm, 8 μm.

among the SA II units. The stimuli were manually delivered by using a pair of sharp tweezers hooked in the superficial layer of the epidermis. Care was taken to ensure that the neuronal response was not caused by indentation of the tweezers. The SA II units could readily be separated into three groups on the basis of their sensitivity to these types of stimuli. Examples of units of the three types named A, B and C are schematically illustrated in Fig. 6. The location of the zone of maximal sensitivity is indicated by the dots in the figures for each unit respectively. The A type shown in the left part of Fig. 6 was characterized by excitation when the skin was stretched from the zone of maximal sensitivity in two opposite directions as indicated by the arrows with plus signs. When stretching the skin at right angles to the excitatory directions, as indicated by arrows with minus sign, the ongoing discharge was frequently inhibited. The approximate area of effective stimulus is indicated by the length of the arrows. Skin stretch in the proximal and/or distal direction increased the discharge rate of those units which were located in the phalanx and the area of effective stimulus always extended transjointally. For units located in the palm excitation was produced by stretch either roughly in

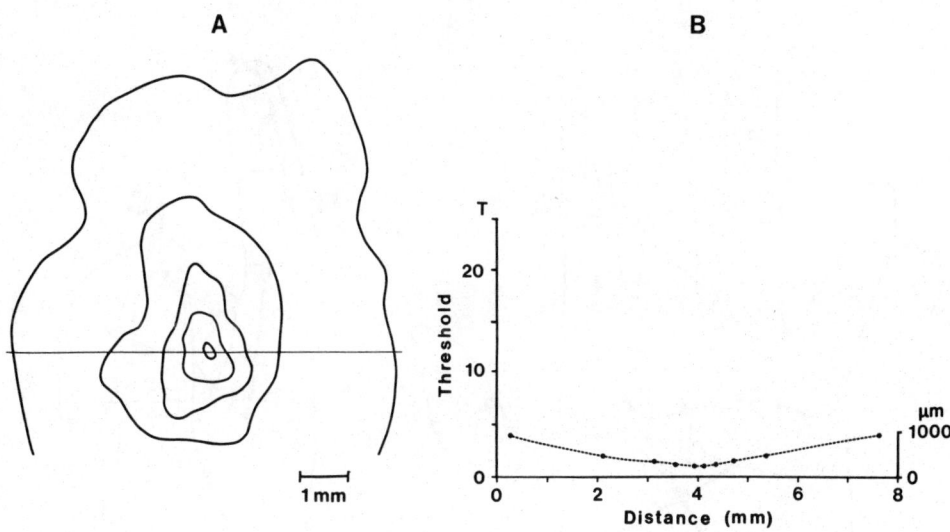

FIG. 5. Receptive field characteristics of an SA II mechanosensitive unit. A and B as in Fig. 1. The iso-sensitive lines refer to the following thresholds amplitudes: 962 μm, 482 μm, 362 μm, 282 μm, 242 μm.

the proximal-distal or ulnar-radial directions. Examples of the B type is shown at the index in the right part of Fig. 6. This type was characterized by excitation when the skin was stretched in one direction from the zone of maximal sensitivity whereas inhibition of the ongoing discharge occurred when the skin was stretched in the opposite direction. All of the B type units had their zones of maximal sensitivity located on the phalanges, and the area of effective stimulus extended transjointally in proximal or distal direction. The A and B type units were frequently spontaneously disscharging when the recordings started, but most of them could easily be stopped by adjustments of the joint positions. These adjustments resulted in a hand position similar to that of the comfortably relaxed hand. The effects of joint movements appeared to be secondary to changes of the skin tension. The C type was characterized by a high sensitivity to mechanical stimulation of the nail. Sometimes a single zone of maximal sensitivity located close to the proximal or lateral borders of the nail could be

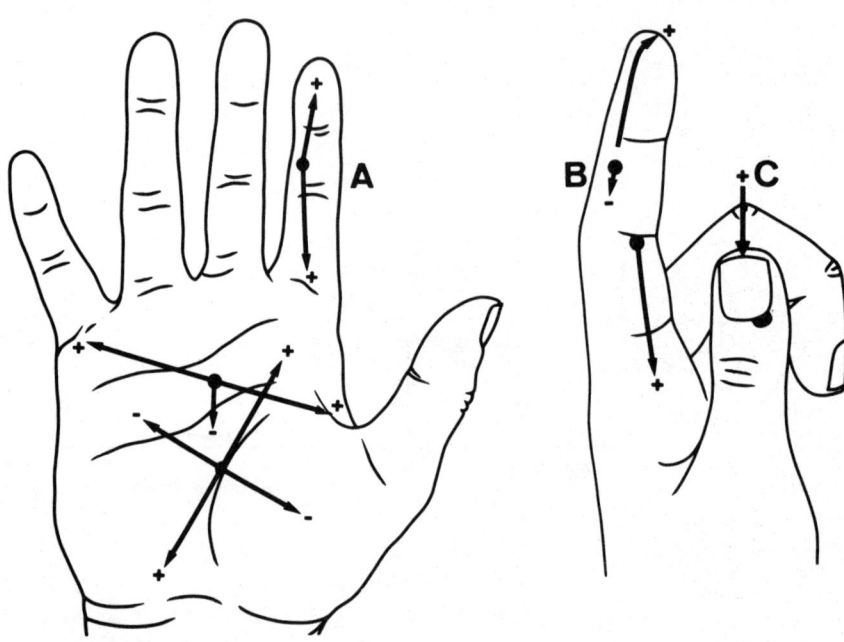

FIG. 6. Schematic illustration of the sensitivity of SA II units to skin stretch and mechanical stimulation of the nail. A, B and C in the figure refer to three different types of SA II units. The location of the zone of maximal sensitivity to local indentation is indicated by a dot for the individual unit. Arrows marked with plus and minus signs indicate directions of skin stretch or pressure upon the nail which gave rise to, respectively, increased and decreased discharge of the unit. The approximate area of effective stimulus is indicated by the lengths of the arrows.

defined. These units responded particularly well when pressure was applied at the distal nail edge in proximal direction and in some cases also when the distal edge of the nail was pressed dorsally. The sensitivity to skin stretch and joint movements was generally poor.

Skin Mechanoreceptors in the Human Hand

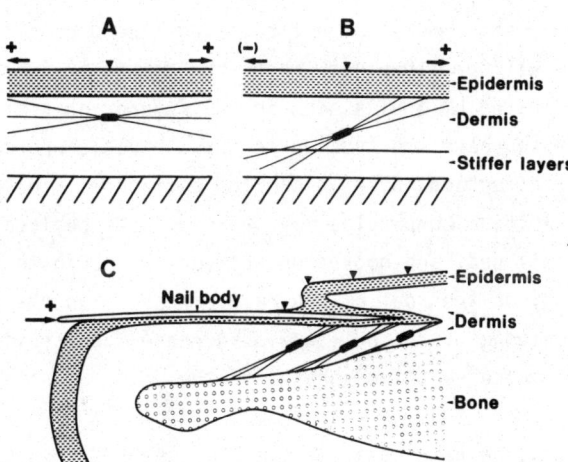

FIG. 7. A, B and C illustrate three hypothetical modes of fixation of the spindle shaped Ruffini corpuscle. The end-organs are anchored to the surrounding tissues by means of the collagenous fibres (thin lines) extending from the two poles of the corpuscle. Skin stretch or nail pressure in the directions of the arrows would increase (+ sign) or decrease (- sign) the tension in the corpuscle. The filled triangles indicate the assumed locations of the zones of maximal sensitivity.

It has been shown by Chambers et al. 1972, that the Ruffini corpuscle constitutes the end-organ of the SA II unit in the hairy skin of the cat. If this is true also for the human glabrous skin, the three different types of responses among the SA II units, as described above, may be explained by three different types of fixations of the spindle shaped end-organ to the surrounding tissues. It may be assumed that the end-organs are anchored to the surrounding tissues by means of the collagenous fibres extending from the two poles of the receptor as schematically illustrated in Fig. 7 A, B and C respectively.

As indicated in Fig. 7A the fibres coming from the two poles of the Ruffini corpuscle may be attached to the fibre network of the dermal connective tissue. Skin stretch in the direction of the arrows would raise the tension in the corpuscle and thereby increase the neuronal activity, whereas skin stretch at right angles would unload the corpuscle. A second alternative is indicated in Fig. 7B. The fibres from one pole of the corpuscle may be attached to the dermis whereas the fibres from the opposite pole may be anchored in the stiffer fibre network of the dermis or in the subdermal tissues. As indicated by a plus sign in the figure, skin stretch in one direction would increase the tension in the corpuscle whereas stretching in the opposite direction would unload the corpuscle. Finally, as shown in Fig. 7C the Ruffini corpuscles may be assumed to be located in the dermis of the nail bed, and hooked up between the periosteum and the dermis close to the body or the root of the nail. Pressure in the proximal direction at the free edge of the nail would increase the tension in the corpuscle and thus increase the discharge of the unit.

These assumptions regarding the fixations of the Ruffini endings seem resonable since it is known that there are large amounts of collagenous fibres running in and between dermal and sub-dermal layers as assumed in the above models, and further that the Ruffini endings are found in all the tissue layers between the epidermis and the bone (e.g. Stilwell 1957, Miller, Ralston and Kasahara 1958).

CONCLUSIONS

As a whole the above described results are in agreement with earlier reports regarding the glabrous skin mechanoreceptor units of primates showing that the RA and SA I units have small receptive fields with distinct borders whereas the PC and SA II units have a single sensitive focus and receptive fields which are not sharply delimited (Lindblom 1965, Lindblom and Lund 1966, Talbot et al. 1968, Knibestöl and Vallbo 1970, Knibestöl 1973, Knibestöl 1975). However, in these earlier investigations the receptive fields have been mapped manually by using small blunt probes to deliver gentle stimuli. The results obtained with these crude methods are characterized by a lack of quantitative as well as certain qualitative information regarding the sensitivity profiles of the receptive fields. In contrary to the earlier findings the present ones reveal that the receptive field of a mechanoreceptor unit is a functional concept: its form and size varies considerably when stimulations of various properties e.g. various amplitudes are applied to the skin. The findings also clearly show that the sensitivity profiles of the RA and SA I units consist of several zones of maximal sensitivity. The fact that the receptive fields grow around zones of maximal sensitivity suggests that these zones correspond to well localized endorgans which give rise to the functionalally definable receptive field. The peripheral organization of the RA and SA I fields with several receptors relatively widely scattered permit the receptive fields of these units to interdigitate extensively with preserved sensitivity profiles. The present findings concerning the SA II units and the classification of the SA II units in three groups with regard to their sensitivity to skin stretch and mechanical stimulation of nail may provide a fruitful basis for further investigations on their functional role in mechanisms involved in tactile sensibility as well as in kinaesthesis.

In summary, the present findings emphasize that there are in the glabrous four types of mechanosensitive units which have very distinctive functional characteristics. These characteristics, in turn, offer a natural basis for a classification when two variables are considered: sensitivity to sustained indentation and sensitivity to remote stimuli. Two types of units are clearly well suited for spatial discrimination and accurate localization of stimule, the RA and the SA I units. They have small and well delimited receptive fields. The detailed organization of their fields seems to emphasize the capacity of the system for analysis of spatial aspects: the single sensory unit has a limited number of endings which are located close enough to provide a sensitivity which is practically uniform within a sharply delimited area and, at the same time, the terminal endings are sufficiently well scattered to permit a large number of sensory units to interdigitate with preserved sensitivity profiles. The other two types, the PC and SA II units, seem less suitable for spatial discrimination. Evidence from earlier studies in other laboratories as well as those presented here, indicate that the primary functions of the PC and SA II units are to analyse other aspects of the mechanical events, which the RA and SA I units can not cover due to their well delimited receptive fields: Mechanical vibrations travelling through the tissues and stretching of the skin.

This investigation was supported by Grants from the Swedish Medical Research council (project no. 04X-3548) and the University of Umeå (Reservationsanslaget för främjande av ograduerade forskares vetenskapliga verksamhet).

REFERENCES

Burgess, P.R. & Perl, E.R. (1973). Cutaneous mechanoreceptors and nociceptors. In Handbook of Sensory Physiology, vol. II, ed. Iggo, A., pp. 29-78. Berlin-Heidelberg-New York: Springer.

Chambers, M.R., Andres, K.H., Duering, M. von & Iggo, A. (1972). The structure and function of the slowly adapting type II mechanoreceptor in hairy skin. Quart. J. exp. Physiol., 57, 417-445.

Jänig, W. (1971). Morphology of rapidly and slowly adapting mechanoreceptors in the hairless skin of the cat's hind foot. Brain Research, 28, 217-231.

Knibestöl, M. (1973). Stimulus-response functions of rapidly adapting mechanoreceptors in human glabrous skin area. J. Physiol. (Lond.), 232, 427-452.

Knibestöl, M. (1975). Stimulus-response functions of slowly adapting mechanoreceptors in the human glabrous skin area. J. Physiol. (Lond.), 245, 63-80.

Knibestöl, M. & Vallbo, A. (1970). Single unit analysis of mechanoreceptor activity from the human glabrous skin. Acta physiol. scand., 80, 178-195.

Lindblom, U. (1965). Properties of touch receptors in distal glabrous skin of the monkey. J. Neurophysiol., 28, 966-985.

Lindblom, U. & Lund, L. (1966). The discharge from vibration-sensitive receptors in the monkey foot. Expl Neurol., 15, 401-417.

Miller, M.R., Ralston, H.J. & Kasahara, M. (1958). The pattern of cutaneous innervation of the human hand. Am. J. Anat., 102, 183-217.

Munger, B.L. (1971). Patterns of organization of peripheral sensory receptors. In Handbook of Sensory Physiology, vol. I, ed. Loewenstein, W.R., pp. 523-556. Berlin-Heidelberg-New York: Springer.

Stilwell, D.L., Jr. (1957). The innervation of deep structures of the hand. Am. J. Anat., 101, 75-100.

Talbot, W.H., Darian-Smith, I., Kornhuber, H.H. & Mountcastle, V.B. (1968). The sense of flutter-vibration: comparison of the human capacity with response patterns of mechanoreceptive afferents from the monkey hand.

Vallbo, Å.B. & Hagbarth, K.-E. (1968). Activity from skin mechanoreceptors recorded percutaneously in avake human subjects. Expl Neurol., 21, 270-289.

SKIN MECHANORECEPTORS IN THE HUMAN HAND: AN INFERENCE OF SOME POPULATION PROPERTIES

R. JOHANSSON and Å. B. VALLBO

Department of Physiology, University of Umeå, S-901 87 Umeå, Sweden

The knowledge of the functional properties of peripheral mechanisms involved in tactile skin sensibility has grown considerably in the last years thanks to a large number of investigations on primates, including man, as well as in other mammals. Most of these studies have been devoted to the relationship between well defined stimulus parameters and the activity in single sensory units rather than to the activity of the population as a whole. However, it seems that a thorough knowledge of the population responses is an essential requisite for a further analysis of many aspects of the function of the somato-sensory system.

Population responses of mechanosensitive units have been studied by Gray and co-workers in the sixties (e.g. Fuller and Gray 1966). At that time the information of the functional properties of the different types of sensory units was relatively meagre and in these studies not much weight was put upon the possible significance of the fact that the unit may have different functional properties. Later, as a more clear picture emerged of the different types of sensory units a few analyses of the population responses to mechanical stimuli have been done (Burgess et al. 1974, Johnson 1974). In a detailed study of the responses of the RA units in the monkey glabrous skin, Johnson has computed the population input-output relations for a 40 Hz sinusoidal stimulation on the basis of the distribution of thresholds and the form and size of the receptive fields.

In the present report which mainly concerns the RA and SA I mechanosensitive units in the glabrous skin of the human hand some preliminary calculations will be submitted and discussed regarding the population response to localized tactile stimuli of varying amplitudes. An increase of a localized indentation has the following two effects. (1) A successive recruitment of units with higher thresholds at the actual point of skin indentation. The recruitment may be described on the basis of an increase of the receptive field size of the individual unit as the indentation amplitude raises.
(2) The impulse discharge in units already recruited raises. Only the former of these two effects will be discussed in the present report. More specifically, the following questions will be considered: (1) How closely are the receptive fields distributed on the glabrous skin? As an expression for the receptive field density the average distance between the center points of neighbouring receptive fields was calculated as a function of the indentation amplitude. (2) How many units will respond to a localized indentation of a given amplitude? This type of analysis seems relevant for the understanding of spatial resolution and descrimination as well as intensity coding in the human somato-sensory system.

The approach in the analysis was to reconstruct the population response from a representative sample of single unit responses. A sample of 334 mechanosensitive units was collected by recordings with tungsten needle electrodes percutaneously inserted into the median nerve on the upper arm of healthy adult subjects. The location of the receptive field was determined and the receptor type was assessed on the basis of adaptation and receptive field properties for each units. The indentation thresholds were measured with the stimulator described by Westling et al. (1976). The stimulus probe had a diameter of 400 μm and the tip was rounded to a hemisphere. Triangular indentations with a slope of 4 mm/sec were employed except for units which had higher critical slopes. In these cases a slope of 8 mm/sec or 16 mm/sec was used. The receptive field size of the RA and SA I units was determined with a stimulus corresponding to an indentation amplitude of about four

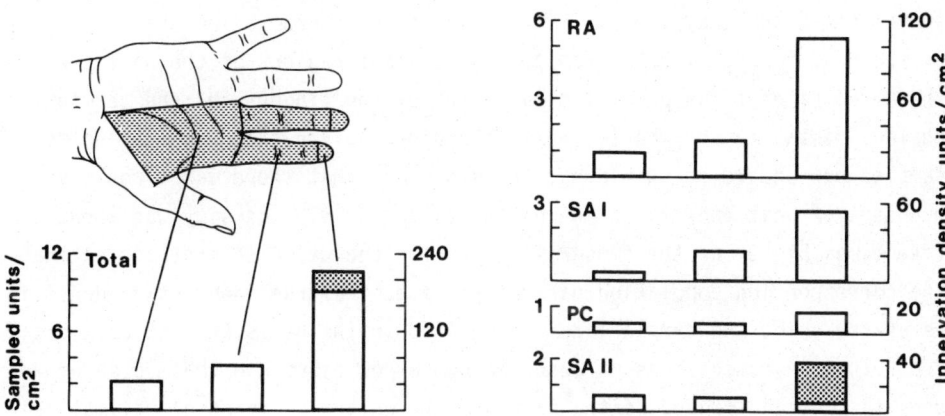

FIG. 1. Diagrams to demonstrate relative and estimated absolute densities of mechanosensitive units in three different glabrous skin regions of the hand innervated by the median nerve as indicated to the left: the palm, the main parts of the fingers and the distal portions of the fingers distally to the whorl. To the left is shown the number of units of all four types taken together and to the right the number of the four types of units separately. The left ordinates in the diagrams indicate the number of units per square centimeter which have been sampled in all the experiment. The right ordinates represent an estimation of the number of units per square centimeter in the human glabrous skin as described in the text. The grey areas of the columns represent those SA II units which were related to the nail rather than to the glabrous skin.

times the lowest indentation threshold of the unit. The following population parameters, derived from the unit sample, served as a basis for the calculations. (1) The density of receptive fields on the skin surface, i.e. the innervation density. (2) The distribution of indentation thresholds. (3) The receptive field size distribution at a given indentation amplitude. These parameters will be considered separately and successively before the calculations will be presented.

INNERVATION DENSITY

The unit sample which constitutes the basis of the innervation density calculations is presented in Fig. 1. In order to exclude sampling bias, due to anatomical variations in the branching of the median nerve, the sampling was limited to the central part of the classical median nerve territory, indicated as the grey area in Fig. 1. In the histogram below the drawing of the hand in Fig. 1 data from three different regions of the hand are shown separately: the palm, the main part of the fingers and the terminal phalanx distal to the whorl. The left ordinate gives the number of units sampled per square cm skin area. It is obvious that there was a positive gradient of unit density in the distal direction. The density was about five times higher on the finger tips than in the palm. In order to estimate the corresponding population parameters, i.e. the true innervation densities of the skin, the sample data were scaled on the basis of available data from other investigations on absolute number of fibres in the median nerve, densities of end organs in the skin and the number of zones of maximal sensitivity in the receptive fields (Sunderland and Bedbrook 1949, Bolton et al. 1966, Buchtal and Rosenfalck 1966, Johansson 1976). The right ordinate gives the absolute innervation densities calculated on this basis. The estimation indicates that there were as many as 212 units per square cm on the distal part of the fingers whereas there were only 43 in the palm of the hand. Although these figures should be regarded as fairly rough estimates, they are probably in the right order of magnitude. This notion was supported by the fact that calculations on the basis of data from different investigations gave roughly similar results. Also from another point of view the exact figures do not deserve too much attention. It is known that the number of fibres in peripheral nerves varies considerably with age and between individuals of the same age (Corbin and Gardner 1937, Gardner 1940, Swallow 1966). Therefore it seems more adequate to give an estimation of the range of normal innervation density. We have reached the conclusion that this range would be between 50 and 200 per cent of the figures given in the histograms.

The four histograms in the right part of Fig. 1 show the separate contributions of the four different types of units:RA, SA I, PC and SA II. The shaded part of the columns in the histograms indicate the contribution of those SA II units which were clearly related to the nails rather than to the glabrous skin (Johansson 1976). These units which constituted as much as 83 % of the SA II units on the finger tips were excluded in the calculations to be presented below. It may be seen in Fig. 1 that the increase in unit

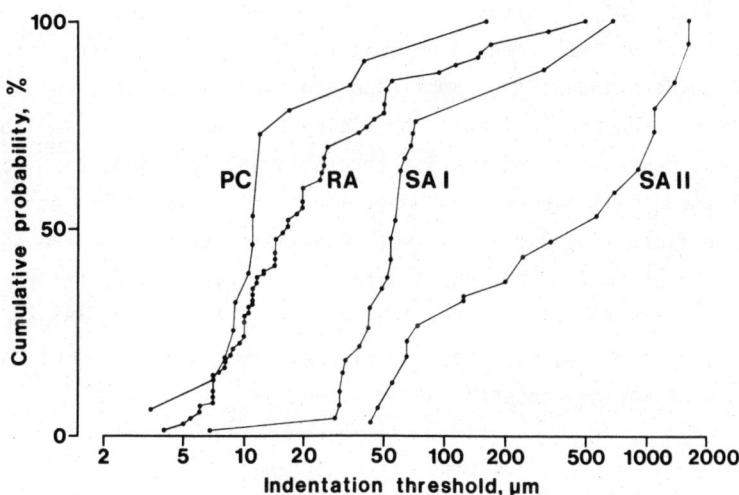

FIG. 2. Indentations thresholds of a sample of mechanosensitive units of the glabrous skin randomly sampled from the median nerve. Separate cumulative probability plots are shown for the four different types of units.

density in the distal direction was accounted for mainly by the RA and SA I units, whereas the PC and the SA II units were approximately evenly distributed over the entire hand.

INDENTATION THRESHOLDS

The indentation thresholds of a unit sample is shown in Fig. 2 as separate cumulative distributions for each one of the four unit types. It may be seen that the PC and RA units were very sensitive, their indentation thresholds extending down to between 3 μm and 4 μm, whereas the slowly adapting units, and especially the SA II units, had much higher thresholds. Fifty per cent of the PC units and just 5 per cent of the RA units had critical slopes above 4 mm/sec. It may be worth pointing out that there was no statistically significant difference between the indentation thresholds from the different regions of the glabrous skin (P>0.05 Wilcoxon-Mann-Whitney test).

RECEPTIVE FIELD SIZE DISTRIBUTION

In a previous study it was shown that the receptive field of any unit was larger the higher the indentation amplitude. It was also shown that the relation between indentation amplitude and field size was predictable for the individual RA and SA I units providing information was available on two points: the lowest indentation threshold and the field size corresponding to a known multiple of the lowest indentation threshold. As described above, the field size and the lowest indentation threshold were determined for a sample of units. From these data the distribution of the receptive field sizes as a function of the indentation amplitude was obtained. This distribution, in turn, was used to calculate the recruitment of the RA and SA I units at various indentation amplitudes.

CENTER POINT DISTANCE

The purpose of the calculation to be presented below was to produce an estimate of how closely the receptive fields are located on the skin surface in various regions of the hand. As an expression for this aspect of the spatial distribution of the units a calculation was done of the average distance between the imaginary center point of a receptive field and that of its closest neighbor.

The calculation required an assumption concerning the spatial pattern of center point distribution. The simplest one was adopted: a hexagonal array of equidistant center points was assumed. It seems reasonable to take this assumption as the calculation would give a good approximation of the average center point distance providing that the distribution of the units is uniform over the skin area. It should also be pointed out that the calculation is based upon the innervation densities presented in a previous section and it refers to local indentations with a slope of 4 mm/sec. Account has been taken of the proportion of units having higher critical slopes. The center point distance was calculated as a function of indentation amplitude thus providing not only a figure for the spacing of the total number of fields but a curve relating the stimulus amplitude to the center point distance between those units which were excited by a given indentation amplitude. The results of the calculations are shown in the diagrams of Fig. 3 where the average center point distance is given as a function of

Skin Mechanoreceptors in the Human Hand

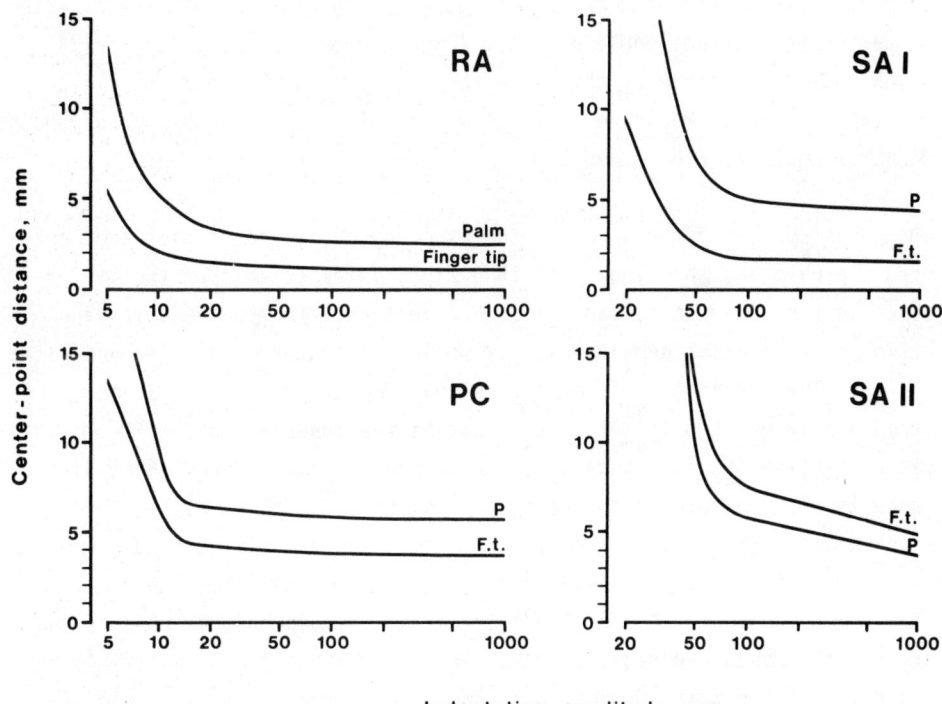

FIG. 3. Estimated average distance between the center point of any mechanosensitive units in the glabrous skin and that of its closest neighbor of the same type, as a function of stimulus amplitude. The calculations were done on the basis of sampled data and the assumption given in the text. Separate diagrams are shown for the four different types of units. The two curves in the diagrams refer to the finger tip and the palm respectively.

the indentation amplitude. An increase of the indentation amplitude exites more units which results in a lower average center point distance. In the RA population this decrease was most pronounced in the amplitude range below 20 μm where the main part of the RA thresholds were located. The corresponding value for the SA I population was about 100 μm. The center point distance attains a minimal value as the stimulus intensity reaches the thresholds of the most insensitive units. The interpretation of the curves in the diagrams may be further illustrated with an example. If the finger tip is mapped with an indentation amplitude of 100 μm, the expected center point distance would be about 1 mm between the receptive fields which would be excited by this indentation amplitude whereas the distance for the SA I units would be just below 2 mm. In the palm, the corresponding distance would be 2.5 mm and 5 mm.

There are smaller differences in the expected center point distances between the palm and the finger tip than might be expected from the differences in the innervation densities. For instance, for the RA units the ratio of innervation density was 5.7 while the center point distance ratio was 2.4. The explanation is of course that the center point distance is reciprocally related to the square root of the innervation density. This basic relation is of obvious interest inasmuch as the center point distance is closely related to the spatial discrimination capacity. The relation suggests that this capacity will not be appreciably altered by moderate variations in the total number of fibres in the peripheral nerve. It is known that considerable variations are present among normal subjects and, of course, pronounced reductions may occur in pathological conditions. A reduction of the total number of sensory units by as much as 75 % would give rise to not more than a doubling of the average center point distance.

RECRUITMENT OF UNITS

When a localized skin indentation is delivered the number of units responding is obviously a function of the stimulus amplitude, as the units having their end organs in the vicinity or directly below the point of indentation represent greatly varying thresholds at this very point. In order to elucidate this aspect of the population response the mean number of units recruited as a function of indentation amplitude was calculated when localized stimuli were delivered randomly to the appropriate skin area. The mean number of units defined in this way is equivalent to the expected receptive field overlap as a function of stimulus amplitude. The calculation was limited to the RA and SA I population and it was based upon two population parameters: innervation density and distribution of receptive field sizes as a function of the indentation amplitude. Strictly the inference is valid only for an indentation slope of 4 mm/sec since the underlying sample parameters were collected with this stimulus slope.

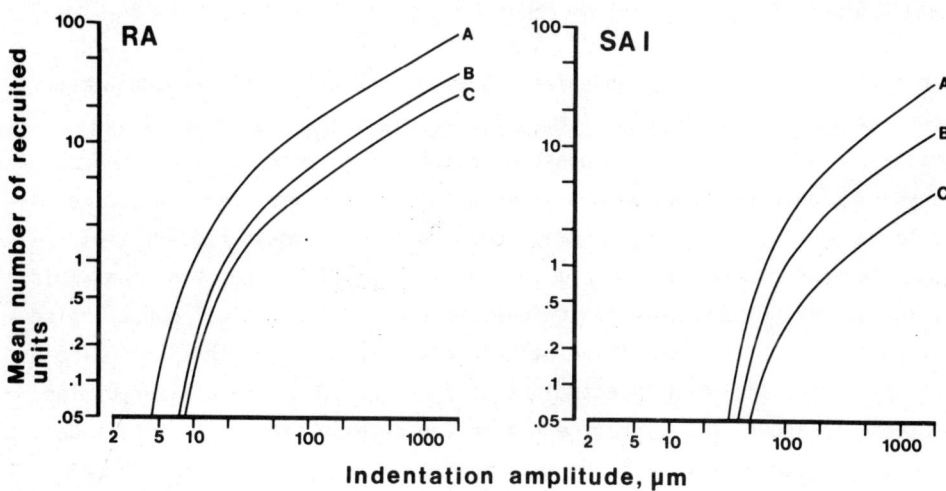

FIG. 4. Estimated mean number of units of the RA and SA I type responding to a localized indentation, as a function of indentation amplitude. The curves A, B and C refer to three different regions of the glabrous skin: the finger tips, the main parts of the fingers and the palm.

The diagrams in Fig. 4 show the mean number of units recruited in the RA and SA I populations as a function of the indentation amplitude. The three curves labelled A, B and C refer to the finger tip, the main part of the finger and the palm respectively. It may be seen that a localized indentation of 2 mm which is quite a strong stimulus would, on the average, excite nearly 100 units in the RA population on the finger tip. The corresponding value for the SA I population is about 30. The overlap was considerably lower in the other regions of the hand. The lowest figure was found in the SA I population of the palm, where on the average just 4 units would be excited by a 2 mm indentation. On the other hand, it may be seen that amplitudes as low as 50 μm would give a surprisingly high recruitment in the RA population, but almost no response from the SA I population.

As may be seen in Fig. 4, there is a very steep increase of the receptive field overlap with stimulus amplitude in the low range for the RA population

A doubling of the indentation amplitude from 5 to 10 μm results in a 10 times higher recruitment of RA units at the finger tip.

In the low range of skin indentations where the population response may consist of a single impulse from a few single units a skin sensitive pattern may be described composed of patches from which a response from any unit would be induced by a stimulus of a given amplitude. Experimental data to provide a correct description of this type would require the simultaneous recording from all the units innervating the skin area. This is of course not possible to achieve. However, a theoretical construction of this type of skin sensitive pattern has been done for the RA population at the finger tip when indentations of 7 μm and 10 μm are delivered. The outcome is shown in Fig. 5. The reason for choosing these low amplitudes, was to illustrate how well the skin surface is covered by units which detect even the weakest stimuli. The four figures in Fig. 5 show a piece of glabrous skin from a finger tip with the grooves between the papillary ridges marked by solide lines. In the two figures above, the filled and the open circles represent Meissner's corpuscles, i.e. the RA receptors. This pattern of end-organ distribution was extracted from a figure in a paper by Cauna (1965). The filled circles in Fig. 5 A and B indicate end-organs which would be excited by an indentation of 7 μm and 10 μm respectively. The number of end-orgnas which would be excited and their locations in relation to the total set of end organs have been selected on the basis of previous findings concerning the distance between high sensitive zones in the receptive field maps (Johansson 1976) and the proportion of units which would be excited at the appropriate indentation amplitudes according to the threshold distribution shown in Fig. 2.

The hatched zones in the figures below indicate the receptive fields accounted for by the responding end-organs in the figures above. In Fig. 5 which refer to the higher stimulus amplitude, a larger number of end-organs would be excited and, in addition, the individual receptive fields of the end-organs already excited by the weaker stimulus as shown in Fig. 5 A would be larger and more confluent. The cross hatched zones indicate overlap of receptive fields belonging to different units.

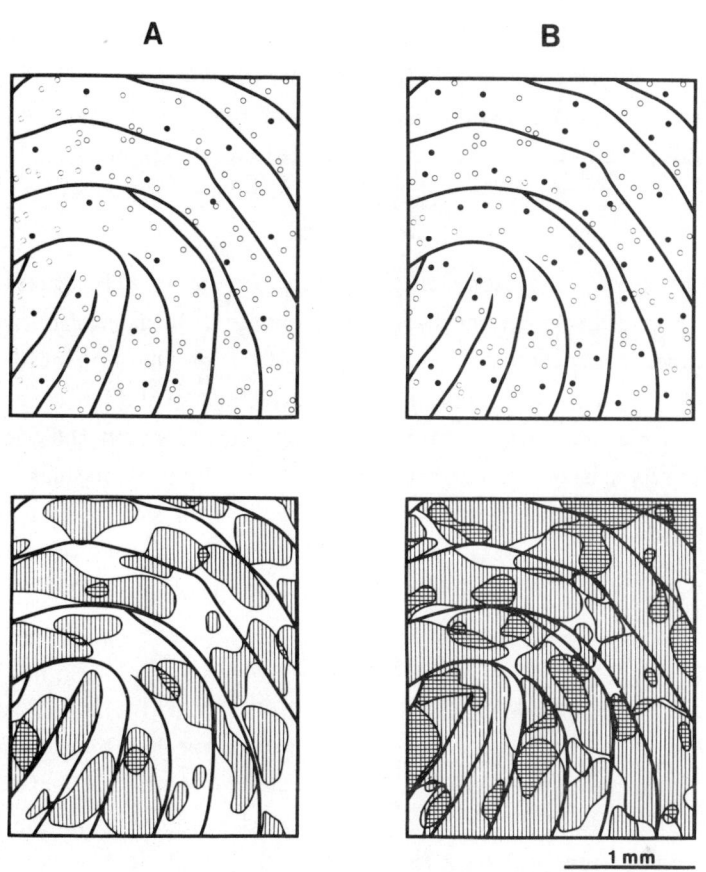

FIG. 5. Plausible maps of the distribution of RA end-organs (upper figures) responding to indentations of 7 μm in A and 10 μm in B, and their receptive fields on the skin (lower figures). The figures represent a small part of the glabrous skin area close to the whorl of a finger tip, the lines indicating the grooves between the papillary ridges, open and filled circles the RA end-organs. Filled circles represent those end-organs which would respond to the stimulus. In the lower figures the hatched areas represent the skin areas from which these end-organs would be excited by a localized indentation of the respective amplitude. The maps were constructed on the basis of sampled data, the assumptions given in the text and a morphological study by Cauna (1965). See text for further details.

The hatched zones in the two figures constitute 50 and 100 per cent of the total skin surface implying that an indentation of 7 μm gives a mean number of 0.5 recruited units and an indentation of 10 μm a mean number of 1.0. However, blind spots may exist despite a mean overlap of one unit, as multiple excitation, i.e. overlap of receptive fields, is assumed.

CONCLUSIONS

It is obvious from the data presented that practically all naturally occurring tactile stimuli to the human hand excite a large number of sensory units, setting up a pattern of neural activity from the population of mechanosensitive units. In addition, even the smallest variation of a suprathreshold stimulation, e.g. variations in the location and the magnitude will appreciably change this pattern. Therefore it seems obvious that the population response must be considered rather than a single unit response in most attempts to correlate the primary neuronal response with the behaviour of the subject, e.g. the psychophysical response.

Considering the performance in the classical tests of tactile spatial capacity, i.e. the two point discrimination and the point localization, it is well known that there are large differences between the palm and the finger tip (e.g. Weinstein 1968). It seems obvious that the performances in these tests are clearly related to the innervation density of the RA and SA I units which have small and well delimited receptive fields. Pritchard (1931) found that localization of a stimulus is independent of stimulus strength, whereas Bishop (1948) states that two point discrimination "depends so much on strength of stimulus that this may be the controlling factor in the causal tests". These findings suggest that there are two different mechanisms involved. However, it would be interesting to reinvestigate this point in the light of the present results as these allow the design of more critical experiments on these problems. The present preliminary results concerning units of the two types which have interdigitating receptors, i.e. RA and SA I units, suggest that these populations are capable of carrying information in excess of what is required for the normal performance in point localization and two point discrimination tests. It was found that the distance between the center points of the receptive fields is pratically constant in a large range of indentation amplitudes and, in addition, largely independent of moderate variations in the total number of sensory units which are known to occur among normal subjects. On the other hand, there were clear and definite variations between skin regions and between different types of units. These considerations suggest that it would be particularly interesting to study performances in spatial tests which may be assumed to be closely related to the center point distance.

The present study was mainly limited to a discussion concerning the recruitment of units with varying amplitudes. However, it is obvious that the variations in the discharge of the single units with stimulus amplitude is an additional factor of great importance in most situations, probably including the spatial discrimination capacity.

REFERENCES

Bishop, G.H. (1948). The skin as an organ of senses with special reference to the itching sensation. J. invest. Derm. 11, 143-154.

Bolton, C.F., Winkelmann, R.K. & Dyck, P.J. (1966). A quantitative study of Meissner's corpuscles in man. Neurology 16, 1-9.

Buchthal, F. and Rosenfalck, A. (1966). Evoked action potentials and conduction velocity in human sensory nerves. Brain Res. 3, 1-122.

Burgess, P.R., Howe, J.F., Lessler, M.J. and Whitehorn, D. (1974). Cutaneous receptors supplied by myelinated fibres in the cat. II. Number of mechanoreceptors excited by a local stimulus. J. Neurophysiol. 37, 1373-1386.

Cauna, N. (1965). The effects of aging on the receptor organs of the human dermis. In Advan. Biol. Skin, ed. W. Montagna. Vol. VI, 63-96. London: Pergamon Press.

Cauna, N. and Mannan, G. (1958). The structure of human digital pacinian corpuscles (Corpuscula lamellosa) and its functional significance. J. Anat. 92, 1-20.

Corbin, K.B. and Gardner, E.D. (1937). Decrease in number of myelinated fibres in human spinal roots with age. Anat. Rec. 68, 63-74.

Fuller D.R.G., and Gray J.A.B. (1966). The relation between mechanical displacements applied to a cat's pad and the resultant impulse patterns. J. Physiol. 182, 465-483.

Gardner, E. (1940). Decrease in human neurons with age. Anat. Rec. 77, 529-536.

Johansson, R.S. (1976). Skin mechanoreceptors in the human hand: Receptive field characteristics. In Sensory Functions of the Skin in Primates, with special reference to Man, ed. Y. Zotterman. Oxford: Pergamon Press.

Johnson, K.O. (1974). Reconstruction of population response to a vibratory simulus in quickly adapting mechanoreceptive afferent fibre population innervating glabrous skin of the monkey. J. Neurophysiol. 37, 48-72.

Miller, M.R., Ralston III, H.J. and Kasahara, M. (1958). The pattern of cutaneous innervation of the human hand. Am. J. Anat., Philadelphia. 102, 183-217.

Pritchard, E.A.B. (1931). Cutaneous tactile localization. Brain 54, 350-371.
Stilwell, D.L., Jr (1957). The innervation of deep structures of the hand. Am. J. Anat. 101, 75-92.
Sunderland, S. and Bedbrook, G.M. (1949). The cross - sectional area of pheripheral nerve trunks occupied by the fibres representing individual muscular and cutaneous branches. Brain 72, 613-624.
Swallow, M. (1966). Fibre size and content of the anterior tibial nerve of the foot. J. Neurol. Neurosurg. Psychiat. 29, 205-213.
Westling, G., Johansson, R.S. and Vallbo, Å.B. (1976). A method for mechanical stimulation of skin receptors. In Sensory Functions of the Skin Primates, with special reference to Man, ed. Y. Zotterman. Oxford: Pergamon Press.
Winkelmann, R.K. (1965). Nerve changes in aging skin. Advan. Biol. Skin, ed. W. Montagna. Vol. VI, 51-61. London: Pergamon Press.

This investigation was supported by grants from the Swedish Medical Research Council, project no. 04X-3548.

Discussion:

Hagbarth: Did you compare the conduction velocities of the different types of units? If the mean fiber diameters are different, this will probably give a sampling bias affecting the estimation of innervation density.

Johansson: No, we have not measured it in this investigation. But it has been studied by Knibestöl. He has shown it to be quite a narrow range. I do not have the exact figures. I do not think that a large bias could have entered for this reason. Other investigations in monkeys have given about the same proportions between rapid-adapting and slow-adapting units and between RA and PC in the slowly adapting group. They have not shown the difference in slowly adapting units in the monkey.

Iggo: In hairy skin it is typical that the hair follicle afferent units there is an overlapping of the territories innervated by the different afferent fibers. I take it from your results that you find this also with the rapidly-adapting receptors or Meissner corpuscles. What is the situation with regards to the slowly-adapting type one units which in hairy skin tend to have separate small spots? I have not seen any reports on attempts in glabrous skin to whether you can have a mosaic formation for the different terminals for the different local cells on separate slowly-adapting type afferent fibers. Do you have any ideas on that?

Johansson: I have mapped five slowly adapting type I receptive fields and there was a mean of five high-sensitive zones. The range was four to seven. Calculations indicate that there has to be a similar interdigitating as for the RA units.

SKIN MECHANORECEPTORS IN THE HUMAN HAND: NEURAL AND PSYCHOPHYSICAL THRESHOLDS

Å. B. VALLBO and R. JOHANSSON
Department of Physiology, University of Umeå, S-901 87 Umeå, Sweden

The concept of a sensory threshold has been discussed extensively in psychophysical literature (for reviews see Corso 1963, Green and Swets 1966). If a distinct sensory threshold existed, the proportion of yes-responses related to the stimulus magnitude would be a step function. It is a general experimental finding, however, that this proportion follows a smooth curve which is often S-shaped. In psychophysical literature, a number of theories have been developed to account for this finding. Practically all of them put the emphasis upon central mechanisms: it has been assumed either that a central threshold level varies over time or that a noise is superimposed upon the afferent signal. As a consequence, these theories predict that the physiological events in the threshold zone of stimulus magnitude are a continuous change in a large number of sensory units and nervous elements, and hence that the probability would be low that a subject would detect a minimal afferent signal, e.g. a single nerve impulse in a single afferent fibre.

On the other hand, there is some support, partly from neurophysiological studies, for the notion that a human observer very likely may detect an input which consists of only a few nerve impulses, maybe just one (Hecht,

Shlaer and Pirenne 1942, Bouman and van der Velden 1947, Hensel and Boman 1960) and also that the response variability to a nominally constant stimulus, in fact, may be accounted for by a genuine variation in the input to the central nervous system (Hecht, Schlaer and Pirenne 1942). However, these notions have been based upon rather indirect evidence and/or very meagre experimental support.

Thus, there seems to be a large gap between neurophysiology and psychophysics with respect to the current ideas as well as the amount of available experimental evidence with regard to the threshold concept which is a cornerstone in sensory physiology and psychophysics.

The present study is a preliminary analysis of the relation between minimal responses in first.order afferents and minimal responses of the human mind: the absolute thresholds at the two levels of the somatosensory system were compared, when tactile stimuli were delivered to the glabrous skin of the human hand. The purpose was to disclose some of the basic principles according to which the central nervous system of man produces a sensation of touch out of nerve impulses in first order afferents.

MECHANICAL STIMULATION

The mechanical stimulus employed in the present experiments was designed to produce minimal neural responses in the population of first order tactile afferents against a silent background. In order to achieve this a small stimulus probe was used, pre-indentation was avoided as well as any mechanical stimulation of the surrounding skin area by, for instance, devices for fixation of the hand. It was judged that pre-indentation might favor the spreading of the mechanical disturbance through the tissues and would thereby raise the probability of exciting a relatively large number of PC units which are known to be very sensitive to remote stimuli. Further, it might give rise to accidental excitation from noise in the driving electronic circuits. Mechanical stimulation of the surrounding skin area might interfere with the detection of the test stimulus through lateral inhibition. It seemed essential to eliminate these effects as they might obscure the picture of the relation between the threshold of single sensory units and the perceptive threshold.

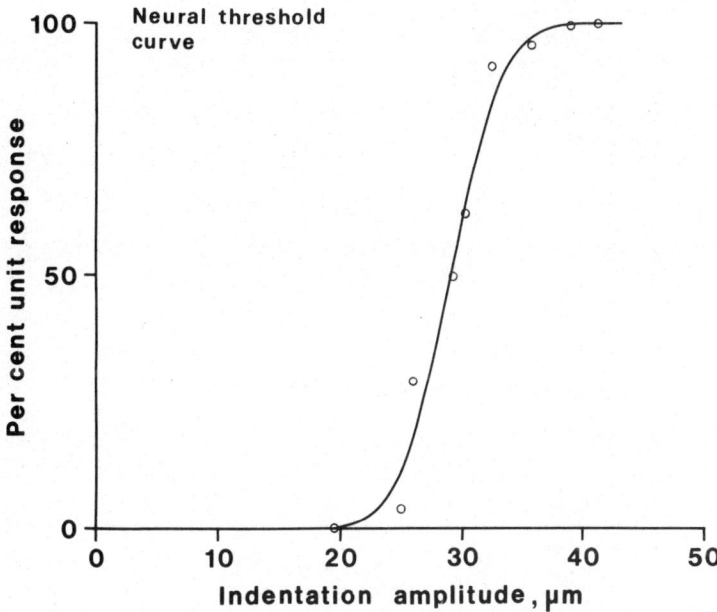

FIG. 1. Neural threshold curve. Open circles represent experimental data and continuous line the best fitting normal distribution function. SA-I unit located on the distal phalanx of the long finger.

The stimulus probe had a diameter of 0.4 mm and ended with a half sphere. Triangular indentations were delivered with an indentation velocity of 4 mm/s. The method of indentation amplitude control has been described in detail in a separate paper (Westling, Johansson and Vallbo 1976). The target point on the skin was carefully controlled manually while the target area was continuously observed through a binocular microscope at a magnification of 40x.

CONSTRUCTION OF THRESHOLD CURVES

Single unit impulses were recorded from low threshold skin mechanoreceptors in the glabrous skin of the human hand with tungsten needle electrodes in the median nerve (Vallbo and Hagbarth 1968, Vallbo 1972) and the perceptive threshold was determined with the method of limits employing the two alternative forced choice (2AFC) and yes-no (Y/N) procedures. Neural and psychophysical responses to the same type of stimulus were studied. The two types of observations were done either simultaneously, or successively when the same point on the skin was stimulated. In addition, neural and psychophysical

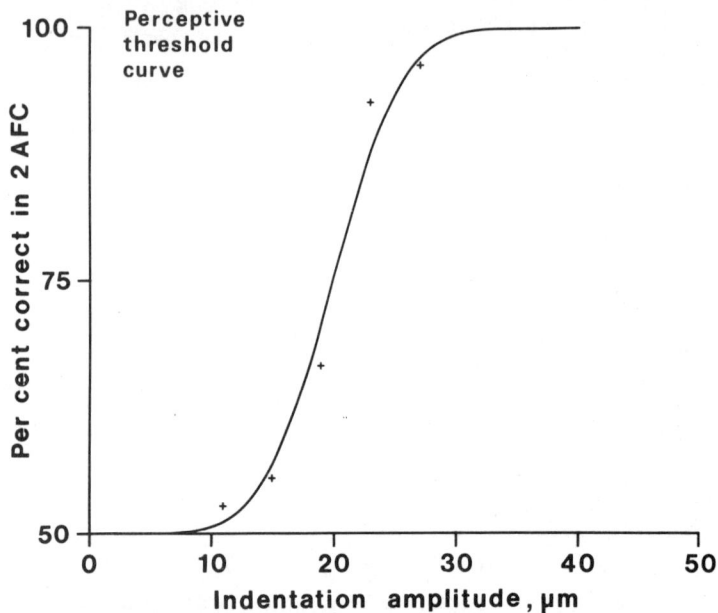

FIG. 2. Psychophysical threshold curve. The crosses represent the experimental data from a two alternative forced choice experiment and the continuous line the best fitting normal distribution function. The test point was located on the distal phalanx of the thumb.

threshold data were collected from different points. Normal cumulative probability curves were fitted to the threshold data by a method of maximum likelihood estimation (Uvell 1975). It might be worth pointing out that the weight of the individual point in this procedure is not invariant but dependent upon the number of tests behind the point. A curve might therefore have a course which does not appear to be the optimum in relation to the positions of the points.

Data from a neural threshold experiment are shown in Fig. 1. The per cent of tests in which an impulse appeared is given by the ordinate and the indentation amplitudes by the abscissa. According to convention the threshold was defined as the midpoint of the normal cumulative probability curve fitted to the data. It should be pointed out that the position of the midpoint along the abscissa is determined quite accurately even if only a few points are available and in many experiments the amount of data collected was much less

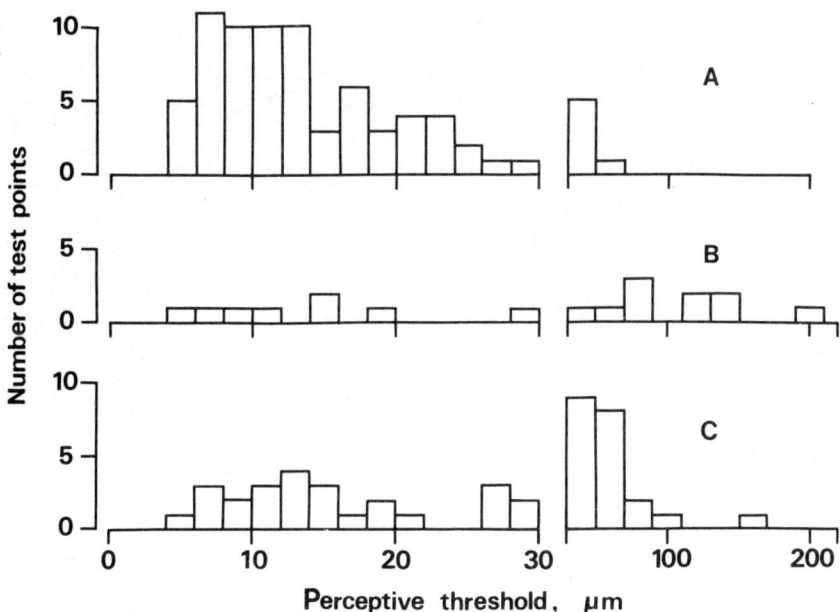

FIG. 3. Histograms showing the distribution of the perceptive thresholds at test points from three different regions of the glabrous skin. A: volar aspects of the fingers with the exception of the flexure lines. B: lateral aspects of the fingers and the flexure lines. C: palm of the hand. Note that the abscissae are compressed by a factor of ten in the right hand part of the figure.

than those shown here. The perceptive threshold data generally fell along similar lines and the same procedure was adapted to define the psychophysical threshold. An example is shown in Fig. 2. The average false alarm rate in the yes-no experiments was only 0.7 % indicating that the psychophysical threshold measured with this method was not inappropriately low. In addition, there was no obvious difference between the thresholds obtained with the two procedures, i.e. two alternative forced choice and yes-no.

PSYCHOPHYSICAL THRESHOLDS

Considering first the distribution of the perceptive thresholds in the glabrous skin area. The three histograms of Fig. 3 show the perceptive threshold data from three different regions of the skin: in A from the volar aspect of the fingers with the exception of the flexure lines, in B from the lateral aspects of the fingers and the flexure lines and in C from the palm of the hand.

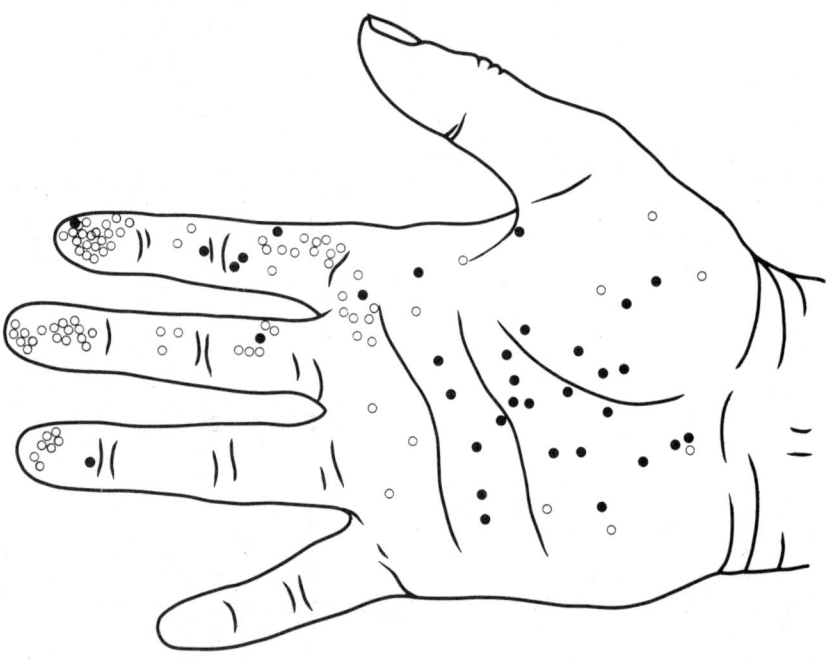

FIG. 4. Locations of test points at which the perceptive thresholds were determined in the palm and on the volar aspects of the fingers with the exception of the flexure lines. Open and filled circles represent perceptive thresholds below and above 25 µm respectively.

On the volar aspects of the fingers the minimal perceptive threshold was 4.4 µm and the majority, or 76 % of the observations fell below 20 µm (Fig. 3 A). It might further be seen that some perceptive thresholds were about ten times higher than the minimal ones. It should be pointed out, however, that the data were collected from untrained and unselected subjects under experimental conditions which, in some cases, probably involved a certain amount of strain upon the subjects. Hence, a suboptimal performance is to be expected in quite a few sessions which may account for many of the high threshold points.

Data from the other two regions exhibited larger scatter and higher medians (Fig. 3 B and C) and it seems obvious that the three samples could not have been drawn from the same population. Considering the data from the palm of the hand, it was found that a certain pattern was emerging when the percep-

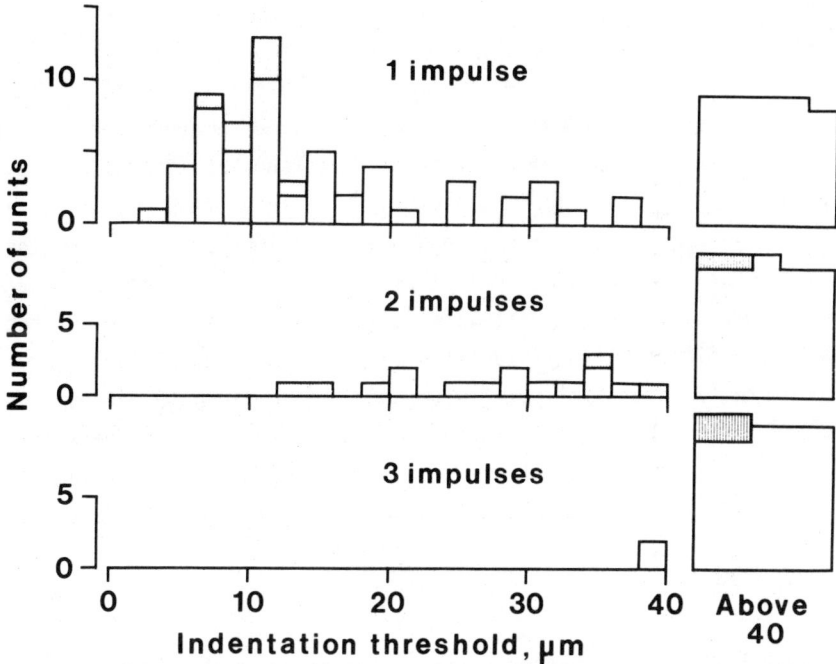

FIG. 5. Histograms showing the distribution of minimal indentations required to produce neural responses consisting of one impulse (A), two impulses (B) and three impulses (C) from a sample of semi-randomly collected mechanosensitive units. Hatched areas represent PC units whereas white areas represent RA, SA-I and SA-II units. Fifty per cent of the PC units and five per cent of the RA units had a critical slope above 4 mm/sec which was the indentation velocity used in the psychophysical tests.

tive threshold was related to the location of the test point. This is illustrated in Fig. 4 where data from the two histograms in Fig. 3 A and C are shown. Open and filled circles represent perceptive thresholds below and above 25 µm respectively. There is clearly an accumulation of high threshold points in the center of the palm in relation to the data from the peripheral parts of the palm and the volar aspect of the fingers. Thus, two fairly distinct regions may be defined: one low threshold region covering the volar aspect of the fingers with the exception of the flexure lines and one high threshold region in the center of the palm.

NEURAL THRESHOLDS

On the basis of recordings from primary afferents innervating the glabrous skin it might be possible to define the quantity and quality of the afferent input which was required to produce a perceptive threshold response. Figure 5 shows histograms of the minimal indentations required to evoke one, two and three impulses from a sample of low threshold mechanosensitive afferents, randomly collected from the median glabrous skin area. It is obvious that stimuli above 38 μm were required to produce three impulses even from the most sensitive units, whereas stimuli above 20 μm were required to produce two impulses except for three units, two of which were of PC type. On the other hand, the minimal stimuli required to produce a single impulse are distributed from a lower limit of 3.4 μm and up to quite high values, but there is obviously an accumulation of observations in the range between 4 μm and 20 μm, which is the range of the majority of the perceptive thresholds in the low threshold region. Thus, it is obvious that a perceptive threshold response is readily produced by a single impulse in a small number of afferent units innervating the volar aspects of the fingers.

Another basic question is whether activity from a particular type of receptor or a particular combination is responsible for the perceptive response. A clear, although incomplete, answer to this question is provided by the experimental finding demonstrated in a previous study that the thresholds of the two types of slowly adapting units, SA-I and SA-II, do not extend below 20 μm, except for a single outliner. On the other hand, there are fairly large proportions of the RA and PC units which have thresholds below this value (Johansson and Vallbo 1976).   Thus, it may be concluded that a sensation of touch may be produced by activity in either or both of the two types of rapidly adapting units and does not require activity in any of the slowly adapting units. From these findings it is not possible to state whether the PC or the RA units or both account for the minimal sensation of touch. However, it should be pointed out that as many as fifty per cent of the PC units had a critical slope above 4 mm/sec and therefore could not possibly be candidates for the detection of the stimuli used in the psychophysical studies.

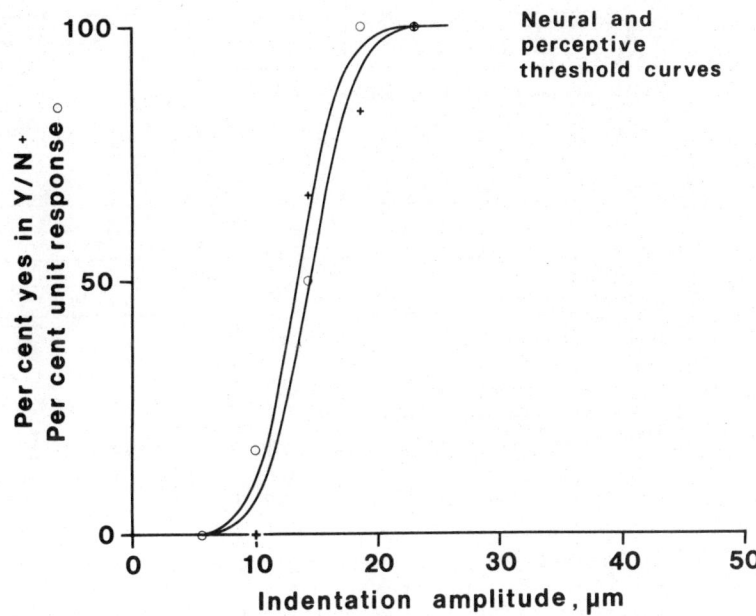

FIG. 6. Neural and perceptive threshold curves from the same test point. The stimuli were delivered to the most sensitive point of a RA unit located on the distal phalanx of the thumb. Symbols and curves as in Fig. 1 and 2.

COMPARISON BETWEEN NEURAL AND PSYCHOPHYSICAL THRESHOLDS

It was shown above that the minimal perceptive threshold in the total sample of observations was almost exactly the same as the minimal threshold of the sample of mechanosensitive units: in the two samples there were a few observations around four micrometers. This suggests that a single impulse in a single unit would be enough to produce a sensation of touch, as the likelihood would be very low of exciting more than one unit by a well localized indentation of only four micrometers (Johansson and Vallbo 1976). Supportive evidence for this conclusion is given by the fact that the distributions of the neural and the perceptive thresholds were broadly similar between four and twenty micrometers.

A more direct evidence and a more complete picture of the relationship between neural and psychophysical thresholds is provided by an analysis of the psychophysical and the neural responses recorded simultaneously when stimuli

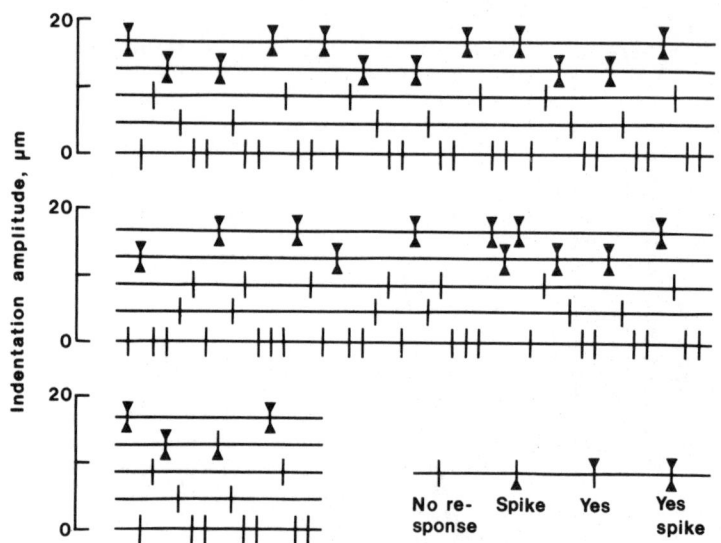

FIG. 7. Neural and psychophysical responses of individual tests delivered in succession, from above left to below right, at the most sensitive point of an RA unit located on the distal phalanx of the ring finger. Indentation amplitudes are given by the ordinate values corresponding to the horizontal lines.

were delivered at a point of maximal sensitivity of a low threshold unit. Fig. 6 shows findings from an experiment of this type with an RA unit which had a threshold of 13.6 μm. The perceptive threshold was very close to that of the unit (14.6 μm) as seen from the curves fitted to the data.

A close agreement between the neural and the psychophysical threshold curves has been found for a fairly large number of test points on the volar aspect of the fingers when the unit activated was of the RA-type, in a few cases when it was of the PC-type but never when it was a slowly adapting unit. However, in most cases the probability of a neural response and the probability of detection did not agree perfectly well as shown by the example of Fig. 6: the two sets of experimental points do not have exactly the same position along the ordinate. Discrepancies of this type were invariably found when a large series of tests was done and there were indications that the discrepancies were not due to random variations but rather to the processes involved being non-stationary. In fact, there were in many cases an almost perfect agreement between neural and psychophysical responses of the indi-

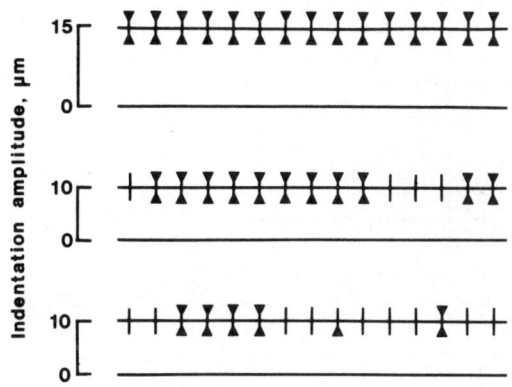

FIG. 8. Neural and psychophysical responses as in Fig. 7. Stimuli delivered at the most sensitive point of an RA unit located on the distal phalanx of the index.

vidual tests during limited periods of a long lasting test series. Examples from two different RA units are shown in Figs. 7 and 8 where the short vertical lines represent tests delivered in succession from left to right. The amplitudes of the indentations are given by the ordinate values corresponding to the horizontal lines. Neural and psychophysical responses are indicated by the filled triangles partly covering the short vertical lines, a nerve impulse by the lower triangle and a yes response from the subject by the upper triangle. In the test series of Fig. 7 consisting of 105 tests, 45 % of the tests were blind trials, i.e. no indentation was delivered, just the warning signal. It may be seen that the subject did not respond psychophysically to any of the catch trials indicating that his yes responses were based upon impulses in primary afferents and not upon internally generated activity. In all but one of the tests, either the two responses appeared together or none of them did. At the end of the series the subject failed to detect one stimulus which evoked an impulse. A similar test series from another subject is shown in Fig. 8 but in this case the stimulus amplitude was the same in successive tests and it was very close to the threshold value of the unit in the last thirty tests. Also in this case the agreement was perfect between neural and psychophysical responses except for one test at the end of the series in which the subject failed to detect a stimulus which elicited an impulse. It seems justified to conclude that it was the single

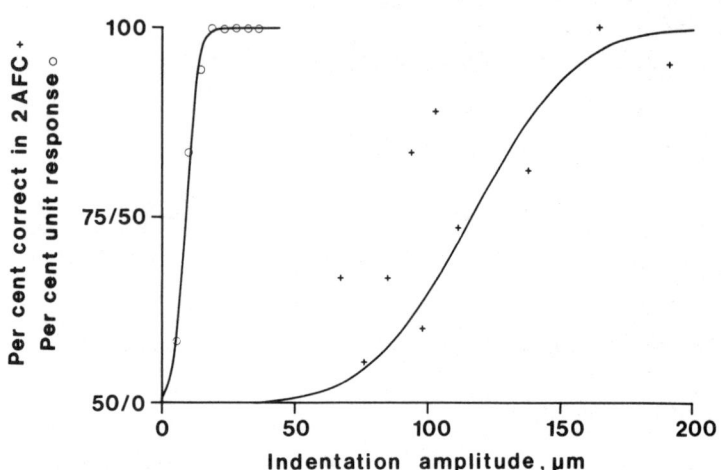

FIG. 9. Neural and perceptive threshold curves from the same test point. The stimuli were delivered to the most sensitive point of an RA unit located in the palm of the hand.

impulses of the particular units recorded from, which accounted for the detection of the stimulus when the agreement was that good between the responses at the two levels of the system. These findings indicate that under optimal conditions the probability of detection was high when a single impulse from a single RA unit reached the central nervous system from the low threshold region of the glabrous skin. A similar agreement has not been found for any of the PC units.

The above findings are in marked contrast to those from the high threshold region in the center of the palm. It has been pointed out in another study that there were no differences in mechanoreceptor sensitivity in the two regions (Johansson and Vallbo 1976), suggesting that the high perceptive thresholds were not accounted for by less sensitive mechanoreceptor units but rather to a different information processing by the central nervous system. This conclusion is supported by experiments in which single unit impulses were recorded from a sensitive mechanoreceptive unit and the psychophysical response was studied at the same point. A representative set of data from an RA unit are shown in Fig. 9. It is obvious that the threshold of the unit was much lower than the psychophysical threshold as defined by the midpoints of the curves. It is also obvious that the slope of the psychophysical curve was much more shallow than that of the neural threshold curve. It must be assumed that additional units besides the one seen by the electrode were excited and that many of them fired several impulses to stimuli between 50 μm and 200 μm, i.e. the approximate range of the perceptive threshold curve (Johansson and Vallbo 1976).

These findings indicate that the probability of detection was low in the high threshold region of the glabrous skin when a single unit impulse reached the central nervous system and, further, that the probability of detection increased but slowly with the number of impulses produced by the stimulus.

CONCLUSIONS

The main conclusions of the present study may be summarized as follows. The limit of detection is not set universally by a single factor. In some regions of the somato-sensory system it is obviously set by the properties of the central nervous system as has been emphasized in psychophysical literature. In other regions, the detection is set by the sensitivity of the peripheral receptors and the absolute threshold of the central nervous system approaches a step function. Further, it was shown that in the regions where this was valid the probability was high for a minimal input signal consisting of an indivisible neural quantum to produce a sensation of touch.

In relation to the signal detection theory (Green and Swets 1966) which has dominated the concepts related to the sensory threshold in the last decades, the findings from the low threshold region imply that a minimal neural input produces a large step change of the activity in the relevant parts of the central nervous system. The findings are not consistent with a basic prediction of the theory: that there is a considerable overlap between the distribution of activity prevailing in the absence of any stimulation and the distributions associated with weak stimuli.

This investigation was supported by grants from the Swedish Medical Research Council, project no. 04X-3548, and by Gunvor och Josef Anérs Stiftelse.

REFERENCES

Bouman, M.A. and van der Velden, H.A. (1947). Two-quanta explanation of the threshold values and visual acuity on the visual angle and the time of observation. J. Opt. Soc. Am. 37, 908-919.

Corso, J.F. (1963). A theoretico-historical review of the threshold concept. Psychol. Bull. 60, 356-370.

Green, D.M. and Swets, J.A. (1966). Signal detection theory and psychophysics. 1-455. John Wiley and Sons, New York, London, Sydney.

Hagbarth, K.-E. and Vallbo, Å.B. (1968). Activity from skin mechanoreceptors recorded percutaneously in awake human subjects. Exptl. Neurol. 21, 270-289.

Hecht, S., Shlaer, S. and Pirenne, M.H. (1942). Energy, quanta and vision. J. Gen. Physiol. 25, 819-840.

Hensel, H. and Boman, K.A. (1960). Afferent impulses in cutaneous nerves in human subjects. J. Neurophysiol. 23, 564-578.

Johansson, R. and Vallbo, Å.B. (1976). Skin mechanoreceptors in the human hand: An inference of some population properties. In Sensory Functions of the Skin in Primates, with special reference to Man. Ed. Zotterman, Y. Pergamon Press.

Uvell, S. (1975). Maximum likelihood estimates based on a general form of partial grouping. Techn. Rep. from Inst. Math. and Statist., Univ. Umeå, Sweden. 5, 1-22.

Vallbo, Å.B. (1972). Single unit recordings from human peripheral nerves: muscle receptor discharge in resting muscles and during voluntary contractions. In Neurophysiology studied in man, pp. 281-295. Ed. Somjen, G.G. Excerpta Medica, Amsterdam.

Westling, G., Johansson, R. and Vallbo, Å.B. (1976). A method for mechanical stimulation of skin receptors. In Sensory Functions of the Skin in Primates, with special reference to Man. Ed. Zotterman, Y. Pergamon Press.

Discussion:

Paintal: I would like to know how it is possible to exclude the fact that you may not be stimulating more than one receptor and the impulse is going up in a number of fibers. I think a possible experiment that you could do would be to produce procain blocks in two parts of the nerve some distance away. Then, when you apply your indentation for rapidly-adapting receptors, you should get an all-or-none response as the person recovered from the procain block. That would mean that two sites were blocked. You would then be quite sure that you have got one fiber active. What do you think about this suggestion?

Vallbo: Many thanks for your suggestion of a method to restrict the input from a skin area to one or a few fibers by double blocking of the nerve with local anaesthetics. I think that it would be very interesting to try. I can see one difficulty, however, if you wanted to really demonstrate that only one fiber is conducting passed the two blocking sites. This would require a recording which sees the activity from a single fiber and at the same time covers the whole nerve trunk to exclude that more than one fiber is conducting. This seems not easy to obtain with this recording method.

Hensel: I am very pleased about your findings suggesting that a single impulse in a single fiber might correspond to the threshold for conscious mechanical sensations. Your findings confirm the conclusion we arrived at sixteen years ago (Hensel and Boman, J. Neurophysiol. 23, 564, 1960), in our first experiments with afferent single fiber records from human cutaneous nerves.

Vallbo: I would like to give a comment in relation to Professor Hensel's remark which implied that it has now been confirmed that a human observer detects a stimulus which gives rise to only a single impulse in a single fiber, as suggested in the paper by Hensel and Boman (1960). One of the main points which we wanted to communicate in our report was that the question of detection of a minimal input cannot be answered with either yes or no but it is clearly different in different parts of the somato-sensory system, in that the information processing within the central nervous system varies with the skin area. It seems that a minimal input from the volar aspects of the fingers, which is a very important area in tactile sensibility, is very carefully considered in the central nervous system and might give rise to a sensation of touch, but this is not true for the center of the palm.

In the light of these findings it would be of great interest to have more experimental data from the hairy skin than those presented by Hensel and Boman. Their conclusion on the relation between neural and psychophysical thresholds was based upon recordings from one single fiber in one single subject without controlled stimulus magnitude and velocity of deformation. Further, there were no indications of how many low threshold sensory units innervated the single hair follicle. Primarily, one would not expect that the information from the hairy skin is handled as carefully in the central nervous system as the information from the volar aspects of the finger and the finger-tips.

Granit: I thought of the concept that the psychologists have introduced "the psychological refractory period". Here you have a good chance of getting at it. They maintain that it has to be the time of one or often five seconds for two impressions to be sensed separately. This would be an elegant way of looking at this question.

Franzén: Yes, take a look at the work of Libbet and his colleagues and you may note that they reported that they recorded a primary low-potential below the threshold of perception. Also, I may refer to my own experiments which I have carried out with other colleagues. If you plot the amplitude of the primary evoked potential against the subjective estimates you will see that the curve is intersecting to the right of the origo. That means, at least in this experiment, that you have a certain amplitude of the evoked response before any sensation is reported. So our data are consistent with those of Libbet. On the problem of psychological refractory periods, Dr Lindblom and I have carried out such an experiment recently and we will report on that.

Vallbo: I would like to point out that Libbet's data referred to the minimal stimulus of the cortex giving rise to sensation. When he uses stronger stimulus to the cortex, the subject notices the stimulus much earlier. We do not know, of course, if a single impulse from a single primary afferent might give rise to the same activity in the cortex as the minimal stimulus induced by Libbet's stimulation of the cortex. We have to be clear about what we mean by minimal stimulus.

STIMULUS-RESPONSE FUNCTIONS OF PRIMARY AFFERENTS AND PSYCHOPHYSICAL INTENSITY ESTIMATION ON MECHANICAL SKIN STIMULATION IN THE HUMAN HAND

M. KNIBESTÖL and Å. B. VALLBO

Department of Physiology, University of Umeå, and
Department of Clinical Neurophysiology, University Hospital, S-901 87 Umeå, Sweden

Since long ago the relation between the intensity of a stimulus and the magnitude of the subjective sensation has interested neurophysiologists and psychologists. Evidence has accumulated from several sensory systems that this relation can be described by a power function. This so called Stevens´ power law has largely replaced the old Fechner´s logarithmic law. Neurophysiologists have been searching for the basic sensory mechanisms behind this psychophysical law, and during the last decade important contributions have come from studies of the skin senses, in particular cutaneous mechanoreceptors sensitive to touch and pressure. Werner and Mountcastle (1965) showed that the stimulus-response relation for slowly adapting cutaneous mechanoreceptors in cat hairy skin could be described by a power function, and they pointed out the obvious parallel to Stevens´ power law. In later studies Mountcastle and coworkers (Mountcastle et al. 1966, Mountcastle 1967, Mountcastle and Darian-Smith 1968, Werner and Mountcastle 1968, Harrington and Merzenich 1970) have extended these concepts, and suggest an even closer parallelism between psychophysical and neural stimulus-response functions. They present evidence that both functions are negatively accelerating power functions on hairy skin, whereas in the glabrous skin, both types of functions are linear. From this evidence Mountcastle (1967) has made the important generalization that the shape of the psychophysical function which represents the final behavioral output of the organism, is determined already at the receptor level, and that all intervening transformations in the central nervous system are in sum linear. The evidence in favour of this hypothesis has been based on neurophysiological experiments in animals and psychophysical studies in man. With the introduction of the percutaneous microelectrode technique of Hagbarth and Vallbo (1967) for recording from human nerves, the possibility has been opened up for studies of human skin receptors. In our laboratory we have concentrated on the glabrous skin area of the hand and collected data concerning the basic physiological properties of the low-threshold cutaneous mechanoreceptors in this area. In the present report we will summarize some of the main findings from these earlier studies, with particular emphasis on the stimulus-response functions of these receptors and present some additional new data. We will also present some preliminary data from psychophysical studies which have been conducted in parallel with the neurophysiological studies and discuss to what extent these new data from human subjects support the concepts and theories which have been hitherto developed on the basis of comparative neurophysiological studies in animals and psychophysical studies in man.

METHODS

Afferent single nerve fibre impulses were recorded with tungsten microelectrodes inserted in the median and ulnar nerves. The electrodes and the recording technique have been described in detail elsewhere (Vallbo and Hagbarth 1968, Knibestöl and Vallbo 1970). Precisely controlled skin displacements were provided from an electro-mechanical skin stimulation system, the details of which have previously been described (Knibestöl 1973). The stimuli were skin indentations usually of 1 second duration linearly rising to a plateau. The indentation velocity and the final amplitude could be independently varied. Maximal amplitude was in different experiments 2, 3 or 4 mm. Stimulus-response functions of the rapidly adapting receptors were constructed by relating impulse frequency to the indentation velocity of the rising phase of the stimulus. For slowly adapting receptors the neural response was studied in relation to skin displacement amplitude and it was measured either as the total number of impulses or as the mean frequency during the last half of the stimulus. When studying stimulus-response functions of the slowly adapting receptors psychophysical functions were obtained simultaneously in a group of 18 subjects by the method of magnitude estimation, i.e. the subjects assigned numbers to the stimuli in proportion to the intensity experienced.

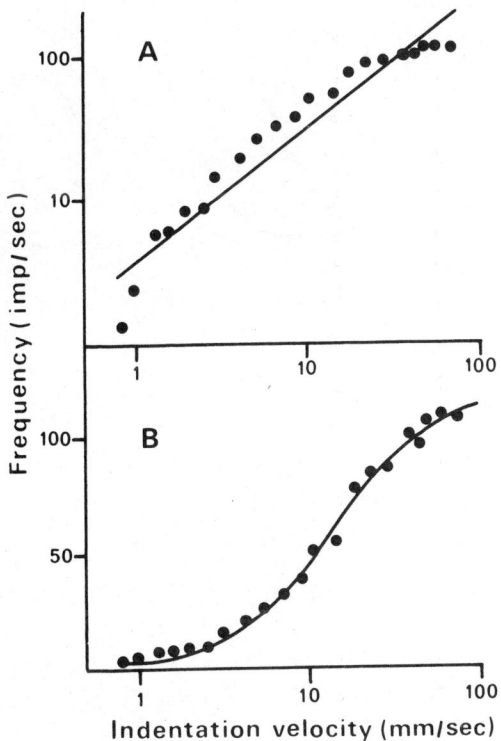

FIG. 1. Stimulus-response function of a RA-receptor. A, data plotted on log-log co-ordinates. The straight line is the best fitting power function (r = 0.96). B, the same data on a semilogarithmic plot. The curve is the best fitting log tanh function (r = 0.99).

STIMULUS-RESPONSE FUNCTIONS OF PRIMARY AFFERENTS

Low-threshold mechanoreceptors in the human glabrous skin area of the hand have been studied extensively and characterized with regard to their basic physiological properties in an earlier series of investigations. Knibestöl and Vallbo (1970) described four different receptor types in this area, two rapidly adapting types (RA- and PC-receptors) and two slowly adapting types

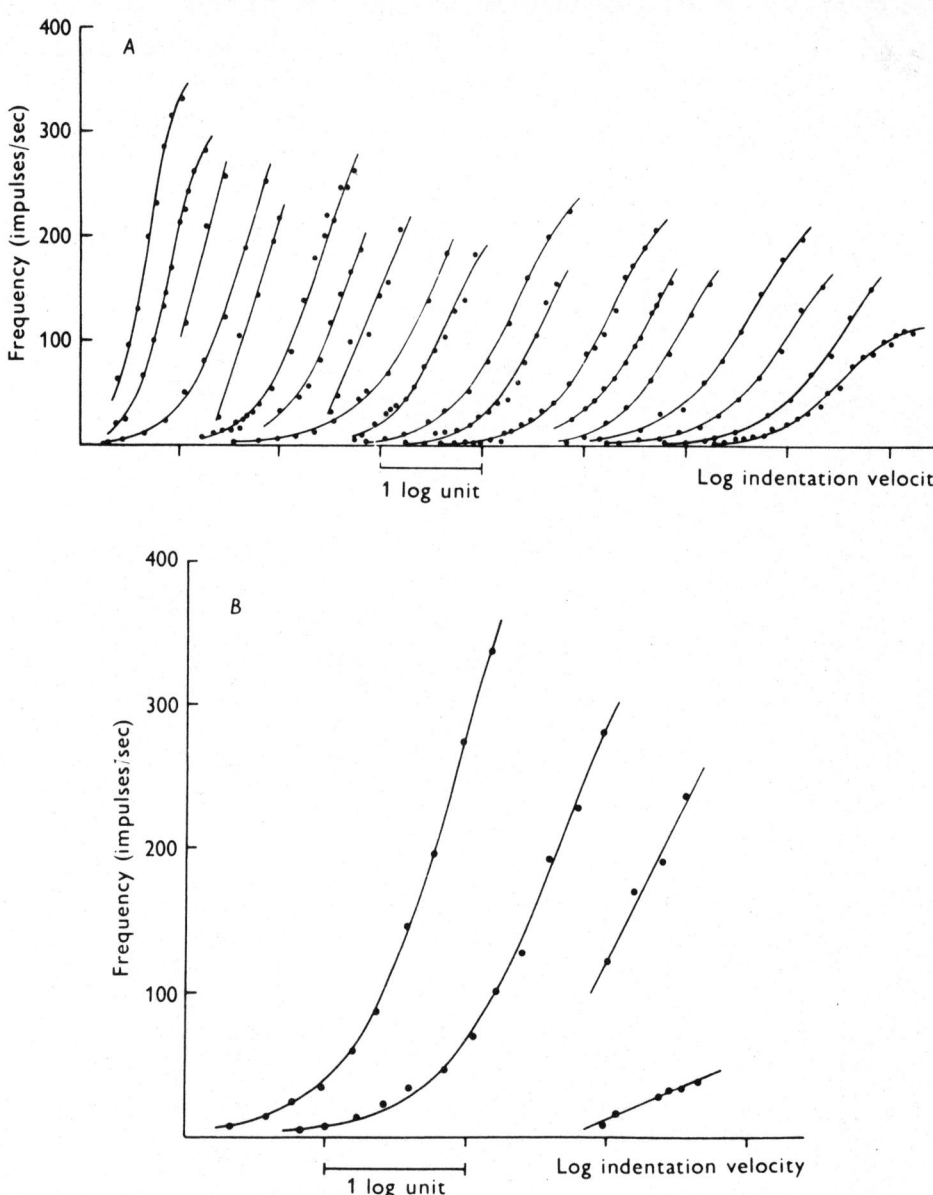

FIG. 2. Stimulus-response functions of nineteen RA-receptors (A) and four PC-receptors (B). The abscissae represent indentation velocity on a logarithmic scale, and the ordinates nerve impulse frequency on a linear scale. The individual plots are arbitrarily shifted along the abscissae. The curves entered over the points are the best fitting log tanh functions or logarithmic functions. (From Knibestöl 1973, J. Physiol. 232, 427-452)

(type SA-I and SA-II). In two subsequent reports Knibeström (1973, 1975) subjected these four types of receptors to further quantitative studies, analysing particularly their stimulus-response functions. Several simple mathematical functions were tested as possible descriptions of the stimulus-response relationships. For the rapidly adapting receptors it was found that a power function, which until then had been the function mostly used to describe the stimulus-response relationships in studies of skin mechanoreceptors in animals was a rather poor description. This is shown in Fig.1 A where in a log-log plot the data points deviate systematically from the best fitting power function. On the other hand, the points described a smooth sigmoid curve in a semi-logarithmic plot (Fig. 1 B), and it was found that in most cases the data could be well described by a log hyperbolic tangent function, which was first used by Naka and Rushton (1966) for transfer functions in the visual system. In all, 19 RA-receptors and 4 PC-receptors were studied, and in most cases the log tanh function was the best description over the total range of indentation velocities, but in a few cases a logarithmic function was adequate (see Fig. 2 A and B).

For slowly adapting human receptors the situation was somewhat more complicated (Knibeström 1975). One problem here was to define a proper measure of the neural response. In Fig. 3 are shown two alternatives of representing the stimulus-response function of these receptors. The upper plot (circles) represents the total number of impulses in response to the stimulus (termed TS-plot) and the lower plot (squares) represents the mean frequency during the last half of the indentation time (termed MF-plot). The upper plot may be separated into two parts: a dynamic part (open circles) and a static part (filled circles) below and above respectively the static threshold. The figure is representative in showing that the MF-plot and the static part of the TS-plot are very similar in shape, and in the following reasoning the same arguments are valid for the two. The total TS-plot could be satisfactorily described only by a log tanh function. However, if only the static TS-plot is considered, several functions seemed reasonable. A power function was a very good description for most units, but it was found that other non-linear functions (logarithmic, log tanh, exponential) were equally good or even better in many cases. Furthermore, the difference in goodness of fit between several functions was negligible in many cases. This is demonstrated in Fig. 4, where several functions have been fitted to the same data points (both TS-plots and MF-plots).

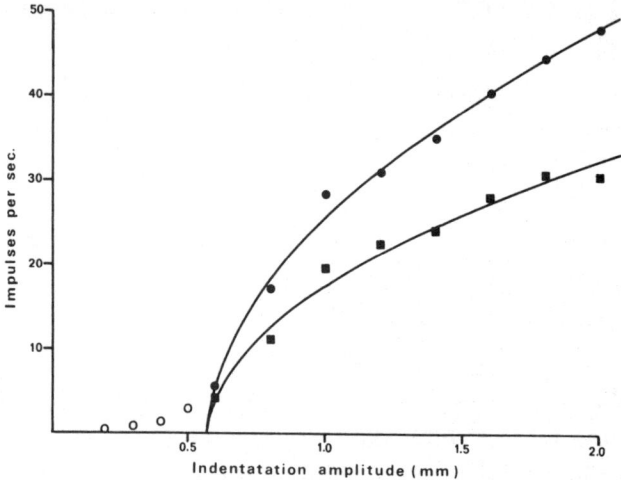

FIG. 3. Stimulus-response plot for a SA-I receptor. The circles represent the TS-plot (ordinate: total number of spikes during an indentation lasting one second) and the squares are the MF-plot (ordinate: mean impulse frequency of the sustained discharge during the last half of the indentation time). In the TS-plot two parts are indicated: a static part (filled circles), and a dynamic part (open circles). The static part of the TS-plot and the MF-plot are fitted with power functions of the general form $R = a \cdot S^b$ (where R is the neural response and S is the stimulus intensity, and a and b are constants). The exponents b of the power functions were 0.52 for the static TS-plot and 0.53 for the MF-plot.

Although the power function could not be considered as the only possible description, it is nevertheless convenient for purely descriptive purposes of the MF-plot and the static part of the TS-plot. The exponent of the power function describes the main shape of the function, whether it is positively or negatively accelerating, or approximately linear. When the power function was used as a tool for comparison between the MF-plot and the static part of the TS-plot, it was found that there was for the individual unit a very good correlation of the power function exponents, as illustrated by the example shown in Fig. 3, where the exponents of the power functions fitted to these plots were nearly identical. An analysis of power function exponents also provides an opportunity to compare the present data from humans with similar data from animals. For most units in the human glabrous skin the plots were clearly negatively accelerating, the mean power exponent being 0.65 (Knibestöl 1975). This is in some contrast to findings reported for similar receptors in the monkey glabrous skin, as Mountcastle et al. (1966) find power exponents close to 1.0, i.e. linear or nearly linear functions.

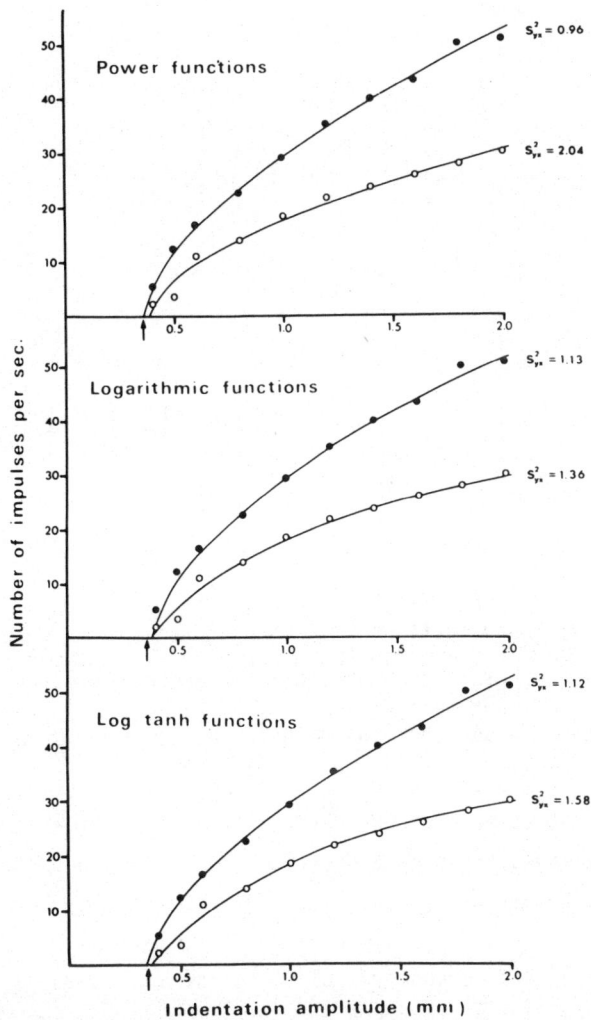

FIG. 4. Stimulus-response plots for a SA-I receptor. Three different types of non-linear functions (power, logarithmic and log tanh functions) are fitted to the same data points of the TS-plot (filled circles) and the MF-plot (open circles) in order to show the small difference in fit of these functions. The residual variance (s^2_{yx}) for each fit is indicated at the right ends of the curves.

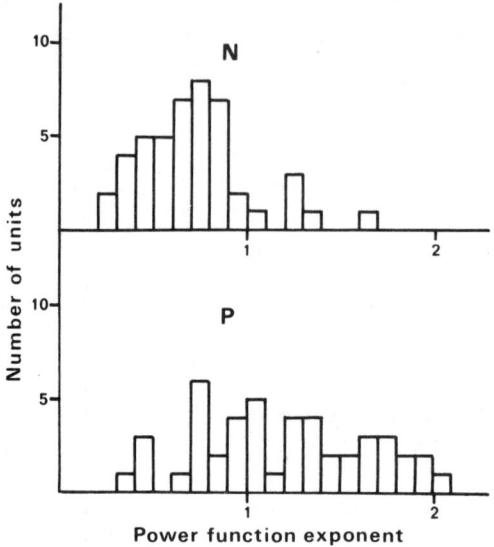

FIG. 5. Histograms showing the distributions of exponents of the power functions fitted to neural and psychophysical data from 18 subjects. The upper part (N) shows the exponents of the stimulus-response functions for 46 SA-I units, and the lower part (P) shows the exponents of the individual psychophysical functions obtained at the same test points.

COMBINED NEURAL AND PSYCHOPHYSICAL STUDIES

The finding that the stimulus-response functions of human slowly adapting glabrous skin receptors were mainly negatively accelerating does not support Mountcastle's hypothesis, as one of the central elements of this hypothesis is that both neural and psychophysical functions are linear on the glabrous skin. We therefore decided to try a more direct approach, producing neural as well as psychophysical stimulus-response functions in the same group of subjects: whenever a SA-receptor was identified, neuronal stimulus-response data were collected, and at the same time the subject estimated the magnitude of the stimulus intensity. From 46 test points in 18 subjects these type of data were obtained. Power functions were fitted to both sets of data and the exponents are shown in the two histograms of Fig. 5. It may be seen that there was a rather large range of variation in the power function exponents within the two sets of data, but the distributions are clearly differently centered. Most of the neural functions have exponents below 1.0 (mean = 0.72) in close agreement with earlier findings (Knibestöl 1975), whereas a large proportion of the psychophysical functions have exponents above 1.0 (mean=1.2).

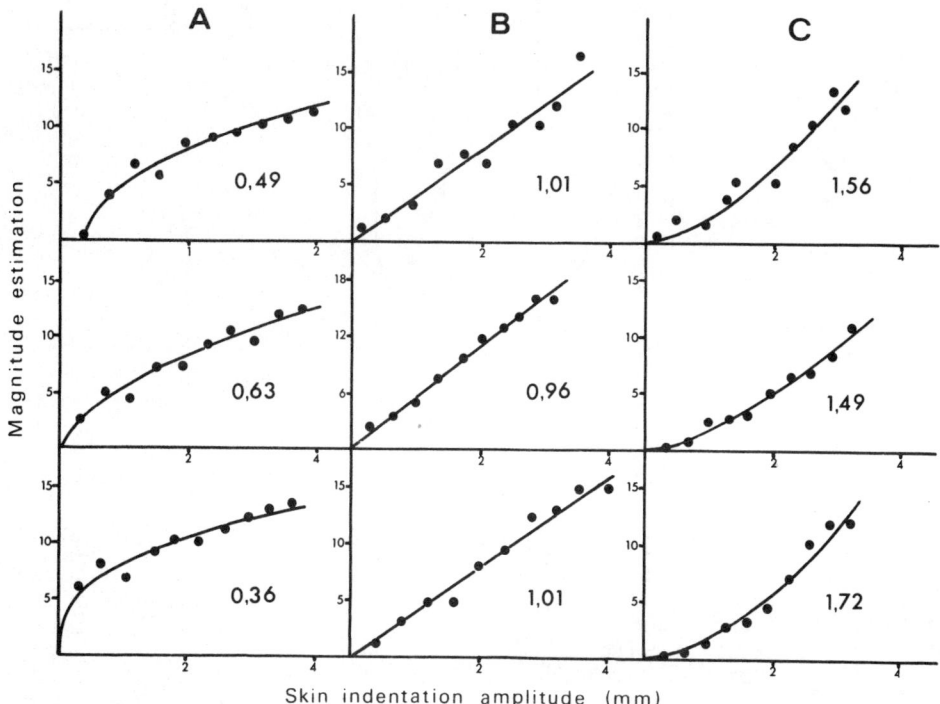

FIG. 6. Psychophysical functions produced by three different subjects in A, B and C respectively, to demonstrate on the one hand, the great inter-individual variability in the type of function produced, and on the other hand, the remarkable intra-individual constancy. For each subject three different magnitude estimation series were performed. In A the subject produced consistently negatively accelerating functions, in B another subject produced approximately linear functions, and in C a third subject produced positively accelerating functions. The exponents of the power functions fitted for each test series are indicated.

A closer look at the individual psychophysical functions revealed interesting properties which are relevant for the main problem of a correspondence between neural and psychophysical stimulus-response functions. In Fig. 6 are shown individual psychophysical data from three subjects, fitted with power functions. Two basic trends are obvious here. One is that different individuals might produce power functions of highly variable shape. The other trend is that the shape of the function produced by the individual subject was

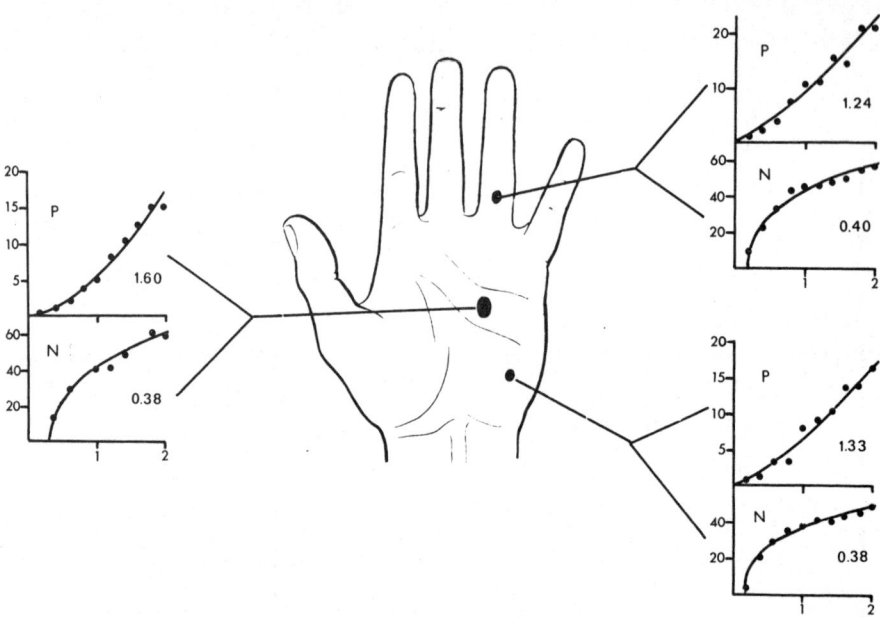

FIG. 7. Neural and psychophysical functions obtained at three different test points in the same subject. The test points were located in the center of the receptive fields of three SA-I units (indicated by black dots). For each test point are shown the psychophysical function (P) as well as the neural stimulus-response function (N) of the unit. This subject produced positively accelerating psychophysical functions at all points, whereas the neural functions were all negatively accelerating. The numbers entered indicate exponents for the fitted power functions.

fairly constant when the test series was repeated several times: it was either positively accelerating, approximately linear or negatively accelerating. This finding seems highly relevant in relation to Mountcastle's hypothesis, which involves the assumption that the neural and the psychophysical functions have the same general shape. It seems reasonable that this principle should also apply to the individual subject. A subject who produces only positively accelerating psychophysical functions would thus have receptors producing similar functions. In order to test this point, neural stimulus-response functions were collected from several test points in some subjects. A typical example is shown in Fig. 7, where three units were studied, and psychophysical functions were obtained at the same three points. This subject showed positively accelerating psychophysical functions at all points, but the neural functions were all negatively accelerating, as expected from the general distribution (see Fig. 5). Similar findings were obtained in several other subjects. Thus, were no indications that the subjects who produced positively accelerating psychophysical functions differed significantly from the average group.

COMMENTS

Since Werner and Mountcastle (1965) introduced the power function description of the stimulus-response relationship for slowly adapting cutaneous mechanoreceptors, most subsequent investigators of slowly as well as rapidly adapting skin mechanoreceptors have used the power function to describe stimulus-response data for these classes of receptors (e.g. Tapper 1965, Brown and Iggo 1967, Merzenich 1968, Harrington and Merzenich 1970, Pubols et al. 1971, Kenton et al. 1971, Munger and Pubols 1972, Chambers et al. 1972, Kruger and Kenton 1973). However, in recent years some reports have appeared which indicate that the power function description may not be generally valid. In particular, there is strong evidence that this description is rather poor for rapidly adapting receptors, and that the best one is a log tanh function (Knibestöl 1973). Also for slowly adapting receptors other functions have recently been discussed (Kenton et al. 1971, Chambers et al. 1972, Knibestöl 1975). It is possible that some of the discrepancies between the various reports may, at least partly, be due to methodological factors, as discussed by Kruger and Kenton (1973) and Knibestöl (1975). Anyhow, for the human glabrous skin slowly adapting receptors, a power function seems to be a fairly good description, useful as a tool for comparison between various kinds of experimental data in this field.

We find that the slowly adapting receptors in human glabrous skin have clearly negatively accelerating functions (Knibestöl 1975, and the present report), whereas Mountcastle et al. (1966) report that similar receptors in monkey glabrous skin display approximately linear functions. This finding from humans is not consistent with Mountcastle´s hypothesis, which requires that the receptors in the human glabrous skin should have approximately linear functions. There might be a possibility that the discrepancies are due to methodological difference, although we do not see where the differences would be.

More difficult to reconcile with Mountcastle´s hypothesis are the findings from studies when neural as well as psychophysical stimulus-response functions were obtained in humans, from the same subjects and, in addition, from the very same tests. First, we found that the distributions of neural and psychophysical functions were clearly different: most psychophysical functions were positively accelerating, whereas the neural functions were largely negatively accelerating. Further, it was evident that the psychophysical functions may vary from one subject to the other, whereas on the other hand the individual subject produced functions of fairly constant shape. However, there was no indication that the subjects who produced positively accelerating psychophysical functions had receptors differing significantly from the whole group of receptors, which were characterized by negatively accelerating stimulus-response functions.

REFERENCES

Brown, A.G. and Iggo, A. (1967). A quantitative study of cutaneous receptors and afferent fibres in the cat and rabbit. J. Physiol. 193, 707-733.

Chambers, M.R., Andres, K.H., Duering, M. and Iggo, A. (1972). The structure and function of the slowly adapting type II mechanoreceptor in hairy skin. Q. Jl exp. Physiol. 57, 417-445.

Hagbarth, K.-E. and Vallbo, A.B. (1967). Mechanoreceptor activity recorded percutaneously with semi-microelectrodes in human peripheral nerves. Acta physiol. scand. 69, 121-122.

Harrington, T. and Merzenich, M.M. (1970). Neural coding in the sense of touch: Human sensations of skin indentation compared with the responses of slowly adapting mechanoreceptive afferents innervating the hairy skin of monkeys. Exp. Brain Res. 10, 251-264.

Kenton, B., Kruger, L. and Woo, M. (1971). Two classes of slowly adapting mechanoreceptor fibres in reptile cutaneous nerve. J. Physiol. 212, 21-44.

Knibestöl, M. and Vallbo, Å.B. (1970). Single unit analysis of mechanoreceptor activity from the human glabrous skin. Acta physiol. scand. 80, 178-195.

Knibestöl, M. (1973). Stimulus-response functions of rapidly adapting mechanoreceptors in the human glabrous skin area. J. Physiol. 232, 427-452.

Knibestöl, M. (1975). Stimulus-response functions of slowly adapting mechanoreceptors in the human glabrous skin area. J. Physiol. 245, 63-80.

Kruger, L. and Kenton, B. (1973). Quantitative neural and psychophysical data for cutaneous mechanoreceptor function. Brain Res. 49, 1-24.

Mountcastle, V.B., Talbot, W.H. and Kornhuber, H.H. (1966). The neural transformation of mechanical stimuli delivered to the monkey's hand. In Touch, Heat and Pain, pp. 325-345. Eds. de Reuck, A.V.S. and Knight, J. Ciba Foundation, London: Churchill.

Mountcastle, V.B. (1967). The problem of sensing and the neural coding of sensory events. In The Neurosciences, pp. 393-408. Eds. Quarton, G.C., Melnechuk, T. and Schmitt, F.O. New York, Rockefeller Univ. Press.

Mountcastle, V.B. and Darian-Smith, I. (1968). Neural mechanisms in somesthesia. In Medical Physiology, pp. 1372-1423. Ed. Mountcastle, V.B. Mosby, Baltimore.

Munger, B.L. and Pubols, L.M. (1972). The sensorineural organization of the digital skin in the raccoon. Brain, Behavior and Evolution, 5, 367-393.

Naka, K.I. and Rushton, W.A.H. (1966). S-potentials from colour units in retina of the fish (Cyprinidae). J. Physiol. 185, 536-555.

Pubols, L.M., Pubols, B.H. Jr. and Munger, B.L. (1971). Functional properties of mechanoreceptors in glabrous skin of the raccoon's forepaw. Expl Neurol. 31, 165-182.
Tapper, D.N. (1965). Stimulus-response relationships in the cutaneous slowly-adapting mechanoreceptor in hairy skin of the cat. Expl Neurol. 13, 364-385.
Vallbo, Å.B. and Hagbarth, K.-E. (1968). Activity from skin mechanoreceptors recorded percutaneously in awake human subjects. Expl Neurol. 21, 270-289.
Werner, G. and Mountcastle, V.B. (1965). Neural activity in mechanoreceptive cutaneous afferents: Stimulus-response relations, Weber functions, and information transmission. J. Neurophysiol. 28, 359-397.
Werner, G. and Mountcastle, V.B. (1968). Quantitative relations between mechanical stimuli to the skin and the neural responses evoked by them. In The Skin Senses, pp. 112-137. Proc. 1st Int. Symp. Tallahassee. Ed.Kenshalo, D.R. Springfield, Illinois: C.C. Thomas.

Discussion:

Zimmermann: A comment concerning the disagreement between the type of intensity functions of single SA receptors and psychophysical magnitude estimation: Is it possible to solve this problem by accounting for recruitment of many receptors of various types, with increasing stimulus strength? Would it be possible to fit the type of psychophysical function by a neurophysiological population response, accounting for excitation of RA and SA receptors?

Knibestöl: Yes, I think it must be explained on the basis of the recruitment phenomena.

MECHANORECEPTIVE UNIT ACTIVITY IN HUMAN SKIN NERVES CORRELATED WITH TOUCH AND VIBRATORY SENSATIONS

T. JÄRVILEHTO, H. HÄMÄLÄINEN and J. KEKONI

INTRODUCTION

Unit activity has been recorded by the method of percutaneous microelectrode recording (Vallbo and Hagbarth, 1968) from the following types of peripheral afferent fibers in man: Pacinian corpuscle (PC) afferents, rapidly adapting (RA) fibers, Type I slowly adapting (SAI) fibers, Type II slowly adapting (SAII) fibers, specific warm fibers, and polymodal C afferent fibers (Knibeställ and Vallbo, 1970; Hagbarth et al., 1970; Knibeställ, 1973, 1975; Torebjörk, 1974; Konietzny and Hensel, 1975). Except for PC afferents which obviously transmit information on fast periodic displacements of the skin (Talbot et al., 1968; Merzenich and Harrington, 1969; Mountcastle et al., 1972), little data are available concerning the perceptual functions of the other types of mechanoreceptive fibers.

On the basis of indirect evidence it has been proposed that RA fibers code low-frequency ("flutter") vibration (Talbot et al., 1968; LaMotte and Mountcastle, 1975). For coding of touch PC afferents, RA fibers, and SA fibers are all suitable candidates (Gybels and van Hees, 1971; Knibeställ, 1973, 1975; Lindblom, 1974) and pressure may be mediated by activity in SAII afferents (Harrington and Merzenich, 1970). These hypotheses need, however, confirmation by direct recording of activity from peripheral mechanoreceptive fibers in man with simultaneous measurements of cutaneous sensations.

Our purpose is to study characteristics of single nerve fibers in the superficial branch of the radial nerve innervating the hairy skin of the human hand and to examine perceptual correlates of activity in mechanosensitive fibers when using a combination of psychophysical measurements and unit recording technique. In the present report tentative correlations between mechanoreceptive unit activity, and touch and vibratory sensations are presented.

METHODS

We have obtained unit recordings by percutaneously inserted microelectrodes from 129 single fibers in the radial nerves of 8 subjects (Ss; 3 female, 5 male; age range 12 - 28 yrs.). The electrodes and the recording procedure have been described elsewhere (Järvilehto et al., 1976).

When unit activity was encountered the fibers were tested as follows (only for a few fibers all testing steps could be carried out):
1) Determination of the type and the receptive field of the fiber.
2) Measurement of conduction velocity of the fiber by applying either electric or mechanical pulses (duration 0.5 and 1 ms, respectively) to the receptive field.

3) Measurement of the mechanical threshold of the receptor for one impulse to appear by mechanical pulses (100 Hz sine-wave, half-cycle) with simultaneous measurement of sensation threshold. Mechanical thresholds were determined also by v. Frey hairs calibrated for weight.

4) Determination of responses of the fiber to mechanical pulses of varying amplitudes (100 Hz sine-wave, half-cycle, peak displacement range 0 - 600 µm) with simultaneous estimation of the stimulus magnitude by S.

5) Determination of the tuning curve of the fiber (cf. Talbot et al., 1968) with simultaneous measurement of absolute sensation threshold for stimulus movement and of the threshold for pitch of vibration (cf. LaMotte and Mountcastle, 1975). The amplitude of the vibratory stimulus was gradually increased from zero at frequencies between 30 and 300 Hz (sine-wave) while S was instructed to respond when he had sensation on slightest movement of the stimulus probe ("absolute threshold") and when he clearly experienced the vibratory stimulus ("pitch threshold").

Vibratory stimuli were delivered to the skin by means of a probe (diameter 2 mm) fixed to the moving coil of an electromechanical vibrator which was driven by a function generator. The signal from the function generator was amplified by a power amplifier. The vibrator was fixed to a micromanipulator to allow exact positioning of the stimulus probe. The probe was adjusted to the receptive field under inspection through a binocular microscope so that it touched the skin without visible deformation and it was then indented by about 500 μm into the skin. The indentation caused weak sensation of pressure. Movements of the probe were recorded by a miniature piezoelectric accelerometer fixed between the probe and the moving coil of the vibrator. The output of the accelerometer proportional to the acceleration of the stimulus probe was amplified by a preamplifier with calibrated **integrating** circuits for velocity and displacement measurements. The signal from the preamplifier was stored on magnetic tape with response signals, reports of Ss and unit activity. Measurement of the displacement of the probe was carried out by displaying the signals on a storage oscilloscope (accuracy of measurements about 10 μm).

In addition to the experiments with unit recording, psychophysical experiments were **carried** out to control possible effects of the recording situation on sensation thresholds, magnitude estimation, and vibratory sensitivity. The testing procedures were otherwise identical as above, but a sensitive spot searched by a v. Frey hair of 0.3 g was used as a stimulation point and its surrounding was fixed by a ring to allow more stable stimulation. Additionally, white noise was given to S in order to mask the sounds caused by the vibrator.

RESULTS

Characteristics of the fiber sample

The total sample amounts to 129 single fibers. Relatively many fibers (23) had no receptive field on the skin and they were spontaneously firing in bursts or with a regular discharge. Some of these fibers had characteristics similar to the sympathetic units described by Hagbarth et al., (1972). According to the response to sustained pressure, 31 fibers could be classified as RA fibers and 74 as SA fibers. One fiber responded to mild warming of the skin (cf. Konietzny and Hensel, 1975).

RA fibers had usually large receptive fields (a few cm in diameter) with obscure borders. Five fibers, however, had spot-like fields (about 1 mm in diameter) and one fiber innervated a hair-follicle. Conduction velocities determined for 7 fibers ranged from 10 to 41 m/s (mean = 26.9 m/s).

SA fibers had usually spot-like receptive fields (about 1 mm in diameter) and 6 fibers innervated at least two spots. However, also larger fields were encountered. No systematic classification of the subtypes of fibers was carried out, but several fibers were identified as SAI or SAII afferents on the basis of sensitivity to stretching the skin (Chambers et al., 1972). SAII fibers had larger receptive fields than SAI fibers whose receptive fields were always spot-like. Conduction velocities of 23 SA fibers ranged from 10 to 73 m/s (mean = 30.2 m/s).

Unit activity correlated with touch sensations

Mechanical thresholds of single mechanoreceptive fibers were in general similar to sensation thresholds. When tested by v. Frey hairs the thresholds of 25 SA fibers ranged from less than 0.1 g to 1.7 g (mean = 0.5 g) which corresponds well to detection thresholds of Ss. Four fibers, however, had threshold values exeeding 4.5 g. Simultaneous testing of the receptor and sensation thresholds with tactile pulses for 9 SA fibers revealed identical thresholds in 4 cases (range of threshold values 10 - 40 µm peak displacement). The thresholds of the other fibers were on the average 20 µm higher than the sensation thresholds. For the unit innervating a hair-follicle, movements of the hair causing 6 - 9 impulses to appear elicited a weak sensation of touch.

In a separate series of psychophysical experiments magnitude estimation of tactile pulses was determined for 6 Ss. For each S three magnitude estimation functions were obtained by using three different stimulation spots on the back of the hand. All functions could be described by power functions ($y = ax^b$) whose exponents varied between 0.61 and 1.53. Fig. 1 shows pooled data for all Ss and the best fitting power function is plotted by the continuous line. The exponent of the function is 0.87. This exponent is somewhat higher than that obtained by Franzén and Offenloch (1969) for magnitude estimation of similar pulse stimuli applied to the glabrous skin.

Magnitude estimates of tactile pulses with simultaneous unit recording were obtained for three SA fibers. Fig. 2 shows an example of responses of one fiber. The response consists of quite a few impulses; for the three fibers the maximal number of impulses evoked was five. The number of impulses was, however, in monotonic relation to the magnitude estimates of the

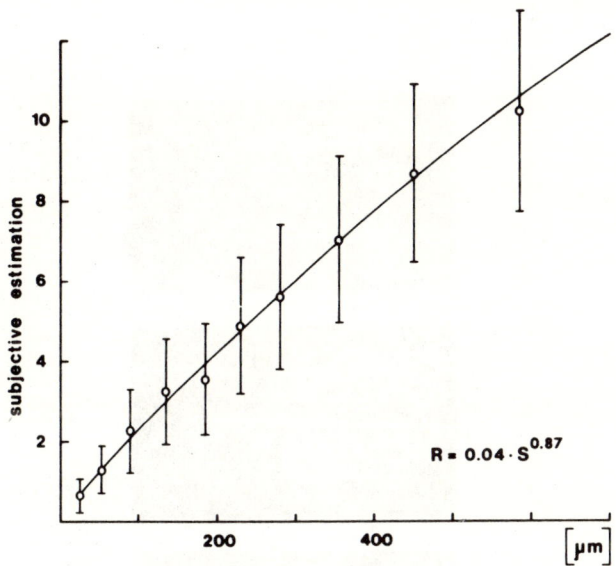

Fig. 1. Subjective magnitude estimation of tactile pulses as a function of peak displacement in μm. Each point is mean of 24 estimates. Bars show standard deviations of means. Continuous line is a power function whose equation is shown on the right.

stimulus intensity as shown in Fig. 3. The data can be described by a linear function ($E = 1.6 \cdot I + 1.1$; F-ratio for slope = 38.8, $p < .01$; for the symbols see the figure) plotted by the straight line. This relationship resembles the functions reported by Gybels and van Hees (1971) for the dependence of sensation magnitude on the neural response. For one fiber positive estimates were obtained in absence of fiber response indicating that also other fibers participate in the coding of the stimulus. The relation between pooled magnitude estimates and stimulus amplitude could be described by a power function with an exponent of 0.82 which is nearly identical to the exponent of the function in Fig. 1. Consequently, the data suggest that magnitude estimation of fast tactile pulses may be based on activity in SA fibers. It is, however, probable that

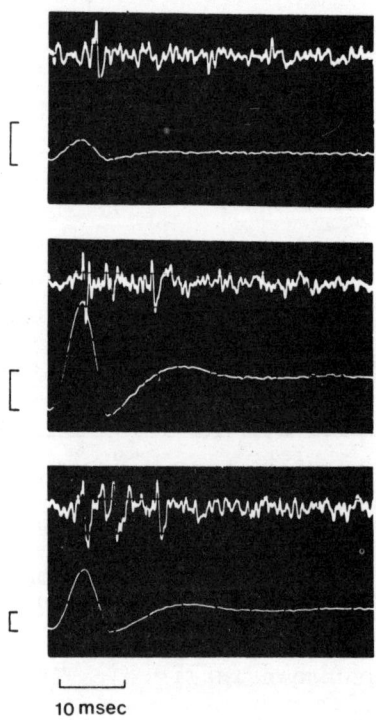

Fig. 2. Responses of an SA fiber to tactile pulses. Lower trace in each photograph shows acceleration of the stimulus probe. Corresponding displacement calibrations (100 µm) on the left.

fiber populations are involved in the coding as five impulses could hardly cover the whole magnitude estimation function.

It is a common opinion that also RA fibers participate in coding of intensity of tactile stimuli (e.g. Gybels and van Hees, 1971), although they probably do not contribute to threshold sensation (Lindblom, 1974). We have determined simultaneous estimation of stimulus magnitude for one RA fiber and in this case no monotonic relation was obtained between the number of impulses and estimate values. The fiber responded rather with 2 - 4

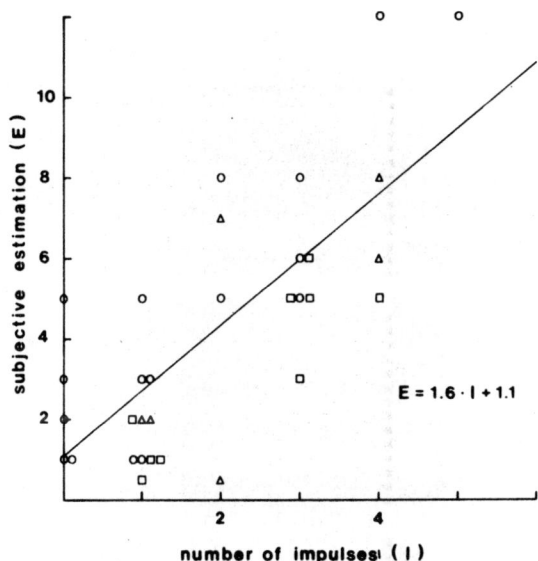

Fig. 3. Subjective magnitude estimation of tactile pulses as a function of the number of impulses evoked in 3 SA fibers. Fibers are shown with different symbols. The equation of the straight line on the right.

impulses in an all-or-nothing fashion.

Unit activity correlated with vibratory sensations

Twelve RA and 26 SA fibers were tested by vibratory stimulation. Four RA and 8 SA fibers could not be entrained at stimulation frequencies between 30 and 300 Hz. Most RA and SA fibers fired synchronously with the vibratory stimulus at low frequencies by discharging once during each stimulus cycle, but when the stimulation frequency exceeded 100 Hz no SA fibers could be entrained (see Fig. 4). This limit of entrainment correlated with a change in the quality of the vibratory sensation described by Talbot et al. (1968) as transition from "flutter" vibration to vibratory "hum". One RA unit could be entrained by vibratory stimuli up to 400 Hz. Other RA fibers had similar response characteristics as SA fibers.

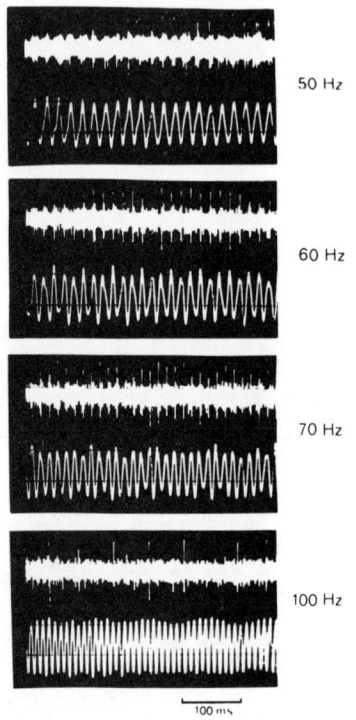

Fig. 4. Responses of an SA fiber to vibratory stimulation. Stimulation frequency indicated on the right. Lower trace in each figure presents acceleration of the stimulator tip.

These qualitative observations suggest that both RA and SA fibers contribute to vibratory sensation, in contrast to the opinion of Talbot et al. (1968) and Merzenich and Harrington (1969) that only RA fibers are involved. This controversy can be solved by determining the quantitative response characteristics of the fibers with simultaneous testing of vibratory sensibility. Fig. 5A presents tentative threshold data for entrainment of 3 RA and 8 SA fibers with simultaneously measured subjective thresholds. Open dots show tuning points (1:1 entrainment thresholds) of RA fibers and filled dots tuning points of SA fibers. Average absolute thresholds of Ss are plotted by

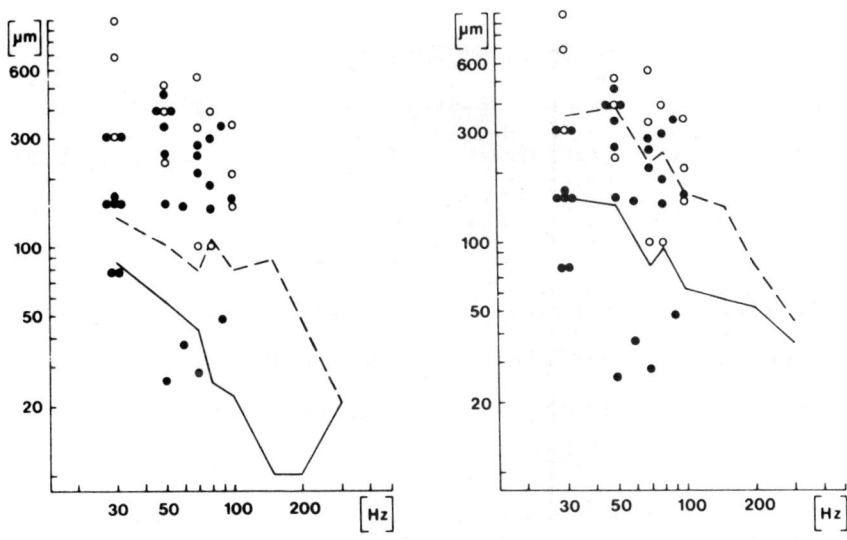

Fig. 5. Tuning points of 3 RA (open dots) and 8 SA (filled dots) fibers compared with subjective thresholds for vibration which are determined (A) simultaneously with recording of unit activity and (B) in separate psychophysical experiments with 10 Ss. Abscissa: stimulation frequency; ordinate: vibration amplitude in μm. Continuous lines are average absolute thresholds, broken lines average pitch thresholds.

continuous lines and average pitch thresholds by broken lines

No fibers could be entrained with vibratory stimuli exceeding 100 Hz. In general, the thresholds of fibers are higher than subjective thresholds and the correspondence between subjective and fiber thresholds is close only for SA fibers at 30 Hz.

In Fig. 5B the tuning points of the fibers are compared with average absolute and pitch thresholds determined in a separate series of psychophysical experiments with 10 Ss. In these experiments the skin around the stimulation site was fixed by a ring. The correspondence between the subjective thresholds and the tuning points of the fibers is now quite close up to 100 Hz.

DISCUSSION

The tentative correlations between unit activity and cutaneous sensations presented in this work indicate that SA fibers may have significance in coding of both tactile pulses and vibratory information in man. Subjective thresholds as well as magnitude estimation of tactile pulses were explicable in terms of responses of SA fibers and low-frequency entrainment thresholds of the fibers were comparable to vibratory sensation thresholds.

The correspondence between subjective thresholds and mechanical thresholds of the receptors is in agreement with earlier findings (Hensel and Boman, 1960; Knibestöl and Vallbo, 1970). However, the sensation evoked by a few impulses seems to have a diffuse character related rather to itch than touch. When stimulating by v. Frey hairs distinct touch sensations were not reported until the afferent discharge exceeded about 40 imp/sec, except for the hair-follicle unit the stimulation of which clearly evoked weak touch sensations.

The comparisons of magnitude estimation functions with responses of SA fibers support the hypothesis of Mountcastle (1967) stating that the brain operates upon information arriving from mechanoreceptors in a linear manner. Our correlations do not solve the problem concerning the types of receptors on which the brain is operating when tactile stimuli are presented. The results render, however, SA fibers as likely candidates

for coding of tactile pulses. RA fibers presumably do not code
tactile pulses at least at threshold intensities as their
mechanical thresholds are relatively high (cf. also Burgess
et al., 1968; Lindblom, 1965, 1974). PC afferents, on the other
hand, are hardly responsible for coding of tactile stimuli
applied to the hairy skin as they seem to be infrequent in the
subcutaneous tissue below these skin areas (Merzenich and
Harrington, 1969).

If RA fibers do not contribute to the detection or intensity
discrimination of tactile pulses what could then be perceptual
correlates of their activity? It is a common observation in
our experiments that RA fibers are readily excited by stroking
of the skin; some fibers seem even to respond exclusively to
gentle stroking. One could therefore speculate that RA fibers
act as detectors of stimuli moving along the skin and their
main function would be the coding of active touch during which
the hand is purposively moved over objects.

Vibratory characteristics of human receptors in the hairy skin
have not been studied earlier. Knibestöl and Vallbo (1970)
present related data for glabrous skin units. Comparison of
the present results with their data seems to indicate that
functional differences exist between units in the hairy and
in the glabrous skin. The authors were able to entrain both
RA and SA fibers by stimulation frequencies up to 400 Hz; however, quantitative threshold data were not presented. Our results are in agreement with the conclusion of Talbot et al.

(1968) that vibratory sensations cannot be explained by a single receptive system. Comparison of tuning points of the fibers with subjective thresholds in the present work suggests that in addition to RA fibers and PC afferents, also SA fibers are able to mediate vibratory information, especially in the low-frequency range. This finding is in agreement with the evidence suggesting that the tactile pad receptors in the hairy skin which are supplied by SAI fibers would correspond to spots described by Geldard (1940) as highly sensitive to both pressure and vibratory stimulation (Lindblom and Tapper, 1967). This dual sensitivity of SA fibers indicates that they may be able to transmit two kinds of information, presumably on the basis of the interval structure of the afferent discharge. We have carried out interval analysis of responses of 9 SA fibers to vibratory stimulation and Fig. 6 shows a typical example. It is evident that the standard deviations of the interval histograms are very small during vibratory stimuli with the exception of exceeding the entrainment limit (200 Hz). Consequently, the codes by which the two kinds of information are transmitted could be based on the variability of the spike intervals. It may be noted that the functions of SA fibers may still be more complicated as they are additionally sensitive to temperature changes of the skin (Burton et al., 1972).

Our psychophysical results on vibratory sensibility of the hairy skin are comparable to those reported by Merzenich and Harrington (1969). It is interesting to note that the vibratory thresholds were in general higher when the skin around

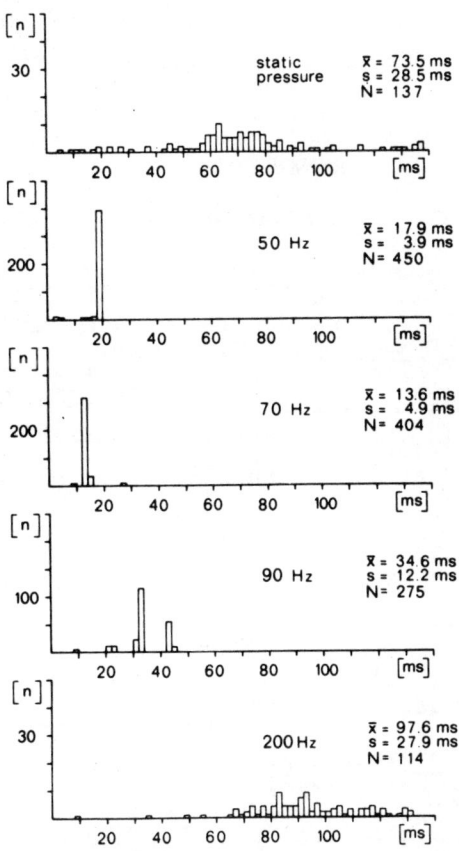

Fig. 6. Interval analysis of vibratory responses of an SA fiber. The uppermost diagram presents the analysis of the static response of the fiber to a steady pressure by the stimulator tip. Abscissa shows the interval class (class width = 2 msec) and ordinate the number of intervals belonging to each class. Vibration frequency is indicated on the right in each diagram. $\bar{X}$ = mean, s = standard deviation, N = total number of intervals.

the stimulation site was fixed. There are of course quite many differences between the recording and psychophysical experiments which might cause such a difference, but one could speculate that the lower thresholds in recording experiments were mainly due to the spread of the vibratory stimulation to areas supplied by sensitive PC afferents when the skin was not fixed. Analogous effects of skin fixation on tactile magnitude estimation functions have been reported by Verrillo and Capraro (1975).

REFERENCES

Burgess, P.R., Petit, D. and Warren, R.M., J. Neurophysiol. 31, 833 (1968).
Burton, H., Terashima, S. and Clark, J., Brain Res. 45, 401 (1972).
Chambers, M.R., Andres, K.H., v. Duering, M. and Iggo, A., Quart. J. Exp. Physiol. 57, 417 (1972).
Franzén, O. and Offenloch, K., Exp. Brain Res. 8, 1 (1969).
Geldard, F.A., J. Gen. Psychol. 22, 243 (1940).
Gybels, J. and van Hees, J., Excerpta Med., Int. Congress Series No. 253, 198 (1971).
Hagbarth, K.-E., Hongell, A., Hallin, R.G. and Torebjörk, H.E., Brain Res. 24, 423 (1970).
Hagbarth, K.-E., Hallin, R.G., Hongell, A., Torebjörk, H.E. and Wallin, B.G., Acta Physiol. Scand. 84, 164 (1972).
Harrington, T. and Merzenich, M.M., Exp. Brain Res. 10, 251 (1970).
Hensel, H. and Boman, K.K., J. Neurophysiol. 23, 564 (1960).
Järvilehto, T., Hämäläinen, H. and Laurinen, P., Exp. Brain Res., in press (1976).
Knibestöl, M. and Vallbo, Å.B., Acta Physiol. Scand. 80, 178 (1970).
Knibestöl, M., J. Physiol. 232, 427 (1973).
Knibestöl, M., J. Physiol. 245, 63 (1975).
Konietzny, F. and Hensel, H., Pflügers Arch. 359, 265 (1975).
LaMotte, R.H. and Mountcastle, V.B., J. Neurophysiol. 38, 539 (1975).
Lindblom, U., J. Neurophysiol. 28, 966 (1965).
Lindblom, U., Brain Res. 82, 205 (1974).
Lindblom, U. and Tapper, D.N., Exp. Neurol. 17, 1 (1967).
Merzenich, M.M. and Harrington, T., Exp. Brain Res. 9, 236 (1969).
Mountcastle, V.B., In: The Neurosciences. Ed. by G.C. Quarton, T. Melnechuck and F.O. Schmitt. New York: Rockefeller Univ. Press, pp. 393-408 (1967).
Mountcastle, V.B., LaMotte, R.H. and Carli, G., J. Neurophysiol. 35, 122 (1972).
Talbot, W.H., Darian-Smith, I., Kornhuber, H.H. and Mountcastle, V.B., J. Neurophysiol. 31, 301 (1968).
Torebjörk, H.E., Acta Physiol. Scand. 92, 374 (1974).
Vallbo, Å.B. and Hagbarth, K.-E., Exp. Neurol. 21, 270 (1968).
Verrillo, R.T. and Capraro, A.J., Percept. Psychophys. 17, 91 (1975).

DIFFERENCES IN TIMING OF CORTICOCUNEATE AND CORTICOGRACILE ACTIONS

J. D. COLE and G. GORDON
University Laboratory of Physiology, Oxford, U.K.

It may seem out of place to present data from experiments on anaesthetised cats at a symposium specially directed to the skin senses of Primates and especially to those of Man. Nevertheless the present experiments are carried out much more easily upon the cat than the monkey and appear to involve systems that are at least structurally similar; and further, if our inferences from what we have seen are right, one might expect them to apply with even greater force to the Primates.

Corticofugal influences on subcortical sensory nuclei are extremely well known, and a great deal of attention has been given to the particular path from somaesthetic cortex to dorsal column nuclei which we deal with here. This path, which contains both excitatory and inhibitory components, has recently been reviewed in detail by Towe (1973). We have worked exclusively on the actions of the first somaesthetic cortex (Sm 1) on the contralateral nuclei: these actions are much more powerful than those of any ipsilateral projections. The ascending lemnisco-thalamocortical projection from these nuclei to Sm 1 is generally regarded as entirely crossed. Some years ago Gordon and Miller (1969) identified a number of crossed corticonuclear cells by recording from single cells in the cortex - mainly the medial part of Sm 1 - and stimulating their axons near their presumed terminations in the gracile and cuneate nuclei. The positions of the antidromically excited cells could then be determined in the cortex and their latency of response measured. More recently this work has been extended to include the whole of Sm 1 (Brech, Gordon and Powell; in preparation), and has allowed a separation of the cells projecting to the two nuclei, using as criterion the lower threshold for antidromic excitation in one or other nucleus. Corticocuneate cells were found to lie consistently lateral to corticogracile cells, on the convexity or in the upper bank of the coronal sulcus, in the cytoarchitectonic areas 3 b, 3 a and 4, with a concentration in 3 a and its boundaries.

Corticogracile cells lay medially, on the convexity or in the upper bank of the cruciate sulcus, mainly in 3 a, some on its boundary with area 4 or in area 4. The region studied was all caudal to the surface marking of the cruciate sulcus; and the regions of greatest concentration of corticocuneate or corticogracile cells have been used as a guide in the present experiments in positioning the unipolar macroelectrode which was inserted into the cortex to activate the path to the appropriate nucleus. Final adjustments of electrode position were made to obtain maximal effects at lowest threshold.

One surprising and interesting fact which emerged from the experiments just described was that in spite of some overlap between the two populations, the mean latency for the antidromic response of corticocuneate cells (3.7 msec) was strikingly shorter than that for corticogracile cells (7.2 msec) in spite of the length of the two paths being almost identical (see Fig. 1). In this respect the descending fibres are in marked contrast to the <u>ascending</u> paths from these nuclei to the cortex, in which the latencies for single fibres ascending to the thalamus in the lemniscus - studied by antidromic stimulation - are exactly similar in distribution for the two nuclei (Gordon and Jukes, 1974; Kleider, 1974), and for which the minimal nucleocortical latency is identical when one or other nucleus is directly stimulated so as to cause a focal response in the appropriate part of Sm 1, an assumption we have recently verified. This actual nucleocortical time is approximately 4 msec in a cat of average size.

The implication of all this is that there is a marked asymmetry between the corticocuneate and corticogracile "loops". But misinterpretation is possible in identifying corticofugal cells projecting to a particular nucleus, if the part of the fibre excited antidromically was not its terminal region and the fibre simply passed through the stimulated region to end elsewhere. The very exact medial and lateral separation of the corticogracile and corticocuneate cells, respectively, suggests that this error occurred rarely if at all: nevertheless it seemed important to see whether a corresponding difference in latency of action on the two nuclei occurred when the corticofugal system was activated orthodromically and the test therefore a more direct one.

In all our experiments the animals were anaesthetised with sodium pento-

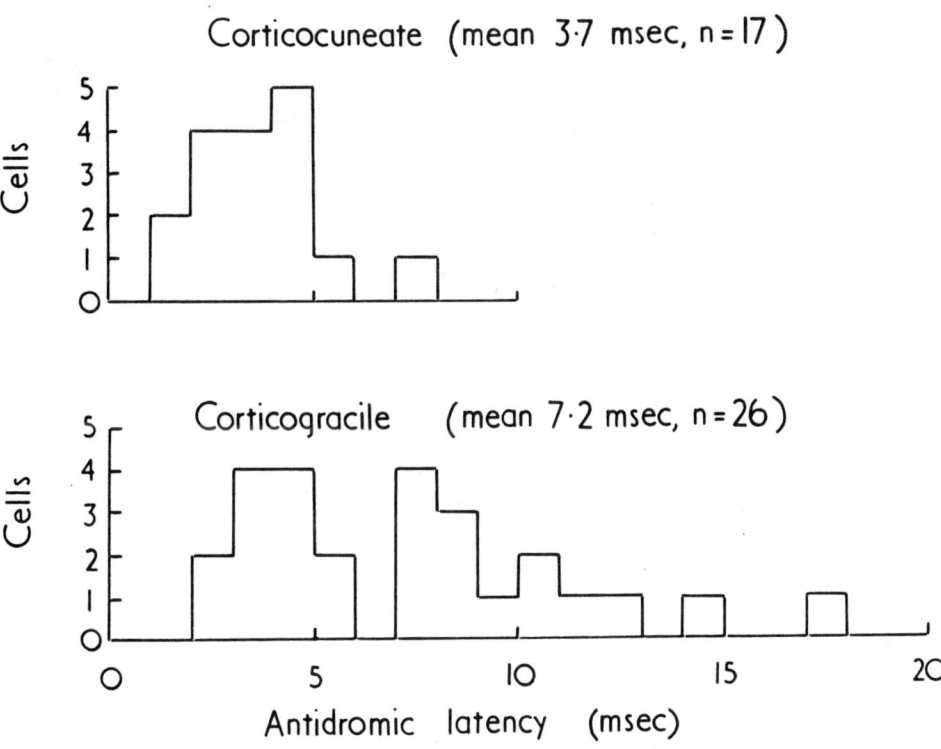

Fig. 1. Histograms showing the latencies for antidromic excitation of cortical cells following stimulation in the contralateral cuneate or gracile nucleus. Data in the upper histogram are taken from cells excited at lower threshold in the cuneate, and those in the lower histogram in the gracile nucleus. Stimuli were of twice-threshold size.

(Data from Gordon and Miller, 1969; and from Brech, Gordon and Powell, unpublished)

barbitone throughout the experiment: some were also given gallamine triethiodide intermittently to improve mechanical stability by inducing paralysis during single unit recording. The dorsolateral fascicle was always divided with forceps at C 4 on the relevant side to eliminate any input through the spinocervical or other lateral tract.

The experiments were of two kinds. In one, transmission through each nucleus was studied by recording the monophasic mass potential in the crossed medial lemniscus generated by a single shock to either the superficial radial nerve (for the cuneate) or the medial plantar nerve (for the gracilis). These are both cutaneous nerves and the twice-threshold shocks we used activated

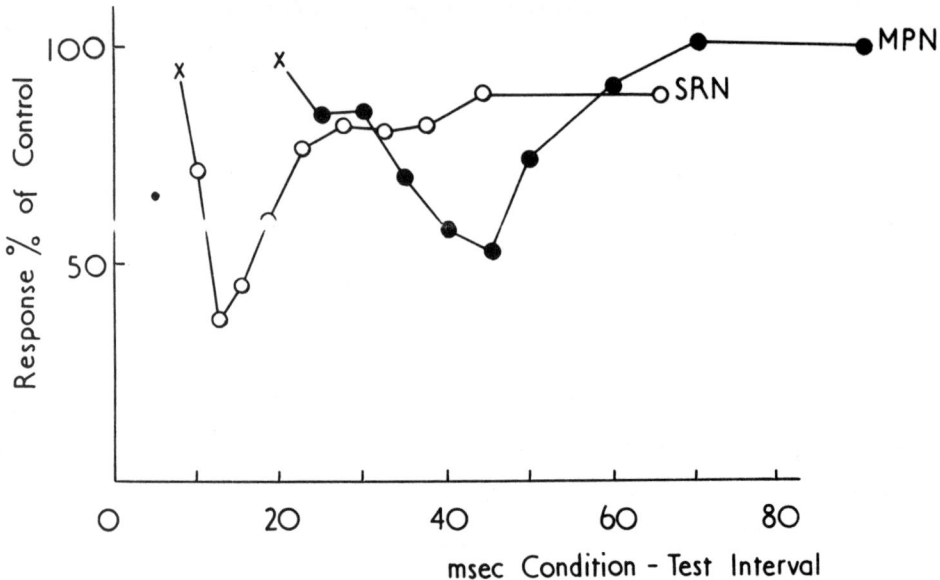

Fig. 2. Time courses for depression of lemniscal response by cortical stimulation. Test responses were elicited by stimulating the superficial radial nerve (SRN, open circles) or the medial plantar nerve (MPN, solid circles). Measurements of response are based on the area under the monophasic lemniscal mass response. See text for further explanation.

the large A fibres maximally without exciting A delta fibres. Time-courses of inhibition of transmission by the cortical conditioning stimuli were obtained (Fig. 2), in which the size of the response to the test shock was always plotted at the time of arrival of the test volley at the nucleus, relative to zero which marks the time of the cortical stimulus. One can see from these graphs that the inhibition of transmission through the cuneate nucleus started earlier and fell off sooner than that through the gracile nucleus, following a double shock (see later) to the cortex. Our main conclusion from these experiments is that the latency of the corticofugal inhibition of the cuneate nucleus is less than half that for the gracile nucleus, which agrees with the prediction from the earlier antidromic studies. Any early facilitation (see later) would have been difficult to quantitate in these studies of mass potentials in the presence of the stimulus artefact.

Naturally any estimate that is based only on the height - or, as in our ex-

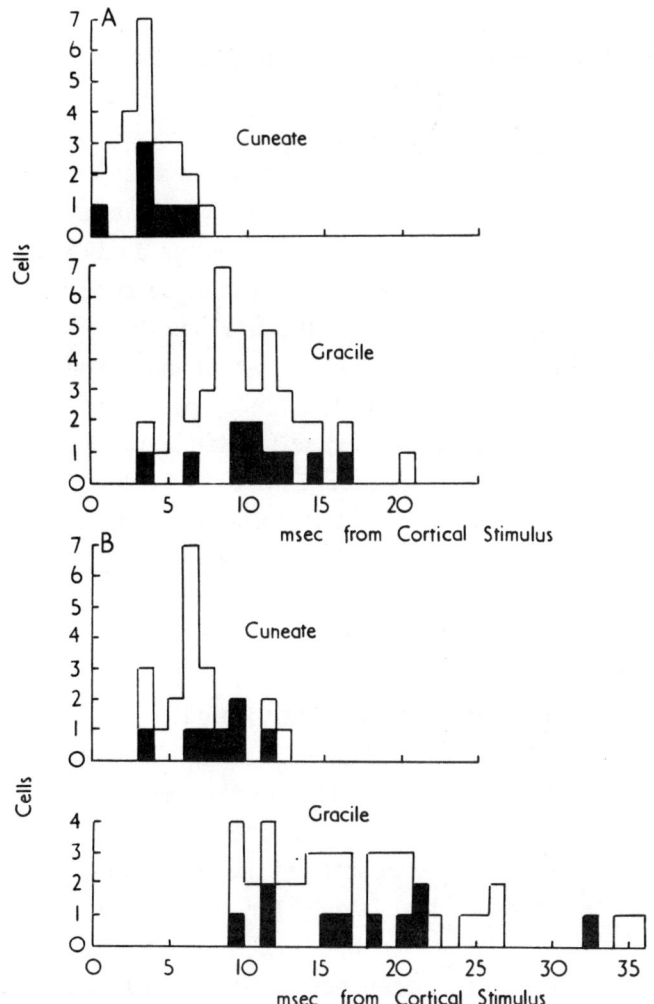

Fig. 3. Comparison of latency of onset of facilitation (A), and of onset of inhibition (B), for single cells in the cuneate nucleus with those in the gracile nucleus. Cells identified by antidromic stimulation in the contralateral upper midbrain as relay cells projecting in the lemniscus are filled in black: their number is certainly an underestimate because of the use of fixed stimulating electrodes not having access to the whole lemniscus. See text for further explanation.

periments, the area - of a mass potential gives information that is limited by ignorance of the differing effects on individual cells, which may be inhibited or facilitated, or both, at differing times after the cortical stimulus. So in our second type of experiment we recorded from "spontaneously" discharging single cells in one or other nucleus and observed the effect of a double stimulus in the appropriate cortical area upon this discharge. To get a statistically meaningful result we superimposed up to 100 oscilloscope sweeps, with the stimulus time-locked to the sweep, while the cell continued to discharge in the absence of any peripheral stimulus. These data were recorded on tape to allow various forms of analysis. Many cells showed a clear break in their discharge several msec after the conditioning stimulus, continuing often for 100 msec or more (inhibition). Records from many of these cells also showed a greater density of spikes, compared with control values, in the first few msec, preceding the inhibition (facilitation). The latencies of onset of facilitation and of inhibition, respectively, are shown in Fig. 3 A and Fig. 3 B. Each figure compares the latencies for cuneate cells and gracile cells, and it is clear that for each effect the mean latency of onset is much longer for gracile cells, without much overlap with the values for cuneate cells. The duration of inhibition of gracile cells was also on average significantly longer than that of cuneate cells. The upper range of durations of inhibition seen among populations of single cells was not apparently detected by the comparatively insensitive mass recording technique (see Fig. 2). Otherwise the observations on single cells, for the dominant inhibitory effect, confirm what was to be expected from the work on mass responses. It should however be noted that the leading edge for depression of the mass potential occurs later, for each nucleus, than the shortest latency for onset of inhibition in the corresponding nucleus measured by the single-cell method. One possible explanation for this apparent discrepancy depends on the cells contributing to the mass potential having been excited by stimulating cutaneous nerves very distally, at wrist or ankle, and therefore having distal receptive fields; whereas the single cells studied, which were picked at random from the region between about 2 and 4 mm caudal to the obex, had more distributed receptive fields, some in the gracile nucleus lying quite proximal. We have some evidence which suggests that, for gracile cells, those with proximal receptive fields are inhibited at shorter latency than those with distal fields; and this, if supported with more evidence, could go some way to explain the discrepancy.

DISCUSSION

Although figures have been quoted by a number of authors for latencies of corticofugal action upon one or other of these nuclei, or upon both, it does not appear that a systematic comparison has been attempted before. The variation among figures previously quoted may partly depend on the tendency to use a repetitive train of cortical shocks for conditioning - a type of stimulation which, though very effective, makes estimates of latency ambiguous. We have used two shocks separated by 2 msec as a satisfactory compromise between effectiveness and accuracy of timing.

The asymmetry we have found is at first sight very surprising, because it does not fit the commonly accepted idea of these corticofugal paths just as components of simple nuclear-cortical-nuclear feedback loops - in these the added time in the descending path to the gracile nucleus would have no relevance. It seems to us that the relevance of the asymmetry of the corticofugal paths may well lie in the corresponding differences in length of the corticomotor paths to forelimb and hind limb. Corticofugal actions eliciting movement may result in a tactile feedback from forelimb or hind limb which will arrive at the cuneate nucleus or gracile nucleus, respectively, after different intervals. Preliminary experiments are in progress in which a motor nerve is stimulated to produce palmar or plantar flexion against a flat surface and the time for tactile feedback is found by recording from the appropriate nucleus. When coupled with information compiled from various sources, including our own data, about the time occupied in the various pathways, it appears that a centripetal tactile volley resulting from a cortically elicited movement will arrive at the nucleus at a time corresponding quite well with the onset of corticofugal action there. The timing of sensory return is thus well matched to the timing of corticofugal action at each nucleus.

Modification of lemniscal activity, seen as a reduction of the mass lemniscal potential elicited by a peripheral test stimulus, has been described in conscious cats in association with both conditioned (Ghez and Pisa, 1972) and free (Coulter, 1974) movement of the limb from which the test response was elicited. This reduction started up to 150 msec before the movement, and persisted or increased during the movement itself. This prior reduction could not have been predicted from our data, but is certainly compatible with them since the mechanisms of motor initiation may use the existing paths in a whole variety of patterns. The built-in asymmetry we have seen appears on present evidence to be concerned with a later phase of the movement-sequence in which tactile feedback has begun. Its significance might be functionally quite different from that of the depression prior to movement. The mere fact that inhibition occurs within a population of nuclear cells tells us nothing of its functional significance: it may represent an increase in "sharpening" and hence in spatial discriminatory capacity in a particular part of the body, and this might be useful in analysing the feedback from an exploratory movement. It may - and this is by no means exclusive of the first possibility - increase the likelihood of detecting unexpected and interesting features of an explored surface by selectively subtracting that part of the sensory input which could be directly predicted from the central instructions initiating the movement, as Coulter (1974) suggests, using the principle of corollary discharge. It may, as Ghez and Pisa (1972) point out, be used to attenuate and reduce the significance of the feedback before and during pre-programmed ballistic movements. This all depends on the nature of the movement, and the cat has little capacity for exploratory tactile behaviour compared with a Primate, which suggests that the difficult task of studying this system in the Primate would be profitable.

A brief note on this work has been published (Cole and Gordon, 1976), and a complete account is in preparation.

ACKNOWLEDGEMENTS

J.D.C. acknowledges the award of an M.R.C. Scholarship, and G.G. that of a Project Grant from the M.R.C. to support this work.

REFERENCES

Brech, A., Gordon, G. and T.P.S. Powell. Paper in preparation.

Cole, J.D. and G. Gordon (1976). Dissimilar timing of corticofugal inhibition of the gracile and cuneate nuclei in cats anaesthetized with pentobarbitone. J. Physiol., Lond. 255.

Coulter, J.D. (1974). Sensory transmission through lemniscal pathway during voluntary movement in the cat. J. Neurophysiol. 37, 831-845.

Ghez, C. and M. Pisa. (1972). Inhibition of afferent transmission in cuneate nucleus during coluntary movement in the cat. Brain. Res. 40, 145-151.

Gordon, G. and M.G.M. Jukes. (1964). Dual organization of the exteroceptive components of the cat's gracile nucleus. J. Physiol., Lond. 173, 263-290.

Gordon, G. and R. Miller. (1969). Identification of cortical cells projecting to the dorsal column nuclei of the cat. Quart. J. exp. Physiol. 54, 85-98.

Kleider, A. (1974). A functional study of some inputs and outputs of the cat's dorsal column nuclei. D. Phil. Thesis, Oxford.

Towe, A.L. (1973). Somatosensory cortex: descending influence on ascending systems. In Handbook of Sensory Physiology, Vol II, Ed. A. Iggo. Berlin: Springer-Verlag.

Discussion:

Odutola: I am tickled by Dr Gordon's presentation and wish to make a few remarks which may bear on his rather unusual results. He has suggested to us that whatever the functional role of the cortical inputs to the cueno-gracile complex is, the nuclei composing this complex make use of the inputs at considerably different time intervals. There is a direct anatomical inference one can draw from the report. This is that populations of corticofugal fibers size which may then account for timing differences. In this respect I draw on the data of Valverde (1966) and Zimmermann, Chambers and Liu (1964) on cortical projections to the rat cuneo-gracile complex. Valverde's report would not seem to justify a difference in the calibre sizes of pyramido-gracile as compared to pyramido-cuneate projections. It is of course possible that this was not specifically looked for by this author. On the other hand, Zimmermann et al observed that cortical inputs to the nuclei in reference occurred over two different pathways. The caudal cuneogracile complex being supplied by pyramidal tract fibers and or collaterals and the rostral cuneo-gracile complex receives input from a dorsal tract arising in part from the basis peduncupli and from longitudinally oriented corticofugal fibers in the rostral pons. Since Dr Gordon claimed to have worked within the rostral regions of both nuclei, the implication of this dual cortico fugal projection to his observations in the cuneate and gracile nuclei is not clear.

I have been looking at the rat cuneo-gracile complex with the Golgi technique over the last two years and have recently formulated (unpublished) operational circuit patterns which seems to have a distinct dorso-ventral organisation within the complex. In relation to Dr Gordon's report therefore, I would like to suggest that it is possible that the timing difference between corticogracile and corticocuneate inputs may be a reflexion of the differential organisation of cortical terminals within these two nuclei. As the details of this is unknown, it would not be unreasonable to suggest that considerable caution needs to be exercised in the interpretation of Dr Gordon's data.

References:

Valverde, F. (1966): Z. Zellforsch, 71, 297 - 363.

Zimmermann, E.A., W.W. Chambers and C.N. Liu (1964):
J. Comp. Neurol., 123, 301 - 324.

Gordon: I agree entirely that it is necessary to be extremely cautious about our particular interpretation, which is entirely hypothetical. It is true that we would expect the mean caliber of the fibers running to the two nuclei to be different: on the other hand the distribution of the latencies for antidromic responses of single fibers entering the two nuclei shows considerable overlap, so the difference in caliber might not be very obvious anatomically. Of course you are right that some part of the difference in timing of corticofugal actions may depend on the mechanisms in the individual nucleus.

CELLULAR MECHANISMS IN THE PARIETAL CORTEX IN ALERT MONKEY

J. HYVÄRINEN
Institute of Physiology, University of Helsinki, Finland

The thalamic projection to the parietal cortex is heaviest to Brodmann's area 3 in the anterior part of the primary somesthetic region (S I) [1] (see Fig. 1). Within S I the various cytoarchitectural regions (3, 1, 2 from anterior to posterior) project to each other [2] and further to Brodmann's area 5 in the posterior parietal association cortex [3]. The posterior parietal association regions (areas 5 and 7) receive cortico-cortical connections and some input from the posterior thalamic nuclei and the pulvinar [4, 5]. Whereas the primary somatosensory cortex in the anterior parietal lobe receives a heavy specific projection from the ventrobasal complex of the thalamus, such specific projection is lacking in the posterior parietal lobe traditionally designated as associative area.

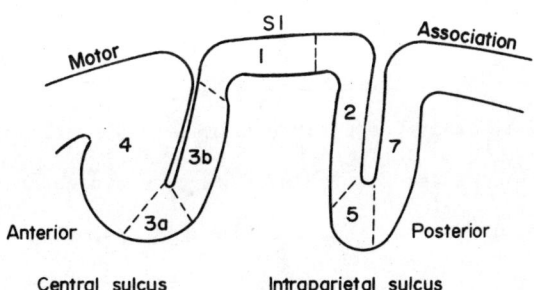

FIG. 1. An idealized sagittal section across the postcentral gyrus on the lateral level of the hand representation. The borders between the cytoarchitectural areas are gradual transitions.

On the basis of this anatomical arrangement the functions of the different parietal areas appear to differ not only in that the anterior part is the primary sensory cortex and the posterior part the associative cortex, but also perhaps in that there are differences in details of function between the various cytoarchitectural regions of S I. One suggestion would be that the anterior part of S I that receives the heaviest projection from the ventrobasal thalamus resembles the thalamus functionally and that a successive stepwise projection from one area to the next caudally within the parietal cortex would lead to a gradual buildup of the associative functions in the posterior parietal lobe. Such an assumption receives some support from the anatomical work of Jones and Powell and from previous studies on the functional types of cells found in anterior S I[6] and in area 5[7, 8]. If such a gradual change in the functional properties of the parietal lobe areas does take place in an antero-posterior succession, this should be discernible in the responses of cells recorded with microelectrodes in these regions. That is why the work reported here was done.

METHODS

A total of 856 cells were studied in the six cerebral hemispheres of three female stump-tailed monkeys (<u>Macaca speciosa</u>) weighing 4-5 kg. They were trained to sit, in a Faraday cage, in a primate chair designed for microelectrode studies. A cutaneous stimulator was positioned on their palms, and they were taught to detect the end of a vibratory stimulus by pressing a lever to obtain a juice reward. In other experiments cutaneous stimuli were applied manually, or the monkeys were allowed to move their arms and reach for objects such as raisins that were offered for them to eat. Recordings were started when the monkeys had become used to the situation and were co-operative. Recordings were made five to six times a week for four to five hours a day, first from one hemisphere and then from the other. In this way recordings from one animal could be extended to several months and the number of animals required was thus reduced. In the histological examination performed afterwards (see below), no distinct signs of damage to the cortex were detected in spite of the long recording periods. As a matter of fact the cortex, protected by the unopened dura, was in better shape than it would have been after an acute experiment with the dura open but covered with saline. To counteract infections in the wound around the recording cylinder and within the cylinder, antibiotics were administered perorally according to the results of resistance determinations of bacterial cultures, and the wounds were kept clean with iodine detergent.

For immobilization of the head during recording sessions, a halo fixation device was used like that employed in human surgery for stabilization of the neck and face[9, 10, 11]. The halo was inserted under intravenous pentobarbital anaesthesia and left in place for the duration of study of each hemisphere.

For extracellular recording of action potentials from the cortical cells, an Evarts[12] type hydraulic micromanipulator base cylinder was implanted under general anaesthesia in the skull above the target area. A burr hole was made but the dura mater was left intact. The day after the cylinder was implanted recordings were started with a transdural mapping of the structures located within it. Metal microelectrodes prepared from platinum-iridum[12, 13, 14] or tungsten[15] and insulated with glass were used. Such electrodes successfully recorded single units in spite of a gradual toughening of the dura during the experiments. Conventional AC-coupled amplification was used to display the discharges on an oscilloscope, to monitor them through a loudspeaker, and to record them on tape. The duration of daily recording was determined by the monkey's co-operativeness, usually four to five hours. The electrode was then withdrawn without making a lesion and the hydraulic manipulator was replaced by a cap which closed the base cylinder, and the monkey was released to its cage.

When the recordings from one hemisphere were completed, a steel electrode was lowered intracortically to points determined with the help of the coordinate system of the Evarts' drive. Iron, that was later stained histologically [16] was electrically deposited from this electrode. After the monkey had been killed with an overdose of intravenous pentobarbital, the brain was perfused first with physiological saline and then with 10 per cent formalin, dissected free and kept in formalin for two to three weeks. Blocks were then cut of the areas studied, and a histological reconstruction of the sites of penetration was accomplished with the help of the known coordinates of the microelectrode penetrations and the iron marks. Since we did not make lesions with the recording electrode, the histological localization of the units given in Table 1 are approximate. The region marked Anterior S I corresponds to the approximate extent of area 3 b, the one marked Central S I to the approximate extent of area 1, and the one marked Posterior S I to the approximate extent of area 2 [17]. In the latter, some units may be included from area 5, since it is difficult to determine the border between these two areas on this level of laterality.

The observations on the cellular responses were documented either on film or as response histograms constructed with the aid of a μ-Linc-computer from data taken on FM-tape. For such analyses the manually presented stimuli were repeated many times, timed by indicator lamps in the timing logic of the data collections system. Usually two different types of stimuli were presented alternately, and the response histograms were constructed separately from the responses to the two types of stimuli.

PRIMARY SOMATOSENSORY CORTEX

Our studies were limited to the hand and face areas in S I. In the anterior part of the primary somatosensory cortex (Brodmann's area 3 b) most cells have simple properties and respond well to any type of cutaneous stimulus on their receptive fields. The receptive fields are small and distinct, often extending only to a portion of a phalanx of a finger. When the electrode moves down in the caudal lip of the central sulcus the receptive fields change in small steps that indicate movement from one cortical column to another [18]. Furthermore when the electrode does not remain in one column during one penetration the groups of cells encountered and the background hash may move stepwise within a relatively small area such as one finger. During downward penetrations such changes occur at some 200- to 1 000-micron intervals which gives a rough idea about the size of the diameters of the cortical columns in this region.

The different types of modalities within the cutaneous sense appear to be segregated in different columns. Some cell groups are slowly adapting and give sustained responses, whereas the majority are rapidly adapting. In area 3 b the rapidly adapting cutaneous cells follow nicely the time course of peripheral cutaneous stimuli such as vibration [6]. Periodicity that matches the vibration period is easily elicited in this part of S I in the rapidly adapting cells. In the paradigm that we used for rewarding the animals, they knew from a light signal whether they would be rewarded for responding correctly to the vibratory stimulus. If a yellow light was on, a correct response within a short reaction time would give them fruit juice; if a red light was on no reward was given. Thus the monkeys were alert and attentive to the stimulus while the yellow light was on. However, in this part of the cortex such changes in the attentive behaviour of the animal seemed to have no influence on most of the cells (Fig. 2). The responses were identical under all conditions. Exceptions to this invariance of the responses were few.

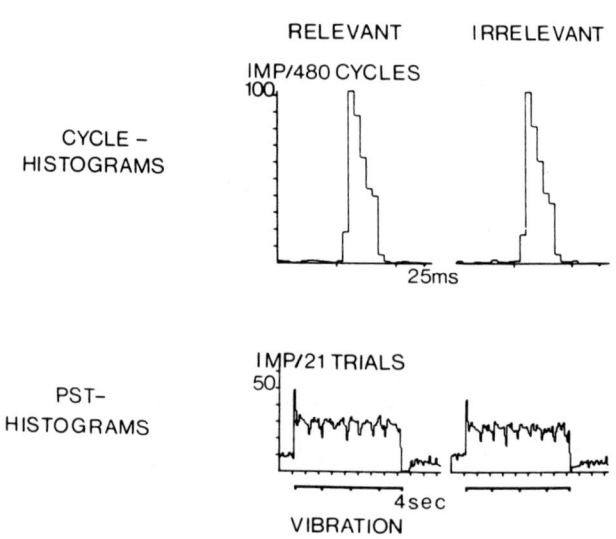

FIG. 2. Responses to vibration of a rapidly adapting cutaneous neuron in area 3. The receptive field was on the glabrous skin of the distal phalanx of the forefinger. There is no difference between the attentive state (relevent) when the monkey responded 100 % correctly to the end of vibration and the nonattentive state (irrelevant) when the monkey did not respond. Vibration 40 Hz, 370 µ p-p (from [31] with permission of the publisher).

When the recording electrode is moved backward along the somatosensory region, an increasing number of cells are found that are not as easy to activate as are those in the anterior part. At the same time the receptive fields tend to increase in size and the thresholds to cutaneous stimulation increase. In many of these cells we got no responses with the type of stimulation that is effective in the anterior part of S I, a light touch on the receptive field nor with stronger pressure on it. To find out whether these cells are simply unresponsive or whether they respond to other types of sensory stimuli, we tried to activate them with movement along the skin, by placing different types of objects on the skin and by letting the animal explore actively with his hands. In several cells unresponsive to simple cutaneous indentation we did elicit a response with these stimuli. Of course this does not mean that the cells responsive to skin indentation would not also respond to these more complex types of stimuli. More meaningful, however, is the fact that the cells unresponsive to simple skin indentation were often responsive to the more complex skin stimuli.

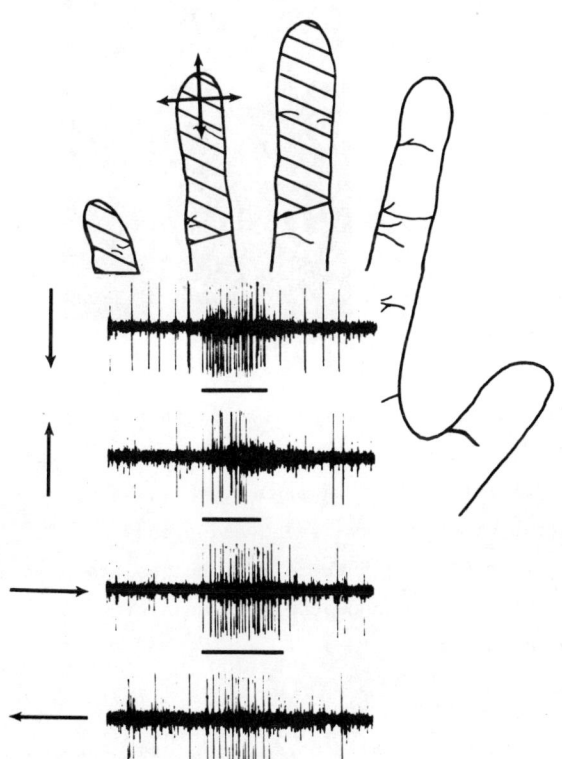

FIG. 3. Responses from a cell recorded in the left area 2. The receptive field (hatched) was the distal volar surface of the third, fourth and fifth fingers. Movement of a small metal probe tip in various directions gave good responses but no responses were seen to skin indentation.

Figure 3 shows an example of a cell that did not respond to punctate stimulation on the receptive field but that did respond well to movement along the skin. This cell was located in Brodmann's area 2. In this case the direction of movement was not critical for the activation of the cell; all directions were equally effective.

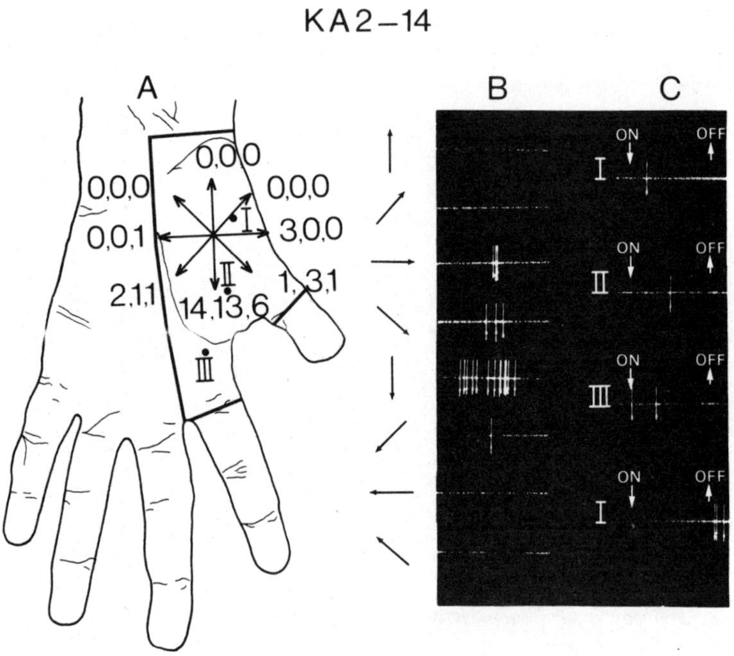

KA2-14

FIG. 4. An example of a directionally selective neuron in the right area 1. (A) shows the receptive field. In (C) punctate stimuli were applied to points I, II, III and I again. (B) shows responses to a manually held stimulating probe moving in various directions with the same speed and pressure. The duration of each record is 2 sec. In (A) the numbers of impulses are plotted for various directions of movement on three consecutive rounds of stimuli (from [32] with permission of the publisher).

For other cells, however, the direction of movement was critical. Figure 4 shows an example of such a cell. In this cell only stimulation from proximal to distal was effective, whereas movement in the opposite direction produced no response. This cell, recorded in Brodmann's area 1, appeared related to the cutaneous rapidly adapting receptors but, as shown in the figure, it was not excited by punctate stimulation on the receptive field. Such cells are not rare in areas 1 and 2. They have also been described by Whitsel et al.[19], who showed that such cells do not exist in the peripheral nerve and are therefore the result of processing in the brain.

Some cutaneous cells were not excited by indenting or moving skin stimulation. In some of these cells we found that edges placed on the receptive field in a particular orientation were effective in activating them. Figure 5 shows an example of such a cell recorded in Brodmann's area 2.

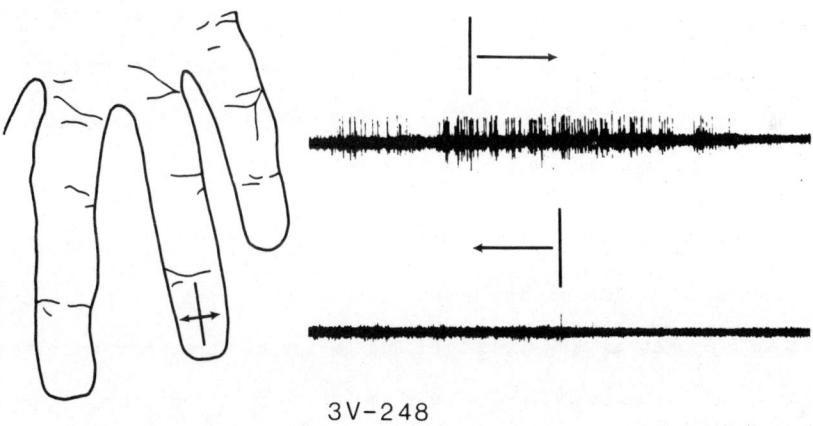

FIG. 5. Responses of a cell recorded in the left area 2. The receptive field was on the distal phalanx of the right 4th finger. The cell was unresponsive to skin indentation and to movement of a small circular probe tip but it did respond to movement of a metal edge in the ulnar direction.

Cells related to the deep modalities, i.e. joints, tendons, fascias and muscles, are interspersed between the cutaneous cell groups within S I. The densest representation of muscle nerves is known to be in area 3 a [20], and it is likely that these cells, too, project backward to the posterior S I and association cortex. For the joint neurons in the posterior part of S I we have found that they can be activated from several joints, for example from the same interphalangeal joint in several fingers. Thus, their receptive fields tend to be larger in the posterior S I than in the anterior, just as are the receptive fields of the cutaneous cells. Furhtermore, in the posterior S I it is not uncommon to observe that a cell can be activated from both skin and joint stimulation. Thus there is some convergence of input from different somatosensory submodalities within the posterior part of S I.

In our material the number of pure joint neurons is small in all parts of S I and the increase in their number toward the posterior noted by previous workers is not conspicuous [18, 21]. This discrepancy might be related to the behavioural state of the animal and reflects our observation that modalities in the posterior S I converge. Here the joint neurons may not be pure joint neurons but may respond to other input as well.

The above studies and considerations take into account all the submodalities of the somatosensory system. Yet we are left with a fairly large proportion of cells in S I that do not appear related to any of these submodalities, not at least if the stimulation is passive (group 5 in Table I). In some preliminary experiments we observed that part of the units that we cannot reliably activate with passive somesthetic stimulation are active during the monkey's self-initiated somatic exploration. It is a difficult task to verify quantitatively the role of active exploration in the responses of such cells, because during active exploratory movement a precise control of the sensory stimulation is difficult. All the cells that are activated by passive skin stimulation, such as simple indentation of the skin, are of course active during exploratory motor behaviour. They alone would already signal a significant amount of information during active exploration. However, for sensory analysis it may be necessary to combine such peripheral information with knowledge of the actions performed during manipulation. Such knowledge of the actions could arrive from deep receptors, notably muscle spindles, or from structures within the central nervous system. In the latter case they would represent the classical concept of corollary discharge. Our preliminary observations suggest that a representation of the corollary discharge might be present in the somatosensory cortex. However, the relation of the cellular responses to self-initiated active exploration is far more pronounced in the posterior parietal association cortex as indicated below.

ASSOCIATIVE AREAS

On the level of laterality of hand and face areas in S I, area 5 occupies very little tissue and is difficult to separate from area 2 on the basis of cytoarchitectural features. We have not studied area 5 but, because of the difficulty in separating area 2 from area 5 at this region, a few of the cells reported above from area 2 may in fact be in a transitional zone between areas 2 and 5. Previous workers have recorded convergence of joint input in area 5 [7] and also convergence of joint and skin inputs [8]. The cutaneous neurons observed by Sakata et al. [8] in area 5 were largely of the directionally selective type. This was recently confirmed by Mountcastle et al. [23].

We have focused our recordings in the parietal association cortex on Brodmann's area 7 (see Fig. 1). The cutaneous modality is not richly represented here, but the cells activated by cutaneous stimuli in this region are interrelated in a particular way to the other modalities represented in this region, namely kinesthesia and vision. We do not find any cells in this region that would be activated like the simple skin cells in the anterior part of S I. Most cutaneous cells require moving stimuli along the skin and many of them are directionally selective. However, a more conspicuous feature in them is a convergence of other modalities, notably vision, into the same cells. Furthermore, there is often some spatial correlation between the cutaneous receptive field and the region in the visual space that activates the cells of area 7. Prior to our work the nature of the visual activation in the neurons of the posterior parietal association cortex had not been demonstrated. Thus our first observations in this region came as a surprise. I quote from Hyvärinen and Poranen [24]: "Cutaneous activation from the contralateral side of the face was an effective stimulus for some area 7 cells, but they sometimes discharged action potentials before their receptive fields had been touched. This ´anticipatory activation´ was abolished when the animal was prevented from seeing the approaching stimulus. As long as vision was blocked only tactile stimuli to the cutaneous receptive field discharged such cortical cells. Thus we concluded that visual activation was capable of driving the cells in area 7. Light stimuli flashing on or off at a distance did not discharge these cells, nor did contoured stimuli approaching from the other side of the face (contralateral to the cutaneous receptive field). It therefore seemed that the visual stimulus had to emerge in a location close to the cutaneous receptive field of the cell."

A large group of cells that we observed in area 7 is related to manual reaching, tracking and manipulation. Most of these cells are related to the opposite hand or to a direction on the contralateral side of the animal. Some of these cells are activated when the arm is extended toward an object, whereas others are activated during the fine finger movements which occur when an object is manipulated. For the latter the contralateral hand is usually effective but occasionally cells are found which are activated from the ipsilateral hand or during similar movement in either hand. It was not possible to relate the discharge to the movement of any single joint or to the tension of any single muscle but rather the discharge was related to the total pattern of movement.

Another common cell type in area 7 was related to visual stimuli and eye movements. Several of these cells were specific to the location of the visual stimuli in the space around the animal or to the direction of eye movements. In visually activated cells we often noted that only stimuli presented close to the animal, within its reach, activated the cells. Spontaneous eye movements not aimed at targets did not activate the cells that were activated by pursuit eye movements. It was often difficult to specify whether the activity was related to the introduction of a visual stimulus in the correct location, to the monkey's subsequent eye movement toward that target, or to mere looking (fixation) at that target.

A smaller group of cells (6 per cent of 193 cells studied in area 7) was related to cutaneous and visual activity. An illustrative, albeit rare, example in a cell with a cutaneous receptive field on the right arm was described in our original report [24] from which I quote: "To study this receptive field in detail, we fixed the arm with leather straps into a handholder and illuminated the arm with a spotlight. During the study of this cell the monkey was seated in a booth from which it could see its own arms projecting through openings out of the booth, but not into the laboratory. Examining the right arm we noticed that the cell discharged when shadows passed across the receptive field in the arm. The monkey was unable to see the moving objects giving rise to the shadows but it could observe the changes in illumination over its arm. Thus a brisk cellular discharge could be repeatedly elicited by shadows moving over the illuminated cutaneous receptive field in the right arm but nowhere else."

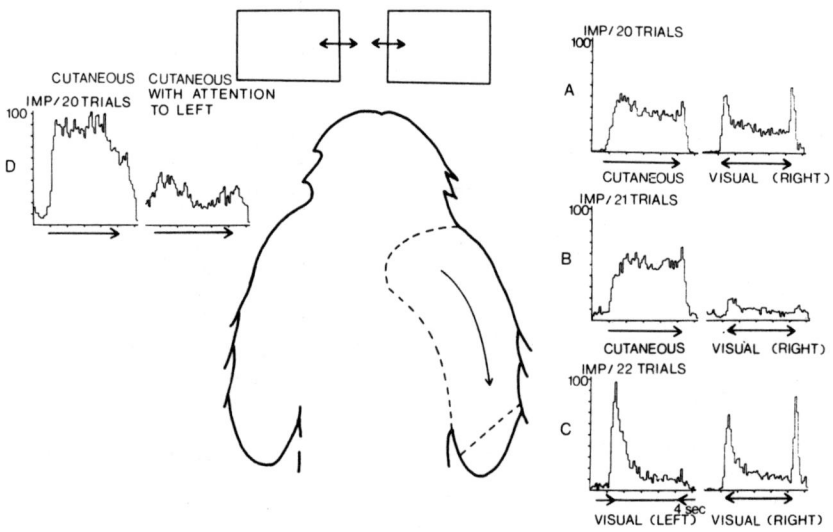

FIG. 6. Response histograms of a cell in the left area 7. (A) Responses to alternating cutaneous stimuli moving distally over the right shoulder and to visual stimuli consisting of a white card brought rapidly into the visual field from the right (on-response), then kept in place (sustained response), and rapidly withdrawn to the right (off-response). (B) Same as (A) but with vision almost totally obstructed. (C) Responses to alternating presentations of white cards from the left and from the right. (D) Responses to cutaneous stimuli moving distally over the right shoulder. During every other cutaneous stimulus orange juice was offered from the left. Visual attention to the left caused a decrease in the cutaneous response. (Reproduced from [24] with permission of the publisher.)

Figure 6 shows an example of a cell activated both cutaneously and visually[24]. The cutaneous receptive field was in the region of the right shoulder and a brisk response was elicited by a movement over this field in the distal direction. Cutaneous movement in the proximal direction did not elicit a response. A white card introduced into the visual field was also an effective stimulus (A) and obstruction of vision (B) blocked this but not the cutaneous response. Withdrawal of a white card from the visual field to the left elicited no response, whereas withdrawal to the right elicited a response (C). That attention toward another object could inhibit the cutaneous response in this cell was demonstrated (D) by offering the monkey, on alternate trials, a spoon from which it could lick orange juice by stretching out its tongue. While the monkey looked to the left and concentrated on this task, the cutaneous response to a stimulus moving over the right shoulder was clearly diminished when compared with the response to the same stimulus evoked when there were no distractions.

Most commonly the cells in area 7 were activated contralaterally (54 % of 193 cells), whereas 7 per cent were activated by stimuli related to the ipsilateral side. Similar cells were encountered in groups, and therefore this region appears to be arranged in columns as are the other cortical areas.

TABLE I. THE DISTRIBUTION OF 856 CELLS STUDIED IN THE PARIETAL CORTEX

Region	Anterior S I	Central S I	Posterior S I	Association
1. Simple skin	69 %	63 %	42 %	0 %
2. Complex skin	3 %	6 %	12 %	0 %
3. Simple deep	9 %	6 %	10 %	1 %
4. Modality convergence	7 %	12 %	19 %	73 %
5. Other	12 %	13 %	17 %	26 %
Total number	113	273	277	193

CONCLUDING DISCUSSION

The problem posed in the introduction concerned the possibility that some sequential processing occurs within the parietal lobe and that part of this processing already takes place within the primary somatosensory cortex before its output is sent to the associative regions. In this series of experiments we find some evidence for this principle. Table I shows that the number of cells activated with simple skin indentation decreases posteriorly within S I, and that a corresponding increase in the number of more complex cells occurs at the same time. A similar increase toward posterior is also observed in the convergence of submodalities. However, within S I the number of cells activated by simple skin indentation is considerable in all subdivisions. Such an increase in the complexity of the cellular properties posteriorly in S I is probably the result of intracortical processing within S I. The same tendency continues into the anterior part of the associative area, Brodmann's area 5, where cells are encountered that have large receptive fields and can be activated from different body regions and different modalities [7, 8]. One step further in the cortical processing pathway, in Brodmann's area 7, another modality, the visual, is added to the cortical processing. For the somatosensory input into area 7 there is the cortico-cortical route from S I to area 5 and further to area 7 [3]. It is more difficult to explain the anatomical pathway of the visual activation in this region since no direct visual projection to this region is known. Such a projection must arrive through a rather complex pathway. From area 7 the activity is relayed to the motor systems, the premotor areas and the pyramidal tract. In this way the sensory information can be used for the guidance of motor performance.

That the different cytoarchitectural areas of S I might have different roles in somatomotor behaviour has recently been shown by selective ablation of areas 3, 1 and 2 [25]. In those experiments ablation of area 3 impaired all somatosensory performance, whereas ablation of area 1 impaired most notably performance involving discrimination of texture, and ablation of area 2 performance involving discrimination of angles.

These results complement the clinical findings in man. Whereas lesions within the primary somatosensory cortex cause a sensory defect [26], those in the posterior parietal regions do not.

A distinctive feature of the unilateral posterior parietal syndrome is the inability of the patient to recognize somatic or visual stimuli opposite to the damaged side. After infliction of an unilateral posterior parietal lesion a sensory defect can only be demonstrated experimentally in a situation of rivalry between two similar stimuli, either somesthetic or visual, presented simultaneously in symmetric locations on the two sides. In such a situation only the one presented opposite to the healthy side will be recognized whereas the other one will pass unnoticed [27]. Thus in a lesion limited to the associative area, the defect is in the attention toward a stimulus rather than an absolute inability to recognize the stimuli.

In bilateral posterior parietal lesions in man defects are present in spatial orientation, in eye movements, in manual reaching, route finding, drawing, etc. [28, 29, 30]. These are functions that depend on the neural structures related to spatial perception and guidance of movements. The cells that we have observed in area 7 in the monkey are related precisely to these functions and may, thus, have counterparts in man.

ACKNOWLEDGEMENTS

The work reported here has been supported by the Foundations' Fund for

Research in Psychiatry and the National Research Council for Medical Sciences, Finland.

REFERENCES

1. Jones, E.G. and Powell, T.P.S., Brain 93, 37 (1970).
2. Jones, E.G. and Powell, T.P.S., Brain 92, 477 (1969).
3. Jones, E.G. and Powell, T.P.S., Brain 93, 793 (1970).
4. Graybiel, Ann M., In F.O. Schmitt and F.G. Worden (eds.), "The Neurosciences, Third Study Program", MIT Press Cambridge, Mass., p. 205 (1974).
5. Jones, E.G., In F.O. Schmitt and F.G. Worden (eds.), "The Neurosciences, Third Study Program," MIT Press Cambridge, Mass., p. 215 (1974).
6. Mountcastle, V.B., Talbot, W.H., Sakata, H. and Hyvärinen, J., J. Neurophysiol. 32, 452 (1969).
7. Duffy, F.H. and Burchfiel, J.L., Science 172, 273 (1971).
8. Sakata, H., Takaoka, Y., Kawarasaki, A. and Shibutani, H., Brain Res. 64, 85 (1973).
9. Perry, J. and Nickel, V.L., J. Bone and Joint Surgery 41-A, 37 (1959).
10. Prolo, D.J., Runnels, J.B. and Jameson, R.M., JAMA 224, 591 (1973).
11. Friendlich, A.R., J. appl. Physiol. 35, 934 (1973).
12. Evarts, E.V., In R.F. Rushmer (ed.) "Methods in Medical Research", Year Book Medical Publishers, Chicago, Ill. p. 241 (1966).
13. Wilska, A., Acta Soc. Med. fenn. "Duodecim", 22A, 63 (1940).
14. Wolbarsht, M.L., MacNichol, E.F. Jr. and Wagner, H.G., Science 132, 1309 (1960).
15. Hubel, D.H., Science 125, 549 (1957).
16. Marshall, W.H., Stain. Tech. 15, 133 (1940).
17. Powell, T.P.S. and Mountcastle, V.B., Bull Johns Hopkins Hosp. 105, 108 (1959).
18. Powell, T.P.S. and Mountcastle, V.B., Ibidem, p. 133.
19. Whitsel, B.L., Roppolo, J.R. and Werner, G., J. Neurophysiol. 35, 691 (1972).
20. Phillips, C.G., Powell, T.P.S. and Wiesendanger, M., J. Physiol. 217, 419 (1971).
21. Whitsel, B.L., Dreyer, D.A. and Roppolo, J.R., J. Neurophysiol. 34, 1018 (1971).
22. Porter, L. and Semmes, J., Exp. Neurol. 42, 206 (1974).
23. Mountcastle, V.B., Lynch, J.C., Georgopoulos, A., Sakata, H. and Acuna, C., J. Neurophysiol. 38, 871 (1975).

24. Hyvärinen, J. and Poranen, A., <u>Brain</u> 97, 673 (1974).
25. Randolph, M. and Semmes, J., <u>Brain Res</u>. 70, 55 (1974).
26. Russell, W.R., <u>Brain</u> 68, 19 (1945).
27. Denny-Brown, D., Meyer, J.S. and Horenstein, S., <u>Brain</u> 75, 433 (1952).
28. Holmes, G., <u>Brit. J. Ophthal</u>. 2, 449, 506 (1918).
29. Balint, R., <u>Monatschrift Psychiatr. Neurol</u>. 25, 51 (1909).
30. Hyvärinen, J., En "<u>Du Controle Moteur á l´Organization Gestuelle</u>", H. Hecaen et M. Jeannerod (eds.), Massion et Cie, Paris (1976).
31. Hyvärinen, J., Poranen, A. and Jokinen, Y., In "<u>The Neurosciences, Third Study Porgram</u>", F.O. Schmitt and F.G. Worden (eds.), Cambridge, Mass., MIT Press, p. 205 (1974).
32. Hyvärinen, J., Poranen, A., Jokinen, Y., Näätänen, R. and Linnankoski, I., In "<u>Somatosensory System</u>", H.H. Kornhuber (ed.), Stuttgart, Thieme (1975).

# THERMOCEPTION

RESPONSE OF CENTRAL TRIGEMINAL NEURONS TO CUTANEOUS THERMAL STIMULATION

D. A. POULOS and J. T. MOLT
Albany Medical College of Union University, Albany, New York 12208 U.S.A.

In the more than forty years since Dr. Zotterman's initial description of thermoreceptors innervating the tongue of the cat (35), peripheral trigeminal thermoreceptors have been studied extensively and their response characteristics described in considerable detail (6,12,14,15,26). It remains unclear, however, as to how the information provided by first-order thermoreceptors is processed and transmitted within the central nervous system. Three types of primary afferent neurons responsive to innocuous levels of thermal stimulation have been identified. Specific "warm" and "cold" fibers are found to innervate the skin in both primate and non-primate forms (12). Both warm and cold primary afferents display: 1) static firing rates over a range of constant temperatures; 2) dynamic rate increases to temperature changes in either the warming direction (warm receptors) or cooling direction (cold receptors); and 3) a relative insensitivity to mechanical stimulation. The third, and more controversial of the neuronal types, are afferents responsive to both mechanical and thermal (usually rapid cooling) stimulation of their receptive fields. The latter group, often described as behaving like slowly adapting Type II mechanoreceptors, are believed by most investigators not to play a role in thermal sensibility (12).

In this summary are described results obtained during studies of thermoreceptive neurons located within the central somatosensory pathway in monkeys and, for purposes of comparison, the cat. All of the findings are based on analysis of extracellular neural discharges obtained by microelectrode recording techniques in anesthetized animals.

Two cell types responsive to innocuous thermal stimuli have been identified and studied in the monkey. One type fits the description of specific cold afferents while the second was responsive to both cutaneous cooling and mechanical deformation of the same receptive field. In the cat medulla, we have found specific cold afferents, and more recently obtained preliminary data on neurons that fit the description of specific warm receptors. The medullary warm afferents had peripheral receptive fields within the 2nd trigeminal division, a region known to have a uniquely dense warm fiber population in the cat (14).

CONSTANT TEMPERATURE STIMULATION

Peripheral Trigeminal Thermoreceptor Input

Primary afferents studied in the gasserian ganglion (31,32) were found to be active over a temperature range of 17 to 41°C with static activity maxima occurring between 33 and 25°C (Fig. 1). Some differences in thermal sensitivity were seen within the population of neurons studied, however individual neurons had reproducible response functions irrespective of factors such as changes in body core temperature (Fig. 1) provided skin temperature remained constant.

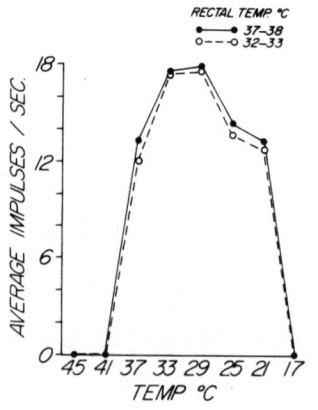

Fig. 1. Constant temperature response profile of a thermoreceptor recorded in monkey gasserian ganglion. Each point represents the averaged number of discharges during the last 90 sec of 3 min test periods. The unit was first studied under normothermic conditions (solid line) and the test repeated 40 min later following induction of hypothermia (dashed line).

Depending upon the rate, direction, and magnitude of a temperature change, several minutes may be required before an absolutely steady rate of firing to a new temperature is attained. The hysteresis seen in the primary afferent curves of Fig. 2 is due to the failure of complete adaptation after 3 min constant temperature stimulation following 4° changes in the warming and cooling direction.

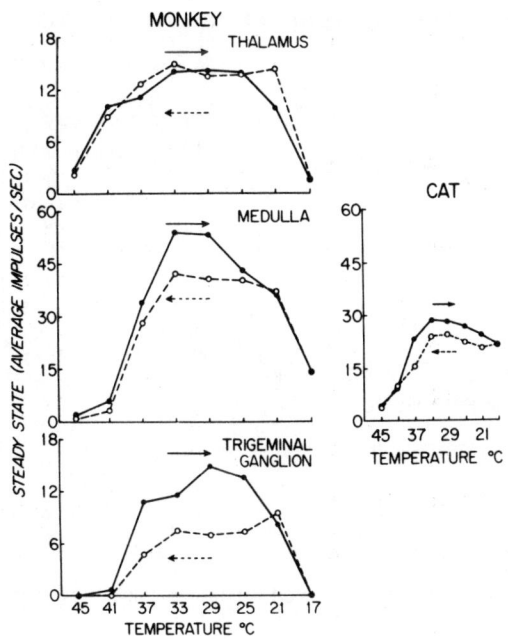

Fig. 2. Constant temperature response profiles of trigeminal neurons recorded at successive synaptic levels in the monkey and in the cat medulla. Each point represents the averaged number of discharges per sec recorded during the last 90 sec of 3 min test periods following changes in the cooling direction (solid line) and warming direction (dashed line).

Medulla

Monkey medullary neurons have static response profiles that are similar to those of primary afferents. Two differences that appear to exist are: 1) medullary units have increased discharge frequencies over much of the responsive temperature range, and 2) medullary units respond over a wider range of temperatures in that activity is seen at 17 and 41°C where primary afferent neurons are usually silent. An interesting comparison can be made with neurons recorded in the cat medulla (Figs 2 and 3). Cat medullary neurons behave much like those in the monkey, however they are responsive over a wider range of temperatures which is especially evident at colder temperatures where little supression of activity is seen at 17°C.

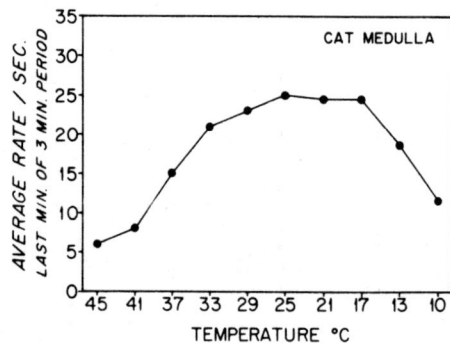

Fig. 3. Averaged constant temperature response profile obtained from 6 neurons recorded in cat medulla. Each point represents the average rate per sec during the last 60 sec of each 3 min test period. Compared with monkey, cat medullary neurons show greater activity over the colder temperature range.

Thalamus

Thalamic neurons responded to an even broader range of constant temperatures than did first and second-order trigeminal neurons in monkey (Fig. 2). In addition, thalamic neurons displayed activity that approached the steady state maxima (29°C in all units) over a broader range of temperatures, e.g., compared with first-order neurons the response profiles of thalamic units were less peaked although the temperature range that elicited rates approaching the steady state maxima did vary (30). Thalamic neurons displayed tonic discharge rates equivalent to those of first-order neurons and appeared to reach absolutely steady rates of firing more quickly following a temperature change (note the absence of a hysteresis in the Fig. 2 curves).

GROUPED DISCHARGE ACTIVITY

A general feature of all peripheral cold receptors and one especially prominent among primate thermoreceptors is the appearance of grouped discharge activity (15,27). That is, with progressively colder constant temperatures unit discharges occur more in groups (Fig. 4), separated by increasingly longer silent periods (Fig. 5). The grouped discharge activity of trigeminal thermoreceptors and speculations about the potential significance of such neuronal behavior are described in detail elsewhere (27). Grouped discharge activity has been observed in medullary recordings (Fig. 6) and there is some evidence for grouped discharge activity at the thalamic level. An evaluation of discharge grouping at the thalamic level is made difficult however by the presence of thalamic spindling activity seen in all thalamic neurons in the anesthetized preparation (Fig. 7).

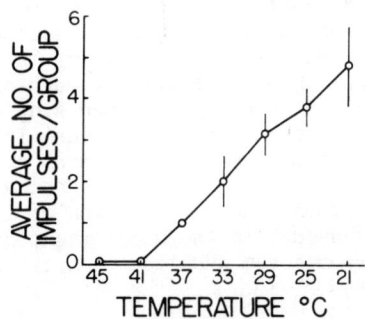

Fig. 4. Averaged number of spike discharges occurring in groups separated by silent periods as a function of steady-state temperature. Data obtained from seven peripheral trigeminal thermoreceptors recorded in monkey. Vertical lines indicate standard errors (SE) (from Poulos, 26).

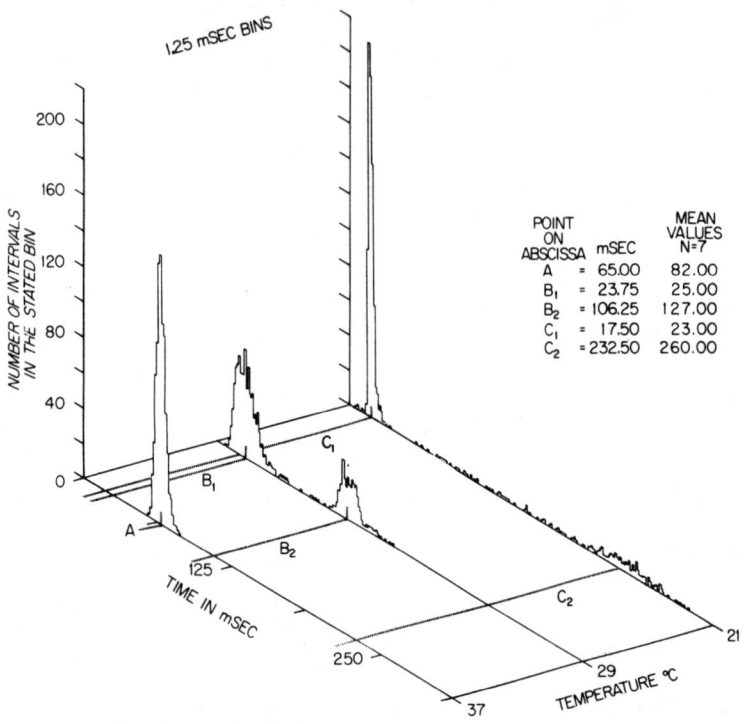

Fig. 5. Interspike interval histograms of a first-order trigeminal thermoreceptor recorded in monkey. The distribution of intervals shown were obtained during the last 90 sec of 10 min of stimulation with 37, 29, and 21°C stimuli. Abscissa: time in milliseconds, bins = 1.25 msec each. Ordinate: number of intervals occurring in each bin. Points on abscissa A to C_2 indicate mean interval for each distribution of interspike intervals. At 37°C the unit displayed single action potentials that occurred at fairly regular intervals (mean interval = 65 msec). At 29°C the unit fired in groupings (mean interval = 23.75 msec) separated by silent periods (mean interval = 106 msec) and at 21°C the number of impulses occurring in groups and the duration of silent periods between groupings further increased. In the upper right are shown comparable mean values obtained from seven additional units (from Poulos, 26).

TEMPERATURE CHANGE STIMULATION

Peripheral Trigeminal Thermoreceptor Input

The dynamic response of the two first-order neuronal types found to be sensitive to rapid temperature changes in monkey are shown in Fig. 8 and may be summarized as follows: (1) The averaged thermoreceptor response to the

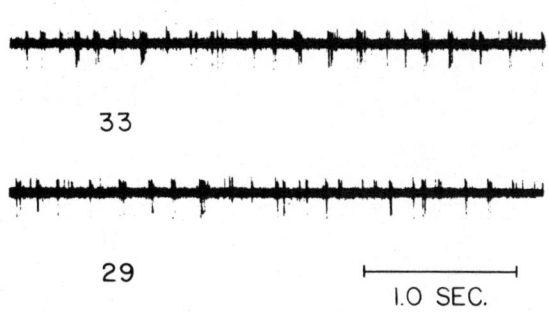

Fig. 6. Records obtained from a medullary trigeminal thermoreceptor in monkey showing grouped discharge activity during constant temperature stimulation at 33 and 29°C (from Poulos, 28).

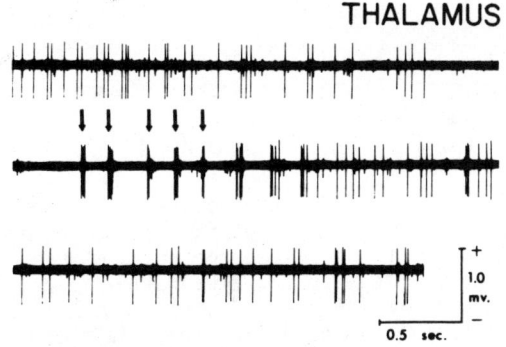

Fig. 7. Record from a monkey thalamic trigeminal thermoreceptor responding during a 29°C constant temperature stimulus. Arrows indicate typical bursting activity attributed to thalamic spindling (from Poulos and Benjamin, 30).

first sec of cooling showed a progressive increase with increased cooling over only a limited range, e.g., from 35 to 27°C. Further cooling (27 to 15°C) did not elicit activity significantly different from that seen at 27°C. By contrast, thermal plus mechanical units showed progressive first sec response increases over the entire range of 35 to 15°C. (2) The average thermoreceptor response to cooling during sec 2 to 5 formed nonmonotonic functions. They reached peak values at 25 to 23°C, and declined steadily with further increases in stimulus intensity. Unlike the thermoreceptors, thermal plus mechanical units continued to show rate increases during sec 2 to 5 that were related to increasing stimulus magnitudes. (3) Temperature changes in the warm direction produced rate decreases in both unit types.

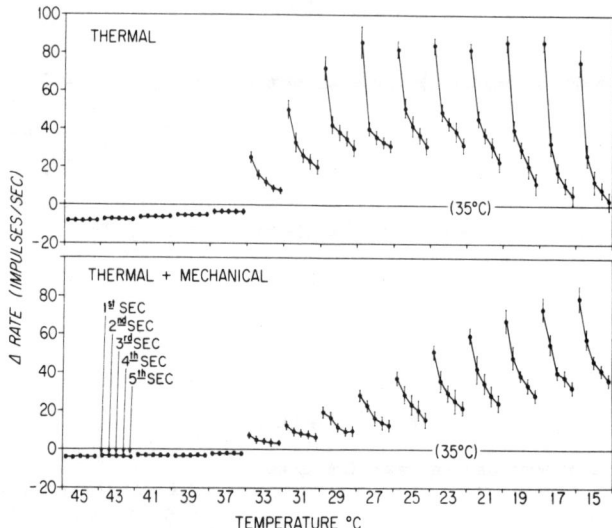

Fig. 8. Dynamic response functions relating the change in rate of discharge to the magnitude and direction of temperature change. Each point represents the difference in discharge rate between a 35°C standard (zero on the ordinate) and the rate following rapid temperature changes. Rate differences are given for each sec of the initial 5 sec of the response. Pooled data are from sixteen thermoreceptors and seven thermal plus mechanical units recorded in monkey gasserian ganglion. Standard errors are indicated by vertical lines through each point. (from Poulos and Lende, 32).

(4) The magnitude of thermoreceptor responses were greater than those of thermal plus mechanical units for small temperature changes. However, the thermal plus mechanical unit responses were equivalent to those of thermoreceptors over the colder temperature range.

While there were some observed differences in thermal sensitivity within the population of specific thermoreceptors studied, all responded to small thermal changes (less than 0.5°C) and all appeared capable of providing information on temperature change over only a limited range (32). When compared with thermal plus mechanical neurons, the latter behaved like higher threshold thermoreceptors, yet their response profiles better approximated that of an "absolute thermometer" over the entire range of cooling stimuli tested.

Medulla

Records of temperature change responses obtained from a medullary thermoreceptor in monkey are reproduced in Fig. 9. The more dynamic aspect of the unit response that occurs during the first sec following rapid cooling is masked by the 5 sec analysis times represented in Fig. 7. Note however, the general supression of activity seen over the lower range of temperatures. The reduction in thermoreceptor activity resulting from increased cooling intensities can more readily be seen in Fig. 10 where the initial 5 sec of the responses are shown.

In the previous description of thermoreceptor responses to temperatures held constant, it was shown that cat medullary neurons appeared to respond over a colder range of temperatures than did their counterparts in the monkey. A similar result is obtained in response to rapid cooling. By comparing the dynamic response functions shown in Fig. 11 with those of the upper curve of Fig. 8, it may be seen that while the first sec response profiles do not differ appreciably (see also Fig. 12), cat neurons do appear to maintain higher firing rates (during sec 2-5) over the colder temperature range. Had the units been tested at temperatures below 15°C, a more obvious difference in dynamic sensitivity would be predicted. Nevertheless, the general temperature change response characteristics of primate and cat trigeminal thermoreceptors do not differ significantly.

Thalamus

The overall response characteristics of thalamic neurons to rapid temperature change did not differ appreciably from those described for first-order trigeminal neurons. There were, however, differences in the duration of

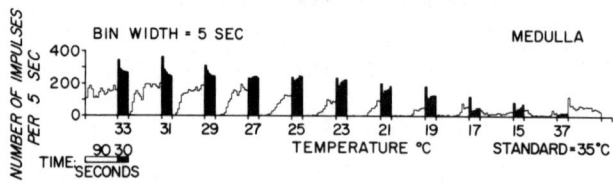

Fig. 9. Rate function of a thermoreceptor (recorded in monkey medulla) to a temperature change sequence. Solid bars indicate rates during 30 sec test stimulus periods and open bars response rates during 90 sec 35°C standard stimulus periods. The height of each bar represents the total number of spikes for a 5 sec interval.

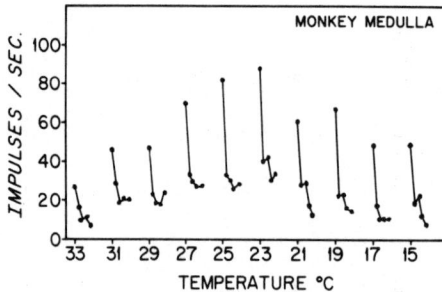

Fig. 10. Dynamic response of a thermoreceptor to steplike temperature changes below a 35°C standard. Data are plotted for sec 1-5 following each cooling stimulus.

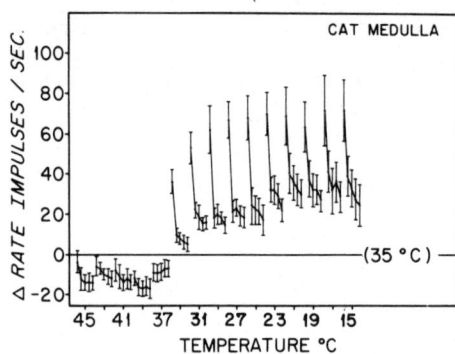

Fig. 11. Averaged dynamic response functions obtained from seven thermoreceptors recorded in cat medulla (see Fig. 8).

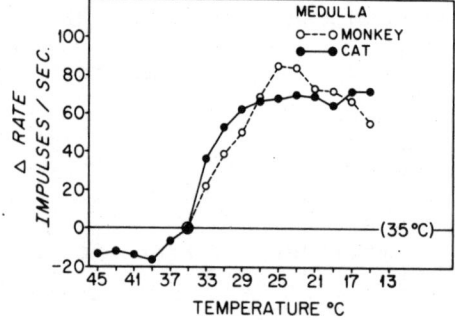

Fig. 12. Averaged curves showing dynamic responses during initial sec following temperature changes (see Fig. 8). Averaged curve for cat taken from Fig. 11 data. Averaged curve for monkey is based on results obtained from two neurons.

phasic rate changes that may be of some significance.

Rate functions of the response of thermal and thermal plus mechanical units recorded in the ventrobasal complex of the monkey thalamus are reproduced in Fig. 13. A summary of the results obtained in the thalamus is as follows: (1) Both thermal and thermal plus mechanical units had dynamic rate increases to rapid cooling. As in the periphery, thermal plus mechanical neurons had dynamic response increases that were proportional to stimulus intensity over the entire range of cooling. Thalamic thermoreceptors had dynamic response functions to cooling characterized by a "best temperature" within the range of 31 to 21°C (the range of "best temperatures" observed in the periphery was 29 to 23°C). (2) The effect of increased warming on thalamic thermal units was a progressive suppression of activity. Unlike peripheral thermoreceptors, thalamic neurons were never completely silenced by warming stimuli, nor was a post excitatory suppression of activity seen

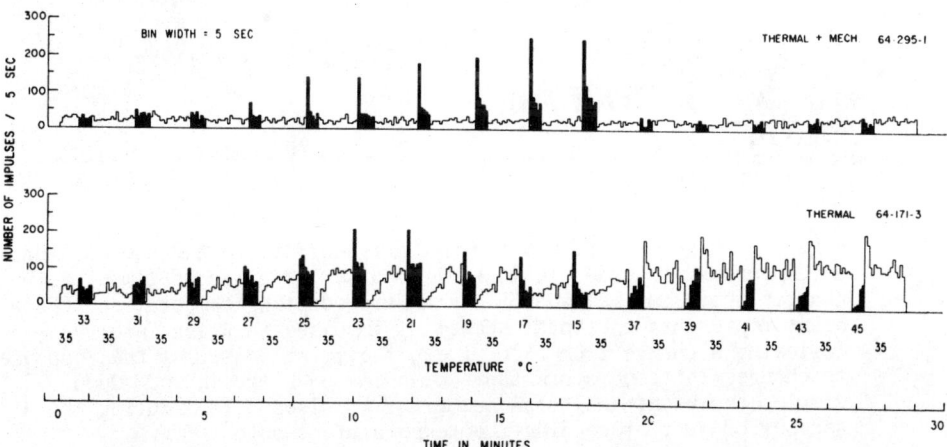

Fig. 13. Rate functions of typical thermal (lower record) and thermal plus mechanical (upper record) units for complete temperature change sequences. Solid bars indicate rates during the 30-sec test stimulus periods and open bars response rates during the 90-sec 35°C standard stimulus periods. The height of each bar represents the total number of spikes for a 5-sec interval. (from Poulos and Benjamin, 30).

in response to colder temperatures as was invariably seen in peripheral thermoreceptors. Indeed, it appeared as if the primary afferent input only transiently modified the ongoing temperature dependent rate of thalamic thermal neurons (Fig. 14).

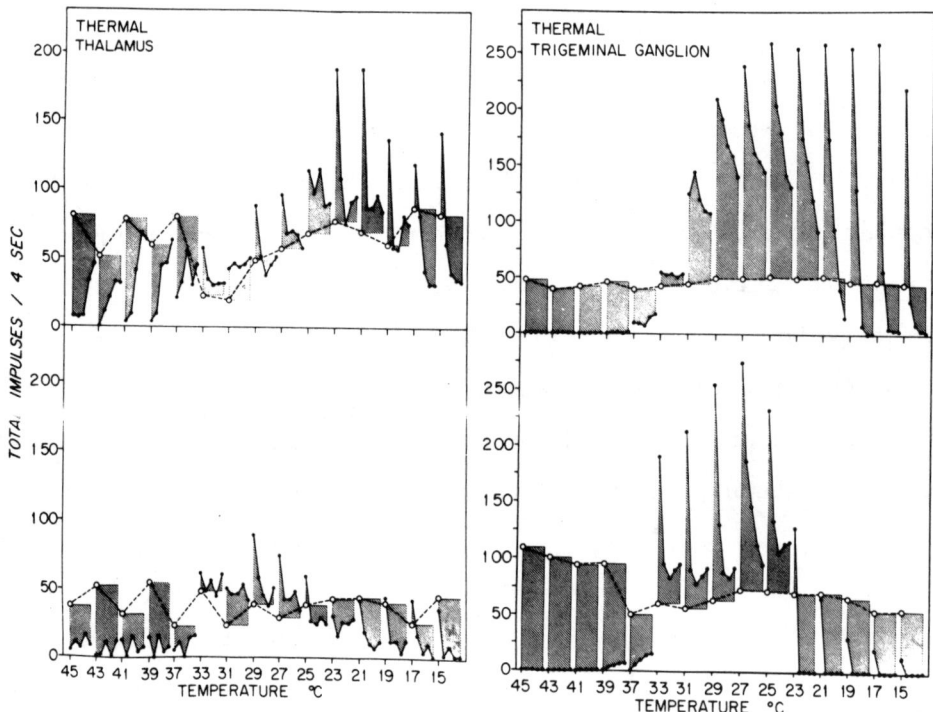

Fig. 14. Responses of two thermal first-order and two thermal thalamic neurons (recorded in monkey) to a series of rapid temperature changes above and below a 35°C standard adapting temperature. Each point represents the total number of impulses in 4 sec intervals following a change from 35°C, i.e., the first 20 sec of the responses to changes in temperature above or below 35°C are shown. Open circles represent the total number of impulses at 35° during the 4 sec period just preceeding the temperature change.

In summary, the dynamic response profiles of trigeminal neurons to rapid temperature changes do not appreciably differ when examined at successive synaptic levels between periphery and thalamus (Fig. 15). Thermal units are particularly sensitive to small thermal changes and show dynamic rate increases to increasing stimulus intensities over a limited portion of the physiological temperature range. Thermal plus mechanical neurons are relatively insensitive to small thermal changes yet respond linearly over the range of cooler temperatures.

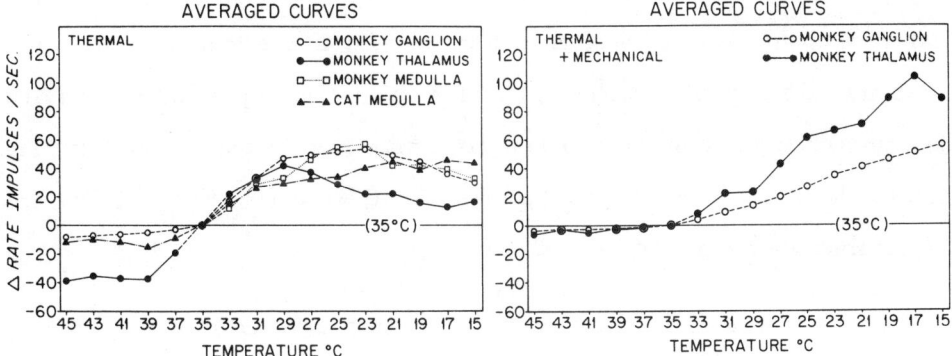

Fig. 15. Averaged curves. Composite graphs showing the change in rate of discharge as a function of the magnitude and direction of temperature change. Data points for monkey ganglion, monkey medulla, and cat medulla represent differences in the mean number of impulses during the initial 4 sec of the stimulus (see Fig. 8). The thalamus curves are based on differences in the total number of impulses during the initial 4 sec of the stimulus. The number of units (n) from which each curve was constructed is: monkey ganglion thermal n = 16; monkey ganglion thermal + mechanical n = 7; monkey medulla thermal n = 2; cat medulla thermal n = 7; monkey thalamus thermal n = 6; monkey thalamus thermal + mechanical n = 9.

CONVERGENCE AND FEATURE EXTRACTION IN THE CNS

The centrally located thermoreceptive afferents described in the preceeding sections demonstrate a rather secure synaptic connection with the periphery. That is to say, the thermal response properties of central neurons did not differ appreciably from those of primary afferent fibers. In addition, central convergence was not evident in that thermal units had single peripheral receptive fields (less than 1 to 2 mm^2) at all synaptic levels studied.

In the cat medulla (unpublished observations) some specific thermoreceptive neurons were found to respond principally to either the dynamic or tonic aspect of thermal stimuli but not both. Some neurons gave only phasic responses to rapid temperature changes in the cooling direction and did not maintain activity to temperatures held constant. The dynamic response profiles of these units did not differ from those previously described. (Similar results are reported by Iggo and Ramsey (17) in the spinal cord). The discharge activity of a second class of medullary neurons could be modified by constant temperature stimuli but was minimally affected by rapid cooling. Again, the steady state response profiles of these cells did not differ from those previously described.

It is perhaps unusual that all of the cells that appeared to extract only certain features of the primary afferent input were found within the central representation of the maxillary division. We have not encountered similar neuronal types in the cat mandibular division nor have similar observations been made in the monkey.

Evidence clearly demonstrating central convergence of thermoreceptive afferents has also been obtained in studies of the cat medulla (unpublished observations). Several neurons studied had two discrete peripheral receptive fields as disparate as the ipsilateral edge of the tongue and the immediately adjacent lip. In the latter case, the tongue could be reflected and the fields easily tested independently. Similar observations have not been made within the monkey CNS, nor have we found central convergence of bilateral receptive fields as reported for the rat scrotum (11).

OTHER NEURONAL TYPES RESPONSIVE TO INNOCUOUS CUTANEOUS THERMAL STIMULATION

Warm Receptors

Specific warm receptors have not been encountered in our studies of the monkey trigeminal pathway. This negative finding is not unusual since, with the exception of neurons innervating highly specialized receptive fields, e.g., the rat scrotum (8-11), warm receptors have been particularly elusive in studies of the CNS.

In recent studies of the cat medulla (Molt and Poulos, unpublished observations), units were found that displayed tonic activity over a range of 29 to 45°C with steady state maxima occurring at about 41°C. These units were silent at 48 and 25°C. Small temperature changes applied in the warming direction produced rate increases, and in the cooling direction, rate decreases, i.e., they fulfilled the requirements of warm receptors (12). Action potentials thus far recorded from such units have been of sufficiently low amplitude to preclude good electrophysiological isolation. The warm unit results are therefore preliminary. We have not for example, satisfactorily established that recordings were indeed obtained from second-order neural elements and not incoming primary afferent fibers. In addition, these observations were limited to units whose peripheral receptive fields were located within the cat nasal region which perhaps makes them unique (14).

Mechanoreceptors

Within the CNS of both cats and monkeys were found a variety of low threshold mechanoreceptive neurons that gave some response to thermal stimulation of their peripheral receptive fields e.g., receptors associated with vibrissae, teeth, cornea, and glabrous skin. However, these receptors gave only meager thermal responses (when compared with their mechanical sensitivities) and are not the type we referred to as thermal plus mechanical or T+M units (30,32). T+M units found in the monkey trigeminal system did not behave like low threshold mechanoreceptors (they could not for example, be activated by slight movements of the thermal stimulator) and they responded equally well to optimal thermal (rapid cooling from 35 to 15°C) and mechanical stimulations (usually moderate pressure or stretch).

ANATOMICAL LOCATION OF TRIGEMINAL THERMORECEPTORS

The functional anatomical organization of the trigeminal system has been a particular concern of neurological surgeons, especially as it relates to surgical intervention for the relief of trigeminal pain. It has been assumed for example, that following partial trigeminal root section the resulting reduction in pain and often seen concomitant decrease in thermal sensibility (while maintaining "normal" tactile sensibility) is due to the selective cutting of anatomically segregated pain and temperature fibers. Experimental evidence obtained in monkeys does not support a functional segregation of trigeminal pain and temperature afferents and it is unlikely that it occurs in man (29). With the possible exception of the medulla, we have not encountered an anatomical region within the trigeminal system of monkeys that appears devoted to subserving a temperature function. In the trigeminal ganglion and root, it was found that thermal and mechanoreceptive afferents innervating a particular field such as the lip, or tongue, were intermingled (21). Similar results were obtained in studies of the thalamic trigeminal representation (30).

In the trigeminal spinal nucleus of both cats and monkeys we have frequently found specific thermoreceptors to be intermingled with light tactile mechanoreceptors innervating adjacent peripheral fields. The region of special interest however, is the dorsal margin of spinal V where we have encountered a relatively dense population of neural elements excited by cutaneous cooling (Fig. 16) and occasionally, innocuous warming. In this same region we have found neurons that are only activated by nociceptive levels of heating (48-60°C) and, at times, extreme cooling (application of ice water following heating to 45°C). The finding that thermoreceptors and neurons specifically responsive to nociceptive levels of thermal stimulation may be found within the superficial zone of spinal V agrees with observations made by Mosso and Kruger (24) and is especially intriguing when considering the location of nociceptive afferents within the superficial margin of the dorsal horn in cat lumbar spinal cord as reported by Christensen and Perl (3).

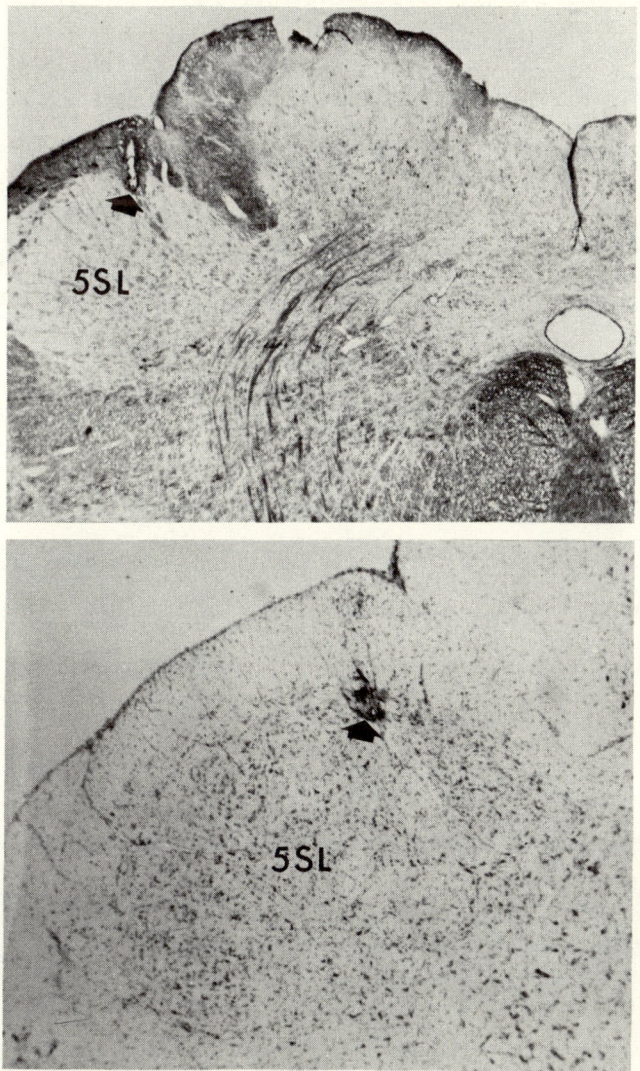

Fig. 16. Photomicrographs of cat medulla showing lesion (arrows) in site from which a thermoreceptor responsive to cooling of the tongue was recorded. The tip of the lesion is within the superficial layer of the laminar spinal trigeminal nucleus (5SL). Upper photomicrograph, Kluver-Barrera X 14. Lower photomicrograph, Thionin X 36. (from Poulos, Molt and Barron, in preparation).

DISCUSSION

Results of investigations into the central somatic thermoreceptive pathways are complex. Most studies of thermoreceptive afferents at the level of spinal cord (1,4,16,34) medulla (33), thalamus (2,20,23) and cortex (18,19), have primarily found neurons responsive to both thermal and some form of mechanical stimulation. The preponderance of central neurons of the thermal plus mechanical type may in part reflect convergence of specific mechanoreceptors and thermoreceptors on common central cells (1) or more simply, the complex behavior of primary afferents innervating different and sometimes highly specialized cutaneous fields (14,25) in different animals. Other investigations of the CNS have found a majority of thermally sensitive cells that appear to be specific thermoreceptors (7,8-10,17,28,30) although some respond to only certain features of "typical" primary thermoreceptor input. Caution is presently warranted in assuming analagous behavior in central thermoreceptive afferents representing such disparate and specialized cutaneous regions as the monkey tongue and rat scrotum, or for that matter, the maxillary and mandibular trigeminal divisions of the cat.

In this summary we have described the behavior of central trigeminal neurons in the monkey and cat that have the capacity to faithfully transmit information about both changing skin temperature and temperatures of the skin held constant. The overall response characteristics of the central neurons did not significantly differ from those of specific primary afferent thermoreceptors that innervate the face (6,31,32) and other fields (5,13) in monkeys. These central neurons are capable of signalling small changes below a wide range of skin temperatures. However, individual thermal units have dynamic response profiles that increase to increased cooling intensities over only a limited range. Since a certain degree of variability in dynamic sensitivity was observed within the population of thermal units studied, it is possible that the integrated responses of a population of thermal units can provide information required for the evaluation of more intense cooling.

Additional information on the degree of cooling is made available by the dynamic responses of thermal plus mechanical neurons. The possible inclusion of neurons having both mechanical and thermal sensitivities into the "thermal afferent" system is controversial. The potential exists however for the organism to perceive thermal plus mechanical unit activity as "touch" in the absence of maximal thermoreceptor activity, and "cold" when thermal plus mechanical unit activity is combined with the maximal activation of thermoreceptors.

The central transmission of information about skin warming must depend upon a class of neurons that have not as yet been adequately studied within the CNS. Similarly, the role played in thermal sensation by more "complex" central neurons that respond preferentially to only certain aspects of a thermal stimulus must await further research.

REFERENCES

1. Burton, H., J. Neurophysiol. 38, 1060 (1975).
2. Burton, H., Forbes, D. and Benjamin, R.M., Brain Res. 24, 179 (1970).
3. Christensen, B.N. and Perl, E.R., J. Neurophysiol. 33, 293 (1970).
4. Courtney, K., Brengelman, G. and Sundsten, J.W., Brain Res. 43, 657 (1972).
5. Darian-Smith, I., Johnson, K.O. and Dykes, R., J. Neurophysiol. 36 (1973).
6. Dubner, R., Sumino, R. and Wood, W.I., J. Neurophysiol. 38, 1373 (1975).
7. Fruhstorfer, H. and Hensel, H., Naturwissenschaften 60, 209 (1973).
8. Hellon, R.F. and Misra, N.K., J. Physiol. London 232, 375 (1973).
9. Hellon, R.F. and Misra, N.K., J. Physiol. London 232, 389 (1973).

10. Hellon, R.F., Misra, N.K. and Provins, K.A., J. Physiol. London 232, 401 (1973).
11. Hellon, R.F. and Mitchell, D., J. Physiol. London 248, 359 (1975).
12. Hensel, H., Ann. Rev. Physiol. 36, 233 (1974).
13. Hensel, H. and Iggo, A., Eur. J. Physiol. 329, 1 (1971).
14. Hensel, H. and Kenshalo, D.R., J. Physiol. London 204, 99 (1969).
15. Iggo, A., Symp. Zool. Soc. Lond. 31, 327 (1972).
16. Iggo, A. In: Advan. in Neurol. (ed. J.J. Bonica) New York: Raven, 1974, vol. 4, p. 1-9.
17. Iggo, A. and Ramsey, R.L., J. Physiol. London, 242, 132 (1974).
18. Kreisman, N.R. and Zimmerman, I.D., Brain Res. 25, 184 (1971).
19. Landgren, S., Acta Physiol. Scand. 40, 202 (1957).
20. Landgren, S., Acta Physiol. Scand. 48, 255 (1960).
21. Lende, R. and Poulos, D.A., J. Neurosurg. 32, 336 (1970).
22. Long, R.R., Brain Res. 63, 389 (1973).
23. Martin, H.F. and Manning, J.W., Brain Res. 27, 377 (1971).
24. Mosso, J.A. and Kruger, L., J. Neurophysiol. 36, 472 (1973).
25. Pierau, F.-K., Torrey, P. and Carpenter, D.O., J. Neurophysiol. 38, 601 (1975).
26. Poulos, D.A. In: Oral-Facial Sensory and Motor Mechanisms (ed. R. Dubner and Y. Kawamura) New York: Appleton-Century-Crofts. 1971 p. 47-72.
27. Poulos, D.A. In: Research in Physiology (eds. F.F. Kao, K. Koizume and M. Vassale) Bologna:Graggi, 1971, p. 441-455.
28. Poulos, D.A. In: The somatosensory system (ed. H. Kornhuber) Stuttgart: Georg Thieme, 1975 pp. 132-147.
29. Poulos, D.A. In: Controversy in Neurosurgery (ed. T.P. Morely) Philadelphia W.B. Saunders Co., 1976 (in press).
30. Poulos, D.A. and Benjamin, R.M., J. Neurophysiol. 31, 28 (1968).
31. Poulos, D.A. and Lende, R., J. Neurophysiol. 33, 508 (1970).
32. Poulos, D.A. and Lende, R., J. Neurophysiol. 33, 518 (1970).
33. Rowe, M.J. and Sessle, B.J., Brain Res. 42, 367 (1972).
34. Zimmerman, M. and Handwerker, H.O. In: Advan. in Neurol. (ed. J.J. Bonica) New York: Raven, 1974, vol. 4, p. 29-33.
35. Zotterman, Y., Skand. Arch. Physiol. 75, 105 (1936).

Acknowledgments

The authors are grateful to E.P. Graham for typing this manuscript.
Dr. J.T. Molt was supported by National Institutes of Health Grant NS11384.
This work was supported by National Institutes of Health Grant NS11384.

Discussion:

Landgren: Your medullary units responding to thermal stimulation seemed to be located in pars caudalis of the spinal trigeminal nucleus. Did you observe any thermal units in pars oralis or part interpolaris of this nucleus?

Poulos: The only area we have explored in medulla is in and around obex. Most of our findings are at that level and just caudal to obex. We have not been rostral to that. At that level we have found specific thermal receptors in the marginal zone and definitely well within the nucleus proper. They are not limited to that marginal zone. However, the frequency of encountering them in that zone is certainly greater.

Landgren: You mentioned thermal units responding also to mechanical stimulation. Did you observe any combinations of thermal and gustatory responses?

Poulos: Yes, we have done that. There was no response to gustatory stimuli unless they were cold.

Hensel: Have you obtained evidence of convergence?

Poulos: Yes we have. In cat medulla there was clear evidence of convergence of two specific cold afferents on common medullary neurons. The peripheral receptive fields were discrete and far enough apart to stimulate independently. We have not made similar observations within the monkey CNS.

Kenshalo: Did you see thermal neurons that received convergent inputs from bilateral receptive fields?

Poulos: We have never seen central thermoreceptive afferents having peripheral receptive fields that are bilateral. Indeed, none have been observed to cross the midline.

Zotterman: In 1937 my friend the brain surgeon Olof Sjöqvist on my instigation studied the size of the fibers in the trigeminal roots and found that the smaller fibers ran down in the descending trigeminal tract while the larger fibers ran upwards. In three patients suffering from trigeminal neuralgia he cut the descending tract at the height of the olive. The patients were relieved of their pain. I examined myself two of these patients and found that there was a complete analgesia and that most of the thermal sensations were lost while touch and pressure were preserved but for the loss of tickling sensations. What kind of mechanoceptive units did you find?

Poulos: We have not really studied the mechanical properties of the response. One does see responses to very light brushing by hairs. I think that our findings would agree with those of Kruger, Kerr and others that one does see the entire range of mechanoceptive units in the descending tract V.

THERMOSENSORY MECHANISMS IN THE SPINAL CORD OF MONKEYS

A. IGGO and R. L. RAMSEY

Department of Veterinary Physiology, University of Edinburgh, Edinburgh, Scotland

Specific cutaneous thermoreceptors

Highly specific cutaneous thermal receptors in the distal part of the hind limb send small myelinated or non-myelinated afferent fibres into the lumbar spinal cord (Iggo [25, 26]; Hensel & Iggo [23]; Dykes [14]) via the lumbar spinal nerves in the monkey as in other mammals. These afferent fibres encode skin temperatures in the normal physiological range by an interspike-interval code. The warm fibres, active in the range 30 to 45°C, typically discharge impulses in a regular stream, at rates that are temperature dependent, with the highest values at 41-45°C (Fig. 1.). The majority of the afferent fibres are non-myelinated (Hensel & Iggo [23]). The cold fibres, in contrast, are active at static temperatures in the range 38 to 15°C with maximal discharges at 25 to 28°C (Iggo [24]; Dykes [14]), and typically carry a discharge of impulses in bursts at skin temperatures from about 32°C to 20°C (Fig. 1). This grouping of impulses varies in number, and intra-burst and inter-burst intervals; the number of impulses/burst has a negative linear correlation with skin temperature (Iggo [26]; Iggo & Iggo [28]; Dykes [14]). This parameter could, therefore, provide an unambiguous index of steady or slowly changing skin temperatures over the range 32-20°C. At high rates of skin temperature change (high dynamic flux) the burst feature may be absent (Iggo [26]), and the mean firing rate may then be linearly proportional to the rate of change of temperature (Dykes [14]). Within the normal rather narrow range of skin temperatures (20-40°C), the cutaneous slowly-adapting mechanoreceptors may act as 'spurious' thermoreceptors (Iggo [26]) and their thermo:sensory rôle will be considered in this article.

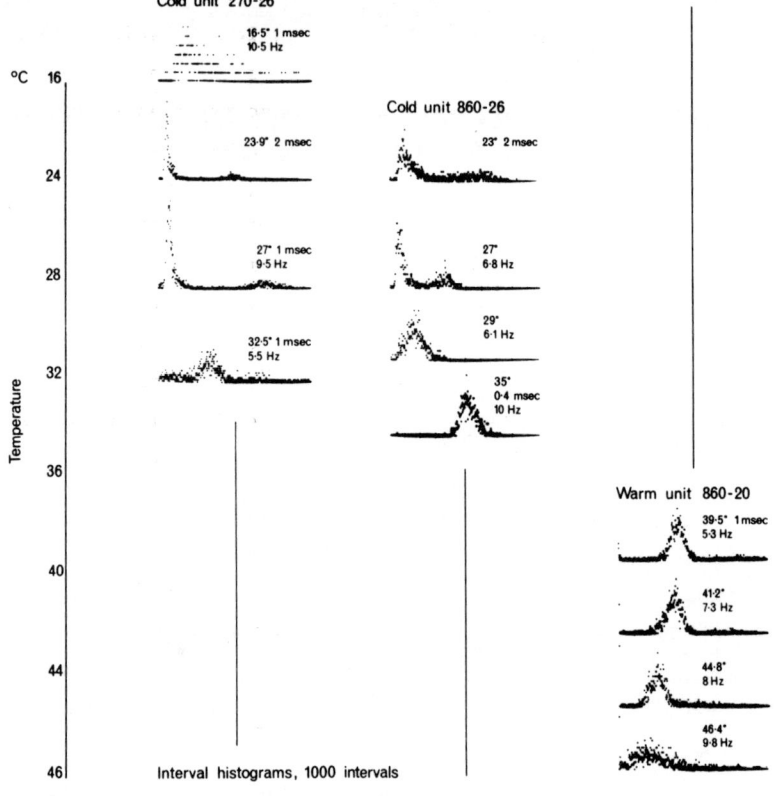

FIG. 1. Interval histograms for 3 monkey thermo-
:receptors. Each histogram, recorded under steady
thermal conditions at the temperature indicated,
was generated by collecting 1000 interspike inter-
:vals. The two cold units had bimodal interspike
intervals at intermediate temperatures (caused by
'burst' discharges) and unimodal distribution (i.e.
uniform interspike intervals) at the extremes,
whereas the warm unit had unimodal distributions at
all effective temperatures (Iggo & Ogawa, unpubl.
obs.)

Nociceptors

Outside the range of skin temperatures encoded by the specific sensitive thermoreceptors there are other cutaneous sensory mechanisms - the nociceptors - that detect the more extreme temperature changes (Zotterman [43, 44]). Single unit studies have established their general characteristics and they are known variously as 'heat receptors' (Iggo [24]; Beck et al [2]; Beck & Handwerker [1]), 'thermal nociceptors' (Iggo & Ogawa [29]) and 'polymodal' nociceptors

(Bessou & Perl [3]). In addition to excitation by skin temperatures above 40°C, these nociceptors can, in contrast to the 'specific' thermoreceptors, also be excited by severe mechanical stimuli [3, 24] and by endogenous or exogenous chemicals such as histamine, brady:kinin, 5-hydroxytryptamine, acetylcholine, (Fjällbrant & Iggo [15]; Burgess & Perl [8]; Beck & Handwerker [1]) or have their sensitivity to natural stimuli and the above chemicals modified by other drugs, such as prostaglandins, aspirin and indomethacin (Handwerker [18]; Chahl & Iggo [11]; Perl [32]). In these latter respects they are like the slowly-adapting mechanoreceptors with myelinated fibres [15]. The afferent fibres from these thermal nociceptors in monkeys are predominantly unmyelinated (Fig. 2) although some are unmyelinated

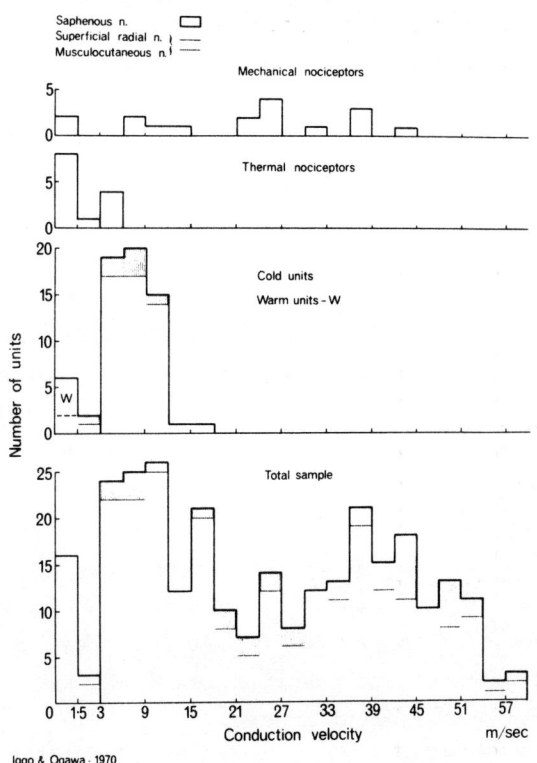

FIG. 2. Conduction velocities of cutaneous afferent fibres in the saphenous, superficial radial and musculocutaneous nerves of monkeys (<u>Macacca</u> spp.). The sensitive mechanoreceptors conducted at velocit:ies greater than 10 m/sec whereas the sensitive thermoreceptors conducted at less than 18 m/sec. (From Iggo & Ogawa, unpubl. obs.).

only in the periphery and have thin myelinated axons more centrally (Iggo & Ogawa [29]). They cannot therefore be distinguished, on this basis, from either the sensitive warm fibres, which have non-myelinated axons (Hensel & Iggo [23]) or the sensitive cold fibres, which have small myelinated or non-myelinated axons (Iggo [26]; Hensel & Iggo [23]; Iggo & Young [30]). They also have thermal sensitivity ranges that overlap those of the sensitive warm and cold thermoreceptors.

The identification of the afferent units can, however, be based on the following criteria
1) maximal static thermal sensitivity
2) excitatory dynamic thermal gradient
3) relative sensitivity to mechanical stimuli
4) size of receptive field (the thermoreceptors have spotlike fields (1 mm diameter) whereas the nociceptors have more diffuse fields, about 2 x 3 mm in hairy skin).
5) a further differentiation may be possible by using a battery of chemical excitants and inhibitors.

A decision whether a particular individual afferent unit or class of afferent units is thermosensory or nocisensory cannot properly be made solely on the basis of their peripheral physiological or biophysical characteristics. Indeed, it could be argued that the central nervous system decides the functional rôles of the cutaneous afferent fibres, although it is probably going too far to suggest that the central nervous system takes the decision alone. There is now overwhelming evidence that peripheral cutaneous sensory systems are highly selective in regard to the natural stimuli to which they respond. Nevertheless, a decision on the functional attributes of the receptors can only be aided by exact and quantitative knowledge of central processing of cutaneous afferent inputs.

DORSAL HORN NEURONES

We chose in 1968 to start our attack on the analysis of the thermosensory input at the dorsal horn in primates since it is known that the small cutaneous afferent fibres terminate there and apparently do not send collaterals to remote parts of the spinal grey matter or spinal cord (Réthelyi & Szentágothai [36]). Furthermore there were reports in the literature, then and since, indicating that neurones in the dorsal horn could be affected by skin temperature (e.g. Brown & Franz [5]; Brown [4]; Burke et al [9]; Christensen & Perl [12]; Gregor & Zimmerman [17]; Hellon & Misra [21]; Poulos [34]; Wagman & Price [39]; Wall [41]).

Categories of dorsal horn neurones

It is now clear that larger neurones in the superficial lumbo-sacral dorsal horn, some of which project into ascending sensory pathways, respond in a highly selective way to afferent input from the skin, muscles and viscera. Several broad categories of units can be made on the basis of a) excitatory natural stimuli, b) kind of effective afferent fibre, c) kind of excitatory afferent unit, d) susceptibility to segmental and descending inhibition and e) location in the dorsal horn. In the anaesthetized reversibly-spinal cat three major categories were made (Iggo [27]; Handwerker, Iggo & Zimmerman [19]; Cerveró, Iggo & Ogawa [10]) - Class 1 are excited only by cutaneous myelinated afferent fibres from mechanoreceptors, but not by thermo- :receptors or nociceptor input; the cells were mostly in laminae IV and V. The responses to mechanical stimulation of the skin were not inhibited from the skin, nor were they suppressed by descending inhibitory systems. Units of Brown's [4] SCT type I units can be assigned to this class. Class 2 units are also excited by an input from cutaneous mechanoreceptors with myelinated afferent fibres but in addition can be powerfully excited by an afferent input from 'thermal nociceptors', but this latter response is selectively inhibited by both segmental and descending inhibitory systems (Handwerker et al [19]). These units do not appear to be excited by an input from the sensitive cutaneous thermoreceptors. They are found in laminae I - V, with a heavy concentration in lamina IV and are probably the most commonly reported kind of dorsal horn neurone (Wall [41]; Wagman & Price [39]; Brown & Franz [5]; Brown [4] types II, III and IV; Handwerker et al [19]; Giessler et al [16]; Cerveró et al [10]). Although there are reports that units of this class can be excited by warming or cooling the skin (e.g. [35, 37, 41]) the possibility could not be excluded that the method of skin-cooling often used (evaporat- :ive cooling caused by spraying the skin with ethyl chloride) is now known to excite cutaneous mechanoreceptors with myelinated afferent fibres. Evaporation of the ethyl chloride can cause very rapid and severe cooling of the skin (see Handwerker et al [19]) which may elicit a brief discharge from the hair follicle afferent units (Brown, Iggo & Miller [7]; Brown & Iggo [6]; Brown & Franz [5]). The rapid cooling of the skin by this means can certainly cause class II dorsal horn neurones to fire, but the latency of the initial excitation is so short that the afferent inflow must be travelling in large myelinated axons. Whether high threshold slowly-conducting afferent fibres also contribute to the response is not known, but from what is already known about the C-thermal nociceptors [24] and their central actions [19] it is quite likely that they do. The lack of any evident excitant effect of skin at 20-30°C, at which temperatures the cold receptor units would be discharging at high rates, is further evidence that the class I-III dorsal horn neurones are not directly affected by cold receptor input. The position with regard to the possible excitatory action of warm receptors is not so clear-cut, and there is some conflict in the literature. Wall [41] reported that 'touch cells' in the dorsal horn responded "to temperature changes in the skin and not to an indirect effect of temperature changes". He illustrates a cell responding to radiant skin heating with a sustained elevation of the firing rate at indicated temperatures of 30-34°C. Subsequent studies do not confirm these results and I attribute the discrepancy to his use of 'imbedded thermometers or thermistors' to measure the skin temperature. In the light of the quantitative studies of Beck et al [2] on skin nociceptors and of Handwerker et al [19] on dorsal horn neurones in the cat responding to radiant heating of the skin, I can only conclude that the skin surface temperatures in Wall's [41] experiments were much higher than the temperatures measured by his imbedded thermistors. In another series of experiments, also on spinal cats, Price & Browe [35] report the existence of a broad class of units in laminae IV-VII excited by pressure and pinch of the skin and also by radiant heat. Most of the units responded in a manner typical of our class II - i.e. by both short and a long latency discharge on electrical stimulation of the skin (i.e. by A and by C afferent volleys). Skin temperature thesholds ranged from 36 to 50°C. Insofar as the thermistors fastened to the skin surface "affixed ......

to various regions of the leg as required" were in the receptive fields of the cells they were testing, their results indicate that both 'warm thermoreceptors' and 'thermal nociceptors' excite the cells. In our later work we have restricted our recording to laminae I-IV but have not found convincing evidence for cells as deep as lamina IV to be excited by other than skin temperatures above $40^{\circ}C$. Since most of Price's and Browe's [35] 'touch-pressure-pinch', 'pressure-pinch' and 'pinch' units were in laminae V and VI there is the possibility that there is greater convergence of different kinds of afferent units on to these deeper cells. The general ineffectiveness of temperatures in the range $20-40^{\circ}$ on dorsal horn cells projecting into the spinocervical tract in cats is reported by Brown & Franz [5]. There was, however, a potent effect at skin/thermode interface temperatures of $40-50^{\circ}C$. Once again the dorsal horn neurones were probably in lamina IV, and the results are in good agreement with Handwerker et al [19] in finding a potent excitatory action only above $40^{\circ}C$ for neurones in the more superficial dorsal horn. In contrast to the foregoing results are the reports of Christensen & Perl [12] and Hellon & Misra [21] that dorsal horn neurones in the lumbo-sacral spinal cord of the cat and rat, with receptive fields in the perineal region and the tail can be excited by small changes in skin temperature. This difference may in part be due to the richer thermosensory innervation of the perineal region (Iggo [26]; Hellon, Hensel & Schäfer [22]). In addition Christensen & Perl [12] reported that many of their units excited by innocuous temperat- :ure changes could also be excited by noxious heating and intense mechanical stimuli, indicating convergence from several kinds of cutaneous afferent units.

PRIMATE DORSAL HORN NEURONES

These results cited above largely refer to detailed studies in cats, which have generally yielded many more results than similar experiment- :al work on monkeys. However, current investigators in several laboratories (Besson and his collaborators in Paris; Willis et al in Galveston, Texas; Price and Dubner in Bethesda at N.I.H.; Perl and colleagues at Chapel Hill and in my own laboratory in Edinburgh) are now yielding new information on the responses of dorsal horn neurones and ascending sensory paths (particularly the spinothalamic) in monkeys.

The general broad classification of dorsal horn neurones into 3 classes (Iggo [27]) which was developed for the cat, also holds for the monkey despite the evident differences in the organisation of the ascending pathways, particularly the major outlet via the spino-cervical tract in the cat in contrast to the spinothalamic tracts in the monkey. Class 1 and 2 neurones project into both contralateral anterolateral (ST) and ipsilateral dorsolateral tracts (SCT) in the monkey and class 3 (nociceptor-driven neurones) into the contralateral anterolateral cord (Handwerker, Iggo, Ogawa & Ramsey [20]). These two routes are thus open to noxious levels of thermal stimulation, although the information carried by class 2 neurones may be inseparable from hair follicle and glabrous rapidly-adapting afferent input in the class 2 cells and from mechanical nociceptors in the class 3 cells.

In the monkey dorsal horn there is an additional kind of neurone which may be similar to some of those reported briefly by Christensen and Perl [12] in the cat, that is excited at innocuous skin temperatures, and which are present in the most superficial levels of the dorsal horn, i.e. in lamina I. In our initial studies it became evident that there is a mixed population of cells in the superficial dorsal horn, when viewed from the aspect of their responses to cutaneous and muscle afferent inputs. All our classes 1, 2 and 3 are present so that attempts to isolate and study units responding to moderate warming or cooling of the skin are hindered by the existence of the units that respond to more severe thermal stimuli. Christensen & Perl [12] in reporting the units excited by innocuous thermal stimuli state that many of the units could be excited by severe mechanical and thermal stimuli, and also by either single and especially by repetitive C volleys in peripheral nerves (or spinal dorsal roots). Their results, indeed, indicate that there may be a convergence of thermoreceptors and nociceptors onto some dorsal horn cells.

Dorsal horn 'cold' neurones in monkeys

In the monkey, using chloralose-anaesthetised, gallamine-paralysed animals, we were attracted by the possibility of testing the hypothesis that the coding of skin temperatures by the temporal coding of afferent discharge, discussed earlier in this paper, might be decoded by the dorsal horn cells. Particular efforts were therefore made to establish the presence of cells excited by innocuous skin temperatures, using receptive fields on the plantar surface of the foot and on the lower leg. Our experience was not comfortable, with severe technical difficulties limiting the yield of extensively studied neurones.

Neurones were examined, as single or multi-unit preparations. They were located in the superficial dorsal horn, and to judge from the vertical distance over which such responses could be recorded, were distributed in a very thin layer, less than 200 μm thick, as a cap on the dorsal horn. In contrast the class 2 and 3 cells in lamina I not only gave larger extracellular action potentials, but could also be recorded only over greater distances. It is likely that included among the latter are Waldeyer [40] marginal neurones, which are relatively large cells.

The 'cold' neurones of lamina I in the monkey dorsal horn, in chloralose anaesthetised preparations, were excited by cooling the skin in their receptive fields, which were on the lower leg or foot and any background activity was reduced when the skin surface was warmed. A characteristic response is seen in Fig. 3. The receptive field was on the great toe. There is a sustained background dis-:charge at a skin temperature of $27°C$, at which the cold receptors would be expected to be firing at a high rate and the warm fibres to be silent. The discharge of the neurone is not, however, at a constant rate, but fluctuates between 4 and 15/sec, using 1 second bin widths for the histogram. This variation was present in all the units examined and is, in this respect, similar to the 'spontaneous' or background discharge of class 2 units, thus adding to the difficulty of distinguishing the two classes while searching for units with the microelectrodes.

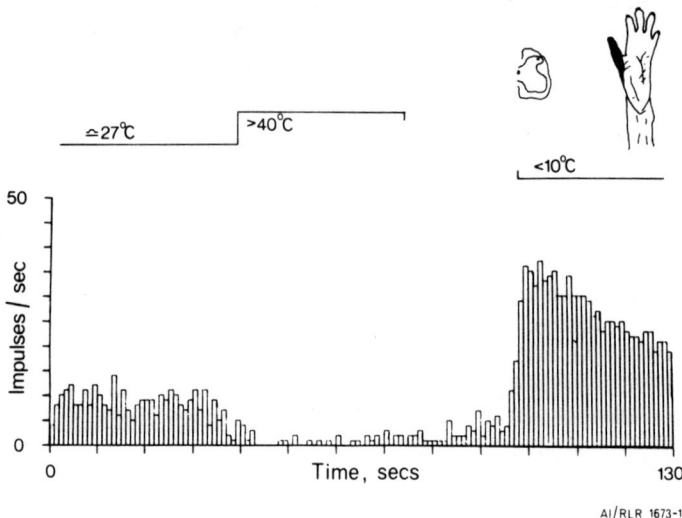

FIG. 3. The responses of a dorsal horn cold neurone in a vervet monkey at different stimulus temperat- :ures of the skin. The inset diagrams show the location of the neurone in lamina I of the lumbar spinal cord and the receptive field (black) on the great toe of the foot. The discharge of the neurone is indicated in histograms of 1 sec, and the stimulus (a moistened cotton swab) temperatures are shown as bars above the histograms.

When the whole surface of the great toe was covered with a warm saline swab, above $40°C$ in temperature, there was an immediate and total arrest of firing in the units for several seconds, with a slow emergence of a very low rate of firing (< 3/sec). When the warm swab was removed and the skin allowed to cool there was a further increase in the firing rate which was greatly enhanced to 40/sec when a cold swab soaked in water at less than $10°C$ was placed on the skin.

Receptive fields. The specific cold afferent units in primate skin typically have very small receptive fields, not more than 1 mm in diameter (Iggo [26]) and in a sample of 58 cold units only 4 were found in which there were two distinct spots, and these were not more than 5 mm apart (Iggo & Ogawa, unpublished data). Duclaux and Kenshalo [13] also found that the receptive field size of individual cold units in the limbs of monkeys were in "a skin area of 1 sq. cm or less". All the dorsal horn cold neurones in our vervet monkeys could be excited from a much larger skin area, at least 10 cm^2, and it is evident therefore that considerable convergence from single afferent units onto each dorsal horn cold cell must have been possible. No exact estimates have been published for the density of cold receptors in the skin of the distal limbs of monkeys but from casual observations made during single unit studies it is likely that there may be at least 10/cm^2, an estimate that is consistent with psycho-physical studies in human subjects (Järvilehto $^{(31)}$). The possible number of converging cold units within the receptive field of a dorsal horn cold neurone is therefore as many as 100. This level of convergence will affect the possibility of any preservation of afferent coding patterns, and makes it highly improbable that there would be any direct relation between, say, the quadruplet discharge in a single cold fibre at 28°C and the discharge <u>pattern</u> of the second order cold neurone. Interspike interval distributions were recorded as in Fig. 4. The afferent unit ISI distribution bears no relation to

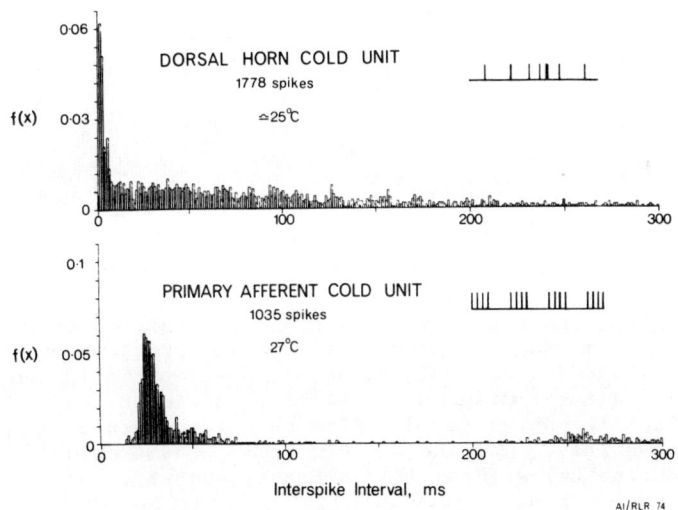

FIG. 4. Interspike interval distributions for a cold receptor (lower) and for a D.H. cold neurone (upper) in vervet monkeys. At 27° there is a clear-cut 'burst' discharge in the cold receptor, (inset diagram), in contrast to the semi-Poisson interval distribution for the D.H. cold neurone at about 25°C. (From Iggo & Ramsey, unpubl. obs.).

the dorsal horn cold neurone ISI distribution. The data available do not permit an analysis of the relation between the probability of firing in the second order cells and the input pattern in the afferent fibres, for these lumbar dorsal horn units.

Relation of cold neurone discharge to skin temperature. A striking feature of the sensitive thermoreceptors is the consistent relation between both static and dynamic skin temperatures and the rate of discharge of the cold units. It was confidently expected that a similar relationship would be found for the dorsal horn units. Fig. 5

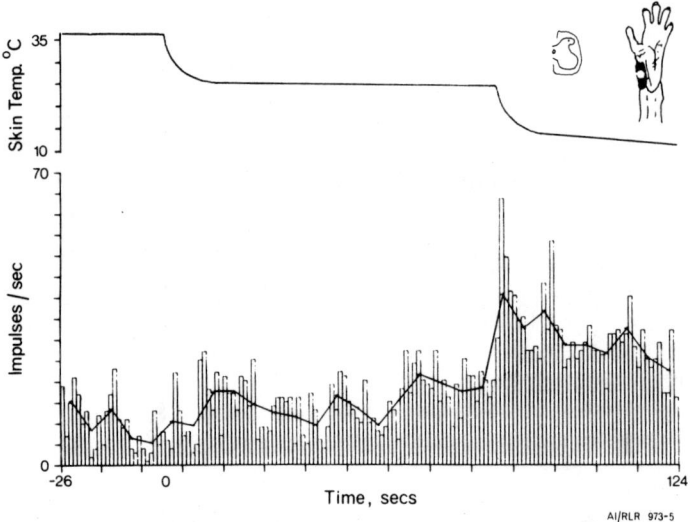

FIG. 5. The responses of a D.H. cold neurone in a vervet monkey to thermal stimulation provided by a thermode (diameter 1 cm) at the position indicated in the inset diagram (as a white circle on the black receptive field). The skin temperature is shown above, and the bar histogram of the cold neurone below (From Iggo & Ramsey, unpubl. obs.).

shows the results of one attempt to test such a relationship. The skin temperature of the centre of the receptive field was controlled by a thermode 1 cm in diameter. In Fig. 5 it was held initially at about $36°C$, a temperature at which both cold and warm receptors would be relatively quiescent. There was a persistent irregular discharge from the D.H. cold neurone. After 26 sec the skin temperature under the thermode was lowered, within 5 sec, to about 25°C. This would cause the cold receptor afferent fibres to fire vigorously at a high rate and then settle down to near the maximum static firing rate. There is only a weak enhancement of the firing of the D.H. cold neurones, which continued to fire at the new rate for the next 70 sec, while the skin thermode was held at 25°C., i.e. there was only a weak dynamic response and very little adaptation. The thermode temperature was then dropped a further 15°C. This would be expected to cause a further dynamic response from the cold receptors under the thermode with a subsequent gradual reduction in the static mean firing rate as the skin temperature fell on the downward leg of the static temperature curve for the receptors. In addition, however, the skin surrounding the thermode would also be cooled and therefore the total cold receptor afferent inflow would, from the general receptive field of the D.H. cold neurone be likely to be greater than when the thermode was at 25°C. The D.H. cold neurone responded with a 2-3 fold increase in discharge while the skin temperature was falling rapidly and slowly declined in firing rate during the next 40 sec. Some relation between skin temperature of a part of the receptive field and the response of the D.H. cold neurone can there:fore be established, but it is much less clear-cut than for the afferent fibres.

The result may be even less well-marked as is illustrated in Fig. 6. In Fig. 6A, in conditions similar to those of Fig. 5, and using the same D.H. neurone, the skin beneath the thermode was cooled rapidly from about 32°C to about 10°C. There was a weak dynamic response, lasting 2 or 3 sec, during the abrupt fall of skin temperature and thereafter a slow decline in the firing rate. On return of the thermode to the starting temperature there was a slight decrease in the firing rate and a post-inhibitory rebound. From a result such as this, it would seem imprudent to conclude that the D.H. neurone was a 'cold' neurone. However, a repetition of the test in Fig. 6B, shows a quite different picture. From a similar starting temperature and firing rate for the neurone, the same change in skin temperature caused a sustained, more than twofold, increase in the rate of firing. The one change in experimental conditions between the two trials was

298   A. Iggo and R. L. Ramsey

that the general temperature of the skin surrounding the cooling thermode was heated in B by a radiator, so that in Fig. 6B it was above 30°C. This would cause a general reduction in cold receptor activity of the receptive field of the neurone, so that the afferent

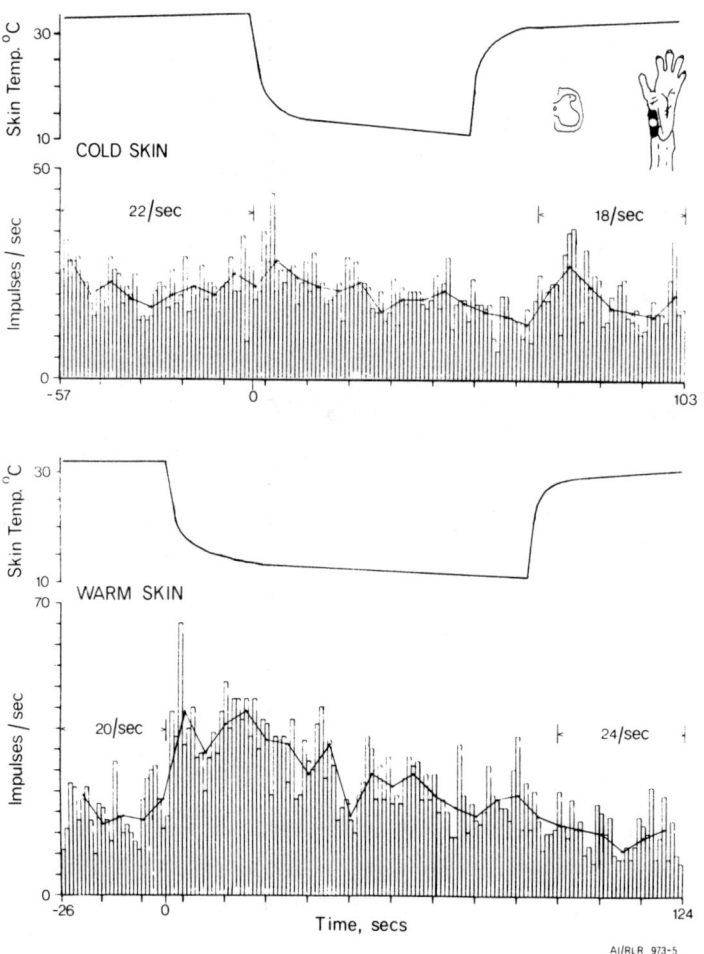

FIG. 6. The same D.H. neurone as in Fig. 5. showing the effect of the temperature of the receptive field surrounding the thermode, on the response of the 'cold' neurone to thermal stimuli delivered via the thermode to the centre of the receptive field. (From Iggo & Ramsey, unpubl. obs.).

inflow from the cold receptors caused by the sudden cooling of the skin under the thermode was now acting against a much lower level of con:current convergent activity, and the 'cold' neurone responds more vigorously, even although the general level of background discharge of the neurone was more or less the same.

The limited results available from these studies do not reveal a mechanism that encodes skin temperature with a great deal of precision, although the system does seem to be fairly specific. The 'cold' neurones in our experiments could not be excited by light or heavy mechanical stimulation of the skin, nor were they found to be excited by skin temperatures in the noxious heat range. It is unfortunate that such great difficulty was experienced in finding and recording from the D.H. cold neurones. Only a small sample (13 units) was studied, and in many of these only fragmentary results are available so that the desirable extensive testing of the characteristics of individual D.H. cold neurones has not been possible.

Location of the D.H. cold neurones. All the recordings were in the lumbar dorsal horn, and recording sites for individual units were marked by the iontophoretic deposition of pontamine sky blue from the recording electrodes. Eleven 'cold' neurones were within 0.6 to 1 mm of the surface of the cord dorsum, and when plotted with reference to the white matter/grey matter margin of the dorsal horn were in lamina I. The other two units were between 1.0 and 1.4 mm from the cord dorsum surface. This narrow band of grey matter containing the 'cold' neurones was not caused by the limitation of our search to the most superficial grey matter of the dorsal horn since as a normal routine each microelectrode penetration was carried to depths of 1500-2000 μm, except when we were concentrating on the most superficial laminae.

Rostral projection of the D.H. cold neurones. In man, temperature sensations are classically attributed to pathways in the antero:lateral tracts of the spinal cord, and recent work on monkeys (e.g. Willis et al,[42]; Price & Browe[35]; Trevino & Carstens[38]) has amply confirmed the existence of a projection via this quadrant of the cord to the thalamus. In collaboration with Drs. Handwerker and Ogawa, stimulating electrodes were placed at the appropriate locations in the upper cervical spinal cord of chloralose-anaesthetized and paralysed vervet monkeys, with recording microelectrodes in the lumbar dorsal horn. It was possible to test for projection into the contra-:lateral ventralateral cervical cord (presumed spinothalamic pro-:jection) and the ipsilateral dorsolateral cervical cord (presumed spinocervical tract projection). Three of the 5 D.H. cold units tested were found to project to the contralateral anterolateral spinal cord. Class 3, nociceptor-driven, D.H. neurones which are also present at lamina I of the lumbar dorsal horn in the monkey, were also tested for their rostral projection. Two of the 5 units tested, like the 'cold' neurones, projected into the crossed ventro-lateral tract (20).

CONCLUSIONS

The D.H. 'cold' neurones are therefore prime candidates for the thermosensory pathway from the skin to the higher levels of the CNS in primates. They offer a mechanism for the onward transmission of information from the specific cutaneous thermoreceptors, even though they appear to lack the precision that might have been expected from the properties of the cutaneous thermoreceptors. At least they have the capacity to send on information that is not contaminated by an input from sensitive mechanoreceptors and their discovery should help to resolve the current controversy on the role of specific and non-:specific afferent contributions to thermal sensation (e.g. Pierau et al, [33]). The thermal responses of the latter, particularly the slowly-adapting I and II mechanoreceptors (Iggo [26]) that are so abundant in primate skin, causes considerable confusion when thermo-:sensory mechanisms are discussed. The present results, which establish that the D.H. 'cold' neurones are not excited by light mechanical stimulation of the skin, is further evidence for the central rôle of the specific thermoreceptors in temperature sensation. At the same time there is good evidence that mechanoreceptive pathways exist, via the dorsal-column system, the spinocervical tract and even through the spinothalamic tract, in neurones other than those with a thermosensory or nociceptive input.

Additional mechanisms exist to handle the thermal nociceptor inputs. Most information currently available deals with the responses to noxious heating of the skin - the class 3 D.H. neurones provide one pathway for this information [10] subject to descending and segmental inhibitory actions. An alternative, and very problematical system could operate via the class 2 neurones [19, 20] which, although excited by light mechanical stimulation, can in certain conditions be powerfully excited by an input from the nociceptor, both thermal and mechanical. These class 2 neurones are present, but do not at first sight seem to be necessary at least for the transmission of information concerning either innocuous or noxious thermal stimuli to the skin.

ACKNOWLEDGEMENTS

The original work reported in this article was supported by grants to A.I. from the Science Research Council and the Wellcome Trust.

REFERENCES

1. Beck, P.W. and Handwerker, H.O., Pflüg. Arch. 347, 209 (1974).
2. Beck, P.W., Handwerker, H.O. and Zimmermann, M., Brain Res.67, 373 (1974).
3. Bessou, P. and Perl, E.R., J. Neurophysiol. 32, 1025 (1969).
4. Brown, A.G., J. Physiol. 219, 103 (1971).
5. Brown, A.G. and Franz, D.N., Exp. Brain Res. 7, 231 (1969).
6. Brown, A.G. and Iggo, A., J. Physiol. 193, 707 (1967).
7. Brown, A.G., Iggo, A. and Miller, S., Exp. Neurol. 18, 338 (1967).
8. Burgess, P.R. and Perl, E., In: Handbook of Sensory Physiology Vol. II. Ed. A. Iggo. Heidelberg: Springer, p.29. (1973)
9. Burke, R.E., Rudomin, P., Vyklický, L. and Zajac, F.E., J. Physiol. 213, 185 (1971).
10. Cerveró, F., Iggo, A. and Ogawa, H., Pain 2, (in press)
11. Chahl, L.A. and Iggo, A., Proc. Aust. Physiol. Pharmacol. Soc. 5, 180 (1974).
12. Christensen, B.N. and Perl, E.R., J. Neurophysiol. 33, 293 (1970).
13. Duclaux, R. and Kenshalo, D.R., Brain Res. 55, 437 (1973).
14. Dykes, R.W., Brain Res. 98, 485 (1975).
15. Fjällbrant, N. and Iggo, A., J. Physiol. 156, 578 (1961).
16. Giesler, G.J. Jr., Menetrey, D. and Besson, J.M., In: Recent Advances in Pain Research and Therapy. Ed. J.J. Bonica. New York: Raven Press. (1976).
17. Gregor, M. and Zimmermann, M., J. Physiol. 221, 555 (1972)

18. Handwerker, H.O., In: *Recent Advances in Pain Research and Therapy*. Ed. J.J. Bonica. New York: Raven Press (1976).
19. Handwerker, H.O., Iggo, A. and Zimmermann, M., *Pain* 1, 147 (1975).
20. Handwerker, H.O., Iggo, A., Ogawa, H. and Ramsey, R.L., *J. Physiol.* 244, 76P (1975).
21. Hellon, R.F. and Misra, N.K., *J. Physiol.* 232, 375 (1973).
22. Hellon, R.F. Hensel, H. and Schäfer, K., *J. Physiol.* 248, 349 (1975).
23. Hensel, H. and Iggo, A., *Pflüg. Arch.* 329, 1 (1971).
24. Iggo, A., *Q. Jl exp. Physiol.* 44, 362 (1959).
25. Iggo, A., *Acta neuroveg.* 24, 225 (1963).
26. Iggo, A., *J. Physiol.* 200, 403 (1969).
27. Iggo, A., In: *Advances in Neurology*. Ed. J.J. Bonica. New York: Raven Press (1974)
28. Iggo, A. and Iggo, B.J., *J. Physiol. (Paris)* 63, 287 (1971).
29. Iggo, A. and Ogawa, H., *J. Physiol.* 216, 77P (1971).
30. Iggo, A. and Young, D.W., In: *The Somatosensory System*. Ed. H.H. Kornhuber. Thieme: Stuttgart (in press)
31. Järvilehto, T., *Ann. Acad. Sci. Fenn. Ser. V.* 184, 1 (1973).
32. Perl, E.R., In: *Recent Advances in Pain Research and Therapy*. Ed. J.J. Bonica. New York: Raven Press (1976).
33. Pierau, F.K., Torrey, P. and Carpenter, D.O., *J. Neurophysiol.* 38, 601 (1975).
34. Poulos, D.A., In: *Oral-facial sensory and motor mechanisms*. Eds. R. Dubner and Y. Kawamura. New York: Appleton-Century-Crafts (1971).
35. Price, D.D. and Browe, A.C., *Brain Res.* 64, 425 (1973).
36. Réthelyi, M. and Szentágothai, J., In: *Handbook of Sensory Physiology* Vol. II. Ed. A. Iggo. Heidelberg: Springer, p. 207 (1973).
37. Taub, A., *Exp. Neurol.* 10, 357 (1964).
38. Trevino, D.L. and Carstens, E., *Brain Res.* 98, 177 (1975).
39. Wagman, I.H. and Price, D.D., *J. Neurophysiol.* 32, 803 (1969).
40. Waldeyer, H., *Abh. preuss. Akad. Wiss.* 3, 1 (1889).
41. Wall, P.D., *J. Neurophysiol.* 23, 197 (1960).
42. Willis, W.D., Trevino, D.L., Coulter, J.D. and Maunz, R.A., *J. Neurophysiol.* 37, 358 (1974).
43. Zotterman, Y., *Acta med. scand.* 80, 9 (1933).
44. Zotterman, Y., *J. Physiol.* 95, 1 (1939).

Discussion:

Paintal: Do you think that these motor reactions of the skin could modify the responses that you are studying?

Iggo: We have not tried to exclude that there is a motor reaction in the skin. We are using anaesthetized animals. We try to keep them in as good condition as we can. But as it is a common experience with monkeys that they just get worse and worse as the experiment goes on, rather more rapidly than cats do. We have not looked at the basal-motor responses directly nor have we tried, for example, stimulating the sympathetic supply to change the conditions of the skin.

Kenshalo: Dr Iggo, in these cold units that you found in the spinal cord, have you tested for bilateral fields as well as the ipsilateral?

Iggo: We had a great deal of difficulty finding the things anyway. We could only hold them for a rather short time. However, we did not find a bilateral representation. We did not test for it very extensively. One might have expected more in the central region but these were working on the foot. We did test for inhibitory effects on these neurons. We did not find any. But we did not test extensively for contralateral excitatory fields.

Zotterman: It must ve very difficult to get into these cells, especially those which send out C-fibers. Is that right? Is there any difference in that respect between the A-delta and C-fiber units?

Iggo: The ones we were looking at were probably driven by the A-delta fibers. They certainly do seem to be much smaller than the other neurons which are driven by the C-fibers by the thermal nociceptors. They seem to be rather larger. They are the kind that Allen Brown was talking about yesterday, by the cervical tract. From our results, we cannot say anything about the actual size of cells that the A- and C-fibers to to. Poulos might have a little more information about this. These thermosensory cells do seem to be very small and seem to be distributed in a very thin sheet because the penetrating microelectrode would go very rapidly past them. At the best of times we had only very small spikes.

Zotterman: The majority of fibers mediating thermal information are, of course, C-fibers. Or do you think there are A-delta fibers responding to warming in the monkey?

Iggo: In the monkey they are mostly A-delta for the cold and C-fiber for warm. We had one cell that was rather like a warm responding central cell.

Zotterman: It is harder to find cells responding to warming in the central nervous system, is that right?

Iggo: We did not really find any that responded to warming. I am extremely frustrated and am giving this up.

Paintal: What do you think is the mechanism for the bursts of impulses in your cold receptors?

Iggo: One quite likely peripheral mechanism although it has not been established experimentally, is some kind of sinusoidal oscillation in the generative potential which then drives the cell to fire the bursts as it goes on and then the temperature change may simply alter the amplitude and frequency of this sinusoidal oscillation. Something of that kind would certainly account for the bursting activity. I did some experiments when I was out in Japan this last year where we stimulated the terminals electrically by just putting electrodes across the skin one underneath and one on the surface of the skin to try and pass DC currents. Although the cells may have been showing a pulsitile discharge, group discharge, to a steady DC current the preresults we obtained indicated that there was, in fact, a steady discharge in response for a steady DC current.

Paintal: But what is the mechanism responsible for the sinusoidal generator potential with constant temperature?

Iggo: I have what is probably not a very helpful answer: I did not invent them. This is a mechanism which the biochemists at the end of the day will have to work out.

Perl: Dr Iggo, I wondered whether you had any comments about the possibility that some of your recordings could have come from axons of cells.

The reason that I ask that question is that when we examined the characteristics of cells in those more superficially it was evident from time to time that we had axonal recordings by the usual criteria of relatively spike positive going and no evidence of associated slope potentials or diphasic spikes as the electrode was moved. Our units of the thermal type did, in fact, behave quite like yours. Our data are quite consistent with your description. But I would think that our cells are not very small, in fact. They are rather thin in the dimension from which the microelectrode approaches them from the dorsal surface and that may give the impression of being small. But we have evidence for those instances of recording when we had diphasic spikes that were over very extensive regions of the spinal cord suggesting perhaps, a rather extensive dendritic tree.

Iggo: We used the usual criteria of spike form to try to distinguish axons from cells. And certainly with the microelectrodes that we were using we would often in tracking down come across quite large primary afferent fiber spikes and they were typical monophasic. These ones we were looking at were not a clean-looking monophasic response. They were recorded from areas of the cord medulla that were getting focal potentials to the electrical stimulation to the peripheral nerves. When we tried on a few occasions to search around, having got rather small spikes then hunted around by using electrodes in 50-micron steps in a grid, we could never succeed in making the responses very much larger. Occasionally we did get larger spikes but they certainly did not survive nearly as long as the cells which got the flat, clear-cut response from mechanical and noxious thermal stimuli. The spikes certainly seemed to be smaller. It was in the vertical direction that they seemed to be a very narrow band the extent to which there may have been an expension of ventral field spreading horizontally across on the cord. We cannot answer this although we did test for it occasionally.

CORRELATIONS OF TEMPERATURE SENSITIVITY IN MAN AND MONKEY, A FIRST APPROXIMATION

D. R. KENSHALO

Psychology Department and Psychobiology Research Center, Florida State University, Tallahassee, Florida 32306

The aim is to draw those correlations that appear reasonable between human thermal sensations and neural activity in the thermal primary afferents of rhesus monkeys. Such correlations rest heavily on the assumption that the results of sensory measures in humans result from the same set of neural events observed in the infrahuman species. Greater confidence attends such correlations when behavioral measurements of the sensory capacity of the infrahuman species demonstrate a close correspondence to those of humans for as nearly identical conditions of stimulation as it is now possible to achieve. This is not the only approach. It is now possible to make both types of measurement on humans by the method pioneered by Hagbarth and Vallbo (1967). Konietzny and Hensel (1975) have recently successfully recorded from human warm fibers by this method.

It is important, regardless of the method employed, to identify those aspects of thermal sensations that can be accounted for at the receptor level. But, of even greater importance is the identification of those aspects of thermal sensations that cannot be accounted for by the thermal receptor activity and beyond that, specification of the nature of the difference between them.

The principal variables of human thermal sensations are identified here and candidate neural codes of the primary thermal afferents that may account for these variables are sought. The lack of receptor correlates is also noted. These correlations represent, at this time, only first approximations, however, they provide a framework from which hypotheses may be deduced and tested.

QUALITY ENCODING

In the realm of thermal sensation there are but two qualities--

warm and cold sensations of graded intensities. Two classes of specifically sensitive thermal afferents that innervate the skin have been identified--warm and cold fibers. Other classes of receptors account for the pains experienced at extreme skin temperatures (Burgess & Perl, 1973). In addition to their role in thermal sensation, activity in warm and cold fibers must also account for the strong thermoregulatory responses that are known to occur when the skin temperature is maintained between approximately 20° and 40°C (Hensel, 1973a).

Electrophysiological studies have shown that only some primary axons show neural activity or changes in neural activity that can be correlated with moderate changes in the temperature of the skin. There are two main classes of these primary axons. The first, warm fibers, respond with an increase in frequency to tissue warming, a decrease in frequency to tissue cooling, and no change in activity to other forms of moderate stimulation. The second class responds with an increase in frequency to tissue cooling and a decrease in frequency to tissue warming. There are two subclasses based on their sensitivity to mechanical stimulation. Some are bimodal and respond at least as readily to mechanical as to thermal stimulation (Burton, Terashima & Clark, 1972; Chambers, Andres, v.Düring & Iggo, 1972; Duclaux & Kenshalo, 1972; Iggo & Muir, 1969; Tapper, 1965). Others, cold fibers, are refractory to mechanical stimulation (Hensel, 1973b). Examples of the activity produced in rhesus single warm and cold fibers are shown in Fig. 1.

The possible contribution of these thermally sensitive slowly adapting mechanoreceptors (types SAI and SAII) to thermal sensations is not clear. It has been maintained that activity of the SAI type does not affect thermal sensations (Harrington & Merzenich, 1970), that they have insufficient channel capacity in response to thermal stimulation to account for thermal sensations (Johnson, Darian-Smith & LaMotte, 1973), and their change in sensitivity as a function of adapting temperature is contrary to what would be expected of receptors involved in thermal sensitivity (Duclaux & Kenshalo, 1972). The thermal

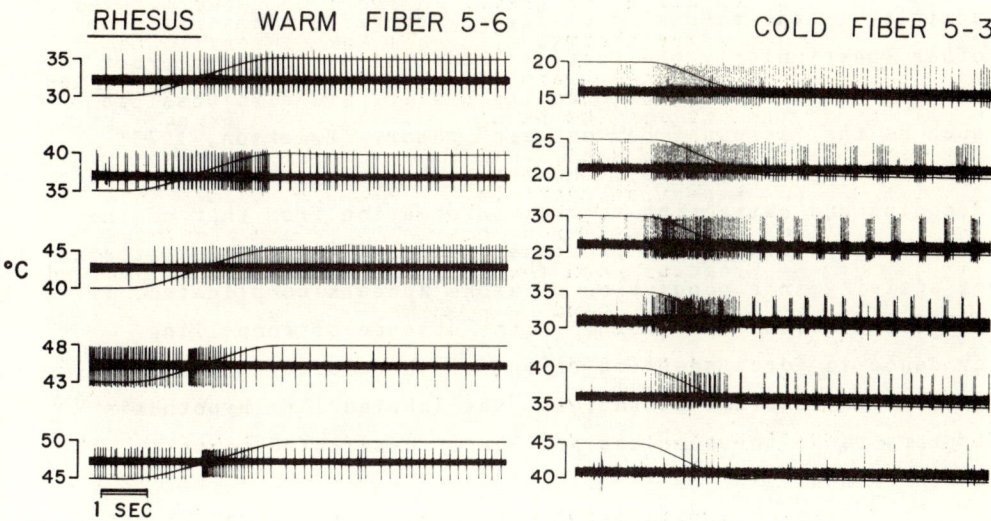

FIG. 1 Examples of the activity seen in primary, specifically sensitive, warm (left) and cold fibers of the rhesus monkey. The dynamic responses are to a 5°C intensity change at a rate of 2°C/sec.

sensitivity of the SAII mechanoreceptors has not been extensively investigated (Burton, Terashima & Clark, 1972; Chambers, Andres, v.Düring & Iggo, 1972).

There is, at this time, no direct evidence that the activity in specific thermoreceptors is the necessary condition for thermal sensations (Melzack & Wall, 1962), nor is there evidence that it is not. It is parsimonious, however, to maintain that activity in the specifically sensitive thermal afferents convey information to the central nervous system about cutaneous skin temperatures and that their absence would be accompanied by an absence of thermal sensations.

As a first approximation, the temperature sensing system is considered to be a "labeled line" system so that cool sensations result primarily from activity of cold receptors and warm sensations result from activity of warm receptors. The two systems may interact although evidence of this is scarce.

Bimodal receptors may contribute to thermal sensations and the activity in the thermal modality may converge with that from other (particularly the tactile) modalities at higher order centers. Other means of encoding quality are also possible such as the "across fiber pattern" theory (Erickson, 1973; Erickson & Poulos, 1973). However, the processes required for decoding and extracting thermal information from that of the other modalities or the processes required to analyze patterns of activity in a population of axons appears complicated, if not formidable. Therefore, in the absence of compelling evidence to force adoption of one of these alternatives to account for thermal sensations, the labeled line hypothesis appears to be the simplest and least complicated place at which to start.

PRINCIPAL VARIABLES OF THERMAL SENSITIVITY

Thermal sensitivity can be considered as static or dynamic depending on whether the sensations arise from a maintained temperature or from changes in temperature. Under static sensitivity are considered the codes for sensations that occur when the skin is maintained at static temperatures within the physiological range. These are the temperature zone of physiological zero where thermal sensations adapt completely, the persisting warm and cool sensations that occur when the skin temperature is maintained outside the zone of physiological zero, and the temporal course of thermal adaptation.

Dynamic sensitivity includes the influence of maintained skin temperature on warm and cool thresholds, the effect of rate of the skin temperature change on threshold and suprathreshold sensations, and the effect of area (spatial summation) on threshold and suprathreshold warm and cool sensations.

Static Temperature Responses

Physiological Zero and Persisting Thermal Sensations. Physiological zero is a range through which skin temperature may be changed, if done sufficiently slowly (0.007°C/sec), without producing a thermal sensation (Hensel, 1950; 1952). The upper and lower temperature limits of physiological zero are approximately 36° and 30°C for an area of approximately 15 cm^2. The zone is narrower when larger areas of skin are exposed, i.e. the whole body. Within this zone, thermal sensations adapt completely. When the skin is maintained at temperatures above or below these limits sensations of warm or cold, after some adaptation, persist no matter how long the temperature is maintained.

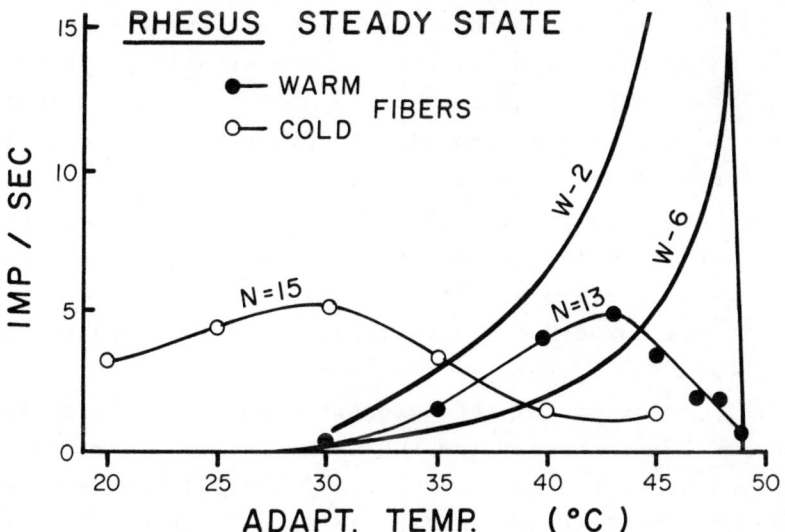

FIG. 2. Mean steady-state responses of specifically sensitive warm and cold fibers found in primate skin. There appear to be two types of warm fiber steady-state responses. Two fibers of this population (W-2 and W-6) were markedly different from the majority of fibers in the population.

Electrophysiological studies have shown that both warm and cold fibers show steady-state responses that vary as a function of skin temperature, as shown in Fig. 2. The mean steady-state responses for cold fibers and for a majority of warm fibers are more-or-less "bell-shaped." The maximum activity in cold fibers occurred at an adapting temperature of approximately 28° to 30°C, while that for the majority of warm fibers occurred at an adapting temperature of approximately 43°C. There appear to be two types of warm fibers: (a) those that showed an increasing level of activity up to a 43°C adapting temperature followed by a decline at higher adapting temperatures, and (b) those (W-2 and W-6 in Fig. 2) that attained higher levels of activity at higher adapting temperatures and a dramatic "shut-off" when the adapting temperature was increased only slightly above that at which the peak frequency was attained (Duclaux & Kenshalo, in prep.; Hensel & Iggo, 1971).

As can be seen in Fig. 2 there was a considerable steady activity in primate warm and cold fibers at skin temperatures between 30° and 36°C--the zone of physiological zero identified in humans. Activity in warm or cold fibers, at least at low levels, does not necessarily result in thermal sensations. Sensations occur only when relatively larger number of nerve impulses arrive in the central nervous system. The density of impulses is a function of the activity in the peripheral fibers and the number of active fibers. Activity in the peripheral temperature fibers is, in turn, a function of the static skin temperature, the intensity, and the rate of the temperature change, while the number of active fibers is primarily a function of the area of skin stimulated and, to some extent, the intensity of the stimulus. Thus, thermal sensations result from the integration of peripheral nerve activity rather than activity of single peripheral fibers (Hensel, 1973a). This "central integrator," as will become apparent later, is not a linear operator. It has a time constant of its own and some of its operating characteristics can be assessed by comparisons of peripheral nerve activity with sensations.

A persisting warm sensation occurs when the mean steady-state response rises above that which occurs at 36°C and it increases in intensity as the mean steady-state response increases. At approximately a 43°C to 44°C skin temperature, heat sensitive nociceptors become active (Burgess & Perl, 1973) and the experience loses its warm quality and changes to one of pain.

A candidate code for the persisting warm sensation is the mean frequency of activity in warm fibers above the frequency that occurs at a 36°C skin temperature for an area of stimulation of 15 cm^2.

The situation is different for cold fibers. The lower limit of physiological zero, for a 15 cm^2 area, coincides with the maximum steady-state response of cold fibers. There are, for example, equal mean steady-state response frequencies at skin temperatures of 25° and 33°C, yet cold sensations persist at the lower temperature and complete adaptation occurs at the higher temperature. An additional code of the cold fiber activity is apparently involved. The spikes of the steady-state responses at adapting temperatures of 35°C and lower are grouped in bursts for a considerable proportion of the primate cold fibers. As the adapting temperature is lowered from 35° to 25°C the number that discharge in bursts increases, the number of spikes per burst increase, and both inter- and intra-burst intervals increase in length (Kenshalo & Duclaux, in prep.; Iggo, 1969; Iggo & Iggo, 1971; Poulos & Lende, 1970). At the 20°C adapting temperature the number of bursting cold fibers decreases, but other burst features continue to increase in those that burst (Kenshalo & Duclaux, in prep.). While bursting does not increase the mean frequency of the steady-state activity it provides a temporal code that removes the ambiguity as to which side of the bell-shaped steady-state response curve the skin temperature is maintained. But, a combination of the static discharges from both warm and cold fibers also provide clear information at any temperature (Hensel, 1973a). The temporal code is required, however, to account for the increasing intensity of the persisting cold sensation as skin temperature is lowered. It also provides sufficient information to account for the strong thermoregulatory responses activated by these low skin temperatures (Dykes, in press).

The temporal code, the frequency code, as well as an interaction of the static discharges of both warm and cold fibers may all cooperate to provide the central integrator with exact information about skin temperature and hence, provide for persisting warm and cold sensations outside the range of physiological zero and initiate thermoregulatory responses.

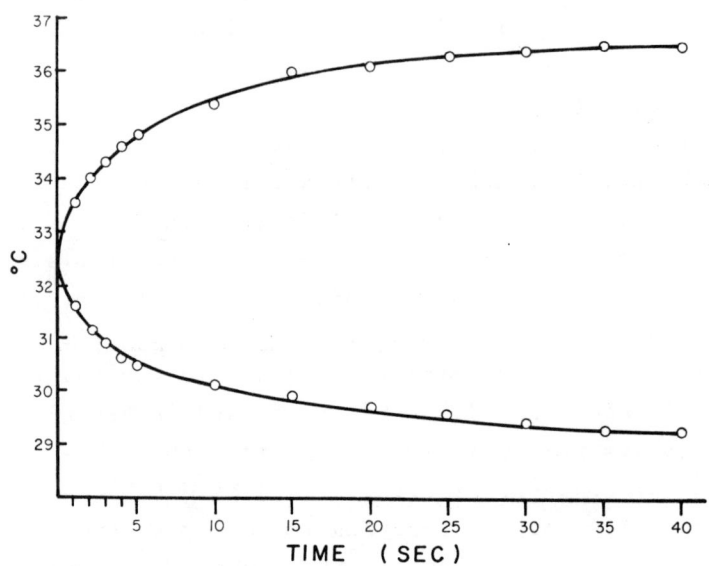

FIG. 3. The temporal course of adaptation. Subjects were instructed to keep the 14.4 cm^2 stimulator placed on the forearm just noticably warm or cool by moving a switch. Periodic readings of the graphed stimulator temperature constitutes the plotted points. (Redrawn from Kenshalo & Scott, 1966)

Adaptation. The temporal course of complete adaptation to a change in skin temperature is slow within the zone of physiological zero. Complete adaptation to a 5°C change in temperature requires tens of minutes (Hensel, 1952; Kenshalo & Scott, 1966). The temporal course of adaptation of warm and cool sensations is shown in Fig. 3.

In primary warm and cold fibers the analog of sensory adaptation is the establishment of a new steady-state response following a change in temperature. When warm and cold fibers are stimulated by a 5°C change in temperature, as shown in Fig. 4, new steady-state response levels are established within 15 sec for warm fibers and within 20 secs for cold fibers. Adaptation of thermal receptors is complete within a matter of seconds, whereas, complete adaptation of sensations required minutes.

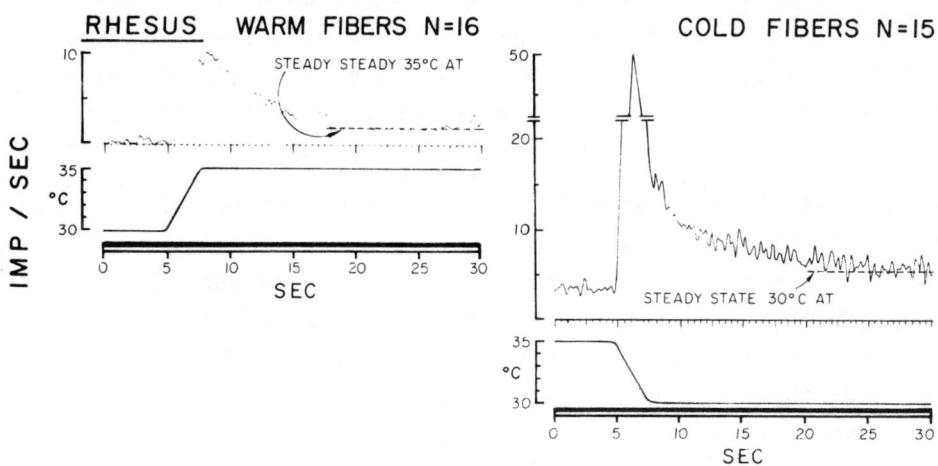

FIG. 4. Mean poststimulus time histograms of the responses of warm (left) and cold (right) fibers to a 5°C temperature change at a rate of 2°C/sec. The mean steady-state responses at the final temperature, obtained from Fig. 2, are shown as dashed-lines toward the end of the histogram.

The persistence of the sensation long after the apparent establishment of a new steady-state in the thermal receptors suggests that a central integrator has a long time constant for decay of activity. The after-effect in the central integrator of the receptor activity far out lasts the activity itself.

Electrophysiological evidence supports the importance of the recent history of thermal events in second and higher order neurons. Responses of second order warm units in the dorsal horn to warming are markedly different when preceded by cooling than by warming steps (Courtney, Brengelman & Sundsten, 1972). A similar hysteresis-like phenomenon has been reported in cold units of the primate thalamus to cooling (Poulos & Benjamin, 1968). In this case the effect became negligible within 80 to 90 sec following the temperature change. It should be noted, however, that similar though smaller effects have been observed in primary cold fibers (Poulos, personal communication).

Dynamic Responses

There are three principal stimulus variables that influence human thermal sensations. These are the effect of skin temperature on threshold, rate of temperature change, and the size of the area to which the stimulus is applied (Hensel, 1950; Kenshalo, 1970).

Skin Temperature. The effect of skin temperature on threshold warm and cool sensations is shown in Fig. 5. At low skin temperatures, e.g. 28°C, the threshold for a warm sensation is large while that for a cool sensation is small. As the adapting temperature was increased the warm threshold decreased and the cool threshold increased until at a 40°C temperature the warm threshold was small and the cool threshold was large.

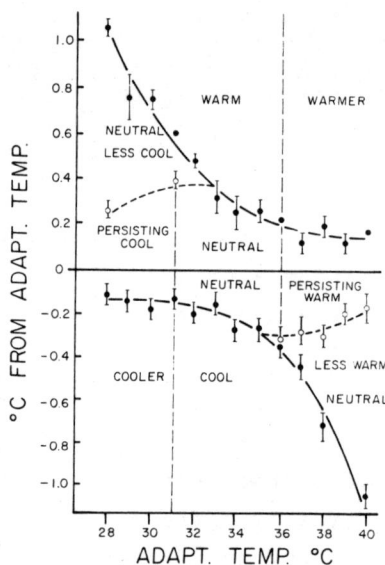

FIG. 5. Warm and cool thresholds as functions of the adapting temperature. Warm and cool thresholds are shown by the filled circles and change thresholds by the open circles. See the text for a detailed explanation. (Redrawn from Kenshalo, 1972).

The relative response magnitudes (imp/4 sec) of warm and cold fibers to a 0.5°C intensity of warming (for warm fibers) and cooling (for cold fibers) at several adapting temperatures are shown in Fig. 6. The response magnitude of cold fibers is relatively large and constant at the 25° to 35°C adapting temperatures and decreased at higher adapting temperatures. The response magnitude of the warm fibers was relatively small at the 30°C adapting temperatures but increased markedly at the higher adapting temperatures. The similarity in shapes of these and the threshold curves of Fig. 5 is striking.

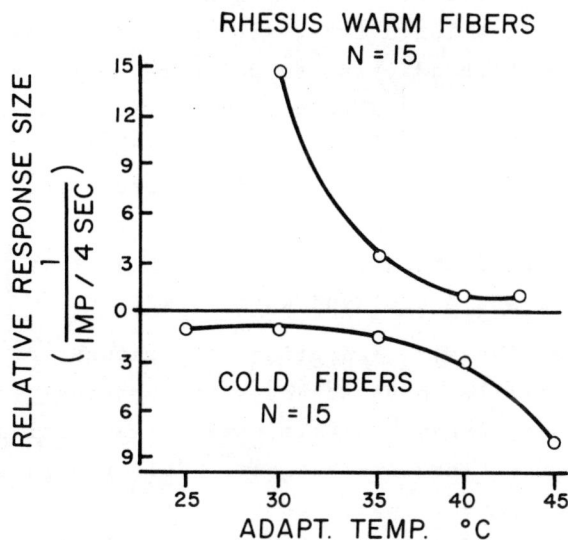

FIG. 6. Relative response magnitudes (cumulative impulse during the first 4 sec following stimulus onset) of warm and cold fibers in response to a 0.5°C temperature change at a rate of 2°C/sec. The reference response magnitude was that of warm fibers at the 43°C adapting temperature. The reciprocal of impulses/sec was used in order to present the vertical axis in a more convential style. Thus, the response magnitude of warm fibers at the 43°C adapting temperature is 15 times that at the 30°C adapting temperature.

A candidate code for near threshold warm and cool sensations is an increase in the frequency of neural activity in the primary afferent warm and cold fibers. But, as will be seen later, this simplistic code encounters difficulties when suprathreshold sensation magnitudes are related to the rate and intensity of the temperature change.

A second feature of the psychophysical thermal sensation threshold measurements is also seen in Fig. 5. Beyond the limits of physiological zero (30° and 36°C) the subject experienced either persisting cool or warm sensations that did not adapt completely no matter how long the temperature was maintained. In measuring the warm threshold from a 28°C adapting temperature, for example, the subject first experienced a reduction in the persisting cool sensation, then thermal neutrality, and finally a warm sensation. Likewise, when measuring the cool threshold from a high adapting temperature, for example, the subject first experienced a reduction in the persisting warm sensation, then thermal neutrality, and finally a cool sensation (Kenshalo, 1970). Detection of the decreased intensity of the persisting cool or warm sensations are called 'change' thresholds and are distinctly different in quality from those described as threshold cool and warm sensations.

In primary warm fibers, at adapting temperatures of 30°C and below there is little to no steady-state response (see Fig. 2). Furthermore, their dynamic sensitivity to warm stimuli is less than at higher adapting temperatures. Cold fibers show a considerable steady-state response as well as bursting. It has already been proposed that the bursting discharge is a temporal code associated with the persisting cold sensations experienced at these low adapting temperatures. The response of cold fibers to warm stimuli of as little as a few tenths of a degree is an immediate suppression in the steady-state response, as shown in Fig. 7.

In the same way, at adapting temperatures of 40°C and above, there is little steady-state activity in primary cold fibers and their sensitivity to cooling is reduced (see Fig. 6). However, there is a considerable steady-state response in primary warm fibers at high adapting temperatures (see Fig. 2). They respond with suppression of the steady-state response when cooled by a few tenths of a degree, as shown in Fig. 7.

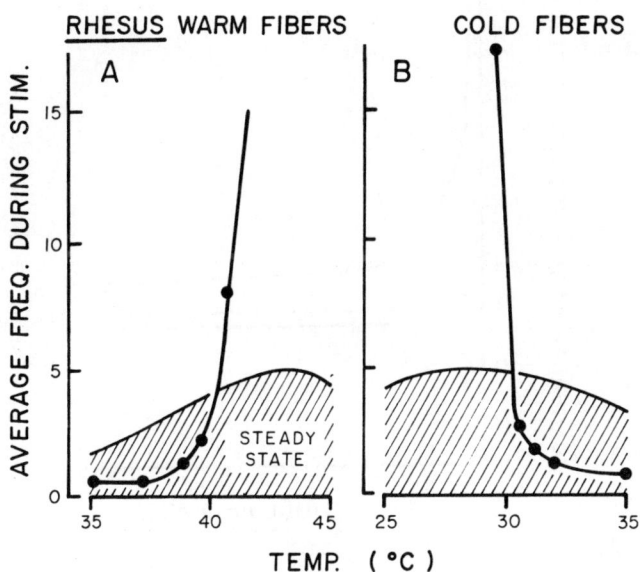

FIG. 7. The responses of warm (A) and cold (B) fibers to cooling and warming, respectively. The response is an immediate suppression of the steady-state response that is curvilinearly related to the intensity of the temperature change. The rate of change was 2°C/sec. Data points above the steady-state response levels are to 0.5° warming and cooling, respectively.

A candidate code for the change threshold is a reduction, rather than an increase, in the frequency of activity of warm and cold fibers. It correlates with the reductions detected by humans in the persisting thermal sensations outside the range of physiological zero.

Rate of Temperature Change. As seen in Fig. 8, the rate of the temperature change has little effect on the size of either the warm and cool thresholds until the rate was less than 0.1°C/sec. At slower rates both thresholds systematically increased (Hensel, 1950; 1952; Kenshalo, Holmes & Wood, 1968). The slow rates of temperature change that resulted in elevated warm and cool thresholds suggest that the effect can be accounted for by adaptation rather than some other feature of the process.

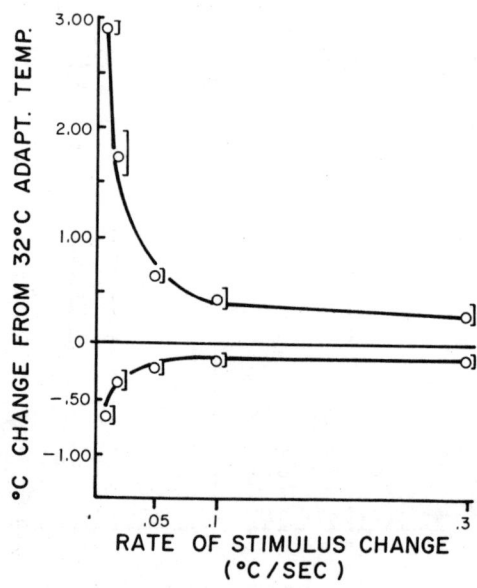

FIG. 8. The effect of the rate of the stimulus temperature change on warm and cool thresholds (Redrawn from Kenshalo, Holmes & Wood, 1968).

The rate of temperature change is without effect on estimates of warm and cold sensation magnitudes. As shown in Fig. 9, the slopes of the magnitude estimates remained the same regardless of the rate at which the temperatures were changed during stimulation. When the fastest rate was used the onset of the sensation was abrupt. When the slowest rate was used the sensation increased slowly in magnitude until it reached a peak near the end of the temperature change, but the subjects judged them equal in magnitude to those produced by the fastest change. The subjects could reliably discriminate the fastest and slowest rate on the basis of the onset and peak of the sensation but frequently confused both with the middle rate (Molinari, Greenspan & Kenshalo, in prep.).

The effect of rate of change of the temperature on the response magnitudes (imp/4 sec) of warm and cold fibers are shown in

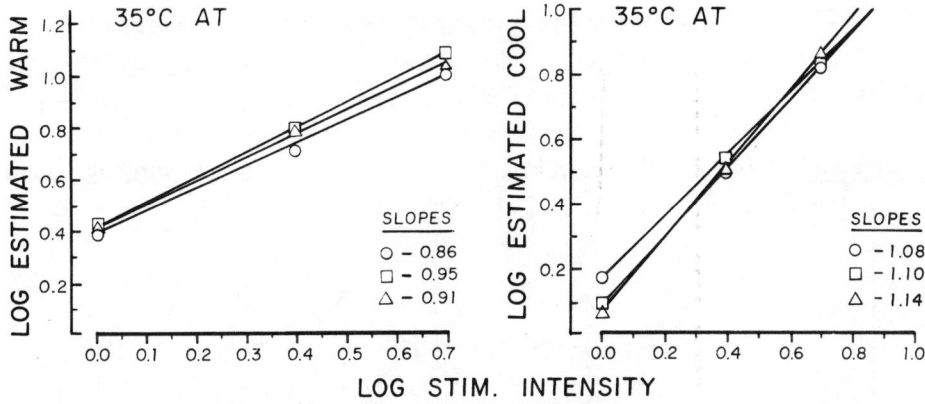

FIG. 9. Estimates of the magnitudes of warm (left) and cool (right) sensations produced by 1°, 2°, and 5°C stimulus intensities presented at rates of 0.4°,1°, and 5°C/sec at a 35°C adapting temperature. The order of the symbols, from the top to bottom correspond to increasing rates. (Molinari, Greenspan & Kenshalo, in prep.)

Fig. 10. The response magnitudes of the warm fibers were small at the 30°C adapting temperature but increased with adapting temperatures up to 40°C. At the 40°, 43°, and 45°C adapting temperatures the response magnitudes to the 0.5° and 1°C intensities, presented at the slow rate, were consistently larger than those produced by the same intensities presented at the fast rate. The decreased activity noted for the 5°C intensity compared to that for 2.5°C at 40°, 43° and 45°C adapting temperature is an artifact of this index of the response magnitude. When peak frequency was used as an index of response magnitude, the response to 5°C warming was as large, but no larger, than that produced by the 2.5°C intensity.

The major effect of rate on the response magnitudes of cold fibers also appears at the 2° and 5°C intensities of cooling (Fig. 10). Cooling by 5°C at a rate of 0.4°C/sec produced responses that were only slightly larger than those obtained from cooling by 2.5°C at the same rate. At the faster rate of 2°C/sec, however, the responses to 5°C cooling were considerably larger than those obtained from cooling by 2.5°C. At the 30°, 35° and 40°C adapting temperatures the responses were almost linearly related to the intensity of cooling at the 2°C/sec, but were not at the 0.4°C/sec rate.

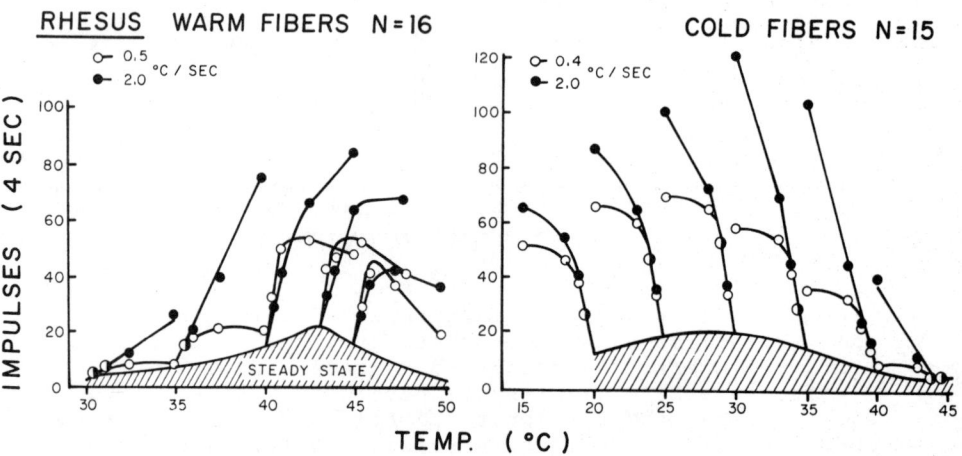

FIG. 10. The dynamic responses of warm (left) and cold (right) fibers to 0.5°, 1°, 2° and 5°C intensities of temperature change at two rates. (Kenshalo & Duclaux, in prep.; Duclaux & Kenshalo, in prep).

In general, the effect of increased rate of temperature change on the responses of primary thermal afferents is to increase the magnitude of their dynamic responses at all adapting temperatures. This effect is larger at the higher intensities of stimulation than at intensities of 0.5 and 1°C.

The effect of rate of temperature change on psychophysical measurements of warm and cool sensation magnitudes and the measures used to represent the dynamic response of primary thermal afferents do not correlate well. Rate of warming and cooling was without effect on the magnitude estimates of warm and cool sensations. Yet, both rate and intensity of cooling affect the response magnitude in much the same way, namely to increase the frequency of the response. If, it is stipulated that sensation intensity is proportional to the activity level in the central integrator and that the central integrator has a long time constant then the apparent contradiction can be accommodated. Slow rates of temperature change require longer time periods to accomplish a given intensity of temperature change, and, in so doing, produce a larger total number of impulses during the change, than do fast changes (Kenshalo & Duclaux, in prep). The time constant of the central integrator must be such that the amount of decay in activity is equal to the difference between the total impulses produced by fast and slow temperature changes.

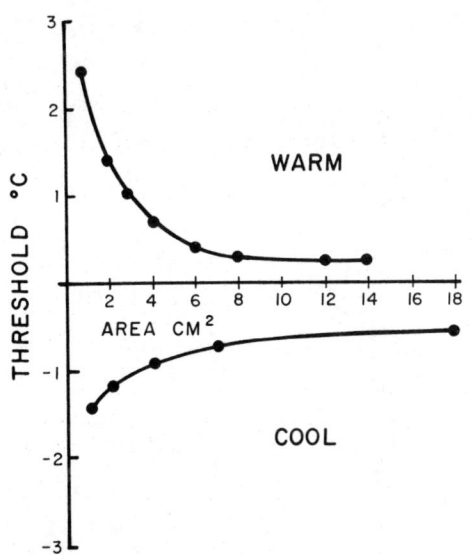

FIG. 11. Areal summations of warm and cool stimuli at threshold (warm summation data from Kenshalo, Decker & Hamilton, 1967; cold summation data from Berg, 1975).

Spatial Summation. At threshold area, (A) and intensity (I) trade approximately equally for warm stimuli, as shown in Fig. 11 (Hardy & Oppel, 1937; Kenshalo, Decker & Hamilton, 1967; Stevens & Marks, 1971). The trading function is expressed as:

$$I = kA^{-1} + C$$

Area does not play so prominant a role in spatial summation for threshold cool stimuli, as seen in Fig. 11 (Berg, 1975). Here the trading function is:

$$I = kA^{-0.5} + C.$$

The slopes of magnitude estimates of warm sensations produced by several intensities of stimulation decrease as the areas of stimulation increased (Stevens & Marks, 1971). They converge at approximately the heat pain threshold. As shown in Fig. 11, the importance of area on warm magnitude estimates diminishes as the intensity of the stimulus is increased.

Magnitude estimates of cool sensations from several intensities of cooling appear to be more straight-forward (Berg, 1975). Cool magnitude estimates for several areas of stimulation are parallel with slopes of approximately one, as shown in Fig. 12. Thus, area retains its importance at suprathreshold as well as at threshold intensities of cool stimulation.

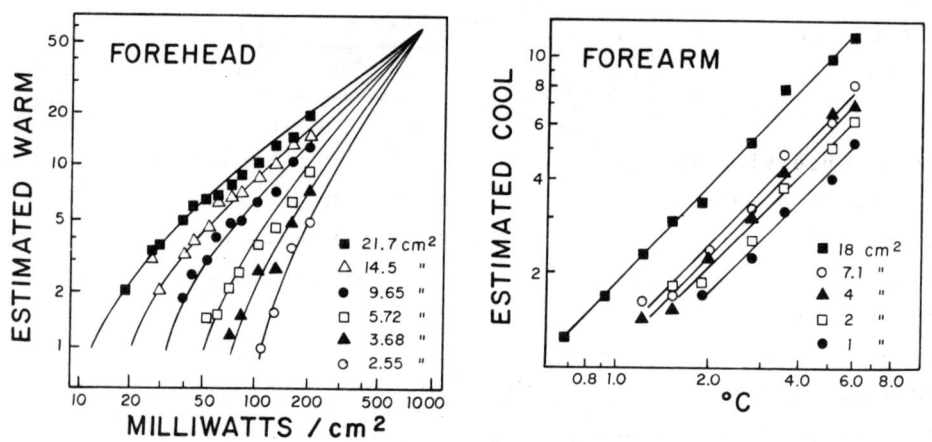

FIG. 12. Magnitude estimates of warm and cool sensations as functions of the area of stimulation (warm data redrawn from Stevens & Marks, 1971; cold data from Berg, 1975).

Even more striking than the summation effect at a single stimulus site is the summation of thermal stimuli presented bilaterally. Warm stimuli presented to the backs of the two hands showed lower thresholds than when either stimulus was presented alone. When presented to the back of the hand and the forehead the threshold was the same as when presented to the forehead alone

(Hardy & Oppel, 1937). Bilateral spatial summation for warmth has also been demonstrated across the body midline on the forehead (Marks & Stevens, 1973). Recently, Rozsa (1975) has shown, using signal detection methods, that cool stimuli applied to the two forearms summate to produce greater detectability than when either forearm was stimulated alone, even after correction for the increased statistical probability of stimulus detection produced by doubling the area, and hence, the number of detectors.

There have been few electrophysiological studies directed toward describing the neural mechanism(s) involved in spatial summation of thermal stimuli. Based on psychophysical evidence, Herget, Granath and Hardy (1941) proposed two mechanisms for spatial summation. The first, involved with small areas (<4 cm^2), is served by endings whose branches converge near the periphery. The second, involved with large areas (>4 cm^2), is served by fibers that converge on common synaptic pools in the central nervous system.

After observing that a single cold fiber might innervate up to 8 spot-like receptive fields, Kenshalo and Gallegos (1967) suggested that this provided the neural analog for the first type of spatial summation proposed by Herget et al. They found that activity from several single spots summated to produce more activity in the primary axon than when a single spot was cooled. A replication of this experiment that employed more sophisticated stimulating equipment (Duclaux & Kenshalo, 1973) showed that the activity in the axon from stimulation of two spots was no greater than that produced by stimulation of the more sensitive spot alone. Thus, the electrophysiological evidence rules out the possibility that spatial summation occurs by virtue of endings whose branches converge near the periphery.

Convergence of the afferent input from thermoreceptors apparently can and does occur at the first synapse in the trigeminal nucleus and in the dorsal horn of the spinal cord. The receptive fields of specific cold units are larger than those of single primary cold fibers in the trigeminal nucleus of the cat

(Fruhstorfer & Hensel, 1973) and in the dorsal horn of monkeys (Iggo & Ramsey, 1974). In both reports the central units were ipsilateral to the site of stimulation. Testing for contralateral receptive fields was not mentioned. In the rat, dorsal horn cells that respond to warming or cooling of the scrotum have large bilateral receptive fields, as do thermally sensitive units in the thalamus and the cortex (Hellon & Mitchell, 1975). In man, bilateral responses, evoked by warming and cooling the thenar eminence, have been recorded in which the ipsilateral response was of reduced amplitude and longer latency than the contralateral response (Duclaux, Franzen, Chatt, Kenshalo & Stowell, 1974; Chatt & Kenshalo, in press a,b).

Spatial summation appears to occur by convergence of primary thermal afferents on second order neurons in the dorsal horn and trigeminal nucleus and perhaps at higher centers. In humans, spatial warmth summation at threshold intensities continues for areas up to about 400 cm^2 (Stevens & Marks, 1971) which suggests that further convergence may also occur at higher centers.

The bilateral receptive fields of the rat scrotum in single dorsal horn warm and cold units (Hellon & Mitchell, 1975) suggest that there are bilateral interacting pathways for thermal information in addition to the commonly accepted simple crossed pathways of the spinothalamic system in the cord (Truex & Carpenter, 1969). The viscera and the anogenital region may be bilaterally represented at single dorsal horn cells (Truex & Carpenter, 1969) but the bilateral responses recorded on the scalp evoked by warming and cooling the thenar eminence (Chatt & Kenshalo, in press, a,b: Duclaux et al, 1974) and the strong bilateral spatial summation of warm (Hardy & Oppel, 1937) and cool (Rozsa, 1975) stimuli in humans supports a more general bilateral representation.

<u>Paradoxical Responses</u>

In 1895 von Frey made the singular discovery that some cold

spots not only gave rise to sensations of cold when cooled but gave similar sensations when touched by a very warm (45° to 50°C) stimulator. This he labeled a "paradoxical" cold sensation.

Electrophysiological studies by Dodt and Zotterman (1952) have described what appears to be the neural analog of the paradoxical cold response. Warming the receptive field resulted in a suppression of activity until it is warmed beyond 45° to 50°C. There followed a discharge in the cold fiber that reached a peak frequency of about 7.5 imp/sec at about 50°C. There was no phasic response to the high heat and the discharge persisted as long as the high temperature was maintained, hence, it was a steady state response.

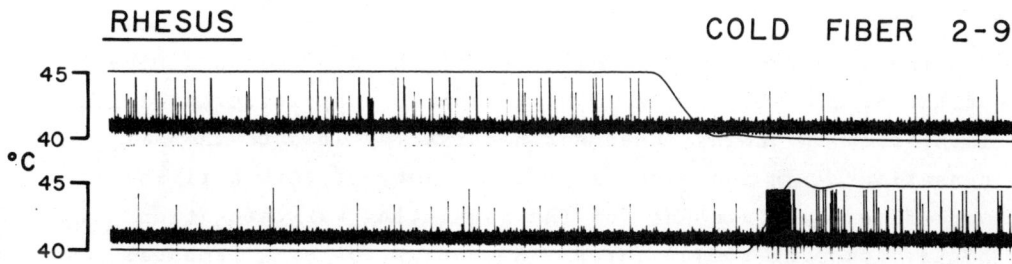

FIG. 13. A paradoxical response of a cold fiber to heating. The receptive field was first cooled from 45° to 40°C which paradoxically resulted in a suppression of the steady-state response. Upon rewarming to 45°C (second spike train) there occurred a phasic overshoot in frequency followed by a return of the 45°C steady-state response. The fiber responded like a cold unit at 40°C and lower adapting temperatures. The biphasic spikes are presumed to be from a polymodal nociceptor.

Some primate cold fibers also show responses to high temperatures. Roughly, 33 percent of a small sample showed a higher steady-state response to a 45° than a 40°C adapting temperature. As seen in Fig. 13, they also showed a phasic response to warming (Kenshalo & Duclaux, in prep.). The entire response process of the receptor appears to be reversed and the activity of the fiber seems more like that seen in warm than in cold fibers. After the fibers had been adapted to 45°C, cooling, even by as little as 0.5°C suppressed the steady-state response and rewarming resulted in a phasic burst of activity followed by a return of the higher steady-state response.

These paradoxical responses of primate cold fibers can account for the paradoxical sensations produced by heating human cold spots.

SUMMARY

1. Thermal sensations, measured in humans, and the responses of primary warm and cold fibers, measured in monkeys, were compared in order to identify possible neural codes.

2. A lack of compelling evidence to the contrary, it is proposed that the temperature sensing system is a "labeled line" system.

3. The low levels of neural activity in warm and cold fibers at the static temperatures in the zone of physiological zero, identified in humans, need not necessarily lead to thermal sensations. An increase in the frequency of this activity in warm fibers may account for the persisting warm sensations at higher adapting temperatures. A combination of a temporal code (bursting) and the frequency code in cold fibers can account for the persisting cold sensation and thermoregulatory responses observed at low skin temperatures. A combination of the steady-state responses of warm and cold fibers can provide accurate information about skin temperature throughout its entire range.

4. Complete adaptation of sensation to a temperature change within the zone of physiological zero requires much more time than the establishment of a new steady-state response in primate warm and cold fibers following a similar change. The concept of a "central integrator," first proposed by Hensel (1973), with a long time constant of decay can accommodate this difference.

5. Thresholds of warm stimuli are large at low adapting temperatures and small at high adapting temperatures. Thresholds

of cool stimuli are the opposite.

The sensitivity of primate warm and cold receptors to a 0.5°C intensity of stimulation vary in a similar way as a function of the adapting temperature and suggests a simplistic frequency code for threshold sensations.

6. The rate of temperature change within the range of 0.5° to 2°C/sec is without effect on estimates of the magnitudes of warm and cool sensations. It has a pronounced effect on the magnitude of the responses of both warm and cold receptors at 2° and 5°C intensities of stimulation but, changes in the intensity of thermal stimuli produce marked changes in the response magnitude of warm and cold fibers. Yet, sensation magnitude follows stimulus intensity and not stimulus rate. The hypothesis of a central integrator with a long time constant of decay can accommodate this apparent contradiction if it is assumed that the activity level of the central integrator is proportional to the sensation magnitude.

7. Neural analogs of areal summation of single stimulus sites or of thermal stimuli presented bilaterally have not yet been described quantitatively.

8. The neural analog in primate cold fibers of the paradoxical cold sensations is described.

ACKNOWLEDGMENTS

This research was supported by USPHS Grant NB-02992 and NSF Grant GB-30610.

REFERENCES

Berg, S. L. (1975) Ph.D. Dissertation, Florida State University.
Burgess, P.R., & Perl, E. R. (1973) In A. Iggo (ed) Somatosensory System, Vol. II., P. 29-78, Handbook of Sensory Physiology. Berlin: Springer Verlag.
Burton, H., Terashima, S. I., & Clark, J. (1972) Brain Res., 45, 401.
Chambers, M. R., Andres, K. H., v.During, M. V., & Iggo, A. (1972) Quant. J. Exp. Physiol. 57, 417.
Chatt, A. B., & Kenshalo, D. R. (in press) Sensory Processes.
Chatt, A. B., & Kenshalo, D. R. (in press) Sensory Processes.
Courtney, K., Brengelman, G., & Sundsten, J.W. (1972) Brain Res., 43, 657.

Dodt, E., & Zotterman, Y. (1952) Acta Physiol. Scand., 26, 358.
Duclaux, R., Franzen, O., Chatt, A. B., Kenshalo, D. R., & Stowell, H. (1974) Brain Res., 78, 279.
Duclaux, R., & Kenshalo, D. R. (1972) J. Physiol. (Lond.) 224, 647.
Duclaux, R., & Kenshalo, D. R. (1973) Brain Res., 55, 437.
Duclaux, R., & Kenshalo, D. R. (in prep.) Steady-state and dynamic responses of primate warm receptors.
Dykes, R. W. (1975) Brain Res., 98, 485.
Erickson, R. P. (1973) Brain Res., 61, 113.
Erickson, R. P., & Poulos, D. A. (1973) Brain Res., 61, 107.
Frey, M. von (1895) Ber: sachs. Ges. Wiss. 47, 166.
Fruhstorfer, H., & Hensel, H. (1973) Die Naturwissenchaften, 60, 209.
Hagbarth, K. E., & Vallbo, A. B. (1967) Acta Physiol. Scand., 69, 121.
Hardy, J. D., & Oppel, T. W. (1937) J. Clin. Invest., 16, 533.
Harrington, T., & Merzenich, M. M. (1970) Exp. Brain Res., 10, 251.
Hellon, R. F., & Mitchell, D. (1975) J. Physiol., 248, 359.
Hensel, H. (1950) Pflügers Arch., 252, 165.
Hensel, H. (1952) Ergebn. d. Physiol., 47, 166.
Hensel, H. (1973a) Physiol. Rev., 53, 948.
Hensel, H. (1973b) In A.Iggo (ed) Somatosensory System, Vol.II P. 79, Handbook of Sensory Physiology. Berlin: Springer Verlag.
Hensel, H., & Iggo, A. (1971) Pflügers Arch., 329, 1.
Herget, C. M., Granath, L. P., & Hardy, J. D. (1941) Amer. J. Physiol., 135, 20.
Iggo, A. (1969) J. Physiol., 200, 403.
Iggo, A., & Iggo, B. J. (1971) J. Physiol. (Paris) 63, 287.
Iggo, A., & Muir, A. R. (1969) J. Physiol. (Lond.) 200, 763.
Iggo, A., & Ramsey, R. L. (1974) J. Physiol. (Lond.) 242, 132.
Johnson, K. O., Darian-Smith, I., & LaMotte, C. (1973) J. Neurophysiol., 36, 347.
Kenshalo, D. R. (1970) In W.D.Neff (ed) Contributions to Sensory Physiology, Vol IV. P. 19, New York: Academic Press.
Kenshalo, D. R. (1972) In J. Kling, L.A.Riggs (eds) Experimental Psychology. Vol I.P. 117. New York: Holt Rinehart & Winston.
Kenshalo, D. R., Decker, T., & Hamilton, A. (1967) J.Comp. Physiol. Psychol. 63, 510.
Kenshalo, D. R., & Duclaux, R. (in prep) Steady-state and dynamic responses of primate cold receptors.
Kenshalo, D. R., & Gallegos, E. S. (1967) Science, 158, 1064.
Kenshalo, D. R., Holmes, C. E., & Wood, P. B. (1968) Perception & Psychophysics, 3, 81.
Kenshalo, D. R., & Scott, H. H. (1966) Science, 151, 1095.
Konietzny, F., & Hensel, H. (1975) Pflügers Arch., 359, 265.
Marks, L. E., & Stevens, J. C. (1973) Amer. J. Psychol., 86, 251.
Melzack, R., & Wall, P. D. (1962) Brain, 85, 331.
Molinari, H.H., Greenspan, J., & Kenshalo, D. R. (in prep.) Rate of temperature change and sensation magnitude.
Poulos, D. A., & Benjamin, R. M. (1968) J. Neurophysiol., 31, 28.
Poulos, D. A., & Lende, R. A. (1970) J. Neurophysiol., 33, 508.

Rozsa, A. J. (1975) Masters Thesis, Florida State University.
Stevens, J. C., & Marks, L. E (1971) *Perception & Psychophysics* 9, 391.
Tapper, D. N. (1965) *Exp. Neurol.*, 13, 364.
Truex, R. C., & Carpenter, M. B. (1969) *Human Neuroanatomy*, 6th Ed. Baltimore: Williams and Wilkins.

Discussion:

Zotterman: What is the reason for this "discrepency"? Is this due to the bursting or nor?

Kenshalo: Intuitively it would appear so. However, I have no evidence that bursting per se is the code although it seems to be an ideal candidate for a temporal code not only for several sensations but also for thermal regulatory process. I think we'll hear a little bit more from Dr Hensel on that.

Zotterman: In order to understand this you should have the integrative response from the total nerve. If you are working on single fibers that gives you very good information about how single units work. But what happens to us is that we have a mass input from various numbers of fibers.

Kenshalo: Our attempt was just exactly that in taking the mean responses of fifteen cold units. That is all we had complete data on. This was the case rather than considering just the activity of a single fiber. But I think you are quite right that certainly the nervous system sees a great deal more than just a count.

von Euler: I would like to ask Dr Iggo whether the secondary neurons and, even more, the subjective sensation is dependent upon the state in which the thermal regulator is operating at the moment?

Iggo: I think it was a waste of time coming up here as Dr Hensel is going to tell us about that in the next paper. But we were using anaesthetized animals in which the further regulatory state was largely out of action. There is evidence, however, from work done in Montcastle's laboratory that the behaviour of the afferent fibers may be affected by the temperature of the animal but these paradoxical discharges seem to become much more prominent in at least Montcastle's lab. Anyway if the animal's deep body temperature is say 38 or $39°$ compared with a deep body temperature of below $37°$, those results are not being confirmed elsewhere. This would suggest that there may be some effect on the general body thermal regulatory condition on the responses of the afferent fibers.

Kenshalo: I think the question included sensation as well. Peripheral ways of constriction is accompanied by an almost total loss of cold sensitivity. We found, for example, in students who were just going into a major examination that you might just as well dismiss them as subjects. In measuring their peripheral rate of motor response it is very restricted and we cannot get a threshold on them. As a matter of fact, almost any kind of physiological stress or psychological stress that will produce such a vasal motor constriction.

Hensel: May I answer your question as to the influence of the thermal rate resistance on the thermal afferents and the thermal thresholds. We have to discriminate between temperature sensation in a strict sense and between thermal comfort and discomfort. These are often confused with each other. As to thermal sensation as expressed by thermal thresholds, we have made experiments with subjects in a climatic chamber under different thermal stress from cold to heat. The thresholds for the local stimulator on the hand and so on remained practically unchanged. So they are highly but not completely independent of the general thermal state of the subject. This was not true of the feeling of comfort and discomfort. This corresponds to everyday experience. If you are overheated and you put your hand into cold water you say "wonderful, comfortable". If your whole body is cooled and you put your hand into the same water you say, "terrible". Comfort changes dramatically with the general state but not temperature sensation in the strict sense.

CORRELATIONS OF NEURAL ACTIVITY AND THERMAL SENSATION IN MAN

H. HENSEL

Institute of Physiology, University of Marburg/Lahn, GFR

Physiology of thermoreception includes various experimental approaches: (a) the phenomenological analysis of temperature sensations, (b) the measurement of thermal stimuli, and (c) the investigation of neural events, mainly by electrophysiological methods. In a wider sense, physiological and behavioral responses belong to this category as well. The relationship between these can be symbolized by a triad (Hensel, 1974) connecting a sensory phenomenon, a physical object, and an object of neurophysiology (Fig.1). The relationship between tempera-

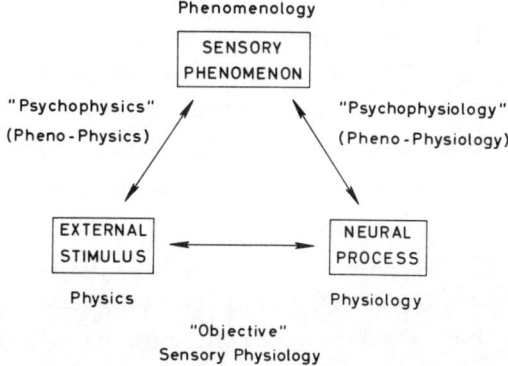

FIG. 1. Relationship between sensory phenomenon, external stimulus and neural events.

ture sensations and thermal stimuli is investigated by "Psychophysics" (or, more precisely, "Phenophysics"), between thermal sensations and neural events by "Psychophysiology" (or "Phenophysiology"), and between thermal stimuli and neural processes by the so-called objective sensory physiology. The latter does not include any thermal sensations but deals only with non--thermal observations.

A direct combination of all three approaches is only possible in human subjects. However, we are far from fully understanding these relationships. This is mainly due to our fragmentary knowledge of neurophysiological processes in man, but more information is also necessary about human temperature sensation, especially in the steady state. The following paper tries to summarize and critically discuss the results of various experimental approaches to thermoreception in man.

SPECIFICITY OF WARM AND COLD SENSATIONS

According to our present knowledge, warm and cold sensations in man are mediated by two different systems, one being specific for the quality of warmth and the other for the quality of cold. The mere existence of receptors in human skin specifically responding either to warming or to cooling would not be sufficient to demonstrate a dual neurophysiological basis for thermal sensations. But there are other facts, old and new ones, which are not compatible with the assumption that both warm and cold sensations are mediated by one system, preferably of $A\delta$ cold fibers (Erickson and Poulos, 1973). Since the fundamental discovery by Blix (1882) of specific warm and cold spots, it has been shown that warm sensations can be elicited only from warm spots and cold sensations only from cold spots. Warming a cold spot is either ineffective or, at higher temperatures, leads to paradoxical cold sensations.

In a series of indirect experiments the activity of cold fiber populations in monkeys was compared with cold sensation in human subjects (Darian-Smith et al., 1973; Johnson et al., 1973). The difference limen of sensation for two cooling pulses was found to be a linear function of intensity. Under the assumption that the neural correlate of the difference limen is a certain statistical difference between the average activities of a cold receptor population, the experimental values imply that only cold receptors, but neither warm receptors nor slowly adapting mechanoreceptors can account for human cold discrimination. On the other hand, warmth discrimination cannot be explained on the basis of cold fiber inhibition alone but requires an additional receptor population sensitive to warming.

Furthermore, measurements of reaction times to thermal pulses in human subjects have revealed lower conduction velocities for warm than for cold sensations (Fruhstorfer et al., 1972). Finally, in recent experiments with nerve blocking, selective inhibition of either cold or warm sensibility has been achieved (Torebjörk and Hallin, 1972; Fruhstorfer et al., 1974).

WARM RECEPTORS IN HUMAN SKIN

While specific cold receptors have long been known to occur in the skin of monkeys (Iggo, 1963) and humans (Hensel and Boman, 1960), specific warm receptors have been found more recently in monkeys (Hensel, 1969; Hensel and Iggo, 1971; Sumino et al., 1975; Darian-Smith et al., 1975).

Afferents of specific warm fibers have now been recorded from the superficial branch of the radial nerve in human subjects (Konietzny and Hensel, 1975). The impulses of these fibers were led off by means of Hostaflon TF coated tungsten microneedles (Konietzny and Hensel, 1974), and the spot-like receptive fields were localized on the basic joint of the forefinger and the inner side of the thumb. Thermal stimuli were applied by a Peltier thermode of 12 mm in diameter delivering constant temperatures as well as linear changes between 0.03 and $2°C/sec$. The warm fibers were not excited by tactile and vibratory stimulation in the physiological range. Conduction velocities of 2 fibers were measured. The values of 0.5 and 0.75 m/sec, respectively, indicate that the fibers were non-myelinated.

The warm receptors were continuously active at constant skin temperatures above 33 to 35°C with a regular sequence of impulses, the frequency of which rose with temperature up to 45°C without reaching a maximum (Fig.2 and 6). Higher temperatures

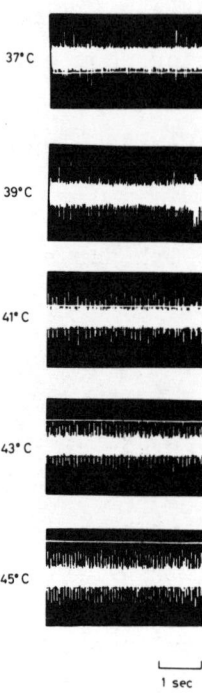

FIG. 2. Discharge of warm-sensitive fiber from superficial branch of human radial nerve at various constant skin temperatures. From Konietzny and Hensel (unpublished).

were avoided in these experiments. Linear temperature rises of 0.8°C/sec starting from an adapting temperature of 35°C caused an overshoot in frequency, while dynamic cooling was followed by a transient decrease in frequency (Fig.3 and 4).

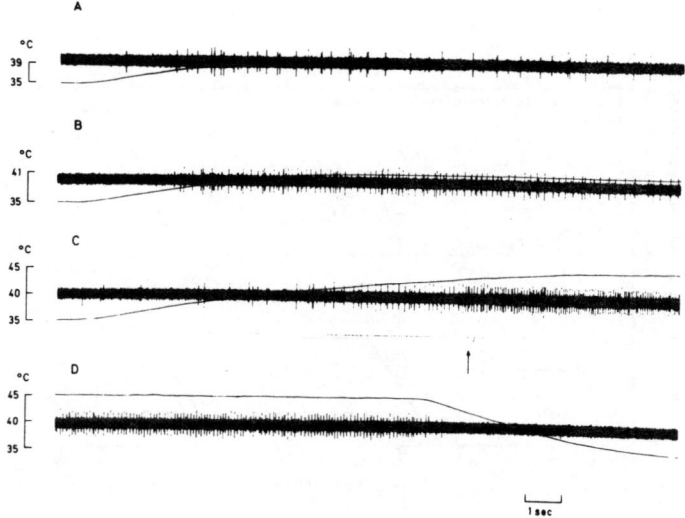

FIG. 3. Discharge of warm-sensitive fiber from superficial branch of human radial nerve and skin temperature when applying thermal stimuli. A, warming from 35 to 39°C. B, warming from 35 to 41°C. C, warming from 35 to 45°C; Arrow indicates threshold of warm sensation. D, cooling from 45 to 35°C; discharge stops at about 43°C. From Konietzny and Hensel (1975).

DYNAMIC THERMAL SENSATION AND NEURAL RESPONSE

There is a straightforward correlation of thermal sensations and neural responses with dynamic temperature changes. Throughout the whole range of activity, warm receptors will always respond with an overshoot in frequency on warming and an undershoot on cooling, while the opposite is true for cold receptors (Hensel, 1973a, 1974). Within a range of about 10°C, the magnitude of the dynamic response of thermoreceptors is approximately proportional to the magnitude of temperature change, as has been shown both for peripheral and central neurons in the thermosensitive pathway (Hensel, 1973a; Darian-Smith at al., 1973, 1975; Johnson et al., 1973; Poulos, 1975; Burton, 1975). The magnitude of temperature sensation corresponds well with the

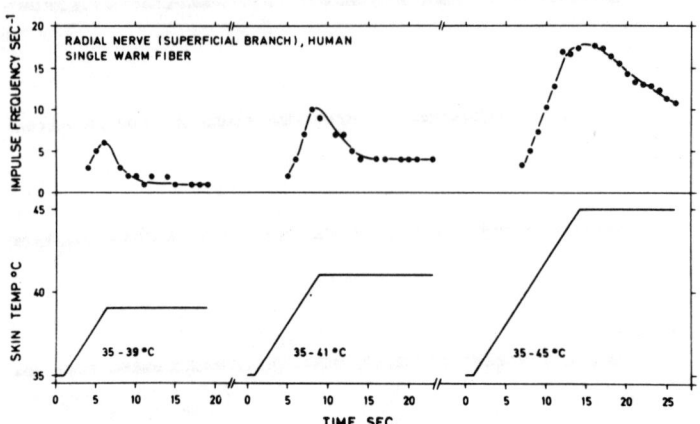

FIG. 4. Impulse frequency of warm-sensitive unit from superficial branch of human radial nerve when applying linear temperature changes and constant temperatures. From Konietzny and Hensel (unpublished).

neural events following dynamic temperature changes (Johnson et al., 1973; Darian-Smith et al., 1973, 1975).

When small areas of stimulation and small temperature changes are used, cold or warm receptors may be excited without conscious thermal sensations. The latter are only observed when a certain number of impulses per unit of time reaches the central nervous system.

Attempts have been made to determine this "central threshold" for single cold spots in human subjects (Järvilehto, 1973). We can assume that usually a warm or cold spot is served by a single fiber (Hensel, 1973a). After having measured the threshold of sensation by means of a micro-thermode, the same stimulus was applied to single cold receptors in the cat's nose, and the activity of the single fiber serving the receptor was recorded. From the results of direct recording of human cold fiber activity as well as of measurements of the thickness of the epidermis, the assumption is justified that the events in man and cat are comparable.

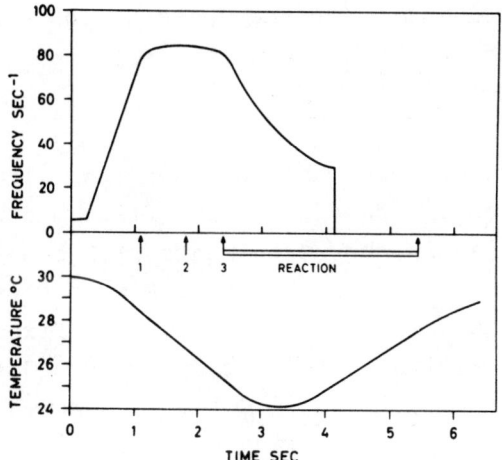

FIG. 5. Comparison between average changes in firing frequency of cold fibers in the cat's nose and reaction in man to a temperature stimulus of $\Delta T = -5.9°C$. Arrows: (1) instant of exceeding the threshold frequency in periphery; (2) instant of exceeding "central threshold" and (3) instant of reaction in man. From Järvilehto (1973).

Fig. 5 shows the relationship between the average reaction in man and the average single fiber activity in the cat to a cold stimulus. The threshold frequency is reached rather early, but this does not yet elicit a reaction in man. This reaction occurs more than 1 sec later. On the other hand, the cold sensation persists even if the peripheral frequency adapts to a value considerably below the maximum. This shows that the neural correlate of the "central threshold" is not simply a certain frequency of peripheral impulses. It seems that the frequency has to be maintained for some time, i.e. that the absolute number of impulses arriving into the CNS may also be significant. Furthermore, if there were a critical threshold frequency, then the cold sensation should disappear during the first period of adaptation. However, this is not the case in human experiments. According to Järvilehto (1973), the results in man are better explained if it is assumed that the "central threshold" is not a threshold in the strict sense, but presents only some kind of limit for the decision process which disappears, once exceeded, and thereafter all impulses arriving into the CNS contribute to the sensation.

Recently we have measured the threshold for warm sensations in human subjects on the same receptive field and with the same stimulator as used in the experiments with single warm fibers (Konietzny and Hensel, unpublished). A warm spot on the back of the hand was localized, and the stimulator fixed on this area. Warming from 35°C with a linear slope of 0.8°C/sec led to an average threshold of 37.8±0.15°C (60 measurements in 6 subjects). According to our limited results, this would correspond to only a few warm impulses per second. Since no more than 1 or 2 warm spots were excited, the central threshold, as expressed by neural parameters, may be smaller for warm than for cold sensations.

STATIC ACTIVITY OF THERMORECEPTORS

It is well known that the static discharge of single warm and cold fibers shows a bell-shaped curve of frequency vs. temperature. The static maxima of various cold receptors are scattered over a temperature range from 17 to 36°C and that of warm receptors over a range from 41 to 47°C. Thus a whole receptor population will cover a broader span of constant temperatures than a single receptor (Fig.6). In the monkey, the mean static frequency of a certain population of warm receptors increased from 30 to 45°C without reaching a maximum (Hensel, 1973a), while the mean static frequency of a cold fiber population increased from 43 to 24°C and then slightly decreased (Dykes, 1975).

As yet we have not enough information about the static activity of cold and warm receptor populations in human subjects. The curve for the warm fiber shown in Fig.6 fits well into the general picture.

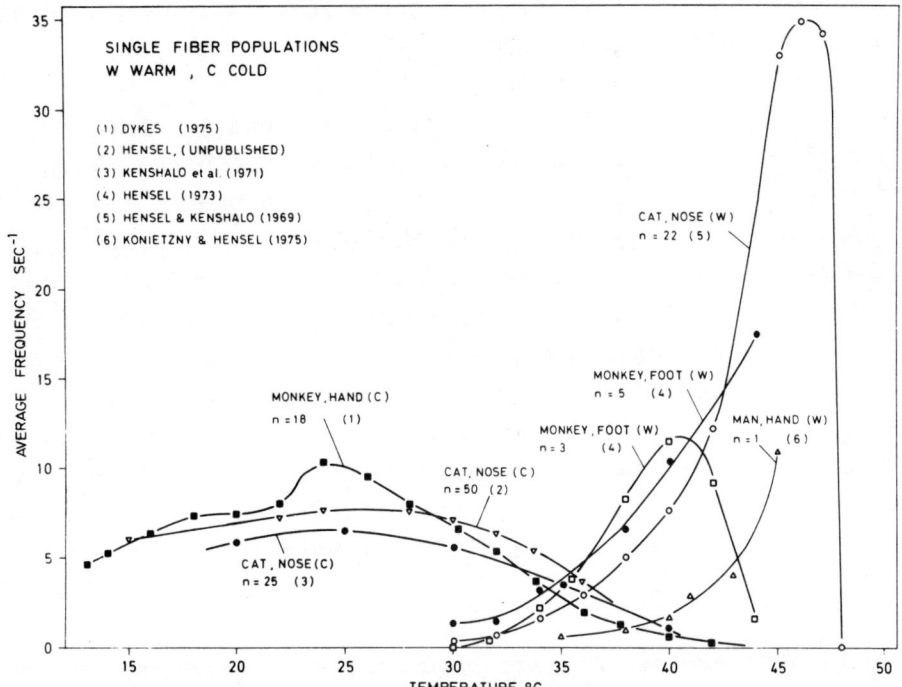

FIG. 6. Average frequency of static discharge of thermosensitive single fiber populations as function of constant skin temperature.

It has been emphasized that, because of the bell-shaped curve, the mean static frequency of thermoreceptors gives ambiguous information of constant temperatures. From a general point of view this is true, although the question remains whether this type of curve would, in fact, be incompatible with the biological function of thermoreceptors. Puzzled by this problem, physiologists have looked for suitable parameters other than mean frequency. A promising candidate is the static burst or group discharge of cold receptors, first seen in the cat's lingual nerve (Hensel and Zotterman, 1951) and later in a number of species. (For references see Hensel, 1973a, 1974; Iggo and Young, 1975). In the monkey certain burst parameters, such as the number of impulses per group, change in a monotonic way with temperature between 35 and 20°C (Iggo and Iggo, 1971; Iggo and Young, 1975; Poulos, 1975; Dykes, 1975) and thus offer a theoretical possibility of unambiguous information about static temperatures within this range.

However, there are difficulties which may lead to some scepticism about the significance of the burst discharge. Static bursting of cold fibers seems to be a common phenomenon only in the monkey. According to an analysis of about 100 cold fibers in the cat's infraorbital nerve, bursting occurred in 80 % of the fibers only during dynamic cooling from 35 to 30°C, whereas at constant temperatures between 30 and 20°C, no more than 2 to 17 % of the fibers showed grouped discharges (Hensel and Schöner, unpublished). Moreover, there was no marked change in the number of impulses per burst between 30 and 20°C, the average values being 2.0 and 3.5, respectively. Here we might ask whether the monkey's hand is a better thermometer than the cat's nose.

Although more experiments are required, a thorough evaluation of our material renders it doubtful whether static bursts occur frequently in human cold fibers. Besides a non-bursting cold fiber already described (Hensel and Boman, 1960), 11 cold-sensitive multi- and few-fiber preparations with clearly visible single spikes have been obtained from human cutaneous nerves (Hensel and Boman, unpublished). When applying static and dynamic temperature stimuli in the range between 38 and 12°C, only one single fiber in a few-fiber preparation showed a typical burst discharge (Fig.7). Ironically enough, this was one of my own cold fibers. During cooling from 38 to 25°C an initial regular discharge of 80/sec gradually transformed into a series of bursts lasting for the remaining period of cooling. The number of impulses per group increased continuously from about 4 to 15, while the interburst interval remained relatively constant (0.04 to 0.05 sec). However, after rewarming for 10 sec to 34°C and repeated cooling to 23°C, only a regular

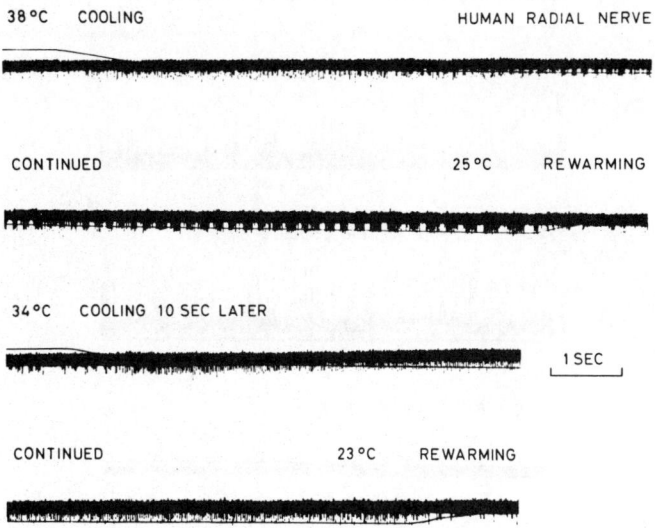

FIG. 7. Discharge of cold-sensitive few-fiber preparation from superficial branch of human radial nerve and skin temperature when applying thermal stimuli. From Hensel and Boman (unpublished).

sequence of cold impulses was seen. Thus the observed burst discharge seems to be a transient phenomenon, similar to that of the cat's infraorbital cold fibers. An example of a few-fiber discharge from the human radial nerve is given in Fig.8. 30 sec after the onset of cooling, the fiber with the largest spikes shows some grouping of impulses but in the steady state at 22.5°C no distinct burst activity is seen.

Sufficient evidence has not been obtained from central neurons in the thermosensitive pathway to either support or reject the hypothesis that the grouped discharge of cold receptors plays a significant role in encoding constant temperatures. In the medulla and thalamus of the monkey (Poulos and Benjamin, 1968;

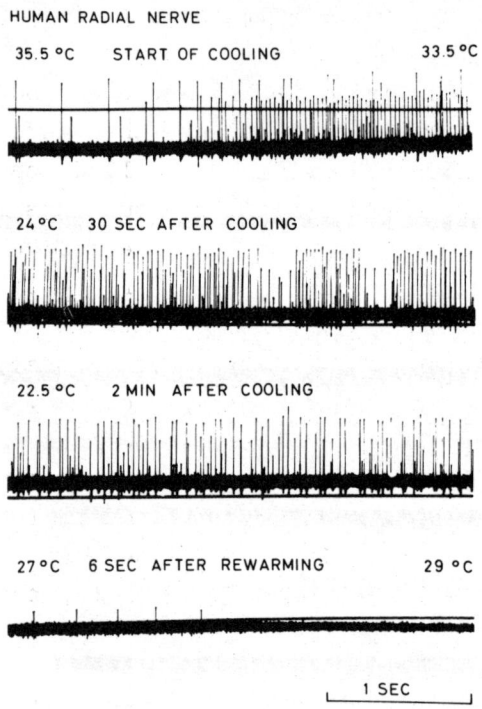

FIG. 8. Discharge of cold-sensitive few-fiber preparation from superficial branch of human radial nerve and skin temperature during cooling to a constant level of 22.5°C and rewarming. From Hensel and Boman (unpublished).

Poulos, 1971, 1975) as well as in the spinal cord of cat and monkey (Burton, 1975), the static response profiles of single neurons remained similar to the bell-shaped curve of mean frequency observed in the periphery. At the thalamic level, some grouped discharges were seen during static thermal stimulation, but the analysis is confounded by the effects of thalamic spindling activity (Poulos, 1975).

STATIC TEMPERATURE SENSATION AND RECEPTOR ACTIVITY

In contrast to numerous studies with dynamic thermal stimulation, thorough investigations of human temperature sensations in the steady state are largely lacking. As far as experimental data in this field are available, many of them have been obtained by using relatively small thermodes and/or adaptation times of only a few minutes. We have therefore started a series of investigations under rigidly controlled conditions (Beste, Hensel and Kaiser, unpublished). The subjects lay in a climatic chamber set at neutral temperature. The palm of the hand was placed on a large water-circulated thermode of 75 cm^2 surface area, or it was immersed in flowing water of controlled velocity and temperature. The temperatures of thermode, water, and skin were recorded by means of thermocouples. The hand was kept on the stimulator or in the water throughout the whole series of measurements, and each steady state was maintained for at least 30 min before observations were made. The sequence of temperatures was started from the highest as well as from the lowest level; this had no significant influence on the estimations in the steady state.

The diagram in Fig.9 shows the estimated static temperatures of the hand on the thermode as a function of constant skin temperature in 18 subjects. The estimations were made both in terms of $°C$ and of a relative scale between the highest ($40°C$) and the lowest ($25°C$) temperature. As can be seen, there is practically no temperature range at which complete adaptation of thermal sensation occurs. The estimation in $°C$ is most correct at $37°C$, while the temperatures above this level are estimated to be higher than the physical value in $°C$ and the temperatures below $37°C$ are estimated to be lower than the corresponding physical value (deviation from the "equal distance" line). Below $27°C$, the curve of temperature estimation becomes practically horizontal and thus the static difference limen relatively large. The qualitative shape of the curve corresponds quite well with the curve of the mean static discharge frequency of cold receptor populations as function of temperature (cf. Fig.6).

In another preliminary series of experiments we have tried to

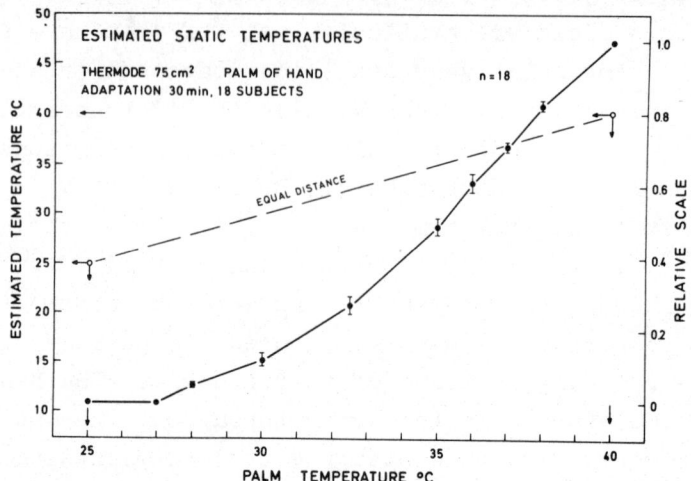

FIG. 9. Estimated static temperatures as function of constant temperatures of the palm on a water-circulated thermode (surface area 75 cm^2, adaptation 30 min). Left scale: estimates in °C. Right scale: estimates in relative units. "Equal-distance" line indicates identity between estimated and physical temperatures in °C. Average values of 18 subjects; bars indicate S.E. of mean. From Beste, Hensel and Kaiser (unpublished).

estimate the magnitude of temperature difference between the left hand continuously immersed in water of 28°C and the right hand exposed to constant temperatures between 28 and 17°C (Fig. 10). No marked difference was experienced until the temperature of the right hand was set below 23°C. Then the hand was clearly judged as being cooler than the other one, but, as some of the 10 subjects spontaneously remarked, this was mainly achieved by a change in quality of sensation becoming more "sharp", "ice-cold" and gradually painful. The measurements by Erickson and Poulos (1973) of static temperature difference limens between the right and left hand, although obtained with different methods (thermodes 36 cm^2, adaptation 5 min), bear at least some qualitative similarity with our results, in that the discriminatory ability was least precise between 29 and 26°C and

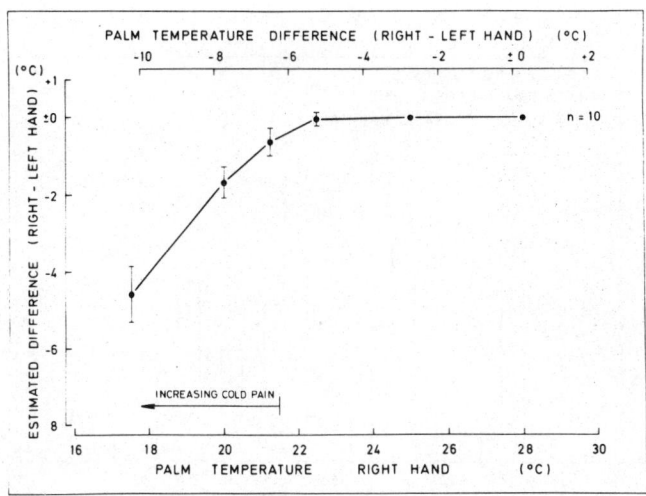

FIG. 10. Estimated difference in °C between left and right hand immersed in flowing water of constant temperature. Left hand was continuously kept at palm temperature of 28°C, right hand exposed for 30 min to palm temperatures indicated on the abscissa. Average values of 10 subjects; bars indicate S.E. of mean. From Beste, Hensel and Kaiser (unpublished).

increased in precision below 25°C.

This brings up the question whether the discrimination of constant temperatures, particularly in the cold range, might have its neurophysiological correlate in a simultaneous pattern of units with different properties. A similar concept of the qualitative aspect of the temperature sense was put forward by Erickson and Poulos (1973), ascribing static thermal discrimination to some kind of across-fiber pattern.

An analysis of static activity curves from cold fibers in the cat's lingual nerve revealed a rather inhomogenous distribution over the temperature range, the static maxima being accumulated at certain temperatures (Fig.11). These findings may give some support for the hypothesis that at lower constant temperatures

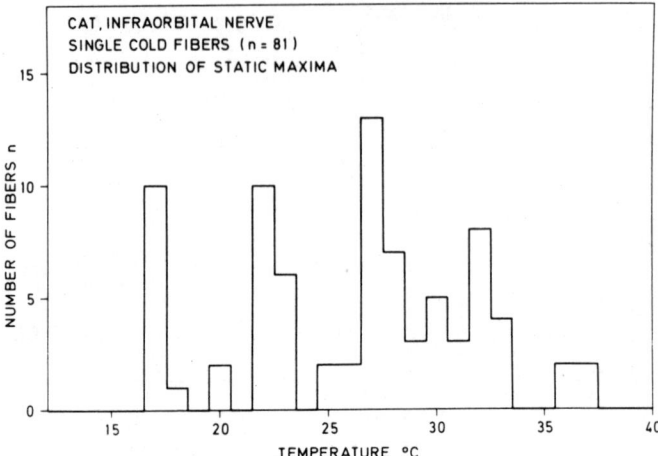

FIG. 11. Relative number of static activity maxima of 81 single cold fibers from the cat's infraorbital nerve as function of constant skin temperature.

receptor populations with different properties may be activated. It seems unlikely that the increasing discriminatory capacity between 23 and 17°C as well as the change in sensory quality may be due to the burst discharge. In the monkey, at skin temperatures below 20°C, the number of impulses per burst decreased again and the organized nature of the discharge deteriorated (Dykes, 1975).

It has been postulated that, in order to maintain constant core temperature, homeotherms must have the capacity to monitor constantly their thermal environment and, therefore, cold receptors must be able to encode unambiguously a wide range of constant temperatures. This is another argument for the significance of the grouped discharge but, to my opinion, it is not convincing. Cutaneous thermoreceptors are involved in the thermoregulatory system mainly by their capacity of signalling rapid temperature changes rather than constant temperatures (Hensel, 1973b). As to the steady state, homeothermic organisms are well equipped with temperature sensors in the CNS, the static characteristics of which will ensure homeothermy, even if the afferents from the periphery are not accurate in the sense of a thermometer. It is true that in humans with constant internal temperature, thermogenetic metabolism in the steady state increases as a function of decreasing average skin temperature (Benzinger, 1969; Nadel and Horvath, 1969). However, when the static skin temperature falls below a level of about 23°C, then the metabolic response decreases again. The curves obtained by Benzinger (1969) for O_2 consumption in humans as a function of average skin temperature correspond relatively well with the curves of the mean static discharge frequency of cold fibers in the monkey, as described by Dykes (1975) (Fig.12).

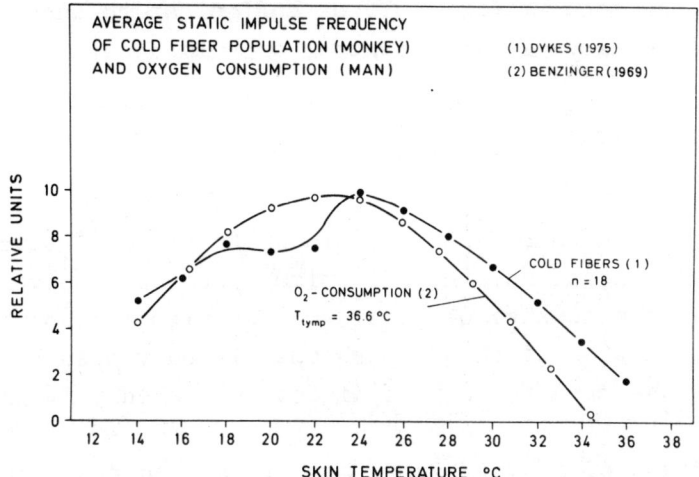

FIG. 12. Comparison of mean static impulse frequency of a cold fiber population in the monkey (Dykes, 1975) as function of skin temperature and oxygen consumption of human subject at 36.6°C tympanic temperature as function of average skin temperature in the steady state (Benzinger, 1969). Skin temperatures are corrected values from the temperature of a water bath in which the subject was immersed.

It should also be emphasized that man, according to his physiological outfit, is a tropical being. In his **tropical** habitat he never reaches low skin temperatures. Even at ambients of 10°C, the average skin temperature of a naked subject will not drop below 26°C in the steady state (Nadel and Horvath, 1969). This is quite unpleasant already and will set up behavioral responses to avoid the cold.

The warm side seems less problematic, as the average discharge of certain warm fiber populations is able to monitor unambiguously the static temperature range between 33 and 46°C (or even more), that is, between thermal indifference and heat pain.

Therefore we may conclude that the mean frequency of cold and warm receptor populations would be sufficient to encode the informations required for the control of human body temperature.

SUMMARY

Physiology of thermoreception includes the investigation of temperature sensations, thermal stimuli, and neural events, in a wider sense also physiological and behavioral responses. A direct combination of these approaches is only possible in humans but the results in this direction are only fragmentary.

The hypothesis of a dual system mediating cold and warm sensations is supported by the presence of separate and specific warm and cold spots, by differential blocking of either warm or cold sensation, and by different conduction velocities in the pathway for these sensations.

In addition to previous knowledge of cold fibers, specific warm fibers have been found in human subjects. These unmyelinated fibers (conduction velocity 0.5 to 0.75 m/sec) show static and dynamic responses to thermal stimuli; their static discharge frequency increases in the range from 33 to 45°C.

The mean frequency of certain warm fiber populations in the

monkey has a static maximum at temperatures above 45°C; the corresponding temperature for the maximum discharge of cold fiber populations is 24°C. Some parameters of the static burst discharge of cold fibers extend the range of unambiguous monitoring of constant temperature until 20°C but it is not known whether bursts are of physiological significance. They seem to be a common phenomenon only in the monkey but not in cats and humans.

Constant temperatures of the hand between 40 and 27°C can be estimated with relatively high accuracy. At lower temperatures, the discrimination decreases but increases again below 23°C, together with a change in quality towards cold pain. The possible significance of cold fiber populations with different properties is discussed.

For the regulation of body temperature the information conveyed by the static and dynamic mean frequency of cold and warm receptor populations would be sufficient.

This work was supported by the Deutsche Forschungsgemeinschaft.

REFERENCES

Benzinger, T.H.: Heat regulation: homeostasis of central temperature in man. Physiol.Rev. 49, 671-759 (1969)
Blix, M.: Experimentala bidrag till lösning af fragan om hudnervernas specifika energi. I. Upsala Läk.-Fören. Förh. 18, 87-102 (1882-1883)
Burton, H.: Responses of spinal cord neurons to systematic changes in hindlimb skin temperatures in cats and primates. J.Neurophysiol. 38, 1060-1079 (1975)

Darian-Smith, I., K.O. Johnson and R. Dykes: "Cold" fiber population innervating palmar and digital skin of the monkey: responses to cooling pulses. J.Neurophysiol. 36, 325-346 (1973)

Darian-Smith, I., K.O. Johnson and C. La Motte: Peripheral neural determinants in the sensing of changes in skin temperature. In: The somatosensory system, ed. H.H.Kornhuber, p.23-37. Stuttgart: Georg Thieme 1975

Dykes, R.W.: Coding of steady and transient temperatures by cutaneous 'cold' fibers serving the hand of monkeys. Brain Res. 98, 485-500 (1975)

Erickson, R.P., and D.A. Poulos: On the qualitative aspect of the temperature sense. Brain Res 61, 107-112 (1973)

Fruhstorfer, H., H. Guth and U. Pfaff: Thermal reaction time as a function of stimulation site. Pflügers Arch. 335, R 49 (1972)

Fruhstorfer, H., M. Zenz, H. Nolte and H. Hensel: Dissociated loss of cold and warm sensibility during regional anaesthesia. Pflügers Arch. 349, 73-82 (1974)

Hensel, H.: Cutane Wärmereceptoren bei Primaten. Pflügers Arch. 313, 150-152 (1969)

Hensel, H.: Cutaneous thermoreceptors. In: Handbook of sensory physiology, Vol.2, Somatosensory system, ed. A.Iggo, p. 79-110. Berlin, Heidelberg, New York: Springer Verlag 1973a

Hensel, H.: Neural processes in thermoregulation. Physiol.Rev. 53, 948-1017 (1973b)

Hensel, H.: Thermoreceptors. Ann.Rev.Physiol. 36, 233-249 (1974)

Hensel, H., and K. Boman: Afferent impulses in cutaneous sensory nerves in human subjects. J.Neurophysiol. 23, 564-578 (1960)

Hensel, H., and A. Iggo: Analysis of cutaneous warm and cold fibres in primates. Pflügers Arch. 329, 1-8 (1971)

Hensel, H., and D.R. Kenshalo: Warm receptors in the nasal region of cats. J.Physiol.(Lond.) 204, 99-112 (1969)

Hensel, H., and Y. Zotterman: Quantitative Beziehungen zwischen der Entladung einzelner Kältefasern und der Temperatur. Acta physiol.scand. 23, 291-319 (1951)

Iggo, A.: An electrophysiological analysis of afferent fibres in primate skin. Acta neuroveg.(Wien) 24, 225-240 (1963)

Iggo, A., and B.J. Iggo: Impulse coding in primate cutaneous thermoreceptors in dynamic thermal conditions. J.Physiol. (Paris) 63, 287-290 (1971)

Iggo, A., and D.W. Young: Cutaneous thermoreceptors and thermal nociceptors. In: The somatosensory system, ed. H.H.Kornhuber, p. 5-22. Stuttgart: Georg Thieme 1975

Järvilehto, T.: Neural coding in the temperature sense. Ann. Acad.Sci.Fenn.Ser. B, 184, 1-71 (1973)

Johnson, K.O., I. Darian-Smith and C. LaMotte: Peripheral neural determinants of temperature discrimination in man: A correlative study of responses to cooling skin. J.Neurophysiol. 36, 347-370 (1973)

Kenshalo, D.R., H. Hensel, P. Graziadei and H. Fruhstorfer: On the anatomy, physiology, and psychophysics of the cat's temperature-sensing system. In: Oral-facial sensory and motor mechanisms, eds. R.Dubner and Y.Kawamura, p. 23-45. New York: Appleton-Century-Crofts, Meredith Corp. 1971

Konietzny, F., and H. Hensel: Hostaflon TF coating of tungsten sensory microneedles. Pflügers Arch. 351, 357-360 (1974)

Konietzny, F., and H. Hensel: Warm fiber activity in human skin nerves. Pflügers Arch. 359, 265-267 (1975)

Nadel, E.R., and S.M. Horvath: Peripheral involvement in thermoregulatory response to an imposed heat debt in man. J.appl. Physiol. 27, 484-488 (1969)

Poulos, D.A.: Trigeminal temperature mechanisms. In: Oral-facial sensory and motor mechanisms, eds. R.Dubner and Y.Kawamura, p. 47-72. New York: Appleton-Century-Crofts, Meredith Corp. 1971

Poulos, D.A.: Central processing of peripheral temperature information. In: The somatosensory system, ed. H.H.Kornhuber, p. 78-93. Stuttgart: Georg Thieme 1975

Poulos, D.A., and R.M. Benjamin: Response of thalamic neurons to thermal stimulation of the tongue. J.Neurophysiol. 31, 28-43 (1968)

Sumino, R., R. Dubner and S. Starkman: Responses of small myelinated 'warm' fibers to noxious heat stimuli applied to the monkey's face. Brain Res. *62*, 260-263 (1973)

Torebjörk, H.E., and R.G. Hallin: Activity in C fibres correlated to perception in man. In: Cervical pain, eds. C.Hirsch and Y.Zotterman, p. 171-178. Oxford: Pergamon Press 1972.

Discussion:

Zotterman: It is commonly known that Europeans cannot go to sleep with cold feet while the Australian aborigenes sleep with cold feet. It is a kind of adaptation which is very well known. How can these Australians surpress this when we cannot? Your idea seems very sound to me. The difficulty is to prove this non-thermal type of impulses that are coming in at low temperatures which are not mediated by specific cold fibers. These fibers are C-fibers, most likely.

Hensel: The temperatures you mentioned in the feet of the Australians are about $12°$ which gives cold pain in ourselves. Not terrible, but quite considerable. Cold pain starts at temperatures of about $17°$. It is higher than one believes.

Zotterman: Having cold feet is not felt as a real pain but a discomfort which prevents you from sleeping.

Hensel: Perhaps we cannot agree on a definition of cold pain.

Zotterman: You know the expression: "I got cold feet".

Hensel: But cold feet are felt at a much higher temperature. Twenty-eight is possible for cold feet in the static state.

Zotterman: I am afraid I can feel that now.

Kenshalo: Dr Hensel, in your data on the zone of physiological zero, the zone of complete adaptation you had about a seventy-five square centimeter area exposed. Is that correct? What was the approximate zone? It was quite narrow.

Hensel: Practically at any temperature the subject could tell you some temperature. Of course, you could say it is thermally neutral. You could tell that this $34°$ or something like that. Mostly we use untrained subjects and just ask them to tell us the temperature of the thermode, not more. The outcome shows that this can be done with relatively good discrimination of the whole range although, of course, the estimated temperatures are not the same as the physical temperatures. But this is not interesting for the first experiments. I would say the zone of neutral temperatures has been in the order of perhaps one or two degrees Celcius near $34°$. Thirty-seven was felt as a nice, pleasant moderate-warm sensation.

Kenshalo: I have forgotten who did the work on it but they were judging thermal neutrality by exposing whole body to a climatic chamber. As I recall, the range there of thermal neutrality was somewhere between 33 and $35°$ which would be quite good agreement with your results.

Hellekant: As I understand you did these experiments over a fairly long period of time because you had thirty minutes for each exposure. What happened with the body temperature of the subjects after three or four hours at this low temperature?

Hensel: The body temperature was practically constant. We saw to it that the subject was lying in the climate chamber in order to avoid larger changes in the external temperature. There might be in some subjects a slight drop in internal temperature during prolonged experiments. For this reason we made our experiments partially starting with the coldest temperatures and in other experiments starting with warmer temperatures. There was no considerable difference between those.

Benzinger: We have changed the central temperature of the subject considerably over wide range and found no measurable influence on the cold reception of the subjects.

CONDUCTION IN THE AFFERENT THERMAL PATHWAYS OF MAN

H. FRUHSTORFER

Institute of Physiology, University of Marburg/Lahn, GFR

In the primate, most classes of cutaneous receptors have been neurophysiologically identified and their biophysical properties have been examined; now interest begins to focus on their significance for conscious sensation.

This is especially true of cutaneous thermosensibility where we well know the different types of receptors but very little about the sensations they evoke. Although there exist several groups of cutaneous thermoreceptors responding either specifically to innocuous or noxious thermal stimulation or, unspecifically, to both thermal and mechanical stimulation (Burgess and Perl, 1973; Hensel, 1973) the hypothesis of a single temperature sensing system in man (Hering, 1877) is still occasionally considered. This is mainly due to the difficulty to trace, in animal experiments, the afferent thermal pathways and to localize their cortical projection areas.

If it were easily possible to correlate in man isolated stimulation of identified receptor neurones with the sensation elicited, the sensory specificity of the different thermoreceptors would be clearer than it is today. An indirect yet practicable approach to this problem is the analysis of their sensory significance on the basis of a characteristic in which they differ. Axon diameter is such a parameter, by which it should be possible to discriminate between specific warm and cold receptors in the primate, as warm receptor neurones seem to have mainly unmyelinated axons whereas those of cold receptor neurones are partly myelinated (Hensel and Iggo, 1971). Due to this fact one could apply methods using conduction velocity or methods which block conduction in one fibre type without affecting the other.

Starting from the assumption that cold sensations are mediated by myelinated cold receptor neurones and warm sensations by unmyelinated warm receptor neurones, one should expect that the information about cold stimuli should reach the brain earlier than the information about warm stimuli and that this latency difference should be the greater the longer the afferent pathway.

BRAIN RESPONSES TO THERMAL STIMULATION

This assumption was first tested by examining cortical reaction potentials to cold and warm stimulation of the skin (Fruhstorfer et al., 1973, in press; Guth, 1975). 57 subjects received pure thermal pulses of 500 msec duration and $10^{\circ}C$ amplitude starting from an adapting temperature of $30^{\circ}C$. The stimuli were presented at a rate of 1 stim/30 sec by a water-circulated thermode of 18 mm diameter (Fruhstorfer and Detering, 1974) resting either on the right upper lip or in 15 subjects, also on the right thenar eminence at the border to the hairy skin. The EEG was recorded from the vertex (Cz-A2) and from a point above the left sensory cortex (C3-F5). During a session 25 responses to both cold and warm stimuli were collected and electronically summated.

Cortical reaction potentials were obtained from 53 subjects (Fig.1). At the vertex they consisted of a negative peak followed by a positive trough. Thus, they resembled in waveform auditory or somatosensory evoked responses (Fruhstorfer, 1971) though they had a longer latency and duration. The peak-to-peak amplitude was for both cold and warm stimuli approximately 15 μV when stimulating the lip and 11 μV when stimulating the hand. The peak latency of both components was significantly shorter (Wilcoxon Signed Rank Test, $p<0.01$) with cold stimula-

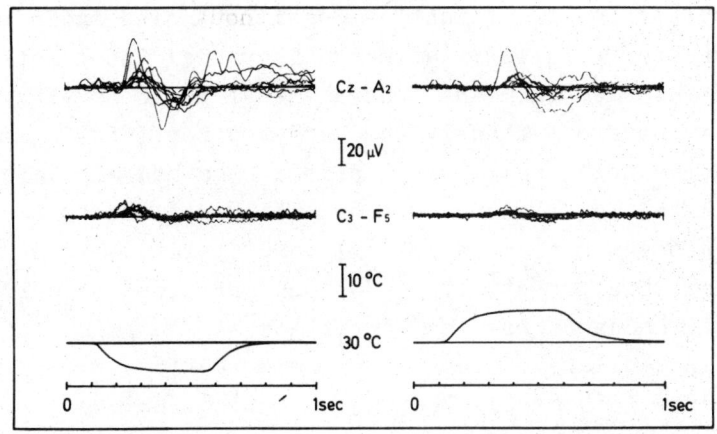

FIG. 1 Cortical reaction potentials from 10 subjects evoked by pure cold (left) and warm (right) stimulation of the right upper lip. The responses recorded from the vertex (upper traces) and from the sensory projection area (middle traces) are given together with the changes in skin temperature (lower traces). Each potential represents the average of 25 single responses.

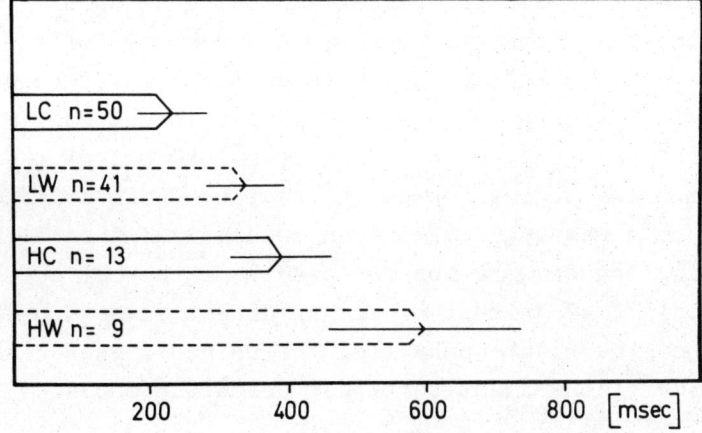

FIG. 2 Average latencies (M±SD) of the prominent negative peak N1 of the vertex potential evoked by cold (C) and warm (W) stimulation of lip (L) and hand (H).

tion than with warm stimulation (Fig.2). Stimulation of the hand resulted in significantly longer latencies and a significantly greater cold-warm latency difference. The reaction potentials recorded from the contralateral postcentral gyrus resembled in waveform closely the vertex potentials though they were considerably smaller in amplitude and had significantly shorter latencies (latency difference approximately 30 msec). These responses differ in polarity and amplitude from those obtained by Duclaux et al. (1974), who recorded on cold stimulation of the hand from the contralateral scalp initially positive potentials of large amplitude (25-36 μV) and long peak latency (325 msec). They did not find, however, responses to warming of the hand. Part of the discrepancies between the results of the two studies can be explained on the basis of differences in stimulation and EEG recording.

SIMPLE REACTION TIME TO THERMAL STIMULI

Our results indicate that the information about cutaneous cold stimulation reaches the cortex earlier than the information about warm stimulation. Similar results should be obtained if one measures the onset of sensation following thermal stimulation of the skin. Therefore, in a second study, simple reaction times to warm and cold pulses were examined in 29 subjects (Fruhstorfer et al., 1972; Pfaff, 1976). The stimuli had the same characteristics as in the study before except that they were terminated by the subject's reaction. Each stimulus was preceded by a warning sound at an interval of 1 sec; 10 % of the warning sounds were not followed by a thermal pulse (i.e. catch trials). 40 stimuli of either direction were presented to the skin of the right upper lip, the thenar eminence and the medial side of the right foot just below the ancle.

All subjects clearly recognized the stimuli and never reacted in a catch trial. The reaction times for cold stimuli were significantly shorter than those for warm stimuli. This corresponds to earlier studies using thermal stimuli contaminated by mechanical components (Bazett et al., 1930; Corson and Crannell, 1970). The cold-warm latency difference increased significantly (Wilcoxon Signed Rank Test, p<0.01) when the hand or the foot was stimulated (Fig.3 and 4). The variability of the reaction

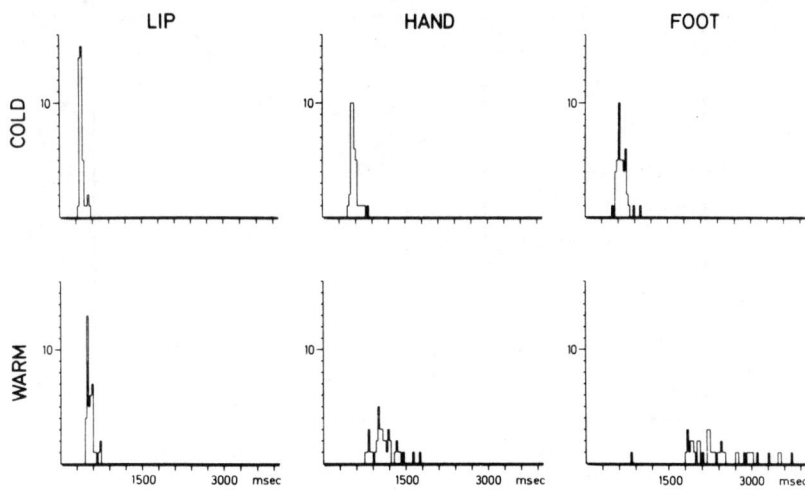

FIG. 3 Distribution of the reaction times of one subject for cold and warm stimulation of lip, hand, and foot.

times for cold stimuli was smaller than that for warm stimuli (Fig.3). This corresponds well to the reports of the subjects that cold sensation had a sharp onset whereas warm sensation was slowly rising in magnitude.

These results indicate that cold stimuli are perceived earlier than warm stimuli and that this time difference increases if the stimuli are applied to sites further away from the brain. Thus, both experiments support the assumption, that cold and warm sensations are mediated by pathways differing in transmission velocity. The conduction velocity can be roughly estimated by calculating the lip-hand latency differences for cold and warm stimulation and relating them to the lip-hand length difference of the afferent pathway, which amounts to approximately 75 cm. Calculated from the latencies of the vertex potentials the cold pathway has a transmission velocity of

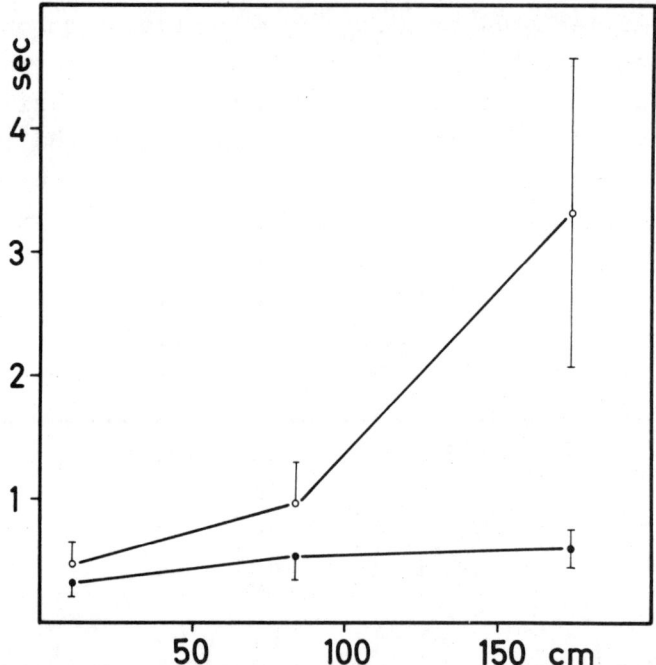

FIG. 4 Average reaction time (M±SD) for warm (upper curve) and cold (lower curve) stimulation as a function of the approximate length of the afferent pathway. Stimulation sites were upper lip, hand and foot. The median reaction times were calculated for each subject and the results of all 29 subjects were then combined.

4.3 m/sec., whereas that of the warm pathway amounts to 2.4 m/sec. Calculated from the RTs the respective values are 4.5 m/sec and 2.1 m/sec. These velocities correspond to those found in cold and warm receptor neurones of the primate (Hensel and Iggo, 1971). Nevertheless, these values have to be taken with care as the method of calculation, though eliminating differences in the receptor localization or in the central processing time assumes a similar receptor density at both stimulation sites. Nevertheless, conduction velocities of about 4 m/sec are so slow that neither evoked responses nor reaction times to cold stimuli could be accounted for by the action of fast conducting cold sensitive mechanoreceptors (Brown and Iggo, 1967).

DISSOCIATED LOSS OF THERMAL SENSIBILITY

If cold sensations were indeed mediated mainly by myelinated axons whereas warm sensations mainly by unmyelinated fibres than it should be possible to block differentially one fibre group leaving conduction in the other one intact. Therefore the loss of warm, cold and pain sensibility was studied during differential chemical block of the ulnar nerve and related to the block of vegetative and motor functions. In 11 subjects, both ulnar nerves were blocked by etidocaine 1 % and 0.5 % and bupivacaine 0.5 % and 0.25 % in two separate sessions (Radtke et al., 1975). Nerve function was tested by a regularly presented cycle of 4 stimuli (cold, pinprick, warm and sound) each preceded by a short warning tone pip. The cycle duration was 1 min. Cold and warm pulses and the pin prick were presented to the hypothenar. The subject had to respond to the stimuli by pressing a key as soon as he perceived them, and the RT was measured. In the case of the pin prick the subject had additionally to report when after the injection of the anaesthetic, the pin prick felt no longer sharp but blunt. During the sound the subject had to abduct his little finger and the maximal force was measured. At the same time the skin temperature difference between index finger and little finger was measured in order to determine the degree of vasodilatation (for details c.f. Fruhstorfer et al., 1974).

Injection of the anaesthetic caused a dissociated loss of warm and cold sensibility in the hypothenar region (Figs. 5 and 6): warm sensibility was lost significantly earlier than cold sensibility (Wilcoxon Signed Rank Test, $p<0.01$). Simultaneously with the warm sensibility block pin prick sensation changed from sharp to blunt. When both warm and cold sensibility were completely blocked, touch was still perceived and the force of the affected muscles was reduced to approximately 55 % of the original value. The loss of a thermal quality was usually preceded by a significant increase in reaction time. This could indicate that, normally, spatial summation occurs in the affer-

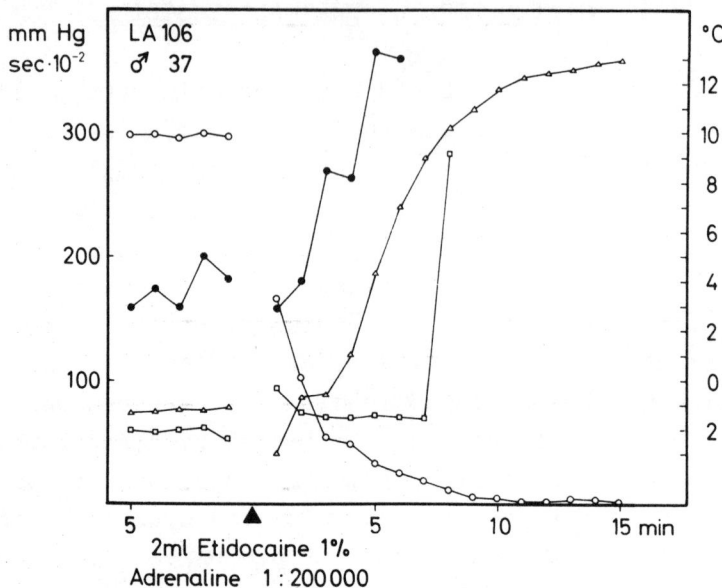

FIG. 5 Onset of a ulnar nerve block. Warm sensation is blocked 7 min, cold sensation 9 min after the injection of the anaesthetic. (Open circles = force in mm Hg; closed circles = warm reaction time; open triangles = temperature difference between index and little finger; open squares = cold reaction time).

ent pathways and that the progressive loss of conducting afferent neurones is compensated by temporal summation. The inability to detect warm stimuli with cold sensibility still intact shows that the decrease in cold receptor activity on warming is not perceived.

Nerve functions tended to recover in the reverse order as they had been lost, warm sensibility block lasting significantly longer than cold sensibility block. None of the subjects reported that a thermal sensation, before being blocked, had changed its quality in the sense that a cold stimulus was perceived as warm, tactile, or painful. As the thick myelinated axons of cold sensitive mechanoreceptors should still conduct

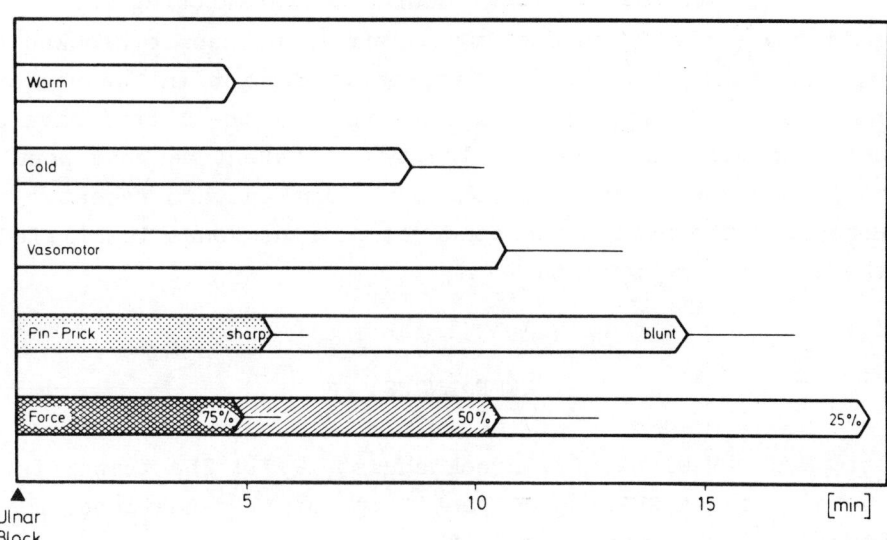

FIG. 6 Average latencies ($M \pm SE$) of differential nerve block. Vasomotor afferents were considered to be blocked when the skin temperature had exceeded 25 % of the final peak amplitude. The results from 44 blocks in 11 subjects are combined. Anaesthetics were etidocaine 1 % and 0.5 % and bupivacaine 0.5 and 0.25 %, both with adrenaline.

at this instant, cold stimulation of these receptors obviously does not lead to conscious sensations. This supports the view that slowly adapting cold sensitive mechanoreceptors have a purely tactile function (Duclaux and Kenshalo, 1972, Johnson et al., 1973). Finally, the block of warm sensibility was never accompanied by a persisting cold sensation, indicating that thermal indifference is not achieved by simply combining the information from both cold and warm receptors.

CONCLUSIONS

The results of the three studies suggest that, in man, the information about cutaneous warm and cold stimulation is transmitted from the periphery to the central nervous system by two different neurone populations. Neurones transmitting warm information are slowly conducting. Their axons can be blocked by local anaesthetics without affecting conduction in the neurones transmitting cold information. The axons of the latter have a higher transmission velocity. The two different neurone populations probably correspond to the unmyelinated warm receptor neurones and the myelinated cold receptor neurones identified in the skin of the primate.

REFERENCES

Bazett, H.C., McGlone, B., Brocklehurst, R.J.: The temperatures in the tissues which accompany temperature sensations. J. Physiol.(Lond.) 69, 87-112 (1930)

Brown, A.G., Iggo, A.: A quantitative study of cutaneous receptors and afferent fibres in the cat and rabbit. J.Physiol. (Lond.) 193, 707-733 (1967)

Burgess, P.R., Perl, E.R.: Cutaneous mechanoreceptors and nociceptors. In: Handbook of sensory physiology, Vol.2, ed.A.Iggo Heidelberg, New York: Springer 1973

Corson, J.H., Crannell, C.W.: Simple reaction time to cutaneous temperature stimuli. Canad.J.Psychol. 24, 305-310 (1970)

Duclaux, R., Franzen, O., Chatt, A.B., Kenshalo, D.R., Stowell, H.: Responses recorded from human scalp evoked by cutaneous thermal stimulation. Brain Res. 78, 279-290 (1974)

Duclaux, R., Kenshalo, D.R.: The temperature sensitivity of the type I slowly adapting mechanoreceptors in cats and monkeys. J.Physiol.(Lond.) 224, 647-664 (1972)

Fruhstorfer, H.: Habituation and dishabituation of the human vertex response. Electroenceph.clin.Neurophysiol. 30, 306-312 (1971)

Fruhstorfer, H., Detering, I.: A simple thermode for rapid temperature changes. Pflügers Arch. 349, 83-85 (1974)

Fruhstorfer, H., Guth, H., Pfaff, U.: Thermal reaction time as a function of stimulation site. Pflügers Arch. 335, R 49 (1972)

Fruhstorfer, H., Guth, H., Pfaff, U.: Cortical responses evoked by thermal stimuli in man. Pflügers Arch. 339, R 88 (1973)

Fruhstorfer, H., Guth, H., Pfaff, U.: Cortical responses evoked by thermal stimuli in man. In: Event-related slow potentials of the brain, eds. W.C.McCallum and J.R.Knott. Bristol: John Wright and Sons, in press

Fruhstorfer, H., Zenz, M., Nolte, H., Hensel, H.: Dissociated loss of cold and warm sensibility during regional anaesthesia. Pflügers Arch. 349, 73-82 (1974)

Guth, H.: Corticale Reaktionspotentiale auf Temperaturreize beim Menschen. Inaug.-Diss. Marburg 1975

Hensel, H.: Cutaneous thermoreceptors. In: Handbook of sensory physiology, Vol.2, ed. A.Iggo. Heidelberg, New York: Springer 1973

Hensel, H., Iggo, A.: Analysis of cutaneous warm and cold fibres in primates. Pflügers Arch.ges.Physiol. 329, 1-8(1971)

Hering, E.: Grundzüge einer Theorie des $T_e$mpertatursinns.Sitzber. K.u.K.Akad.Wiss.(Wien) math.nat.Cl. LXXV/III 1877

Johnson, K.O., Darian-Smith, L., LaMotte, C.: Peripheral neural determinants of temperature discrimination in man: a correlative study of responses to cooling skin. J.Neurophysiol. 36, 347-370 (1973)

Pfaff, U.: Reaktionszeit auf Temperaturreize beim Menschen in Abhängigkeit vom Reizort. Inaug.-Diss. Marburg 1976

Radtke, H., Nolte, H., Fruhstorfer, H., Zenz, M.: A comparative study between etidocaine and bupivacaine in ulnar nerve block. Acta anaesth.scand. Suppl.60, 17-20 (1975).

This work was supported by the Deutsche Forschungsgemeinschaft (Fr 265/2)

Discussion:

Iggo: The conduction velocity of the primates cold fibers is between three or four to nine meters per second. This would fit quite well although there are others that are conducting up to say, twelve meters per second. A very large number of the myelinated fibers in the monkey are conducting at around four to five meters per second. It is always disturbing to find that other peoples's results seem to fit so well with one's own preconceived ideas. I was trying to bring out in my own talk the fact that there appeared to be a semi-sensory pathway carrying information from the periphery about temperatures particularly from the cold fibers. This made it unnecessary to assume that the mechano-receptors play any part in contributing to cold sensation in man. Your results with the differential nerve block where you had preservation of mechanical sensitivity to striking the skin and so on (at the time there was a total absence of thermal sensations) they announced this idea that in fact, the responses among the mechano-receptors to changing temperature had nothing, in fact, to do with thermal sensation.

Zotterman: I would challenge anyone to show that a nonthermal, purely mechanical stimulus applied to the skin evokes a cold sensation.

Fruhstorfer: I think that we have to accept Iggo's elegant results within the limits of the experiment. As I recall, there was about a ten degree cooling change. Those who have postulated a possible role of the nonspecific thermal receptors in this change in quality with extreme cooling that Dr Hensel mentioned are discussing thermal changes in excess of ten degrees cooling. This would only be interpreted if received in parallel with thermal receptor input. In other words (and this is very speculative I agree) if one were to lower the specific thermal input, those channels, then perhaps, with extreme cooling this change in quality the analysis could be made or at least aided with these so called bi-modal cells. I do not know if the experiment really rules that out. If I could finally comment on conduction velocity with mechanical stimulation, I was fortunate enough to have data on vibratory stimulation of finger tips and hands. If I calculate the conduction velocity with the same methods as before I get some thirty meters per second with vibratory stimulation. So those are thickly myelinated fibers.

THE ORIGIN AND PROJECTIONS OF A SPINAL NOCICEPTIVE AND THERMORECEPTIVE PATHWAY

D. L. TREVINO

Department of Physiology, University of North Carolina School of Medicine, Chapel Hill, North Carolina, 27514 U.S.A.

INTRODUCTION

The ventrolateral quadrants of the spinal cord have achieved tremendous clinical importance since it was discovered that surgical transection of the pathways in these quadrants produces analgesia and thermanesthesia of the side of the body below and opposite to the site of the cordotomy (33). This result has been used to support the concept of specific somesthetic systems for pain and for temperature sense, although this concept has come under vigorous attack recently in the case of pain (27,28). However, I will not address myself to the question of the validity of the psychological assumptions of this concept which is under attack. Instead, I am here concerned with an explanation of the changes seen after a ventrolateral cordotomy which requires an understanding of the contribution to somesthesis of the fibers which were cut. My initial efforts are directed at the ascending sensory pathways to the brainstem, particularly the spinothalamic tract. Although a large portion of the ascending fibers in the ventrolateral quadrants terminate in the lower brainstem, a significant number travel all the way to the dorsal thalamus and thus form a direct pathway from the spinal cord to the thalamus. It seems likely that these spinothalamic fibers, especially those which link up with thalamocortical relay neurons, are therefore a significant part of the direct spinal pathways to the higher somesthetic centers of the brain.

What type of sensory information is being carried by individual spinothalamic fibers? With this question in mind, the identification and study of spinothalamic units was undertaken with the use of the technique of antidromic activation with a stimulating electrode in the thalamus (3,35,36,40). With this method the somata of spinothalamic neurons are invaded by the anterogradely traveling action potentials, thereby identifying these units in the spinal cord, which can be found with a recording microelectrode, as projecting to the thalamus. In a series of experiments on 54 rhesus monkeys 180 spinothalamic units were studied (40). While over 50% were responsive to innocuous mechanical stimulation of the skin, 30% responded only to noxious intensities of stimulation. About half of these latter units were located in the marginal zone of the dorsal horn (lamina I) while the remainder were in laminae IV, V and VI. The lamina I units are particularly interesting because they all required noxious levels of mechanical or thermal stimulation for activation. Perl and his co-workers originally reported the nociceptive nature of lamina I responses, although they have also found thermoreceptive lamina I units which respond well to innocuous cooling (or, rarely, warming) and weakly to noxious mechanical or burning stimuli (11, 20).

The physiological specialization of cutaneous afferent fibers is well established, and several types of nociceptive afferents have been documented. The discovery of spinal neurons whose sole excitatory drive is apparently from the nociceptors leads to the question of whether they constitute a 2nd order relay for a direct nociceptive pathway to the brain. In order to answer this question, a determination of the projections of these spinal nociceptive neurons and a physiological analysis of their effects on the neurons on which they terminate would be called for. To this end the technique of the retrograde transport of horseradish peroxidase (HRP) was used to determine the projections of lamina I neurons of the macaque spinal cord. It is recognized that there are also spinal neurons having a "wide dynamic range" (38,39) that are easily excited by gentle stimuli but respond maximally to stimuli reaching noxious intensities. These cells probably have an important contribution to nociception, but they occur in the dorsal horn ventral to the substantia gelatinosa, intermingled with other sensitive mechanoreceptive neurons which do not have a wide dynamic range. Therefore, identification of the areas to which lamina I projects indicates with certainty that they are receiving a nociceptive and/or thermoreceptive input from the spinal cord, but projections to an area from deeper laminae could be from the neurons receiving non-noxious inputs.

The introduction of the method of retrogradely labeling neurons by Kristensson and Olsson (18) has provided a technique with several advantages over an electrophysiological attempt to map the projections of lamina I neurons. A large injection of HRP into the caudal thalamus of a single animal retrogradely labels neurons throughout the spinal cord (34). Subsequent smaller injections in other animals into the various brainstem nuclei known to receive spinothalamic fibers will label only those spinal neurons which project to (or through) each respective nucleus. Information about the size and shape as well as the precise location of the spinothalamic neurons will also be gained since the retrogradely transported HRP fills the somata and proximal dendrites. The results obtained to date after injections of HRP into various brainstem nuclei of 11 cats and 5 monkeys will be described.

METHODS

Injections of 0.2 to 3.0 µl of 30 or 50% HRP in sterile water or saline were made unilaterally under aseptic conditions in animals anesthetized with sodium pentobarbital. The HRP was delivered by means of 1 to 3 penetrations of a 1 or a 10 µl Hamilton microsyringe needle which was placed stereotaxically through a trephine hole in the calvarium. In the later experiments the final placement of the microsyringe needle was determined electrophysiologically by searching for evoked potentials with a recording electrode while stimulating a contralateral forelimb and hindlimb cutaneous nerve percutaneously. For each penetration 0.2 to 1.0 µl of HRP was slowly injected manually over 20 to 45 minutes. After 2 to 3 days survival the animals were reanesthetized and fixed by transcardiac perfusion with saline followed by 0.5% paraformaldehyde - 2.5% glutaraldehyde in 0.1M phosphate buffer at pH 7.2. The brains and spinal cords were then removed, cut into blocks, collected in phosphate buffer and every third section was transferred to an incubation medium containing 0.05% 3,3-diaminobenzidine tetrahydrochloride and 0.01% H_2O_2 in Tris buffer for 30 minutes. The sections were transferred through 2 changes of distilled water or phosphate buffer and mounted on slides with alcoholic gelatin. Slides were either left uncounterstained or were lightly stained with 0.1% cresylecht violet or 1% neutral red. Sections of the spinal cord were scanned microscopically using both dark- and bright-field illumination. Neuron somata containing granular reaction product (16,21,22,30,32,34) were compiled to obtain the distribution pattern of the cells. Sections through the injection site were examined both microscopically and by projection to determine the regions invaded by the HRP.

RESULTS

Monkey

Fig. 1 shows the extent of spread of HRP injected into the brainstem of two monkeys. In M-6 most of the nuclei in the posterior and lateral thalamus were involved due to the amount of HRP injected (2.0 µl in two penetrations). Since most of the thalamic nuclei which receive terminals of the spinothalamic tract were involved, a large number of retrogradely labeled neurons was found throughout the spinal cord of this monkey. In M-12 the HRP remained restricted primarily to the periaqueductal gray and adjacent reticular formation (0.3 µl in one penetration). A large number of labeled neurons was found throughout the spinal cord of this monkey also, but their distribution differed significantly from M-6.

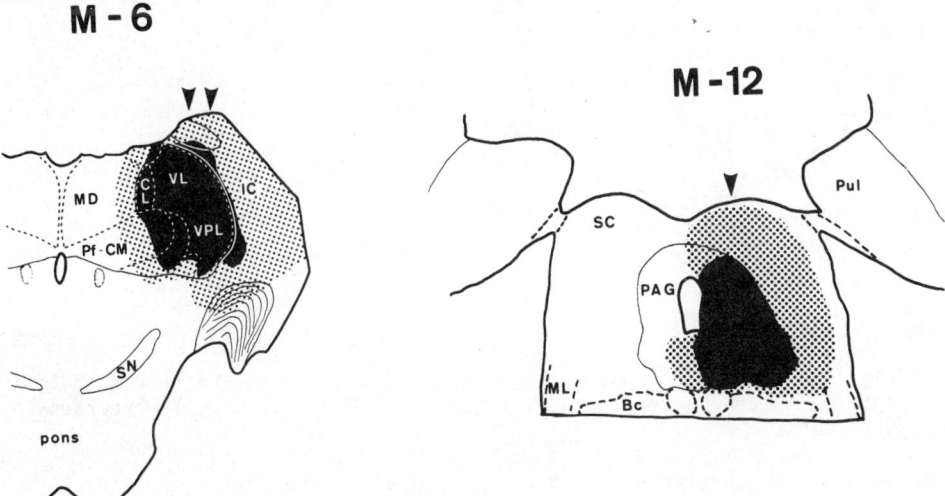

Fig. 1 HRP injection sites in two monkeys. The solid black areas are the regions staining most densely to diaminobenzidine. Arrows indicate the position of the needle tracks.

Fig. 2 shows the distribution of the retrogradely labeled somata seen in the spinal cord of monkey M-6. Contralateral to the injection site labeled neurons were found most commonly at the "neck" of the dorsal horn in lateral laminae V and IV at all levels of the spinal cord. Labeled neurons were also seen in lamina I at all levels. In the caudal spinal cord labeled neurons were also seen ventrally in laminae VII and VIII. Labeled cells in these laminae were rare in the cervical enlargements and upper thoracic cord. Some labeled neurons were also found on the side ipsilateral to the injection site at all levels. The second cervical segment presents a special picture. Since the HRP injection involved most of the nucleus VPL, most of the cells of the lateral cervical nucleus and the dorsal column nuclei on the contralateral side were retrogradely labeled. Cells in the external cuneate nucleus were labeled as well, an observation first reported by Boivie et al. (7). There were many labeled cells in the deeper regions of the contralateral dorsal horn of C2, perhaps equivalent to laminae V and VI of the cat, and in lamina I. The unique aspect of

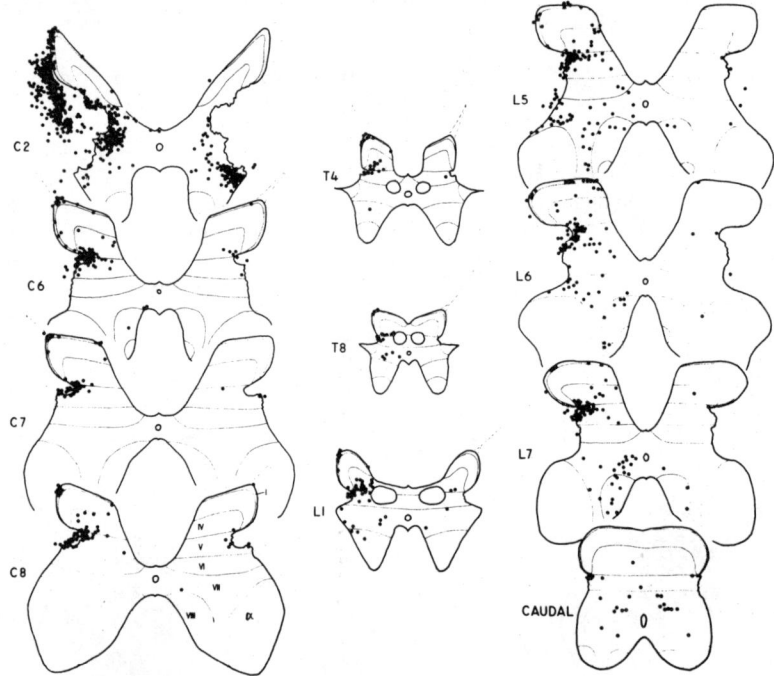

Fig. 2 Composite drawings showing the locations of the retrogradely labeled somata in the spinal cord of M-6. C = cervical, T = thoracic, L = lumbar.

C2, however, is the large number of labeled somata found in the lateral half of the ventral horn on the side ipsilateral to the injection site. Labeled cells in this location have also been found in cats with HRP injections into various thalamic regions (see below). It is believed that this is a previously undescribed source of direct projections to the dorsal thalamus from the upper cervical spinal cord.

In two other monkeys in which the VPL was the thalamic nucleus primarily involved by the HRP injection, there was a very low yield of retrogradely labeled cells in the spinal cord. Those that were present were distributed in the same regions as shown in Fig. 2, including the ipsilateral ventral horn of C2. Although the collection of data is incomplete at this time, a few labeled cells in the ventral horn of C2 have also been found in one monkey in which the intralaminar region was injected with HRP.

Figure 3 shows the distribution of the retrogradely labeled somata seen in the spinal cord of monkey M-12 in which HRP (0.3 µl) was injected into the periaqueductal gray (PAG) of the midbrain. The most conspicuous difference between this monkey and M-6 is the very large number of labeled lamina I cells found at all levels. Because of the overlap of individual dots on these composite drawings it is not possible to judge what the actual number of marginal cells found on the contralateral side is, so the numbers will be listed here. There are 58 in C2, 69 in C6, 72 in C7, 80 in C8, 36 in T4,

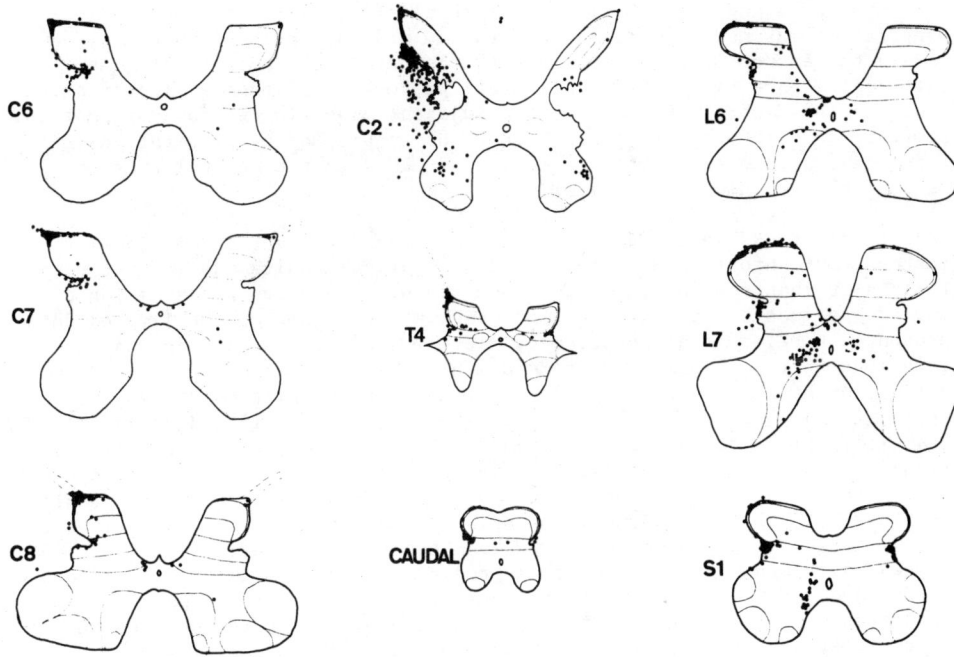

Fig. 3 Composite drawings showing the locations of the retrogradely labeled somata in the spinal cord of M-12. C = cervical, T = thoracic, L = lumbar, S = sacral.

49 in L6, 72 in L7 and 18 in S1. However, these values understate the actual number of labeled marginal cells present in these segments since only every third section from each segment was examined. Other distinguishing characteristics following PAG injection are fewer labeled somata in laminae IV-V (except for the S1 segment where 46 labeled neurons are represented by the overlapping dots in lateral lamina V) and relatively more labeled neurons in laminae VII-VIII in the lumbar segments. Another interesting feature is the consistent presence of a few labeled somata at the ventromedial base of the dorsal horn (medial VI and dorsomedial VII) in the enlargements. Labeled somata at this location are frequently seen in the cat material (see below). In C2 there are fewer labeled cells in the gray matter below lamina I and the heavy concentration that was seen in lateral laminae V-VI of M-6 is virtually absent. There are labeled cells in the ipsilateral and contralateral ventral horns, although much fewer than in M-6. The large number of labeled lateral cervical nucleus neurons presents a problem in interpretation. A possible reason for their presence is that the HRP at the injection site spread far enough laterally to encompass the cervicothalamic tract, ascending in the midbrain to the thalamus (13). This possibility, though, has difficulties associated with it. If the cervicothalamic fibers had picked up the HRP, then a large number of medial lemniscal fibers should also have picked up HRP, since at this level the cervicothalamic tract sits just dorsal to the medial lemniscus (13). This did not occur as there were almost no labeled cells in the dorsal column

nuclei; there were only a few rare cells seen in the very base of these nuclei. Also, in order for there to be significant uptake of HRP by axons, they must be damaged by the injection needle (14,19). Here the needle penetration was made 1.5 mm lateral to the midline (arrow in Fig. 1), hardly far enough lateral to penetrate the cervicothalamic tract. An alternative possibility is a collateral projection of the cervicothalamic tract to the midbrain PAG and/or the adjacent midbrain reticular formation. However, no such projection was seen by Ha in his Marchi preparations. Hopefully, a more restricted injection of HRP into the central gray can be achieved to answer this question

Injections of HRP were made into the brainstems of several additional monkeys, but unfortunately they yielded negative results due to poor perfusions or inappropriately placed injections. Therefore a discussion of the projections of lamina I must be based at this time on the limited data presented here, on that reported by Albe-Fessard et al. (1), and on the locations in the thalamus of stimulation sites which caused the antidromic activation of units having the location and characteristics of marginal cells (4,35). Both the HRP technique (Fig. 2 and ref. 1) and antidromic stimulation (35) confirm a projection of lamina I to VPL. There still remains a possibility that axons of lamina I neurons which pass through VPL on their way to terminate in caudal VL are responsible for the results obtained with both techniques. The spinothalamic projections to VL in the cat is largely represented by axons from cells in lamina I (Fig. 4 C, see below), although the source of this projection in the monkey has not been determined. However, Perl and Whitlock (31) have reported finding a few ventrobasal units which could only be excited by noxious stimuli to a discrete area of the skin in cats and monkeys having spinal lesions which left only one ventrolateral quadrant intact. Perhaps a direct excitatory input to these units from marginal cells, which have been shown to have small receptive fields, was responsible for their activity.

Albe-Fessard, et al. (1) report the retrograde labeling of lamina I cells after a small injection of HRP into the caudal intralaminar region, an area also known to receive spinothalamic terminals. A third brainstem region apparently receiving lamina I projections is the midbrain periaqueductal gray and/or adjacent reticular formation (Fig. 3). There is abundant anatomical evidence for a projection here from the spinal ventrolateral quadrants (17,24,25,26). This is also a very significant area with respect to pain because of the analgesic or strongly aversive reaction produced by local electrical stimulation, depending on the location of the electrode (see 23,29). Therefore, the heavy projection of lamina I neurons to this area is very interesting. Again, there is the possibility that some of the axons of these labeled cells were passing through this region on their way rostrally, perhaps to terminate in the intralaminar area. However, it is unlikely that this possibility could account for the retrograde labeling of all of the lamina I cells seen. It is not possible at the present time to assess whether lamina I projects to the posterior regions of the thalamus (SG, MGmc). Electrical stimulation in this region certainly has resulted in antidromic activation of lamina I units (4,35), but spinothalamic fibers traveling more rostrally also pass through this area. Likewise, an injection of HRP here would likely be picked up by these axons terminating more rostrally, especially if they were damaged by the injection needle. Because of the "throughway" nature of this area a definitive answer may not be forthcoming with these techniques.

Cat

It is of interest to compare these results in the monkey (Fig. 2 and 3) with those in the cat, for which a larger number of successful experiments are available. Fig. 4 illustrates the results from 3 experiments which summarize the projections of spinothalamic tract neurons in the cat. Fig. 4 A shows the locations of retrogradely labeled somata in the C7 and L7 segments after injecting a total of 3 µl of HRP into the caudal thalamus in 3 penetrations. The labeled somata are clustered at 3 sites in the cervical enlargement (laminae I, V and medial VII-VIII). The same distribution of labeled cells was seen in two other cats with similar large injections, one encroaching more caudally into the midbrain and one more rostrally in the thalamus. The spinothalamic neurons in the intermediate region and medial ventral horn of the lumbar segments were previously located with the method of antidromic activation (3,12,36); however the neurons in lamina I and in the dorsolateral funiculus adjacent to the dorsal horn (which were retrogradely labeled with HRP) were not encountered in those studies. In the one study of the cervical enlargement (12) antidromically excited units were found in the region of laminae V and VI (one unit was in lamina I). The results shown in Fig. 4 A therefore confirm these findings.

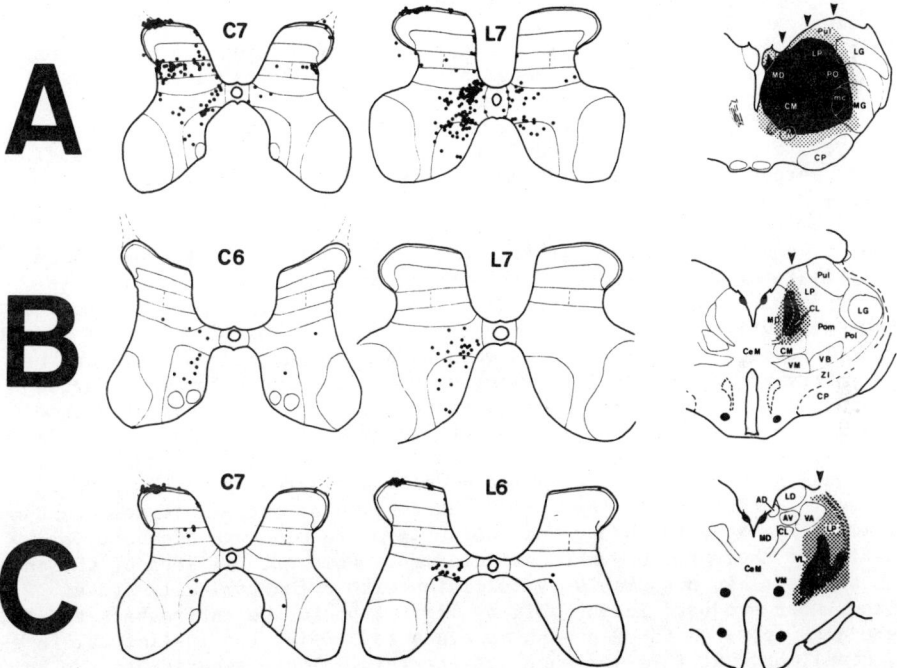

Fig. 4 Locations of retrogradely labeled somata in the spinal cords of 3 cats. Arrows indicate the position of the needle tracks.
    A. 3.0 µl HRP, 3 penetrations
    B. 0.2 µl HRP, 1 penetration
    C. 0.3 µl HRP, 1 penetration

In 4 cats small injections which remained confined to the ventrobasal region labeled cells in the dorsal column nuclei and the lateral cervical nucleus but failed to label cells in the spinal cord below C2, confirming recent reports that the spinothalamic tract does not terminate in VPL in the cat (6,15).

In one cat (Fig. 4 B) a small injection (0.2 µl) was made into the intralaminar region. The number of labeled somata in the spinal cord was very low, but those which were found are located in medial laminae VII-VIII in both the cervical and lumbar segments. Although no labeled cells were seen in lamina I, this negative result should not be taken as definitive without additional confirming experiments.

In two cats a small injection was made into the area of caudal VL - rostral VB in order to label the spinothalamic neurons projecting to caudal VL (6,15). The results from one cat are shown in Fig. 4 C. There are a large number of labeled somata in lamina I of the enlargements (39 in C7, 26 in L6). There were fewer labeled cells in the other cat with a similar injection but their distribution was identical, ie. most were in lamina I with an occasional one in deeper layers. Therefore, since approximately equal numbers of lamina I cells were labeled by a small VL injection as by a massive caudal injection, it can be suggested that caudal VL is a major termination area of lamina I in the cat, especially since no projection to the intralaminar region was demonstrated. Two attempts to label the neurons projecting to another thalamic area receiving spinothalamic terminals, the posterior group, have been negative. Therefore, it is not possible yet to say whether lamina I projects there. One attempt to label the spinal neurons projecting to the mesencephalic central gray was also negative.

As was previously mentioned, there is a projection to the thalamus from the ipsilateral ventral horn of the upper cervical spinal cord in cats. This projection is to many different areas of the thalamus, since most of the HRP injections reported above resulted in the labeling of cells in this area. In some cats labeled cells were also seen in the same area on the side contralateral to the injection, although they were fewer in number compared to the ipsilateral side. The function of this previously undescribed pathway can only be guessed at the present time. An attempt is being made to study these cells electrophysiologically. Two units have been found so far which were antidromically activated from the caudal thalamus. Unfortunately the maximum extracellular potentials seen were not sufficiently above the background noise level to allow an adequate determination of their responses to stimulation. However, failures of the antidromic potential, presumably by collision with orthodromically evoked spikes, were produced in one unit by light taps to the entire back and tail. There also appeared to be a weak response to tapping the ipsilateral fore- and hindlimbs, but this was much less certain. These experiments are being continued in order to determine the characteristics of these neurons.

CONCLUDING REMARKS

The data reported here suggest that there is a direct nociceptive and thermoreceptive input to VPL and the PAG-mesencephalic reticular formation because of the projections here from spinal lamina I in the macaque. The intralaminar region also receives this input (1). Electrophysiological studies have reported finding units responding to noxious mechanical and to thermal stimuli in these regions (2,5,10,31,37). A physiological demonstration of a monosynaptic input to these nociceptive and thermoreceptive units from spinal lamina I remains to be performed. The determination of the projections of spinal lamina I to the brainstem in macaques remains incomplete, however. It is planned to inject HRP into the various other brainstem regions receiving a direct spinal input (6,15,17,24,25,26).

ACKNOWLEDGEMENTS

The data reported here from cats was obtained in collaboration with Earl Carstens of the Neurobiology Program. I would like to thank him for his assistance in the preparation of this manuscript and Dr. C.J. Vierck for his critical review of it. I am grateful to Dr. E.R. Perl for generously providing the use of laboratory facilities and equipment and to Carol Metz, Sharyn Sawick, Gail Burd and Royce Joiner for their technical assistance.

This work was supported by NS 11132, MH 11107 and a General Research Support grant, all from the USPHS, by the UNC University Research Council, by the North Carolina United Community Services and by the Alfred P. Sloan Foundation.

ABBREVIATIONS

AD	n. Anterior Dorsalis	Pf	n. Parafascicularis
AV	n. Anterior Ventralis	PO	Posterior Group
Bc	Brachium Conjunctivum	Pol	lateral division of PO
CeM	n. Centralis Medialis	Pom	medial division of PO
CL	n. Centralis Lateralis	Pul	Pulvinar
CM	n. Centrum Medianum	R	Red nucleus
CP	Cerebral Peduncle	SC	Superior Colliculus
IC	Internal Capsule	SG	Suprageniculate nucleus
LD	n. Lateralis Dorsalis	SN	Substantia Nigra
LG	Lateral Geniculate	VB	Ventrobasal Complex
LP	n. Lateralis Posterior	VL	n. Ventralis Lateralis
MD	n. Medialis Dorsalis	VM	Ventromedial Complex
MG	Medial Geniculate	VPL	n. Ventralis Posterolateralis
MGmc	magnocellular division of MG	ZI	Zona Incerta
ML	Medial Lemniscus		

REFERENCES

1. Albe-Fessard, D., Boivie, J., Grant, G. and Levante, A. Neurosci. Letters 1 (1975) 75-80.
2. Albe-Fessard, D. and Kruger, L. J. Neurophysiol. 25 (1962) 3-20.
3. Albe-Fessard, D., Levante, A. and Lamour, Y. In: Advances in Neurology, Vol. 4. J.J. Bonica, ed. Raven Press, N.Y. 1974, pp. 157-166.
4. Applebaum, A.E., Beall, J.E., Forman, R.D. and Willis, W.D. J. Neurophysiol. 38 (1975) 572-586.
5. Becker, D.P., Gluck, H., Nulsen, F.E., and Jane, J.A. J. Neurosurg. 30 (1969) 1-13.
6. Boivie, J. Exp. Brain Res. 12 (1971) 331-353.
7. Boivie, J., Grant, G., Albe-Fessard, D., Levante, A. Neurosci. Letters 1 (1975) 3-8.

8. Burgess, P.R. Am. J. Chinese Med. 2 (1974) 121-148.
9. Burgess, P.R. and Perl, E.R. In: Handbook of Sensory Physiology, Vol. 2, A. Iggo, ed. Springer-Verlag, N.Y. 1973, Ch. 2, pp 29-78.
10. Burton, H., Forbes, D.J. and Benjamin, R.M. Brain Res. 24 (1970) 179-190.
11. Christensen, B.N. and Perl, E.R. J. Neurophysiol. 33 (1970) 293-307.
12. Dilly, P.H., Wall, P.D. and Webster, K.E. Exp. Neurol. 21 (1968) 550-562.
13. Ha, H. Exp. Neurol. 33 (1971) 205-212.
14. Halperin, J.J. and La Vail, J.H. Brain Res. 100 (1974) 253-269.
15. Jones, E.G. and Burton, H. J. Comp. Neurol. 154 (1974) 395-432.
16. Jones, E.G. and Leavitt, R.Y. Brain Res. 63 (1973) 414-418.
17. Kerr, F.W.L. J. Comp. Neurol. 159 (1975) 335-356.
18. Kristensson, K. and Olsson, U. Brain Res. 29 (1971) 363-365.
19. Kristensson, K. and Olsson, Y. Brain Res. 79 (1974) 101-109.
20. Kumazawa, T., Perl, E.R., Burgess, P.R. and Whitehorn, D. J. Comp. Neurol. 162 (1975) 1-12.
21. Kuypers, H.G.J.M., Kievit, J. and Groen-Klevant, A.C. Brain Res. 67 (1974) 211-218.
22. La Vail, J.H. and La Vail, M.M. Science 176 (1972) 1416-1417.
23. Liebeskind, J.C., Mayer, D.J. and Akil, H. In: Advances in Neurology Vol. 4. J.J. Bonica, ed. Raven Press, N.Y. 1974, pp. 261-268.
24. Mehler, W.R. In: Basic Research in Paraplegia, J.D. French and R.W. Porter, eds. Thomas, Springfield, Ill. 1962, pp. 26-55.
25. Mehler, W.R. NY Acad. Sci. 167 (1969) 424-468.
26. Mehler, W.R., Feferman, M.E. and Nauta, W.J.H. Brain 83 (1960) 718-750.
27. Melzack, R. The Puzzle of Pain, Penguin, England, 1973.
28. Melzack, R. and Wall, P.D. Science 150 (1965) 971-979.
29. Nashold, B.S., Wilson, W.P. and Slaughter, G. In: Advances in Neurology, Vol. 4. J.J. Bonica, ed. Raven Press, N.Y. 1974, pp. 191-196.
30. Nauta, H.J.W., Prinz, M.B. and Lasek, R.J. Brain Res. 67 (1974) 219-238.
31. Perl, E.R. and Whitlock, D.G. Exp. Neurol. 3 (1961) 256-296.
32. Ralston, H.J., III, and Sharp, P.V. Brain Res. 62 (1973) 273-278.
33. Spiller, W.G. and Martin, E. JAMA 58 (1912) 1489-1490.
34. Trevino, D.L. and Carstens, E. Brain Res. 98 (1975) 177-182.
35. Trevino, D.L., Coulter, J.D. and Willis, W.D. J. Neurophysiol. 36 (1973) 750-761.
36. Trevino, D.L., Maunz, R.A., Bryan, R.N. and Willis, W.D. Exp. Neurol. 34 (1972) 64-77.
37. Wagman, I.H. and McMillan, J.A. In: Advances in Neurology, Vol. 4, J.J. Bonica, ed. Raven Press, N.Y. 1974, pp. 171-177.
38. Wagman, I.H. and Price, D.D. J. Neurophysiol. 32 (1969) 803-817.
39. Wall, P.D. J. Neurophysiol. 23 (1960) 197-210.
40. Willis, W.D., Trevino, D.L., Coulter, J.D. and Maunz, R.A. J. Neurophysiol. 37 (1974) 358-372.

Discussion:

Iggo: Do you think that the absence from your electrophysiological data of "specific cold neurons" of the kind that I described in lamina I may be due to the small size of the neurons?

Trevino: I cannot give an answer because we were not using an adequate thermal stimulus to detect cold units. Perl and his co-workers have found them in both cat and monkey. Some of our spinothalamic units in lamina I could have been cold units.

Iggo: In your horse radish peroxidase experiments, you found very few reacting cell bodies in the substantia gelatinosa. Do you think it likely that the units recorded extracellularly by several workers, including myself, and apparently in the substantia gelatinosa, may have had their bodies elsewhere?

Trevino: If I recall Perl's data correctly, the units he studied in substantia gelatinosa were not antidromically activated from the upper cervical spinal cord, so my data are not in conflict with his.

ROLE OF THERMORECEPTORS IN THERMO-REGULATION

T. H. BENZINGER*
National Bureau of Standards, Washington, DC

Historical Remarks

A new epoch of sensory physiology began on a raw November day in Cambridge, 1925, when Zotterman[1] and Adrian set forth the law of sensory receptor action:

> "*Impulse frequencies, not amplitudes, signal the intensity of sensory stimuli.*"

A quarter century later, thermoreceptors were found to act in accordance with this rule, by Hensel and Zotterman[2] in Stockholm. Their classical findings are now the objective basis for understanding the subjective, conscious sensations of temperature by man. However, for the unconscious and unwillful mechanisms that might be activated by thermoreceptor stimulation, electrophysiology could not possibly find the answers alone. Moving separately toward the joint goal was the science of homeostasis, founded by Claude Bernard, with even earlier contributions from Antoine Lavoisier and Benjamin Franklin[3]. Equally indispensable was a new state of a very old art: Human or animal calorimetry, founded by Antoine Lavoisier and Pierre Simon De La Place[4].

Inspite of intensive cultivation during the 19th and the early 20th century by d'Arsonval, Regnault and Reiset, Voit, Rubner, Zuntz, Tigerstedt, Johansson, Atwater and Rosa, Benedict, Du Bois and others the arts of indirect and direct calorimetry were until 1930 or 1942 subject to one severe limitation: They lacked the speed of time-response required to follow the swift and powerful actions by loss or gain of heat which thermoreceptors elicit in response to changing temperatures.

The work reported here was supported under Research Contracts #R-8 and R-38 by the National Aeronautics and Space Administration.

*Collaboration by Charlotte Kitzinger and Arnold W. Pratt in part of this work is gratefully acknowledged.

New Methods

For indirect calorimetry this impediment was first overcome when Hermann Rein[5] (1933) developed his "Gaswechselschreiber" extended 1934-36 by Brauch, Hartmann and myself[6] to direct recordings of alveolar air composition, O_2 consumption and CO_2 production in man.

Direct calorimetry followed ten years later, with the method of gradient layer calorimetry[7], first described (1942) in a letter from me to my late friend, Konrad Buettner. The second world war did not permit construction of more than a crude model with gradient layers of plexiglass for resistance thermometry of the heat flow, which we baptised "Schneewittchen". Five years later, in the U.S.A. 1947, the expensive project was brought to life (fig. 1) by generous funding obtained through tireless efforts of A. R. Behnke, E. G. Hakansson and E. F. Du Bois, who are remembered here with lasting gratitude[8].

Trials and Tribulations

After ten years of planning and engineering, expensive construction and successful calibrations, the results of our first physiological experiments in 1958 were an unmitigated disaster (fig. 2).

> *Neither with skin temperatures in various steady states,*
> *nor with internal temperatures as measured in the rectum,*
> *could any reproducible relationship be found with loss of*
> *heat by sweating.*

However, in transient states under stable external conditions the high time-resolution of the layer calorimeter permitted us to find a definite and reproducible relationship (fig. 3) between the response of sweating and its hypothetical stimulus[9]:

> *Whenever skin temperature rose in these experiments, the*
> *rate of sweating fell; whenever skin temperature fell,*
> *the rate of sweating rose.*

Finding this paradoxical, mirror-image correlation was worse than finding none at all. It meant a dangerous confrontation with the accepted theory, that warm-reception at the skin was the driving stimulus of physical thermoregulation, and that the "heat loss center" in the anterior hypothalamus was a relay station for peripheral warm-impulses, modified in its "sensitivity" by its own temperature (See Pickering[10]. Why such a theory could have been advanced and accepted we could not understand until we found later[11]:

> *When temperatures below 33°C excite the cold-receptors of*

Role of Thermoreceptors in Thermoregulation

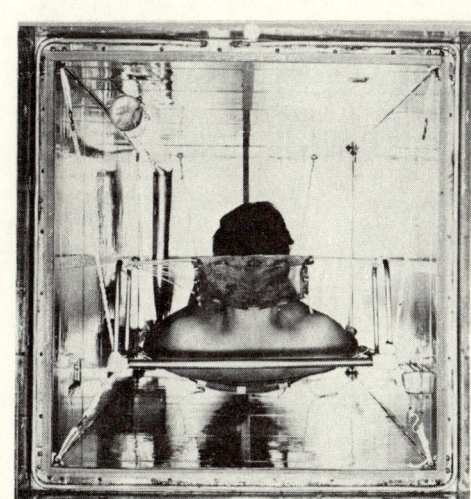

Figure 1.

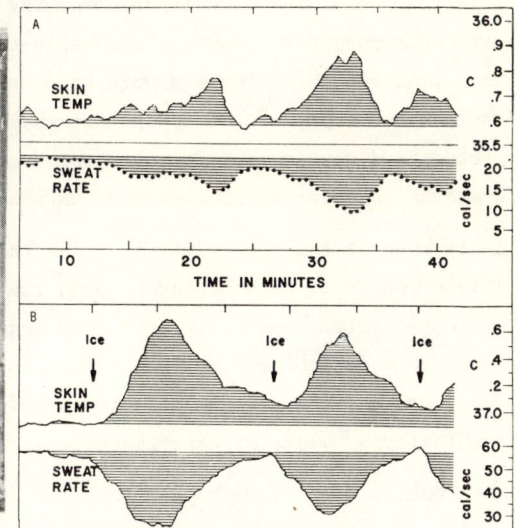

Figure 3.

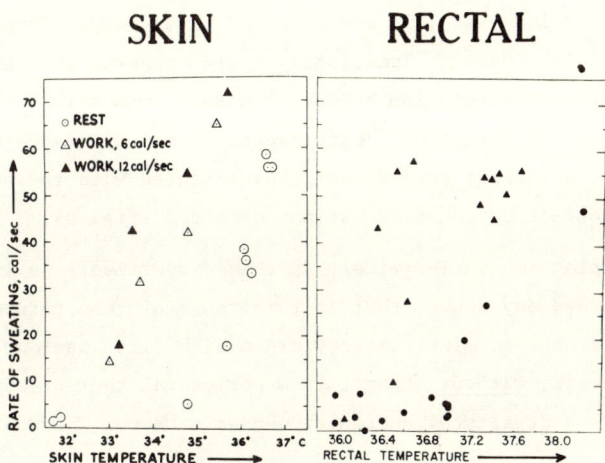

Figure 2.

*the skin while strenuous exercise fires up the central
warm-receptors, sweating is anti-homeostatically inhibited
and may be even abolished.*

This anti-homeostatic action is useful to animals or man, as it prevents useless wetting of fur or skin and freezing afterward when rest follows upon a strenuous physical effort. Since this cold-inhibition of sweating also occurs when athletic physiologists work hard on the ergometer in a cool laboratory-- the favored experimental design for this kind of study--it had been misinterpreted as a requirement for skin warm-reception to elicit sweating, at a time when the receptor thresholds were unknown.

In retrospect one recognizes that the thermal homeostasis of man would be ill-served if it were dependent upon the firing of skin warm-receptors which would be cooled (and their action extinguished) by sweat whenever they would begin to function as required. There would be positive feedback. Nevertheless, at the time, the controversy persisted, a disturbing companion during the following years of experimentation.

The Mechanism of Thermoregulatory Sweating

The calorimeter had disproved a theory. But, the dismal plot of sweating against rectal temperatures (fig. 2, right) offered no constructive replacement. The expensive, ten-year effort seemed to be doomed to failure, unless the courage was found to abandon rectal temperature, the established and trusted method for 100 years, in medicine and physiology. Tympanic thermometry (fig. 4) was introduced. Immediately there appeared in transients (fig. 5) an almost perfect correlation between tympanic temperature and rate of sweating. The previous series of experiments in steady states of rest or exercise in many different environments was repeated with the new technique,[12] and an almost perfect correlation was now obtained (fig. 6).

Since skin temperatures varied widely in these experiments as intended, the graph proved beyond any doubt, that in this range of temperatures a central station operated as a terminal sensory organ with first neurons for the reception of warmth, <u>without</u> support from peripheral thermoreceptors. It proved that this central station functioned as a "Human Thermostat".

By rate control, rates of heat loss are doubled, tripled or quadrupled. Heat gains of that order by radiation or conduction onto and into the body, or heat loads of that magnitude in exercise, are handled smoothly, with insignificant load errors for the thermal homeostasis of man. Another way of

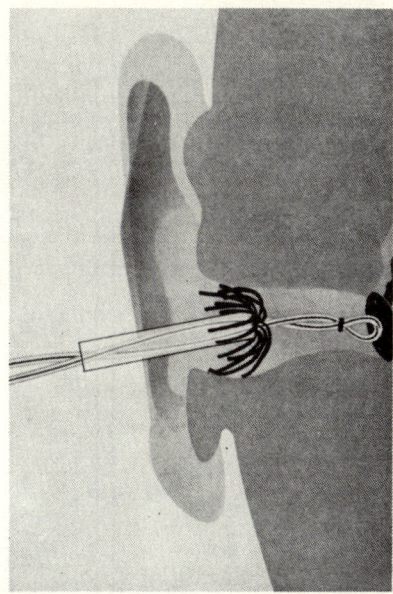

Figure 4.

TYMPANIC

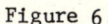

Figure 6.

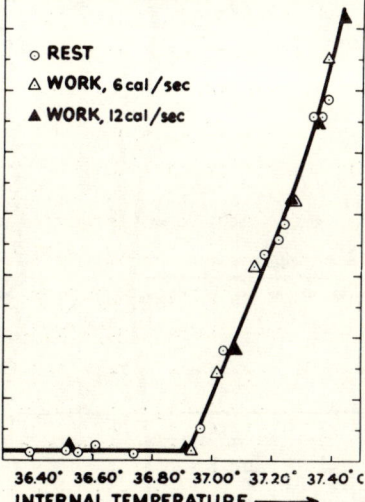

○ REST
△ WORK, 6 cal/sec
▲ WORK, 12 cal/sec

36.40° 36.60° 36.80° 37.00° 37.20° 37.40° C
INTERNAL TEMPERATURE ⟶

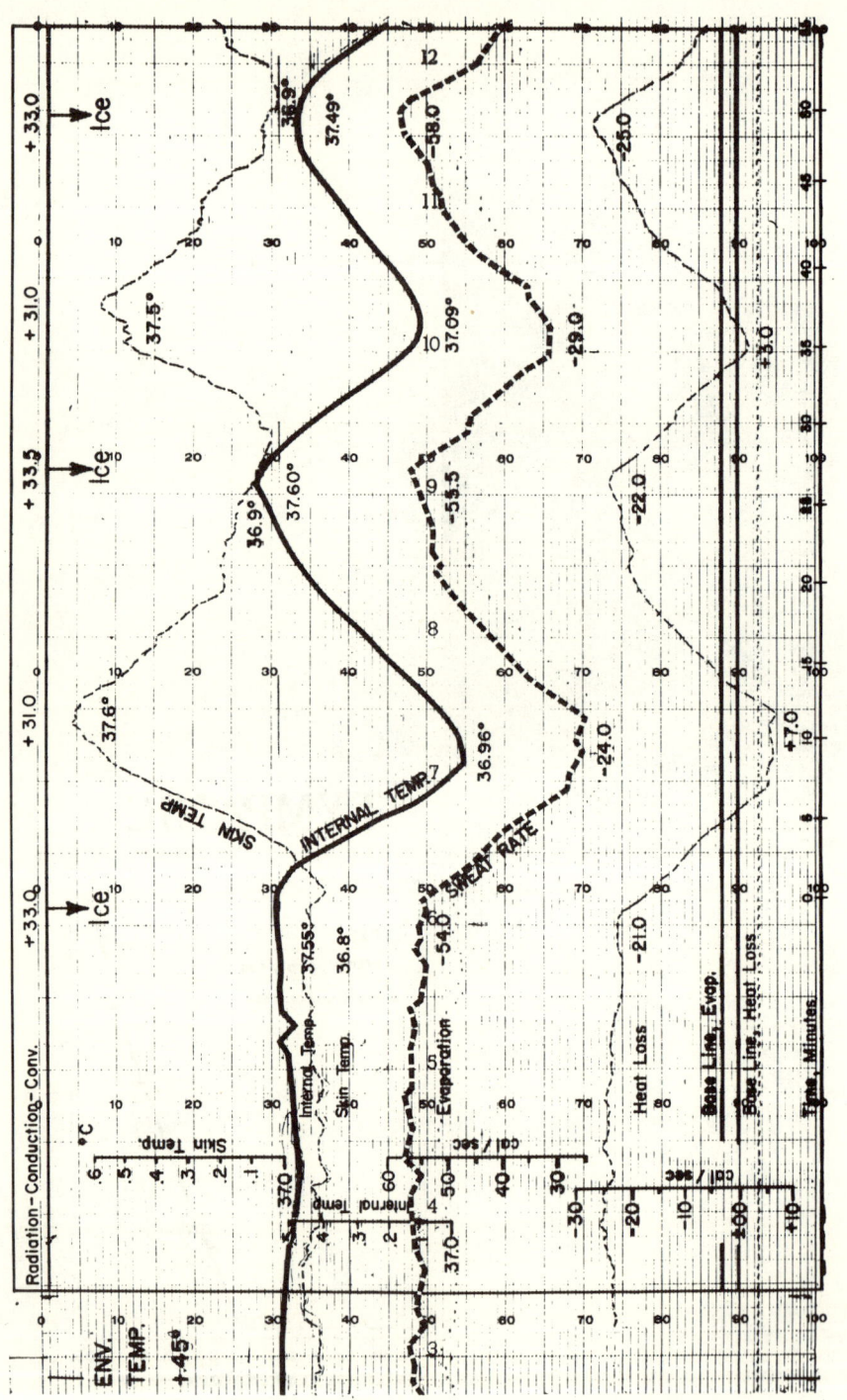

Figure 5.

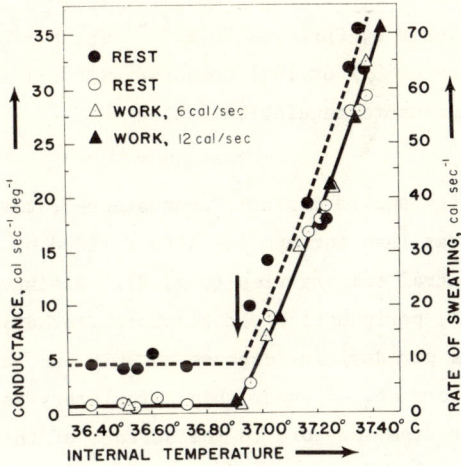

Figure 7.

Figure 8.

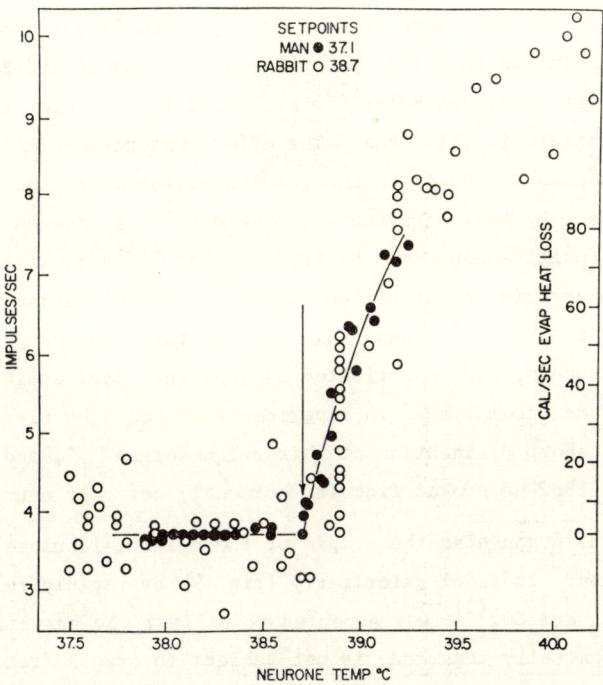

Setpoint characteristics of preoptic warm-sensitive neurons of "Type C." Open circles indicate firing rates plotted against neuron temperature [from Hellon (132)]. Central temperature-dependent rates of human sweating (closed circles) from Benzinger et al. (42) were projected into this plot with superimposition of the respective setpoints—38.7 C (rabbit) and 37.1 C (man).

describing the efficiency of physical thermoregulation, determination of the "open loop gain", was used by Curt von Euler[14] for his own experiments in 1964. He found ratios of 8:1 or 10:1 compared with 1:1 for baroreceptor efficiency in blood pressure regulation.

Vasomotor Responses

The calorimeter permits one to measure "conductance", the index of peripheral blood circulation--heat loss through the skin divided by the difference between skin- and central temperatures (fig. 7). Rising sharply from the setpoint for sweating, peripheral blood flowrate reaches seven times its resting rate (∼3 tons per day) in response to only one half degree C of internal temperature increase. Without this circulatory assistance heat could not move fast enought from the core to the surface of the body; the product of the sweat glands could not evaporate rapidly enough as it must, to fulfill its function of cooling.

The Human Thermostat

It was a fair conclusion[12] in 1959, that the sudomotor and vasomotor responses as observed reflected sensory impulses from the "First Heat Center", discovered 1885 in the anterior hypothalamus by Aronsohn and Sachs. In a pioneering effort, Curt von Euler[15] had found in 1950 slow temperature-dependent potentials in this area. The effort was resumed elsewhere, after a visit by Eisenman and Hardy to the gradient-calorimeter and an exposition of its findings. By 1961 Nakayama and Eisenman[16] succeeded in detecting firing, warm-sensitive neurons. By 1967, Hellon[17] demonstrated setpoints and firing-characteristics of various types of central sensory units (fig. 8). In 1967-68 Wit and Wang[18] found that the central warm-receptors were silenced by pyrogens, and re-activated by aspirin. Earlier, in 1956, Bengt Andersson[19] had accomplished in experiments on goats by electrical stimulation, a sharp delineation of this unique organ[20], and using thermal stimulation in 1962 he evoked from it hormonal, not only neural responses.

Was this central organ also the origin of the driving impulses for chemical thermoregulation? Indirect calorimetry (fig. 9) by rapidly responding gas analysis for O_2 and CO_2[21] was expected to deliver the answer. Heat production, chemically measured, is not subject to errors from storage or loss, with changing heat content of the body. Water baths can be used during indirect calorimetry, for production of any desired combination of skin and central temperatures.

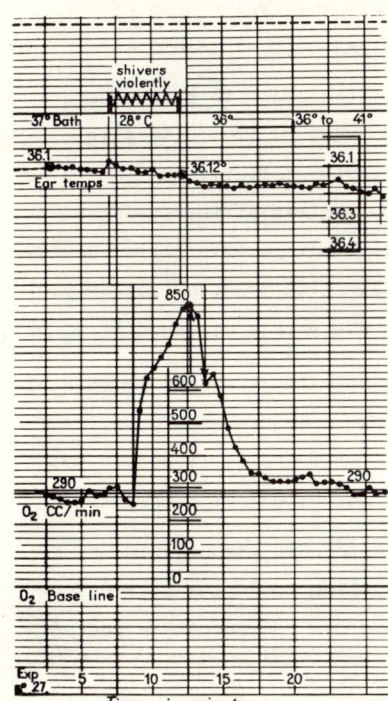

Figure 10.

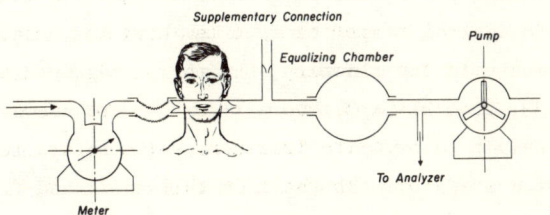

Figure 9.

(From Reference 6)

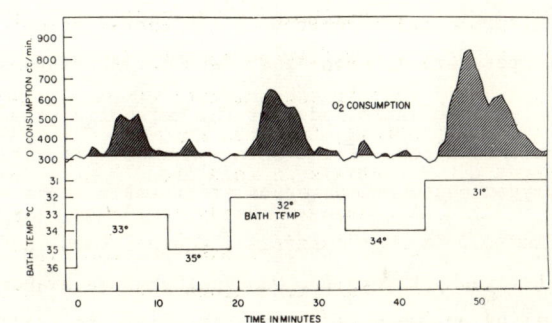

Figure 11.

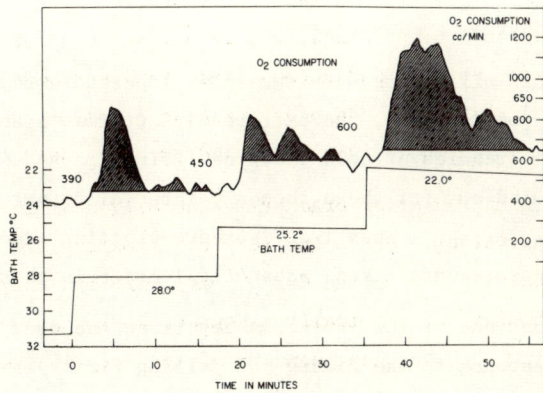

Figure 12.

Chemical Thermoregulation: The Peripheral Drive

Sobered by past experience, when we had expected sweating to arise from skin thermoreception and found that its origin was central, we now expected chemical thermoregulation to originate from central cold-receptors as a parallel to physical thermoregulation. This hypothesis was shaken by the first experiment (fig. 10) with rapidly responding indirect calorimetry.

During a two-minute dip into a cool bath (28°C), too short to be reflected in central temperature, metabolism increased from 200 to 800 cc of oxygen consumed per minute. Similarly, step changes of bath temperature from 37 to 33, from 36 to 32, from 34 to 30 were answered by spikes of increasing height in oxygen consumption, with return to basal levels (fig. 11). However, the steps from 31 to 28, from 28 to 25 and from 25 to 22 produced not only transient spikes but also elevated levels after the spikes declined (fig. 12).

In these oxygen tracings members of this symposium will recognize immediately the characteristics of the cold-receptors as first seen by Hensel and Zotterman, with their peculiar characteristics of thresholds, response to temperature as such, and overshooting responses to changes of temperature.

So we were satisfied that the metabolic response to cold was elicited by cold-receptors of the skin. A smooth regression line in a plot of steady oxygen consumption versus steady skin temperature was confidently expected.

Chemical Thermoregulation: Central Warm-Inhibition

The graph, figure 13, was another rude awakening—a total failure. Before giving up, we decided however, first to utilize the tympanic measurements that had been carefully taken—numbers appear at every point in the scattered diagram.

When all points with tympanic temperature 36.6 were sought out and connected by an isotherm, the pattern of Zotterman's and Hensel's steady-state frequencies of cold-receptor firing emerged. The isotherm-plotting had ruled out for these chosen points, different inputs from central thermoreception. When the "isotherm-plotting" technique was applied to all measurements taken, a beautiful order in this phenomenon appeared (fig. 14).

Each one of the isotherms describes the over consumption of oxygen in response to the rising and falling firing-rates of the skin thermoreceptors, with their maxima near 20°C and their thresholds at 33 to 34°C. And yet, with every increment of 0.1°C in central temperature the curve is shifted,

Role of Thermoreceptors in Thermoregulation

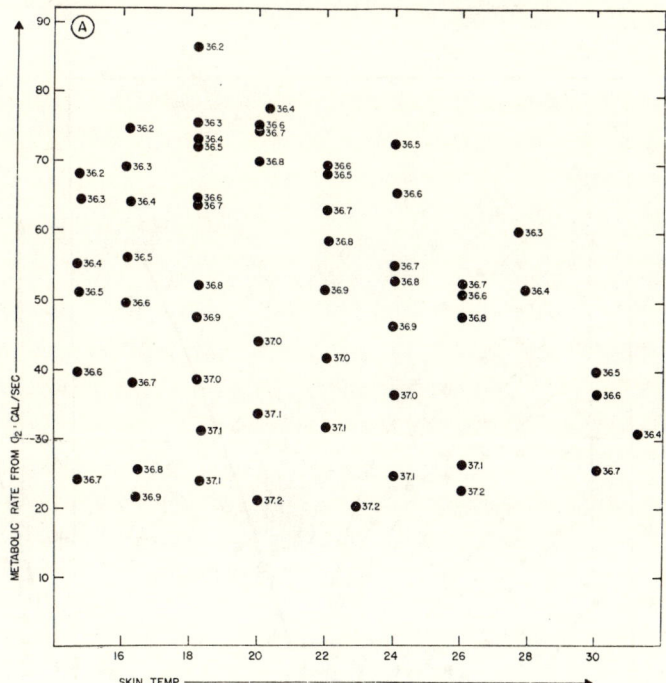

Figure 13.

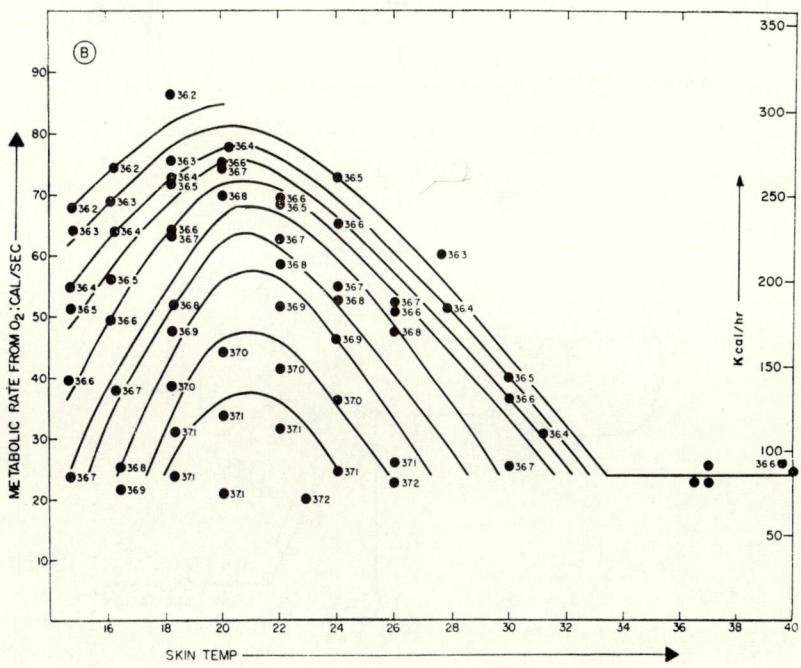

Figure 14.

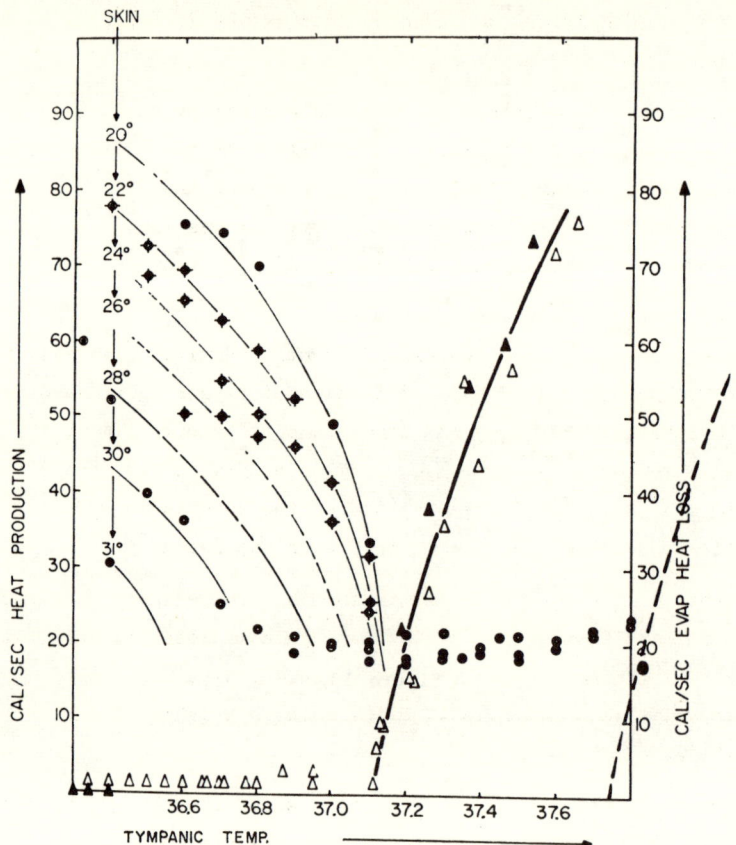

Figure 15.

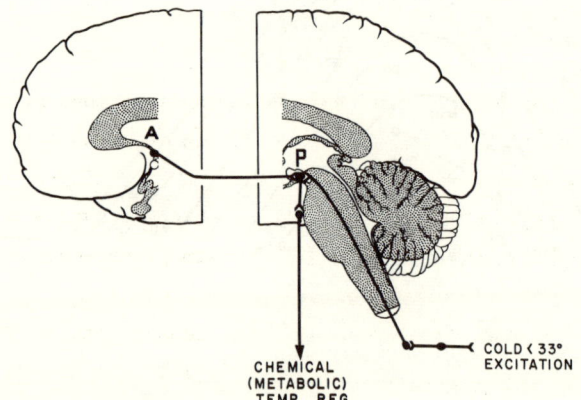

Figure 16.

lowered by 5 to 10 calories per second, that is, by 25 to 50% of a basal metabolic rate.

Clearly, the metabolic response to cold was excited by cold-reception at the skin. It was dramatically inhibited by subtle central warm-reception. It was abolished when tympanic temperature rose beyond the setpoint of the human thermostat, the threshold for sweating. It was the precision of this central control which produced the homeostatic performance by inhibition[22].

The Dual Functions of the Human Thermostat

To visualize the coordinated functions of both, chemical and physical thermoregulation, one can now plot the rates of oxygen consumption against central, not skin temperature, and draw the skin-temperature isotherms (fig. 15). Into the same graph one plots as before, the rates of heat loss by sweating against tympanic temperature of the same individual. The dual thermostatic feedback operations of the human thermostat are now visible.

Whenever central temperature deviates from the pre-set norm to the right or left, such deviation is counteracted by gain or loss of heat at rates controlled by the magnitude of the deviation. One half of one degree suffices to drive either the loss or the gain to heights of four times a basal metabolic rate.

It is important to observe that on the cold side, the phenomenon materializes only when the skin is cold enough to deliver the driving impulses. If such is the case, then the loss of heat will soon exceed the defensive production-- a basic weakness of chemical thermoregulation as compared with physical thermoregulation. In cold, the main defense of man is, therefore, behavioral.

Thermoreceptors and Behavioral Thermoregulation

The behavioral responses of man to conscious sensations of cold are of many kinds: pulling in the arms, crossing one leg over the other, curling-up, putting on some piece of clothing, bundling-up, working-up heat production, avoiding wind, seeking shelter, pulling the blanket over a shoulder in bed, heating the shelter, moving from cool to warm places--occur continuously, and immediately when required, often without our being fully conscious of these actions and their common cause. One reason that the reactions to an "early warning system" for cold are so efficient, is the overshooting response of the cold-receptors at the skin to the onset of cooling. Another reason is the striking fact that conscious sensations, unlike automatic responses to cold by shivering and heat production are not inhibited by central warm-reception (fig. 17).

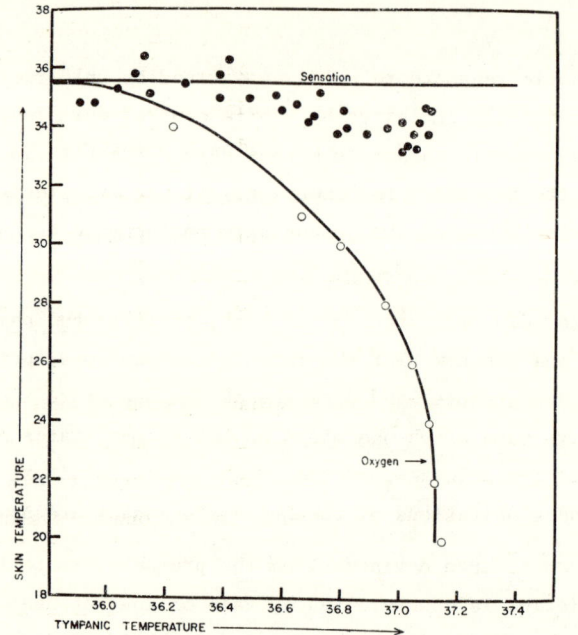

Figure 17.

We found this out in a series of experiments[23] with subjects submersed in a tub (head excepted). Tub temperature was lowered very slowly (1°C per hour) from 38°C to wherever the subject reported the very first impression of a cold-sensation. This threshold is fairly reproducible and, as the figure shows, independent of central temperature in the range under consideration. A correction is required for the gradient of temperature that arises between the warm subcutaneous receptors and the surrounding water when central temperature is substantially higher than water temperature (at right where the thresholds appear to be lower than they are).

For comparison, the dramatic inhibition of the autonomic, metabolic response to cold has been placed into the same graph, with its total elimination of the overproduction of heat at the "setpoint" (see also fig. 14).

For the reasons outlined, the behavioral defense against cooling will tend to keep the central temperature of man just below, right at, or even above the threshold of sweating however faint, and central vasodilation. That means that autonomic control with the superior precision of physical thermoregulation will be almost continuously active, taking over from wherever behavioral protection from cooling has left the condition of the body.

By comparison, behavioral defenses against overwarming are weak, and late in coming, because warm-sensation at the skin is not unpleasant unless it occurs in conjunction with high central temperatures. The latter, however, are perceived as unpleasant, a general malaise, and vague by quantity as well as quality. They are always associated with sweating.

A special role may come to be attributed to warm-receptors in the area of the Vth cranial nerve as investigated more recently by Herbert Hensel. For, these can serve indirectly as sensors for humidity of the inspired air having a major or lesser cooling effect on the mucuous epithelia in the mouth and the upper respiratory tract.

In summary concerning this topic, the dominant system of defense against cold is behavioral, whereas for defense against warmth, it is autonomic. The behavioral systems, particularly when they are supported by heating or cooling-technology, are superior in power. The autonomic systems excel by far in precision.

Functions of the Two Heat Centers

On account of the experiments reported, we have contended (fig. 16) since 1959, that the anterior hypothalamic, "First Heat Center" (A) of Aronsohn and Sachs (1886) is a terminal sensory organ with first neurons for warm-reception, and since 1961, that the posterior hypothalamic, "Second Heat Center" (P) of Isenschmidt and Krehl (1912) is a temperature-blind, synaptic relay station. At that station the action of skin cold-receptors is inhibited by warm-impulses from the First Heat Center.

In recent months, Robert D. Myers[24] at Purdue University has discovered with his ingenious new methods that thermal stimulation of the skin, as well as thermal stimulation of the First Heat Center provoke in the Second Heat Center Phenomena of Ca^{++} efflux or retention, demonstrable by extraction of effluent in push-pull cannulae, followed by analysis with radioactive tracer methods.

This means that at the Second Heat Center which is itself "temperature-blind", messages on temperature arrive from the two main receptor fields for warmth and cold. They provoke ionic changes, which are known from Myers' work to elicit powerful responses of heat loss or gain. In this area, where sensory pathways terminate and effector pathways begin, conclusive findings on thermoregulation may occur in the immediate future.

Concluding Remarks

The efforts at understanding the thermal homeostasis of man date back far in the history of the art, where the successes but not the temporary failures are being recorded. I hope you will forgive me for having discussed both aspects, as far as our own work was concerned. For journeys of this kind, Claude Bernard once offered guidance and comfort to his students, in his First Lecture on the Experimental Method where he said.

> "The verification of a preconceived idea leads only to the confirmation or extension of a known theory, while the appearance of an unexpected fact constitutes discovery par excellence."..."The unexpected is always more fruitful than the expected aspect, because the observation of natural phenomena is more instructive than the idea we make of it for ourselves."

(1) Zotterman, Y. G., Touch, Tickle and Pain, Part I, Pergamon Press, 1969.

(2) Hensel, H. and Y. Zotterman, Acta, Physiol. Scand. 23:291 (1951).

(3) Franklin, Benjamin, Letter dated June 17, 1758 to Dr. Lining of Charles Town, South Caroline, in "Observations on Electricity made at Philadelphia in America, London, 1774.

(4) Lavoisier, A. L. and P. S. De La Place, Mémoire Sur La Chaleur, Mémoires de L'Académie Des Sciences, Paris, 1782.

(5) Rein, H., Ein Gaswechselschreiber. Naunyn Schmiedebergs Arch. 171:363 (1938).

(6) Benzinger, T. H., Ergeb. Physiol. 40:1 (1938).

(7) Benzinger, T. H. and C. Kitzinger, Rev. Sci. Instr. 20:849 (1949).

(8) Benzinger, T. H., R. G. Huebscher, D. Minard and C. Kitzinger, J. Appl. Physiol. 12:51 (1958).

(9) Benzinger, T. H., J. Am. Med. Ass. 209:1200 (1969).

(10) Pickering, G., Lancet 1:1 (1958).

(11) Benzinger, T. H., Proc. Natl. Acad. Sci. 47:1683 (1961).

(12) Benzinger, T. H., Proc. Natl. Acad. Sci. 45:645 (1959).

(13) Benzinger, T. H., Physiol. Rev. 49:671 (1969).

(14) Euler, C. von, J. Cell. Comp. Physiol. 36:333 (1950).

(15) Euler, C. von, Progress on Brain Research, W. Bergman and J. P. Schode, Eds., Elsevier, Amsterdam, 1964.

(16) Nakayama, T. and J. S. Eisenman, Federation Proceedings, 20:334 (1961).

(17) Hellon, R. F., J. Physiol. (London) 193:381 (1967).

(18) Wit, A. and C. S. Wang, Am. J. Physiol. 215:1160 (1968).

(19) Andersson, B., R. Grant, and S. Larson, Acta Physiol. Scand. 37:361 (1956).

(20) Andersson, B., L. Ekman, G. C. Gale, and W. Sundsten, Acta Physiol. Scand. 54:191 (1962).

(21) Pratt, A. W., J. Natl. Cancer Inst. 20:161 (1958).

(22) Benzinger, T. H., Arnold, W. Pratt, and C. Kitzinger, Proc. Natl. Acad. Sci. 47:730 (1961).
(23) Benzinger, T. H. Proc. Natl. Acad. Sci. 49:832 (1963).
(24) Myers, Robert D., Personal Communication, January 1975.

Discussion:

Hensel: I would like to raise the question of the effects of central cooling. You put much emphasis on the warm side, which is surely the more important effect because overheating in many cases starts internal increase in temperature. Cooling starts more on the outside. On the other hand there are also the effects of primary central cooling as we have shown in the unaesthetized cat in 1959. Very recently we have shown that you can also elicit long-term cold adaptation in the rat by isolated cooling of the hypothalamus. This will come out in the American Journal of Physiology next month. Whereas the skin temperature goes up dramatically as an effect of the activity of increased heat production and so on. So the rectal temperature of the rat increases to about 41° C. But when the isolated hypothalamus is cold the animals get long-term adaptation as can be seen by an increased oxygen consumption to adrenalin injection for example. This was only an additional experiment. Central cooling might also have some effect on that temperature regulation system.

Zotterman: One thing that is very intriguing is the "setpoint" for temperature. Have you any idea of the mechanism behind it.

Benzinger: The "setpoint" of the human thermostat is a thermoreceptor threshold. Its anatomic substrate are warm-receptors in the preoptic region. When minute quantities of pyrogens are injected into this area, the setpoint shifts, because the warm-receptors are silenced. They are firing less or not at all. Temperature rises and rises and nothing (no corrective action by heat loss mechanisms) happens.

In answer to Dr Hensel's question, the production of cold-adaptation by cooling of the anterior hypothalamus is well established. Bengt Andersson, in 1956, adapted goats in this way. They grew an enormous fur as a result of the treatment. The figure on next page is shown in response to the question what is the role of central cold-receptors in thermoregulation.

Cold receptors in the preoptic region have been demonstrated by Hardy in 1963. Their contribution to thermoregulation is shown at left (open rings) in the figure (experiments by Downey and Chiodi on a paraplegic patient with his skin receptor system disconnected). The right hand side of the figure (solid dots) shown in a normal person the increased metabolic heat production in response to cold-receptor impulses from the skin, which is enormous (rising to 400 % BMR while central temperature decreases only to 36.3° C). The central system of the paraplegic at left (open rings) begins to respond at 35.8 (!) and reaches only 150 BMR at 34.6 (!) where induced hypothermia for surgery would begin.

The low quantity of the central contribution is explained by the low setpoint of the central cold-receptors, by their small number, and their low ratio of firing-rate over change in temperature. Practically, for regulation of temperature under normal conditions, central cold-reception plays no role in man. (In furred animals, as Hensel rightly points out, its role may be very important because their skin thermoreceptor field is heavily shielded against thermal cold stimulation).

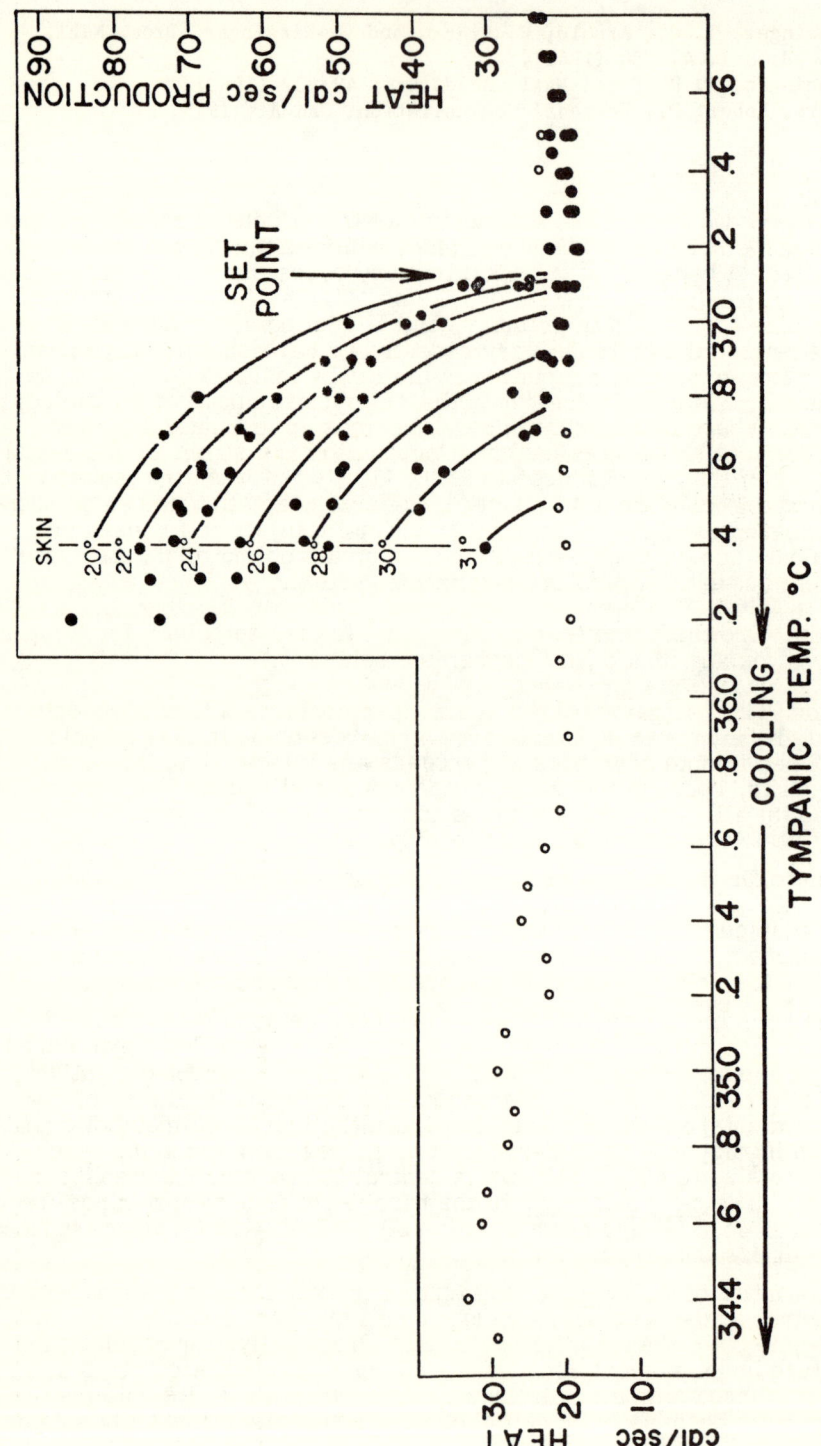

von Euler: I should like to comment on the **role** of cutaneous temperature receptors from different skin areas in thermoregulation, referring to observations that Dr Söderberg and I made in the 1950ies. My comment applies to results which we obtained in rabbits when we studied cutaneous vasomotor reactions and the reflex inhibition of shivering which could be elicited by warming different regions of the skin. We found that the cutaneous thermoreceptors of the ears had very little influence on the thermoregulatory reactions, whereas those of the skin of the trunk were powerful in eliciting such reactions. On the other hand, the thermoregulatory vasomotor reactions and the concomitant changes in skin temperature of the ears were much stronger than those of the skin of the trunk. As you know, the ears of the rabbit are of great importance for heat dissipation in the temperature regulation of the rabbit. Our observation indicates that the cutaneous temperature receptors of a skin area which takes active part in temperature regulation are not projecting to the temperature regulatory mechanism in the same powerful way as the thermoreceptors of skin areas where the vasomotor reactions are of less importance in temperature regulation. This differential organization can be regarded as a mechanism whereby positive feedback in temperature regulation is avoided, yet maintaining full responsiveness to the outer environment.

Benzinger: I am so pleased that you informed us of this radiancy phenomenon and found an explanation yourself. I wish I would have had the ears of the rabbit the other night when it was so cold in Stockholm.

Zotterman: I think we have collected quite a few of the active people in this field who have made some of the most fundamental contributions to thermal reception theory. We all look forward to reading their communications when they appear in the book.

TEMPERATURE SENSATIONS AMONG OTHER SENSATIONS TO THE STIMULI OF FOCUSED ULTRASOUND. THE COMPARISON WITH THE TEMPERATURE SENSATIONS BY MECHANICAL STIMULI

E. M. TSIRULNIKOV and E. E. SHCHEKANOV
Institute of Evolutionary Physiology and Biochemistry, USSR Academy of Sciences, Leningrad

Contents

The sensations provoked by focused ultrasound
Temperature sensations provoked by focused ultrasound
    Methods
    Results
    Note
Temperature sensations provoked by mechanical stimuli in comparison with sensations provoked by focused ultrasound
Temperature sensations provoked from cornea and scleral conjunctiva
Discussion
Conclusion

The sensations provoked by focused ultrasound

High frequency ultrasonic oscillations (MH_z) allow a considerable energy to be concentrated in various organs and tissues on body surface as well as in the deep structures (3).

Stimulation of the man's arm skin spots with short focused ultrasound stimuli results in tactile, tickling, temperature, pain and itch sensations (4,5,7). The biological effect of focused ultrasound may be due to various factors. The medium displacement amplitude was calculated in the focal region (A, μ), sound pressure (P, atm), particle velosity amplitude (V, m/sec) and increase in temperature in the focal region (ΔT, °C). In the Table I are given the values of the above parametres for the stimuli of 1 msec duration. The values were calculated from the lowest threshold intensities observed in two subjects (6).

TABLE I. PARAMETERS OF ULTRASOUND STIMULI OF 1 MSEC DURATION ASSOCIATED WITH APPEARANCE OF THRESHOLD SENSATIONS
(Temperature of water -35°C. f, MH_z - frequency, - I, W/cm^2 - intensity of ultrasound)

Parameters		I, W/cm²				A, μ				P, atm				v, m/sec				ΔT, °C			
f, MHz		0.48	0.887	1.95	2.67	0.48	0.887	1.95	2.67	0.48	0.887	1.95	2.67	0.48	0.887	1.95	2.67	0.48	0.887	1.95	2.67
Sensations																					
Tactile	finger	8	15	80	120	0.1	0.08	0.08	0.08	4.9	6.7	15.5	19	0.3	0.45	1	1.35	$2 \cdot 10^{-4}$	$0.6 \cdot 10^{-3}$	$7.5 \cdot 10^{-3}$	0.015
	palm	10	40	250	350	0.15	0.18	0.15	0.13	6.9	15.5	27	32	0.45	1	1.85	2.2	$4 \cdot 10^{-4}$	$3.5 \cdot 10^{-3}$	$2.4 \cdot 10^{-2}$	0.045
Warm	finger	55	90	1420	3200	0.28	0.2	0.35	0.4	13	16.5	65	98	0.85	1.1	4.3	6.7	$1.3 \cdot 10^{-3}$	$4 \cdot 10^{-3}$	0.14	0.41
	palm	130	820	2940	4500	0.43	0.6	0.5	0.47	20	50	93	116	1.3	3.3	6.1	8	$3.1 \cdot 10^{-3}$	$3.5 \cdot 10^{-2}$	0.28	0.59
Cold	finger	—	—	—	—	—	—	—	—	—	—	—	—	—	—	—	—	—	—	—	—
	palm	130	820	2000	3000	0.43	0.6	0.42	0.38	20	50	78	95	1.3	3.3	5.1	6.4	$3.1 \cdot 10^{-3}$	$3.5 \cdot 10^{-2}$	0.19	0.39
Pain	finger	55	140	2860	—	0.28	0.24	0.5	—	13	21	93	—	0.85	1.35	6.1	—	$1.3 \cdot 10^{-3}$	$6 \cdot 10^{-3}$	0.27	—
	palm	240	850	—	3000	0.64	0.39	—	0.38	29	32	—	—	1.9	2.2	—	6.4	$7 \cdot 10^{-3}$	$1.5 \cdot 10^{-2}$	—	0.39

Stimulation with focused ultrasound of different frequencies and identical medium displacement amplitude in the focal region corresponded to the same threshold sensations. Other parametres varied more significantly, in some cases by several orders (see Table I). We failed to find any connection between caviation and threshold pain sensation. Our working intensities were too low for the cavitation to appear when the threshold sensations of other modalities arose (6,7).

Different sensations were connected with the stimulation of different skin spots. Thresholds of sensations increased with the movement of the focal region from finger skin spots to palmar spots and to forearm skin spots (5). At the same region, e.g. at finger skin, threshold amplitude of displacement increased for sensations observed in the following order: tactile sensations, tickling, warm, cold, itch and pain sensations. Unlike the sensations of the other modalities the pain appeared with the focal region not only in the skin, but also in muscles, bones and joints (6,7).

Temperature sensations provoked by focused ultrasound

Methods

Experiments were performed on the man's arm immersed in a distilled water together with the ultrasound transducer. The water temperature was 30, 35, 40 and 45°C. The arm was placed in a special casting to provide a fixation. The shape of casting repeated the shape of the arm. In the present study used were ultrasound stimuli of various intensity with frequencies 0.48, 0.887, 1.95, 2,67 MH_z and durations 1, 10 and 100 msec. Methods were described in detail elswhere (4,5,22).

Results

It was found that the 1 and 10 msec duration stimuli of focused ultrasound were capable to provoke warm or cold sensations from the same skin spot. 100 msec stimuli associated with the great increase in temperature in focal region were capable to provoke only warm sensations (see Fig 1).

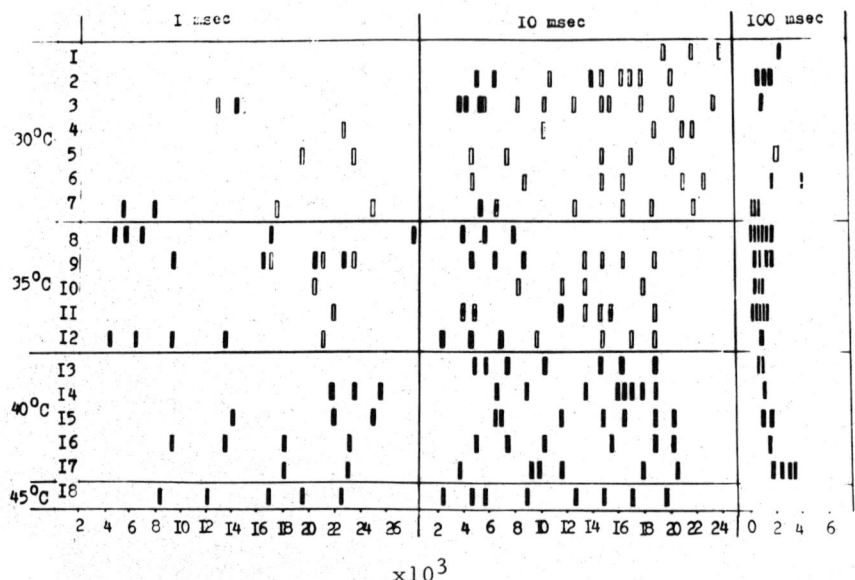

FIG 1. Relations between the modality of the temperature sensations (cold-warm) and water temperature
◻ - cold sensation
▮ - warm sensation
▯ - warm and then cold sensation

The other sensations (tactile, pain, etc.) are not shown 30, 35, 40, 45°C - water temperature, numbers 1-18 - the ordinal number of experiment, numbers below - ultrasound intensity, W/cm^2; 1, 10, 100 msec - duration of stimulus. Subject N 2, The spot is on the forefinger tip skin of the left arm. Ultrasound frequency - 2,67 MH$_z$.

"Warm" and "cold" skin spots were found with thermodes of the Blix type in the finger, palm and forearm skin (with Dr. L.A.Popova's help). Diameter of the thermode tip was about

1 mm, 1 and 10 msec focused ultrasound stimuli provoked warm and cold sensations from the spots having been found with thermodes. With water temperature 30°C there were cold sensations, with 35°C - warm or cold and with water temperature 40 and 45°C - warm sensations. The sensations from the sensitive spots having been found with the focused ultrasound stimuli were of the same character depending on the water temperature (Fig 1). These spots were "warm" or "cold" with the thermodes.

Note

Different sensations with focused ultrasound in the same spot depending on the water temperature lead to the idea that such the spot is the same for warm and cold sensations (22). This idea contradicts traditional point of view about "warm" and cold spots (1,2). There were found electrophysiological data for and against this idea (9,11, 12). But influence outside body temperature and in itself at skin spots was not studied (16). As it is shown later the solution of this question meet some great difficulties. Perhaps it would be simpler to observe temperature sensations provoked by mechanical stimulation of sensitive skin spots and then to compare the temperature sensations to mechanical stimulation and the sensations to focused ultrasound stimulation. We must remind the fact that the main active factor of focused ultrasound stimuli is a mechanical displacement of the medium in the focal region (4).

Temperature sensations provoked by mechanical stimuli in comparison with sensations provoked by focused ultrasound

Cold sensations provoked by mechanical stimulation were known by investigators in the last sentury (8, 23). As for warm sensations the problem is not solved yet (see reviews 16, 27). The aim is to find out if cold sensations provoked by mechanical stimulus in the conditions of the medium temperature, are followed by the warm sensations when the temperature is changed. At the same time it would make a clear idea how to induce a warm sensation by a traditional mechanical stimuli. But the question is not as simple as it may seem. The difficulties naturally may increase when using electrophysiological methods.

In the focused ultrasound experiments most effective were the short stimuli, 1 and 10 msec (see Fig 1). The zone of the ultrasound effect in the sensivity spot depends mostly on the size of the focal region (1,5). Here no displacement of the surrounding tissues and the focal region itself (if the stimulation is repeated) is observed. When using traditional mechanical stimuli, even as "delicate" as Frei hairs, the tension around the spot of contact of stimuli appears, the shortest affecting time grows to 2-3 order, the zone of maximum tissue displacement changes when the stimulation is repeated. The tissue tension could be observed visually by the tissue growing pale around the hair. This phenomena becomes more evident, when the mechanical core is applied. Then the mechanical stimulus is applied the effect of skin vessels tone oscillations is possible too. It is very important temperature factor, taking into consideration the fact, that about $1/3$ of blood volume may accumulate in the skin vessel plexes (25). When the short ultrasound stimulus is applied, these effects are minimal or impossible. Anyhow their role in the skin temperature is not important. Skin has a great number of contracting structures, which react to the changing of medium temperature, intensity and the time of stimulation (26). Besides skin humidity, degree of perspiration, the material of mechanical stimuli and many other reasons may also influence upon the temperature sensations, namely the their frequency and stability. This can make the comparison with sensations provoked by the stimuli of focused ultrasound more complicated.

Cornea and scleral conjunctiva are quite different from the skin because of the absence of epidermis, contract tissue structures and a great number of blood vessels. Therefore corneal and scleral conjuctiva receptor structures, are situated in the more stable conditions than the similar receptive structures in the skin. In the cornea and scleral conjunctiva only free nerve endings and Krause bulbs (in the scleral conjunctiva and limbus of cornea) are found (see review 14, 15). According to Frey cornea and scleral conjunctiva are considered to be the place where the sensations of pain and cold appear. The question of possibility of appearance of the warm sensations is not settled yet (15), though Molter (17) and later Lele a Weddell (14) described them. These authors used temperature-mechanical stimuli (warmed and cooled brushes, glass sticks, etc.). The possibility to provoke the warm sensations to the pure mechanical stimuli is not quite clear yet. The usage of cornea and scleral conjunctiva in our investigations is particularly interesting, because if we could provoke warm sensations on the traditional "cold place" by mechanical stimuli it would support the idea of general temperature spots.

Temperature sensations provoked from cornea and scleral conjunctiva

As stimuli we used wooden or plastic sticks with tip diameter about 1,5 mm. The wooden stick with tip diameter about 0,3 mm and a thick hair are also used. In room temperature cornea is usually warmer than the surrounding air (20). In this conditions touching of the cornea and scleral conjunctiva by the stick with tip diameter about 1,5 mm provokes cold sensations. These cold sensations grows by the decrease in surrounding air temperature. When the temperature was below zero, the touching by the warmed sticks also provoked the cold sensation. It is necessary to mention that Nagel in 1895 (18) payed attention to the fact that the cold sensations in such conditions appear independant of the temperature of the stimulator. Besides the cold sensation, the tactile sensations, tickling and pain with burning component can be provoked by the mechanical stimuli too. Different sensations appear, according to the force of "touch-pressure" (to minimal "touch-pressure" - tactile, then - tickling, after that - cold and pain sensations). With a sertain experience changing "touch-pressure" of the stick, one can provoke the above sensations separately or in combinations. With a stick with tip diameter about 0,3 mm it was possible to provoke only cold and pain sensations, and with a thick hair - only pain. Different data of various authors who used Frey hairs and sticks with tip diameter more than the thickness of the Frey hair can be explained by the dependance of sensations on the tip diameter of the mechanical stimulator. So, Frey, using the hairs, provoked only pain sensations from the cornea (2), but Nagel with metal sticks and air stream could provoke besides pain also tactile and cold sensations (18).

We provoked the some sensations to mechanical stimuli from the cornea and scleral conjunctiva at the air temperature 42 and 44°C. At the very first minute, the subject in the camera with the above mentioned temperature (after the room with 25°C) felt touch, tickling, cold and pain, provoked by stick with tip diameter of 1,5 mm; after that cold sensations disappeared. In a minute and later on among the mentioned feelings warm sensation appeared. Cool stick also provoked warm sensation. Stick with diameter about 0,3 mm or thick hair provoked warm and pain, but thick hair - mostly pain.

Discussion

On provoking temperature sensation from cornea and scleral conjunctiva by mechanical stimuli the same facts as by focused ultrasound stimuli in the sensative spots in the skin are observed: warm and cold sensations appear depending on the medium temperature. So the idea of the same spot for the warm and cold sensations is proved. Apriori one may suggest that different structures or structures of one type may be in the sensitive spots. It may be possible, that free nerve endings in the cornea can be different, as they are described in the skin, which the authors connect with cold reception (10). In the forearm skin the receptor structures are located in less density, that for example in the finger skin (21), and the space between them may be over that the size of focal region of ultrasound (22). But in the experiments with focused ultrasound on the forearm skin the results were the same when the spots on the fingers and forearm skin were stimulated. It proves the idea that one and the same receptor structure can cause cold and warm sensations.

Conclusion

In this report we wanted to dwell upon the importance of the medium temperature in the temperature sensations from sensitive spots. We don't exclude the possible importance of the number of factors, for example, inside body temperature, season, the time of day (26) etc. We don't touch upon these factors. Some of them will be characterised in the separate work. When the sensitive skin spots are stimulated by the focused ultrasound, but cornea and scleral conjunctiva spots - by mechanical stimuli, the influence of the medium temperature becomes evident. Nevertheless it is not clear if the supposed temperature structures in the skin, cornea and scleral conjunctive are the only receptor structures, or there are others, more specific only for warm and cold reception. The experiment showed that mechanical factor takes part in the temperature reception, but the nature of its action is not clear yet. We can suggest not less two types of this action: 1) long-lasting (static) action on the tissues, as a result of medium temperature transformation 2) short-lasting (dynamic) action in the sensitive spot. We don't include the processes of dynamic and static displacement in the receptor structures, as little is known about these structures.

There are many works about the possibility of temperature effects on ion-processes in membranes, having nothing to do with temperature receptors and also non-direct data of temperature effects on hypothetik cold receptor structures (19,24). Mechanic effects on ion-processes in membranes are not touched upon in the aspects of our discussion.

The general range of questions, which appeared in the course investigations includes the questions of resemblance of temperature sensations provoked by focused ultrasound and sensations provoked by mechanical stimulators; the problem of mechanical factor importance for temperature reception; the role of medium temperature in appearance of cold or warm sensations; the ability of one and the same structures to take part in the cold and warm reception. This range of questions should be worked out, described and discussed in future.

References

1. Blix, M., Ztschr. Biol., 21, 3, 145 (1885).
2. Frey von, M., Ber. Verhand. Gesellsch. Wissensch. Math.-phys., 47, 166 (1895).
3. Gavrilov, L.R., Sov. Phys. Acoust., 17, 287 (1972).

4. Gavrilov, L.R., Gersuni, G.V., Ilyinsky, O.B., Popova, L.A., Sirotyuk, M.G. and Tsirulnikov E.M., <u>Sov. Phys. Acoust.</u> 19, 332 (1974).

5. Gavrilov, L.R., Gersuni, G.V., Ilyinski, O.B., Sirotyuk, M.G., Tsirulnikov, E.M. and Tsukerman V.A., <u>Sechenov Physiol. J.</u> 58, 1366 (1972) (in Russian).

6. Gavrilov, L.R., Gersuni, G.V., Ilyinsky, O.B., Sirotyuk, M.G., Tsirulnikov, E.M. and Shchekanov, E.E., <u>Symp. "Tissue reception"</u>, Leningrad, 1974, 33 (in Russian).

7. Gavrilov, L.R., Iljinsky, O.B., Popova, L.A., Sirotyuk, M.G., Tsirulnikov, E.M. and Shchekanov, E.E., <u>Symp."Neuronal mechanisms of pain"</u>, Leningrad, 1973, 23. (in Russian)

8. Goldscheider, A., <u>Arch. f. Anat. u. Physiol. Physiol. Abtheil.</u> Suppl., 1 (1885).

9. Hensel, H., <u>Nova acta Leopold.</u> 37/2, 208, 211 (1973).

10. Hensel, H., Andres, K.H., Düring, M. von., <u>Pflügers Arch.</u> 352 (1974).

11. Hensel, H., Boman, K., <u>J. neurophysiol.</u> 23, 564 (1960).

12. Konietzny, F., Hensel, H., <u>Pflügers Arch.</u> 359, 265 (1975).

13. Kurilova, L.M., <u>Sechenov Physiol.</u> J. 61, 554 (1975) (in Russian).

14. Lele, P.P., Weddell, G., <u>Brain.</u> 79/1, 119 (1956).

15. Millodot, M., <u>Atti Fondaz.</u> 29, 889 (1974).

16. Minut-Sorochtina, O.P., Physiology of the Thermoreception, Moscow, 1972 (in Russian).

17. Molter, A. Ueber die Sensibilitätsverhältnisse der menschlicher Cornea. Dissertation. Cassel. Verlag von Theodor Fischer, 1878.

18. Nagel, W.A., Pflügers Arch. 59, 563 (1895).
19. Pierau, F.-K., Torrey, P., Carpenter, D.O., Brain Research, 73, 156 (1974).
20. Pysä, P., Sarvaranta, J., Acta ophtalm. 52, 810 (1974).
21. Sergeev, K.K., Skin exteroreceptors in man and mammalia. Ref. of diss. Rostow-in-Don, 1963 (in Russian).
22. Tsirulnikow, E.M., Shchekanov, E.E., J. Evol. Bioch. a. Physiol. 11, 479 (1975) (in Russian).
23. Weber, E.H., Temperatursinn. In: "Handwört. der Physiol." Rudolf Wagner, b.3, 2 Abt. Braunschweig, 1866, 549.
24. Winter, Ch., In: Eff. Temp. Ectothermic Organisms. Berlin e a. 45 (1973).
25. Yas Kuno, Human perspiration. Springfield, Illinois USA (1959).
26. Zeveke, A.V., Sechenov Physiol. J. 60, 1740 (1974) (in Russi Russian).
27. Zotterman, Y. In: Handbook of physiology. sec.1: Neurophysiology. v.1: 431, Washington, 1959.

NOCICEPTION

THE DEVELOPMENT IN REGENERATING CUTANEOUS NERVES OF C-FIBRE RECEPTORS RESPONDING TO NOXIOUS HEATING OF THE SKIN

H. DICKHAUS, M. ZIMMERMANN and Y. ZOTTERMAN

INTRODUCTION

Of the many animal experiments performed to elucidate the de-dails of regeneration of nerves and sensory receptors (e.g. YOUNG 1942; MORRIS, HUDSON and WEDDELL 1972; WERNER 1974) only in a few the recurrence of function was studied by electrophysiologically recording from single afferent fibres. In the skin senses the concern of these single fibre studies was the redevelopment of the various types of specific low threshold mechanoreceptors with myelinated afferents (BROWN and IGGO 1962; BURGESS and HORCH 1973).
No reports exist however on the restitution of receptor function in regenerating non-myelinated (C) fibres.

We have therefore studied this subject in cats, subsequent to crushing the plantar nerves. Controlled radiant heat to the cat's foot skin was used as an adequate noxious stimulus to test the reappearance of heat sensitive C-fibres in the regenerating cutaneous nerves. Specific thermal nociceptors (IGGO 1959) with C-fibres have been reported to exist in this skin region of normal animals (BECK, HANDWERKER and ZIMMERMANN 1974). Their well established characteristics served as reference for those of the regenerated C-fibres.

METHODS.

In 9 cats the medial and lateral plantar nerves, that innervate the skin and joints of the hind foot, were crushed over a length of 5 mm, at between 2o and 4o mm proximal to the center of the large footpad. The lesions were performed in a sterile operation under Halothane/N_2O anesthesia. In no case infections occurred during the postoperative period. In a separate experiment it was shown by electrophysiological recording that our procedure of crushing interrupted conduction in quantitatively all myelinated and nonmyelinated fibres.

In subsequent experiments, performed between 1 and 92 days after the nerve crush, the posterior tibial (PT) nerve was exposed in a paraffin oil pool. The plantar nerves, exposed in a separate pool, were put on electrodes for electrical stimulation, at sites proximal to the previous crush. Fine strands were dissected from the PT. When a nerve strand contained not more than six single C-fibres, as identified by stimulation of the plantar nerves, all these C-fibres were tested systematically for peripheral excitability by adequate mechanical and thermal stimulation. Our emphasis was to determine quantitatively the characteristics of thermally excitable units. We used radiant heat to the skin, the skin temperature being measured by a fine thermocouple in firm contact with the skin surface. The heating lamp was controlled by feedback from the thermocouple output. Predetermined constant levels of surface temperature could be produced with this setup; the duration of these heat stimuli was 1o sec. In order to avoid damage to the skin, and sensitization of nerve endings, the repetition rate was 1 per 3 min. The method was identical to that used and described in a previous study in animals with no nerve lesions (BECK et al, 1974).

RESULTS

A total block of conduction was produced by the crush in all types of myelinated and nonmyelinated fibres of the plantar nerves. At regeneration periods longer than 22 days an increasing proportion of C-fibres was excitable by natural skin stimulation. According to the adequate stimulus we could discern redeveloped low threshold mechanoreceptors (IGGO, 196o; BESSOU, BURGESS, PERL and TAYLOR, 1971; ZIMMERMANN, 1975), mechanosensitive nociceptors (IGGO, 196o) and heat receptors (IGGO, 1959; BECK et al, 1974).

The characteristics of redeveloped C-heat receptors.
We tested systematically the responsiveness of C-fibres to radiant heat, since C-heat receptors constitute a class of

nociceptors in the cat's foot with well defined characteristics (BECK et al, 1974). Fig. 1A shows the responses of a regenerated C-fibre to a "square pulse" of radiant heat, 1o sec in duration; the time course of skin temperature is displayed in Fig. 1B.

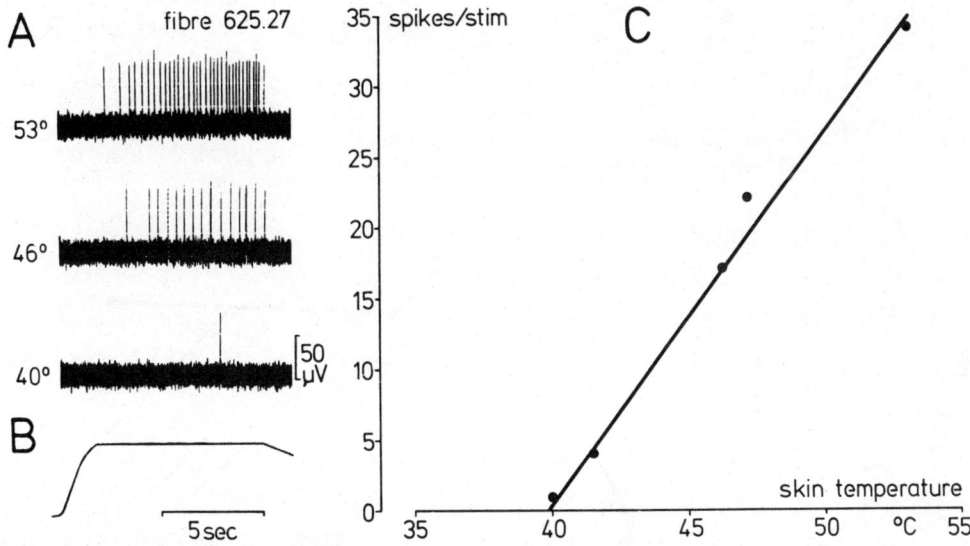

Fig.1. Discharges of a C-heat receptor in the skin of the foot after 51 days of nerve regeneration. A: specimen records of action potentials elicited at 3 different levels of thermal stimuli, as indicated. The skin temperature between stimuli was kept constant at 30°C. B: Time course of actual skin temperature produced by an electrical square pulse signal of 1o sec in duration which controls the heat stimulator. C: receptor characteristic relating the number of spikes per thermal stimulus to the skin temperature. Trials were performed randomly with different skin temperatures at intervals of 3 min.

The total number of impulses per stimulus and the maximum frequency both increase gradually with the skin temperature. The relationship between skin temperature and response is linear. The threshold of this fibre is 40°C. Thus, after nerve crush C-fibre endings redevelop that have the characteristics of heat receptors, i.e. they encode the intensity of the thermal stimulus. However, the thresholds of these C-fibre receptors are lower than in normal nerves (see below, Figs. 3 and 4).

The time course of redevelopment of C-heat receptors.
We tested systematically all the C-fibres found by electrical search stimulation of the plantar nerves, whether or not they could be excited by skin heating. The proportion of heat responsive C-fibres is plotted in Fig. 2 against time of regenreration.

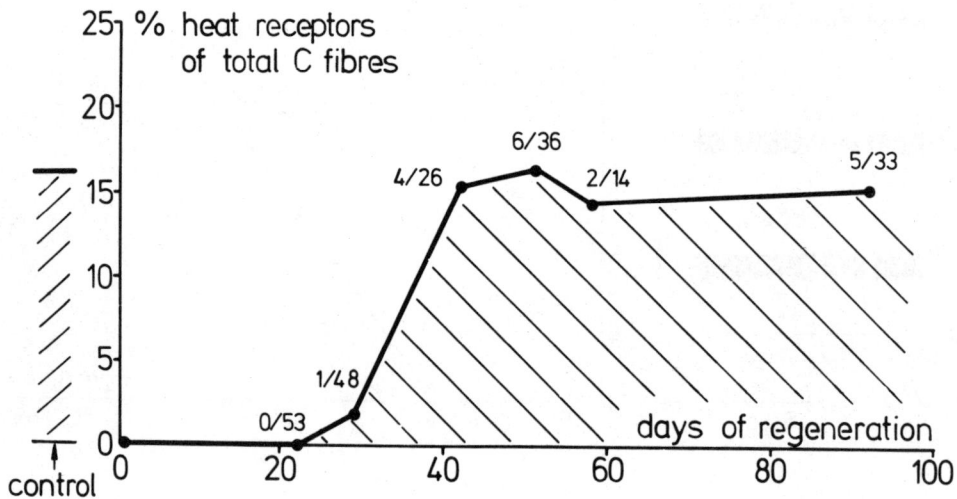

Fig.2. Time course of regeneration of C-heat receptors after nerve crush. The ordinate plots the percentage of heat receptors relative to the total number of C-fibres which were identified by electrical stimulation of the plantar nerves at a site proximal to the crush. Numbers at the points indicate no. of heat receptors/total no. of C-fibres tested for responsiveness to skin heating. Each point contain data from one or two experiments. The control value (16%) is from experiments performed under identical conditions of thermal stimulation (BECK et al, 1974).

At day 28 the first heat receptor appeared, at day 42 and later about 16% of the plantar C-fibres could be activated by skin heating. This proportion is practically the same as in control experiments, indicated on the left of the graph. Thus, the number of heat responsive C-fibres contained in a regenerated cutaneous nerve is identical to that in normal nerve. Although we do not know whether or not these endings are distributed in the original area of innervation, we conclude tentatively that the density of C-heat receptors in the skin is the same after regeneration following crush, as compared with normal skin.

The threshold of the heat response.

The quantitative measurement of response characteristics revealed some differences of C-heat receptors in regenerated compared with normal nerve. The thresholds of 15 regenerated fibres to heating the skin of the receptive field ranged from

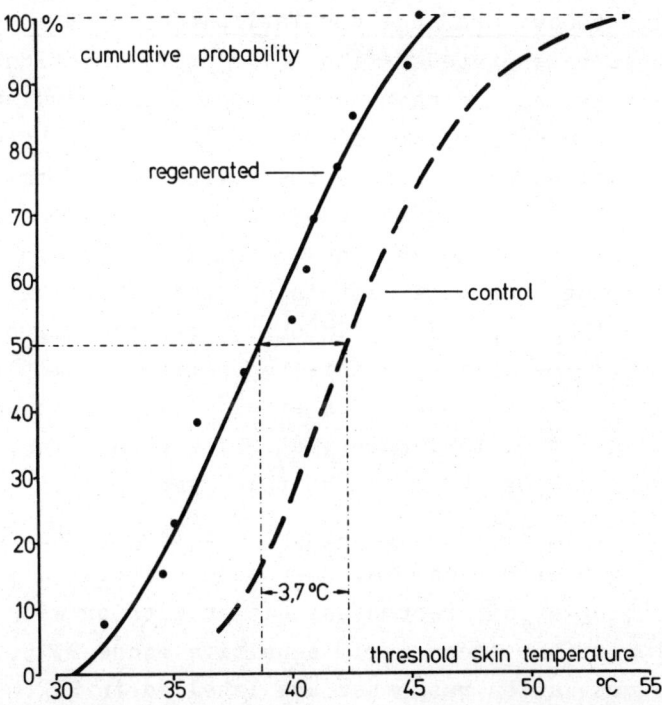

Fig.3. Temperature thresholds of regenerated C-heat receptors. The continuous curve plots the cumulative probability (ordinate) of temperature thresholds (abscissa) for a population of 13 regenerated C-heat receptors; the threshold criterion was the generation of at least one spike during a heat stimulus of 1o sec in duration. The broken line shows the cumulative probability function of 4o C-heat receptors sampled from normal nerves (results from BECK et al, 1974). The indicated median values are $38.7°C$ and $42.4°C$ for the regenerated and control nerves, respectively.

$32°$ to $46°C$. The cumulative probability distribution of the thresholds of 13 of these units is displayed in Fig. 3. The median value is $38.7°C$. The broken line in Fig. 3 is the corresponding distribution of temperature thresholds of a control sample of 4o C-heat receptors: the median of these is $42.4°C$. Thus the threshold distribution of our sample of C-heat receptors found in regenerating nerves is shifted to lower temperatures by about $3.7°C$ relative to the thresholds of the C-heat receptors in normal nerves. The difference is highly significant ($P=o.98$, t-test).

The intensity function of the population of C-heat receptors.
In 12 of these regenerated C-fibres intensity functions as in Fig. 1 were measured. In each case a monotonic correlation was found between the temperature of the stimulus and the number of impulses per stimulus. In Fig. 4 the regression lines of these units are pooled (thin lines). The discharge frequencies, and the total number of spikes per heat stimulus, were in the same range as in normal nerve, except in one unit (fibre 2315.13): in this fibre the slope of the intensity function is extremely steep. Such very sensitive C-fibre receptors have not been found in our previous study (BECK et al, 1974), although there is some evidence that they occur, at a low proportion, in normal plantar nerves (HANDWERKER, this symposium).

The thick lines in Fig. 4 represent two alternatives for the average response of our sample: they were calculated as the mean of the single unit responses, either with or without consideration of the exceedingly sensitive fibre 2315.13. These alternative population responses are labelled in Fig. 4 as "mean" and "mean except fibre 2315.13", respectively. The broken line is the average of a control population.

Either alternative for the sample response is shifted to lower temperatures, as compared to the controls. When including fibre 2315.13 the slope of the average stimulus strength/response relation is steeper for the regenerated C-heat receptors relative to that in normal nerves. In either case, there is a considerable decrease of average threshold compared to normal, as is evident also from Fig. 3.

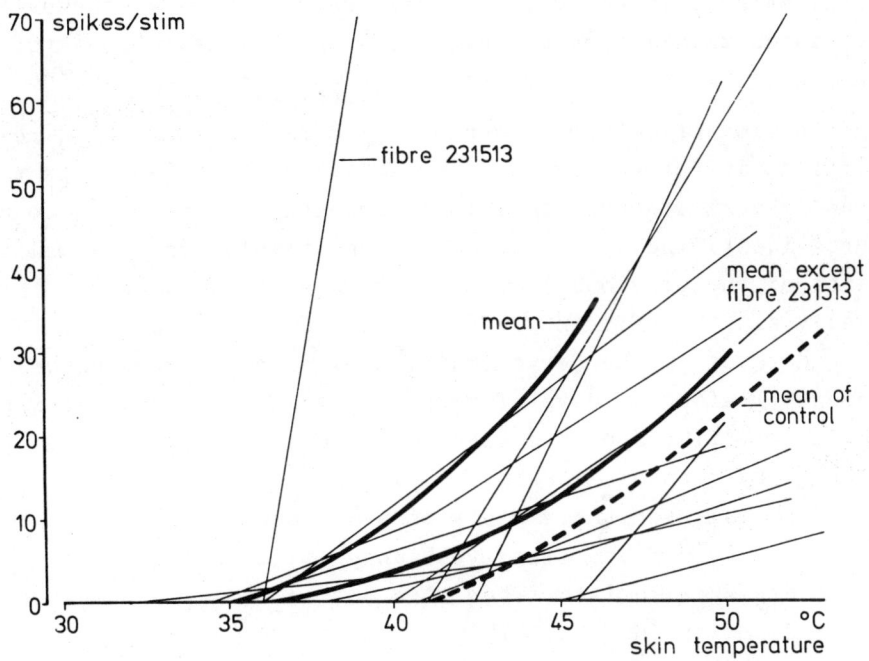

Fig.4. Stimulus strength/response characteristics of a population of 12 regenerated C-heat receptors. Thin lines represent the regression lines of the individual fibres, established by eye fit (see Fig. 1C). The thick line "mean" indicates the mean of the total sample, calculated as the average of the 12 individual responses. The other thick line "mean except fibre 2315.13" is the mean calculated without consideration of this fibre. The broken line "control" plots the mean of a control population of 12 receptors in normal animals (from BECK et al, 1974).

DISCUSSION

Heat receptors with afferent C-fibres, that have been interpreted to constitute a class of specific nociceptors (BECK et al, 1974), redevelop after nerve injury. Under the conditions of our experiments the first responses in C-fibres to heating the skin appeared at 29 days of regeneration. If it is assumed that most of this time was required for the longitudinal growth of the fibre sprouts, and not for development of receptor specificity, the velocity of regeneration is estimated to be about

1 mm/day. Under the same conditions part of the myelinated fibres (Group II or Aβ) can be activated by low intensity mechanical stimuli at day 22; obviously regeneration is faster in these fibres than in the C-fibres (our unpublished observations; see below).

The proportion of C-fibres responding to radiant heat at a regeneration time of 42 days and longer (17 of 1o9 fibres) is the same as in normal nerve: 16%. This percentage is relative to all C-fibres identified by electrical nerve stimulation proximal to the site of the previous lesion. Therefore it is suggested that virtually all the afferent C-fibres have regenerated within less than 9o days after the nerve crush. Myelinated fibres behave differently: after 9o days of regeneration less than half of the Group II (Aβ-)fibres of the plantar nerves can be activated by low intensity mechanical skin stimuli, such as normally are the adequate stimuli for the variety of well known specific mechanoreceptors in this fibre class (our unpublished observations). This deficit still exists after more than 3oo days of regeneration (BURGESS and HORCH, 1973).

The decrease in threshold of the heat response in the C-fibre receptors might provide a neurophysiological basis for the hyperpathia observed in man during nerve regeneration (e.g. HEAD, RIVERS and SHERREN, 19o5; TROTTER and DAVIES, 19o9; SUNDERLAND, 1968). Hyperpathia to thermal skin stimuli has been documented by Sir Henry HEAD in the nerve lesion experiments done on himself; during regeneration of one of his cutaneous nerves his heat pain threshold was at $38^\circ C$, which is well below that normally found in man: $45^\circ C$.

Unfortunately in the descriptions of clinical observations of hyperpathias quantitative data usually are lacking. Therefore it is desirable to introduce methods like those reported by U. LINDBLOM and colleagues (this symposium) for broad clinical application. The correlation of data on pain sensitivity in patients with the information coming from neurophysiological animal models of pathologic states, might help to improve the understanding of pain mechanisms.

REFERENCES

Beck, P.W., H.O. Handwerker and M. Zimmermann (1974): Brain Res. 67, 373-386.

Bessou, P., P.R. Burgess, E.R. Perl and C.B. Taylor (1971): J.Neurophysiol. 34, 116-131.

Bessou, P. and E.R. Perl (1969): J.Neurophysiol. 32, 1o25-1o43.

Brown, A.G. and A. Iggo (1962): J.Physiol. 165, 28P.

Burgess, P.R. and K.W. Horch (1973): J.Neurophysiol. 36, 1o1-114.

Head, H., W.H.R. Rivers and J. Sherren (1o5): Brain 28, 99-115.

Iggo, A. (1959): Quart.J.Exptl.Physiol. 44, 362-37o.

Iggo, A. (196o): J.Physiol. 152, 337-353.

Morris, J.H., A.R. Hudson and G. Weddell (1972): Z.Zellforsch. 124, 76-2o3.

Sunderland, S. (1968): Nerves and nerve injuries. Livingstone, Edinburgh and London.

Trotter, W. and H.M. Davies (19o9): J.Physiol. 38, 134-246.

Werner, J.K. (1974): Am.J.Phys.Med. 53, 127-142.

Young, J.Z. (1942): Physiol.Rev. 22, 318-374.

Zimmermann, M. (1975): Cutaneous C-fibres: peripheral properties and central connections. In: The Somatosensory System. pp. 45-53. Ed. by H.H. Kornhuber. Thieme Verlag Stuttgart.

This work has been supported by the Deutsche Forschungsgemeinschaft, grant Zi 11o/5.

We are indebted to Mrs. A. Manisali for performing the illustrations, to Mrs. U. Nothoff for typing the manuscript, and to Mr. J. Pringle for technical assistance.

Discussion:

Paintal: Did you examine the other ordinary warm fibers and did the threshold also shift to lower temperatures?

Zimmermann: We do not discriminate in the cat´s foot pad between warm fibers and cold fibers. In our original investigation with Beck and Hungerer we believed that there are no warm fibers in the cat´s foot pad. The lowest thresholds of these pain C-fibers to warming were just below fourty degrees in normal animals. This is perhaps too high for a warm fiber because the cat´s foot pad is normally in the range of twenty to thirty degrees when the cat is walking. Therefore we believe that there are no warm fibers in the cat´s foot. Today we have some doubt as to whether or not some of these very steep fibers may be interpreted as warm fibers. We are not sure about that. We are making behavioural experiments in order to decide the question whether the cat can discriminate between warm stimuli. Kenshalo had shown some years ago that the cat can discriminate warm stimuli in the region below the nociceptive threshold.

Paintal: The reason I asked is that in case the warm fibers are effected in the same way you ought to look for the same mechanism. Otherwise, in the case of regeneration you would look for other factors such as blood supply and so on as part of the cause of the change in sensitivity.

Zimmermann: It could be that the blood supply determines the threshold and the response of the heat receptors. But then the blood supply will change the response of the receptors and the sensitibility in animals and in man. In any case, whatever the cause, you get hyperalgesia or hyperestesia to some stimuli.

Lindahl: If you cut or damage human nerve after regeneration, I suppose that in every case you will have hyperpathia. If it is, it will have a tame shelter so in the beginning it will be hyperalgesia and later it will be normal. Can you comment on that in relation to your findings?

Zimmermann: We want to answer this question. The precise time caused the thresholds I had pooled in my diagrams showing the thresholds of all fibers irrespective of the time of regeneration. We want now to make additional experiments in order to see whether there is a certain period of lower thresholds which will then normalize after longer periods, say after half of a year or more. At the moment our sample is too small to allow an answer to your question.

Iggo: It is well known from clinical observations that the regeneration tip of a damaged nerve can be excited by a brief mechanical stimulus (Tinel´s Sign). Could you find any such effect in your regenerating axons? Second, do you have any information on the time that may elapse between the arrival of the regenerating axon at its final destination and the recovery of its normal excitability?

Zimmermann: Our aim was originally also to look for some neurophysiological signs of Tinel´s phenomenon. But the length of regeneration was too short to decide whether locus of adequate excitability was on the farther side or whether this was the real original territory. But nerve length was not long enough. We want to repeat this question in experiments on the sural nerve as you and Brown did. I remember that you described that C-fibers were sensitive to slight mechanical deformations of the skin overlying the regeneration nerve. This would be quite in agreement of the observation of Tinel's Sign in men.

Zotterman: After fracturing my left radial bone in November 1974, a typical hyperalgesic state developed especially on the ulnar side of my left hand where a light stroke caused pricking sensations. This hyperalgesia gradually disappeared in about 7 months. We found in January 1975 that the heat pain threshold on the ulnar side of my left hand was lowered to 37° C while it was 43° C on the normal right hand.

Mense: I enjoyed your paper, Dr Zimmermann, particularly because it seems that this experimental preparation may be used as a model of some kinds of pathological pain. I would like to know if you have tried any type of spinal or supraspinal stimulation to influence this excitability level, since I know you have been working with vibration.

Zimmermann: You could, of course, use these animals with regenerating nerves in a state of presumably hyperalgesia as a model for say chronic pain. We are just going to use these preparations for behaviour experiments. We want to find out whether the thresholds and the responsiveness of animals in the state of regenerating nerves changed compared to normal animals. We have no definite results at the moment. If these experiments are successful, we will certainly try to make some electrical stimulation as used in neurosurgery for relief of pain in man. But we have not done any experiments. In anaesthesized populations as we used here, we did not make any stimulations in order to see whether the thresholds of these fibers are influenced by electrical stimulation of the whole nerve.

PHARMACOLOGICAL MODULATION OF THE DISCHARGE OF NOCICEPTIVE C-FIBRES

H. O. HANDWERKER

INTRODUCTION

For many years the discussion on the physiology of pain was characterized by a controversy on the existence of specific nociceptors. In this controversy the pioneer work of ZOTTERMAN was a break-through, who was in 1939 the first to describe recordings of slowly conducting nerve fibres with specific nociceptive endings. Meanwhile the existence of cutaneous afferent fibres with receptors responding more or less exclusively to noxious stimulation has been well established by means of single fibre recording techniques (HENSEL et al., 1960; IGGO, 1959; BESSOU and PERL, 1969; BECK et al., 1974).

Since the early paper of ZOTTERMAN mentioned above radiant heat was among the favored stimuli in experimental studies on nociceptors. This type of stimulation is assumed not to excite usually low threshold mechano- and thermoreceptors. In addition it has the advantage to provide a distinct and reproducible threshold: pain reactions are elicited in man and in other mammals when the skin surface temperature exceeds $45°C$ (HARDY et al., 1952).

Besides some thin myelinated afferents, which have been described to transmit information on noxious heating in the monkey (IGGO and OGAWA, 1971; SUMINO et al., 1973) most receptors providing information on injurious heating in man and other mammals have unmyelinated (C-) afferent nerve fibres.

In a previous study performed together with P.W. BECK and M. ZIMMERMANN, we have studied characteristics of those "C-heat receptors" in the skin of the cat's hindpaw (BECK et al., 1974). In the present paper modulations of these characteristics by endogenous substances produced e.g. as consequence of skin damage shall be described.

METHODS

The experimental methods are essentially the same as extensively described in previous papers (BECK et al., 1974; BECK and HANDWERKER, 1974). To summarize: Discharges of single cutaneous C-fibres were recorded from the plantar nerves or from the saphenous nerve of cats anesthetized with pentobarbital sodium (Nembutal, 40 mg/kg). Radiant heat was applied using the radiation of a bulb focussed by a lens to the centre of the receptive field of the respective unit. Skin surface temperature was measured by a thermocouple (copper-constantan wires, 0,2 mm ⌀) placed in good contact with the skin in the centre of the focal spot. The output voltage of the thermocouple was fed back to control the heating current of the bulb.

Pharmacological substances were injected into the blood stream of the femoral or popliteal artery through a small cannula inserted through a muscle artery branching off the main artery. The other muscle branches nearby were tied off to lead as much of the blood stream as possible to the skin vessels. Substances tested most frequently were bradykinin[+] (BKN), Serotonin (5-HT), Ca gluconate, and prostaglandins E_1 and E_2.

RESULTS

1. <u>Sample of receptors tested:</u> only "C-heat receptors" are included in this study. I.e. those C-receptors (fibres conducting with velocities below 2 m/sec) which had a high thermal threshold (near $40°$) and were able to transmit quantitative information on heating the skin above the pain threshold. These fibres cannot be excited by slight mechanical stimulation, but some of them are excited by heavy and presumably painful mechanical stimuli (BECK et al., 1974). For pharmacological studies on these fibres it was most important to determine characteristics quickly and with minimal need for repetitive stimulation which might <u>sensitize the receptor. Therefore a standardized heat stimulation</u>

[+] Bradykinin was kindly supplied by SANDOZ, Nürnberg.

program was used, by which the skin surface temperature was adapted first for half a minute to a non-noxious temperature

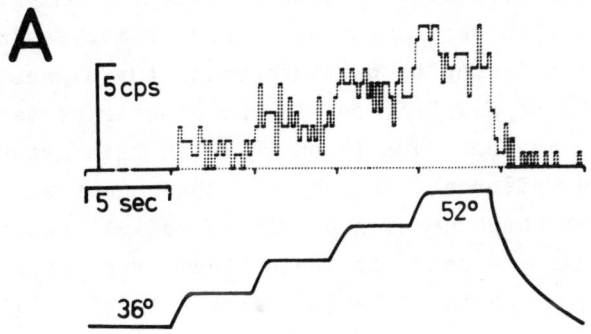

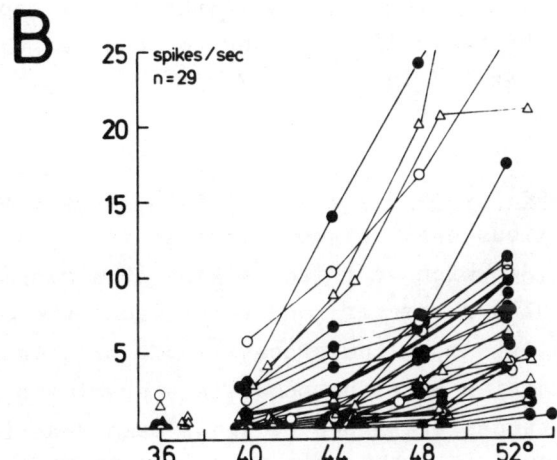

Fig.1: Characteristics of C-heat receptors from the plantar skin region:
(A) Histogram (upper trace) of the discharges of a single unit when stepwise increasing the skin surface temperature (shown by the lower trace) after 30 sec. preadaption to 36°. The histogram shows averaged discharges from 6 consecutive trials performed at 5 min. intervals.

(B) Characteristics of a population of "C-heat receptors" when tested with the same complex heat stimulus as shown in A. The symbols indicate mean frequency of individual units during each one temperature step lasting 5 sec. Each characteristic is taken from one trial. ($\triangle$) indicate receptors in the hairless skin of the cushions, ($\bullet$) those in the surrounding hairy skin, ($\bigcirc$) receptive field at the borderline between hairy and hairless skin. - Heavy line: mean characteristic line of the population.

(36°). Then the temperature was raised in equal steps of 4°, each 5 sec. in duration, to noxious levels. Fig. 1A shows the response of a "C-heat fibre" to such a stimulus. Only those fibres were included in this study which had an increasing discharge rate at increasing temperature up to the highest level tested. About 60% of all C-fibres in the plantar nerves which could be excited by heat were found to be in this group, i.e. about 10% of the C-fibres recorded from these nerves. Other units which might have been C-heat fibres as well had a decreasing discharge frequency at the highest temperature, presumably due to fatigue of the receptor. They are not included in this study.

Fig 1B shows the great variability among characteristics of a population of units. The mean characteristic of the population is represented by the heavy line. It should be noted that the discharge frequency at 40° is about 10% of that at 52° on an average.

2. **Influence of local hormones:** like all stimuli able to elicit pain reactions, noxious heat is known to also initiate the processes of inflammation which we tried to keep at a minimum by selecting the stimulus parameters and repetition rate of heat application carefully. Among the processes of inflammation the production of vasoactive local hormones is a prominent feature. Some of these substances are known to evoke pain reactions themselves when introduced into the skin even in very small concentrations (KEELE and ARMSTRONG, 1964).

We have shown (BECK and HANDWERKER, 1974) that two of the most potent of these substances, BKN and 5-HT, applied intraarterially (single doses 5 µg of BKN and 30 µg of 5-HT) evoke spike responses in most cutaneous C-heat fibres. Though sensitive slowly adapting mechanoreceptors are excited as well, it is likely that the excitation of these and other nociceptive endings is responsible for the pain produced e.g. by i.a. BKN injections. Though we have no direct information whether the action of algogenic substances is direct or indirect, at least one argument is in favor of a specific and independent action of BKN and 5-HT at the receptive endings: tachyphyllaxis developing as consequence of repetitive injections of one substance does not influence the excitation of the receptor by the other substance (BECK and HANDWERKER, 1974).

3. <u>Modulation of heat induced discharges by BKN:</u> To test the modulation of the responses to noxious radiant heat by BKN we used two experimental procedures. The first was designed to test the influence of BKN on the dynamic heat response (Fig. 2).

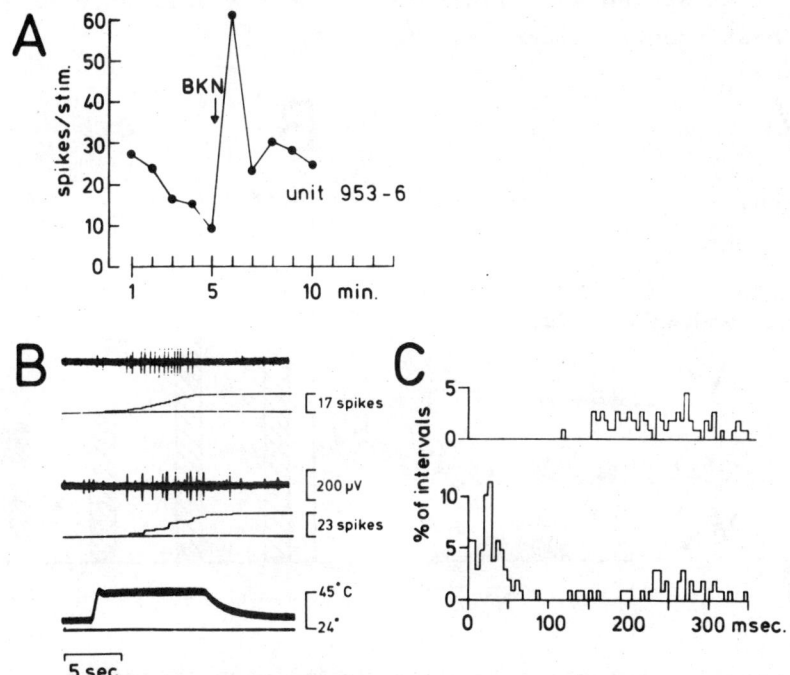

Fig.2: Modulation of heat induced discharges of a single C-fibre by intervening BKN injection.

(A) Total number of spikes (●) counted in the course of 10 sec. heat stimuli of 45° delivered once each minute. I.a. injection of 10 μg BKN after the 5th trial.

(B) Specimen of recordings during a heat stimulus before (above) and after (below) BKN injection. Time course of skin surface temperature at bottom.

(C) Interval histograms derived from the discharges during the 5 trials before (upper histogram) and from the respective recordings after BKN injection (lower histogram).
(Modified from BECK and HANDWERKER, 1974)

For this purpose we applied heat pulses of standard duration and temperature (10 sec., 45°) once each minute. After a single injection of BKN (e.g. 10 µg) the number of spikes / stimulus of C-heat receptors was increased for 5-10 minutes. In contrast the direct excitation of those units by a single BKN injection never exceeded 1 min. Furthermore in many units tested a regular discharge frequency changed to a bursting pattern as a consequence of a BKN injection.

At second we tried to evaluate the influence of BKN on tonic heat induced discharges (Fig.3).

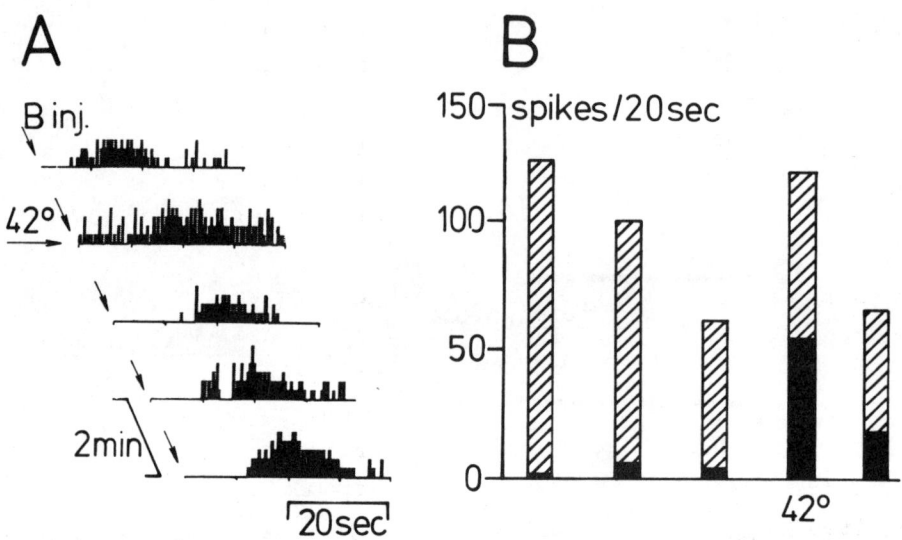

Fig.3: Interaction between the effects of heat and intra-arterial application of BKN.
(A) Histograms derived from the discharges of a "C-heat receptor" following i.a. inj. of 20 µg BKN, first inj. at bottom. The forth dosis was applied when the skin surface was adapted to 42°. The heat stimulation started 45 sec. before BKN application. The other injections were given at a skin temperature of 30°.

(B) The total height of the columns indicates the total number of spikes during 20 sec. after the onset of the BKN effect. The black part of the columns indicates the discharges during 20 sec. before.

The histograms in Fig. 3A are derived from the discharges of a single C-fibre induced by i.a. 20 µg BKN injections (arrows).

BKN was given each 2 min., first injection at bottom of the figure. The 4th injection was given when the skin was adapted to 42°, heat stimulation starting 45 sec. before application of the agent. The total height of the columns in Fig. 3B represents the total number of impulses during 20 sec. after the onset of BKN induced discharges. The black parts of the columns correspond to the discharges during 20 sec. before, thus the hatched parts are estimations of the BKN induced increase in activity. One can see from this figure that heat- and BKN effects seem to be additive. Furthermore the tachyphyllaxis of the BKN response is not influenced significantly by the combination of heat and pharmacological stimulation. This was just so when the tachyphyllaxis was much more pronounced than in the example shown in Fig. 3.

4. Modulation of heat induced discharges by prostaglandins:
Another group of substances which have been described as being synthetized in the skin in the process of inflammatory reactions are E prostaglandins (ARTHURSON et al., 1973; WILLIS, 1969). Prostaglandins are not as potent algogenic substances as BKN, but they have been found to enhance nocifensive reflex hypertension elicited by BKN in dogs (FERREIRA et al., 1973; MONCADA et al., 1975). In order to test the effect of prostaglandins (PGE), experiments have been performed in which the formation of endogenous PGE as a consequence of heat stimulation was inhibited by an initial i.v. application of 180 mg lysin acetylsalicylate^{+} (equivalent to 100 mg acetylsalicylic acid). Prostaglandin E_2 or E_1 was not effective to modulate heat responses when injected in single doses as BKN, but it had to be infused continuously by a pump into the artery (doses 0.5-3 μg/min). With continuous infusion there was no significant difference of the actions of both prostaglandins. Influence of PGE infusions on heat induced discharges of C-receptors were tested by comparison of characteristics determined as shown in Fig. 1 from trials of heating performed once each 5 min. before, during and after PGE infusions. The most frequent effect of PGE application was a parallel shift of characteristics to lower temperatures. When PGE infusion was stopped after e.g. 20 min., the majority

$^{+}$ Kindly supplied by BAYER, Leverkusen.

of the receptors persisted in a sensitized state, but some became less sensitive than during the control heatings before PGE.

The sensitization as consequence of PGE_1 and PGE_2 infusions could be obtained with some C receptors even when the prostaglandin infusion was given not i.a. near the receptive skin field, but into the radial vein (HANDWERKER, 1975). The latter finding is surprising since most of the E prostaglandins infused into the systemic circulation seem to be metabolized in the lungs (FERREIRA and VANE, 1967). Thus one cannot exclude that the sensitization is effected by a metabolite of the infused substance in these cases.

The parallel shift of characteristic lines indicates that - as with BKN - the effect of prostaglandins on heat induced discharges is presumably mainly additive. Since PGE infusions intensify BKN induced discharges of C-heat receptors (HANDWERKER, 1975) and BKN induced circulatory nocifensive reflexes (FERREIRA et al., 1973; MONCADA et al., 1975), the assumption is reasonable that the sensitization of receptive endings by both agents demonstrated in this paper is not independent, but part of one mechanism.

5. <u>Modulation by Ca^{++}ions</u>: Modulations of heat receptor responses by local hormones produced in the process of inflammation are interesting as models of hyperalgesia, no conclusion can be drawn however from the experiments reported above on the receptor mechanism of heat sensitive receptive endings. To study e.g. whether these receptor mechanisms are similar to those of sensitive warm fibres, it is useful to test the influence of Ca^{++}ions. It has been shown by HENSEL and SCHÄFER (1974)that calcium ions excite warm receptors, whereas they inhibit cold receptors. The influence on other receptor types of the skin, such as mechanoreceptors seems to be inhibitory as well. The excitation of warm receptors is as stronger as higher the discharge rate induced by warming the skin. In our experiments some, but not all of the heat receptors were influenced by Ca^{++}ions (single i.a. injections of 0.4-1.6 mEq). The effect was strongly dependent on the temperature at the receptive field. An example of calcium

induced discharges of a C-heat fibre is shown in Fig. 4

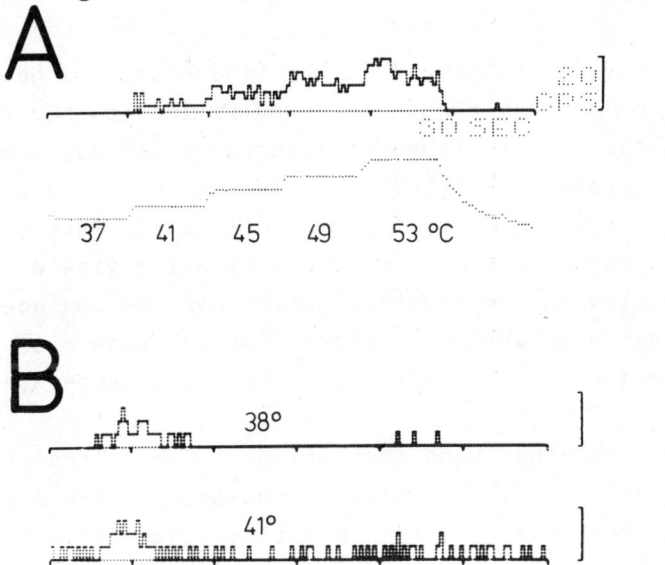

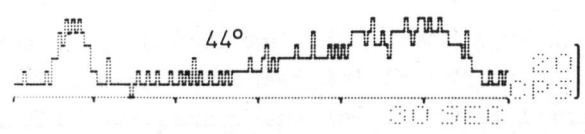

Fig.4: Influence of calcium ions on a C-heat fibre.
(A) Responses of the fibre to stepwise increasing skin temperature.
(B) Modulation of tonic discharges of the same fibre by Ca^{++}. The receptive field of the unit was adapted to different temperatures, adaptation starting 45 sec. before injection of single doses of 0.8 mEq Ca^{++} into the artery. Infusions starting with the histograms.

As all C-heat receptors tested this fibre was not excited by Ca^{++} infusion when the skin temperature at the receptive field was 35° or below. 38° was just below the threshold of a tonic heat response of this fibre. At this temperature a Ca^{++} response appeared which was definitely smaller than the response at 44°. This indicates a more than additive synergistic mechanism of heat and calcium ions.

Calcium responses as shown in Fig.4 might be an indication that the receptor mechanisms of cutaneous warm- and heat fibres - which are still unknown - are similar.

CONCLUSION

Heat responses in presumably nociceptive cutaneous heat receptors are modulated by agents produced in the course of inflammatory reactions. Both types of substances tested, bradykinin and E prostaglandins exerted a mainly additive effect. Since these local hormones play a major role in inflammation, our results might contribute to a more quantitative view of inflammatory hyperesthesia. An additive action has the consequence of a lower threshold of the nociceptors, but the amount of increase of discharges on an increased suprathreshold temperature is not changed.

On the other hand modulation of C-heat receptor discharges by Ca^{++} ions is of interest not so much for a study of nociceptive mechanisms, but it might be a cue for a comparison of receptor mechanisms of C-heat fibres with those of sensitive warm receptors.

In our experiments calcium ions did not act simply additive to the heat. No calcium responses have been observed far below the thermal threshold of the fibres. Calcium induced discharges became more frequent with increasing heat induced excitation of the receptor. These results have a parallel in calcium induced excitations of sensitive warm fibres described previously (HENSEL and SCHÄFER, 1974). In contrast all other types of cutaneous receptors seem to be inhibited by Ca^{++}. This might indicate similar receptor mechanisms of low and high threshold receptors excited by increases of the skin temperature.

REFERENCES

1. Arthurson, F., Hamberg, M. and Johnsson, C.E., Acta Physiol. Scand., 87,270-276 (1973)
2. Beck, P.W. and Handwerker, H.O., Pflügers Arch., 347,209-222 (1974)
3. Beck, P.W., Handwerker, H.O. and Zimmermann, M., Brain Res., 67,373-386 (1974)
4. Bessou, P. and Perl, E.R., J.Neurophysiol., 32, 1025-1043 (1969)

5. Ferreira,S.H., Moncada,S. and Vane,J.R., Br.J.Pharmacol., 49, 86-97 (1973)
6. Ferreira,S.H. and Vane,J.R., Nature, 216, 868-873 (1967)
7. Handwerker,H.O., 1st World Congr. on Pain, Florence (1975)
8. Hardy,J.D., Wolff,H.G. and Goodell,H., "Pain sensations and reactions". Williams and Wilkins, Baltimore (1952)
9. Hensel,H., Iggo,A. and Witt,I., J.Physiol., 153, 113-126 (1960)
10. Hensel,H. and Schäfer,K., Pflügers Arch., 352, 87-90 (1974)
11. Iggo,A., Quart.J.Exp.Physiol., 44, 362-370 (1959)
12. Iggo,A. and Ogawa,H., J.Physiol., 216, 77-78 P (1971)
13. Keele,C.A. and Armstrong,D., "Substances producing pain and itch". Edward Arnold, London (1964)
14. Moncada,S., Ferreira,S.H. and Vane,J.R., Europ.J.Pharmacol., 31, 250-260 (1975)
15. Sumino,R., Dubner,R. and Starkman,S., Brain Res., 62, 260--263 (1973)
16. Willis,A.L., J.Pharm.Pharmacol., 21, 126-128 (1969)
17. Zotterman,Y., J.Physiol., 95, 1-28 (1939)

Discussion:

Hellekant: I have some observations on another receptor which may interest you. I was trying to make some perfusion of the tongue to study the effect of blood circulation on taste receptors. I was advised to inject acetylsalicylate in 72 mg per kilo body weight. When I started to do my recording an hour later I could not obtain any taste response at all. After two or three animals I thought there must be something wrong not just my technique but with the injection I am doing. I developed that and have looked at the effects of salicylate locally, intravenously and intraarterially into the tongue. I found a definite effect of **salicylate**. If you make it in an acute experiment directly into the tongue, it is hard to say exactly how much you give but a few micrograms or less than a microgram will block the taste response within thirty seconds. What doses did you use?

Handwerker: Only in the prostaglandine experiments, not in the other experiments, I gave 100 mg for a cat weighing **3** - **3.5** kilos one to two hours before the experiment, (40 mg per kilo body). Of course I made control experiments with heating first, measuring heat responses and then application of acetylsalicylic acid intraveneously and then I measured the response as well. I did not find significant decrease of the heat response. I did not have a large sample. I did this three or four times and there was no marked effect. I would not like to say that there is no effect at all. But if there is an effect it must be small. Perhaps Dr Hensel can say something on responses of unmyelinated muscle nerve fibers.

Hensel: We have applied bradykinin intraarterially and have recorded the responses of C-fibers from muscle. We have found that by acetylalicylate it is possible to reduce the responses of the mixed receptors to bradykinin.

Handwerker: I never studied the influence on the skin of bradykinin so I cannot say anything about it. But I definitely saw no large effect on heat responses.

Hellekant: Since you mentioned prostaglandine E I tried that too. I thought it might have something to do with this transmission in the synapse or something. I could not obtain any effect of the prostaglandine on the taste response, at least no specific effect. I would like to ask some of these people working on humans to try to look at the effect of salicylate in the human beings on the threshold, for example. Not on taste but on touch.

Lindblom: Perhaps it would be good to clarify, are these units in the category of multimodal nociceptors?

Handwerker: In these pharmacological experiments, I avoided applying high threshold mechanical stimulation but used only low threshold stimulation. None of these units could be excited by low touch. I did some experiments with Evans blue injection into the circulation and I found that the usual test for mechanical stimulation in nociceptors, that is squeezing with forceps even if you take blunt forceps, seems to make heavy damage to the skin. You get a blue spot immediately. This effect is much more pronounced than that of heat stimulation. Therefore, I did not use it in those experiments where I might have a sensitization. But we have studied this in a paper together with Professor Zimmermann previously. We found that if you take as an upper limit, I think, 300 gram test square millimeter stimulus then about half of these units can be excited by mechanical stimulation in the foot sole region. This might be in variance to other body regions where the skin is more tender.

Lindahl: Did I understand you correctly that you injected your substances in the receptor area?

Handwerker: I did it sometimes in the receptor area but the usual type of injection was closed arterially.

Lindahl: Every injection in the tissue will change circulation and the pH will make something with the impulses. Which change in pH was the result following injection?

Handwerker: It is very difficult to control in whole-animal experiments. Therefore, I tried to have control experiments before and after the injection. But I have no direct measurement of the pH in the tissue or so. I cannot tell you much about the mechanism of the bradykinin effect.

Lindahl: What about the pH effect then?

Handwerker: Personally, I do not believe it. There are several arguments. One argument is that 5-hydroxitrytamine and bradykinin as was shown by different people have effects which seem to be different. You do not get contantiphalaxis, for example. These might be two mechanisms which are independent from each other. I do not believe in the pH effect but I cannot exclude it.

Zotterman: I remind you of the box of medicine in the army. It always contained Sebum salicylatum to apply on the blisters the infantrymen get on their heels. It relieves the pain. For this reason, I find it very extraordinary that Handwerker did not find any effect of salicylic acid. The only explanation I can find at the moment is that the acetylsalicylic acid may not effect the specific heat pain fibers. Maybe the acetylsalicylic acid acts only on those pain fibers which are excited by strong mechanical stimulus.

Handwerker: I wanted to say only that I did not see much influence on the heat response. That does not mean that it does not influence the heat fibers or the sensitization of heat fibers or something. So this might be a different thing.

Zotterman: I was once treated with an intravenous injection of CaCl which gave me an enormously strong sensation of warmth in the skin all over the body. After such an injection Hensel (1975) recorded a massive inflow of impulses in the specific cutaneous warm fibers. That is related to what we heard from the presentation of Dr Benzinger. There may be some likeness between warm receptors in the skin and the central cells sensitive to the blood temperature. I find it very plausible that Ca-ions play an important role here.

Handwerker: I would like to add that the way of application may explain the different effect of salicylic acid. It is perhaps not the same to inject it closed arterially and apply it locally as Hellekant described. That is another explanation.

Paintal: I was looking around for Dr Perl because in his paper with Bessou, I recall that he said that the application of a noxious injurious stimulus left the receptor in a state of hypersensitivity. I would like to know from you with regard to the techniques you adopted whether applying injurious heat over a long period could not in itself cause sensitization. What is the difference between the prolonged application of repeated heat and the effects of the drugs you have tested? Secondly, it looks to me that it has not been possible to differentiate between sensitization and stimulation by bradykinin. I think it is mostly a case of slight stimulation and no sensitization of the receptor. Is that right? Or did I not see the graphs properly?

Handwerker: To answer your second question first, if you inject bradykinin you usually get direct response with a defined latency of about twenty seconds. This response has a duration of about twenty or thirty seconds as well. Of course, we saw sensitization in some fibers. And if you have a pronounced sensitization you cannot test for the influence of sensitizing agents. That is clear. That is why I tried to make several control stimuli. At first we tried to find parameters of the stimulation where sensitization seldom happened. But, of course, I saw in several cases a quicker sensitization. These are not included in the sample. But you do not see exclusive sensitization. You must see the contrary as well, the desensitization of the receptor. Both might happen.

Hellekant: I tried salicylate intravenously, intraarterially and by local application. In every case it had a strong effect.

THE EFFECTS OF ANTI-INFLAMMATORY AGENTS ON THE RESPONSES AND THE SENSITIZATION OF UNMYELINATED (C) FIBER POLYMODAL NOCICEPTORS

J. S. KING, P. GALLANT, V. MYERSON and E. R. PERL

Department of Physiology, University of North Carolina, Chapel Hill, North Carolina 27514 U.S.A.

A considerable fraction of the sensory receptors with unmyelinated (C) fibers in cutaneous nerves have elevated thresholds for all forms of mechanical and thermal stimuli in comparison to other skin receptors. The most common of these high threshold, C-fiber receptors are excited to maximal activity by mechanical and heat stimuli of tissue-damaging intensity and by irritant chemicals placed on the intact skin. This spectrum of responsiveness to noxious stimulation led to their designation as polymodal nociceptors (Bessou and Perl, 1969). Polymodal nociceptors are a feature of cutaneous nerves of every mammalian species studied to date (cat, rhesus monkey, rabbit and man) making up 40% to over 90% of the afferent C-fiber population (Bessou and Perl, 1969; Burgess and Perl, 1973; Kumazawa, Boivie and Perl, 1974; Törebjork, 1974).

Polymodal nociceptors show little or no background activity provided that the skin is uninjured; however, noxious stimulation, especially when skin damage results, initiates an ongoing discharge. Moreover, under appropriate conditions, a substantially increased response appears upon repeated testing, particularly with the use of noxious heat. Parenthetically, temperatures high enough to cause gross destruction of tissue, presumably including the nerve terminal, will inactivate these as well as other receptors (Bessou and Perl, 1969). Enhanced responsiveness (sensitization) takes the form of both a lowering of threshold and a higher frequency of discharge at a given temperature; the total response in terms of numbers of impulses on repeated identical tests may be increased by one-third to more than 10-fold from that recorded during the initial trial. The presence of a significant background discharge makes threshold measurement difficult; nevertheless, in some elements with low levels of background activity, the liminal temperature for heat-evoked response was found to decrease 5 - 10°C upon repeated heating (Bessou and Perl, 1969; Perl, Kumazawa, Lynn and Kenins, 1976). On first heating with a contact thermode, the heat threshold typically was in the range of 45 to 50°C; after sensitization responses may occur at temperatures under 42°C and therefore be below usual noxious levels (Bessou and Perl, 1969;

Perl et al, 1976; Kumazawa and Perl, unpublished). Sensitization may last for hours, although the magnitude of the response at a given temperature and the background discharge tends to decrease toward first test levels with time. The C-fiber polymodal nociceptors have characteristics consistent with those expected for sense organs related to pain and pain-like reactions (Bessou and Perl, 1969). Their enhanced responsiveness and background discharge implies that they could be, at least in part, responsible for pain elicited by weak stimulation of damaged tissue and/or pain from injured structures in the absence of stimulation.

The well-known relationship between inflammation and pain and the ease with which cutaneous inflammation may be induced, raises the possibility that the processes associated with inflammation and nociceptor sensitization are correlated. This connection seems particularly likely since there is evidence that the polymodal sensitization can spread to nearby unstimulated skin. Heating the skin with small probes (2 - 3 mm) is not associated with background discharge in a unit with a receptive field 10 mm or more distant (Bessou and Perl, 1969); however, after damage of large areas of the skin, background activity and unusual responsiveness appears in every polymodal unit (Lynn, unpublished). These observations and the associated line of reasoning were points of departure for earlier studies on sensitization of polymodal nociceptors (Perl et al, 1976). The present experiments tested the effects of agents known to modify inflammatory responses either clinically (Goodman and Gilman, 1975) or experimentally (Wilhelm, 1973) upon nociceptor sensitization, in the hope of gaining evidence for additional parallels between the two processes.

METHODS

An isolated perfused rabbit ear was prepared in the general fashion described by Rischbeiter (1913). Under sodium phenobarbital anesthesia the ear and greater auricular nerve (4 - 5 cm length) was removed from a 3 - 4 kg domestic female rabbit and placed on a specially-designed platform. The concha of the excised ear was filled with plasticine, which in turn was placed on the platform so that the dorsal surface of the ear was uppermost. This platform was set at an angle of 45° relative to a horizontally-placed plastic trough. The cut portion of the ear and the nerve lay within the trough and were covered with mineral oil. The proximal end of the nerve was placed upon a dissecting plate and laid across stimulating electrodes located near the base of the ear 20 - 40 mm from the recording site. Modified Kreb's solution saturated with 95% O_2 and 5% CO_2 was delivered to the arterial cannula at static pressures of 120 - 140 mmHg. Efflux from an auricular vein was allowed to run along the nerve to the dissecting plate. This efflux plus that from the cut end of the ear was siphoned off from the bottom of the trough.

Recordings were made from filaments of the nerve cut down with needles, bits of razor blades and sharp jewelers' forceps until the activity of an unequivocably identifiable unit conducting at C velocity appeared in response to single electrical shocks. The cutaneous receptor of the unit was then tested for responsiveness to gentle mechanical stimulation of the skin, pressure with small probes and by innocuous cooling. Units with elevated thresholds for mechanical stimuli which did not respond to cooling were studied using a small, rigidly mounted thermode with a contact surface of approximately 3 mm^2. The pressure of the thermode itself often initiated a low frequency discharge. Discharges of the afferent fibers were filtered (10 Hz to 1 KHz bandpass), amplified and displayed on a multichannel oscilloscope; they were also stored on magnetic tape in parallel with analogue voltages representing the contact probe temperatures by an analogue FM-modulated instrumentation type recorder. After analogue to digital conversion the resultant records were analysed using a DEC PDP-11/45 digital computer in conjunction with a modified E & S LDS-2 digital interactive graphics computer system with a derivative of the general scheme described by Schmittroth (in Bessou and Perl, 1969). The following data are selected from observations made on several hundred units.

RESULTS

In the course of searching for C-fiber units, numerous receptors with myelinated afferent fibers were encountered and generally could be readily identified according to criteria established in other species or other nerve distributions in the rabbit (Brown and Iggo, 1967; Burgess and Perl, 1973). Lynn (unpublished), in a survey of forty C-fiber afferent units of rabbit's ear *in vivo*, found the same general receptor types previously established in cat and monkey; the preponderance exhibited characteristics of either the polymodal nociceptors or C mechanoreceptors; a few had the features of thermoreceptors, particularly the cooling type (Bessou and Perl, 1969; Hensel, 1973; Kumazawa, Boivie and Perl, 1974). In the present search for polymodal nociceptors, an occasional C-fiber unit was encountered with a subcutaneous receptive field which could be excited by manipulation of the ear cartilage. Some other units did not respond to thermal stimulation and were excited only by obvious mechanical stimulation of skin areas along the course of the vasculature. There was no attempt to study either of these latter two types. In many preparations, four hours or more after the ear had been removed from the animal and artificial fluid perfusion begun, differences from the usual receptor behavior in vivo were noted and the proportion of C-fiber units with a considerable background discharge was increased. We interpreted these observations, as well as instances in which a number of units responding to electrical stimulation were inexcitable by natural stimulation of the skin, as indicative of deterioration of the preparation.

When receptors of the perfused ear appeared "normal" (similar to those in vivo), C polymodal nociceptors showed little background activity (< 5 impulses/min) prior to manipulation of the skin, although the mechanical stimulation used to identify the receptive field often was followed by slightly increased background frequency (5 - 10/min). Mechanical thresholds with flexible probes typically were in excess of 20 gm/mm^2; the response incremented with progressively noxious mechanical stimulation in the same fashion as for in vivo receptors. With the small contact thermode, heat-evoked responses typically began at thermode temperatures in excess of 45°C on first trial, although units with thresholds as low as 40°C and as high as 60°C were encountered. Sensitization and an associated increase in background discharge (Bessou and Perl, 1969; Perl et al, 1976) were routine for the units from the isolated ear after one or more suprathreshold heat stimuli.

At the same time, a considerable variability in the behavior of individual units posed a problem for evaluating experimental manipulations. Inasmuch as reversible changes could not be assured for many circumstances and each heat stimulation could be expected to modify future behavior, the data from an individual element could not be used as a basis of comparison. The combination of the problems related to reversibility and variability led us to establish a range of behavior under standard conditions which could then be

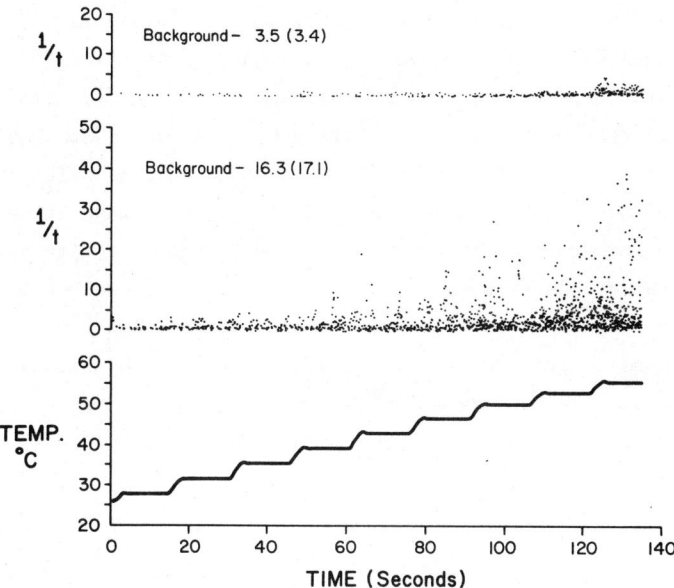

Fig. 1. Sensitization of C-fiber polymodal nociceptors of the isolated, perfused rabbit ear by noxious skin heating. The standardized heating sequence of the thermode contacting the receptive field is illustrated by the lowermost graph. Discharges of ten units from ears perfused with the standard, oxygenated Kreb's solution are shown. Each discharge is plotted as a dot located on the horizontal axis according to its time of occurrence relative to the start of the heating cycle and on the vertical axis as the reciprocal of the interval between it and the preceding discharge (1/t). Uppermost graph: activity recorded for all ten receptors during the first exposure to heating cycles. Background: mean discharge in impulses/min (standard deviation) for two minutes before heating cycle. Middle graph: activity recorded for same 10 units during second heating cycle started 5 minutes after end of the first cycle. Background: as for graph above except that sample taken during the two minutes prior to beginning of second heating cycle.

compared to results obtained with additional variables. The lower trace of Fig. 1 shows the heat stimulation program employed in much of the present work; the temperature was automatically raised in 3°C steps at 1°/sec and held at each level for 12 sec. The heating cycle was interrupted after the first temperature step which evoked an unequivocal increase in impulse frequency above the background rate. This usually occurred at a temperature between 48 and 54°C. The thermode was then cooled to an adapting level of 26°C for five minutes, after which a second heating cycle was allowed to progress to the maximum reached during the first cycle. In some experiments specific temperature limits were chosen (i.e., 51 - 53°C) rather than a termination determined by response. Considerable (occasionally maximal) sensitization usually occurred after a single activation by such a heating sequence. Consequently, the paradigm of two heating cycles separated by a five-minute recovery period was chosen for study of the effects of various chemical agents.

Fig. 1-1 plots every discharge recorded from 10 polymodal nociceptors during the first standardized heating sequence and Fig. 1-2 shows the activity of the same units on a second exposure to an identical heating cycle. A comparison of Figs. 1-1 and 1-2 illustrates the enhanced (sensitized) response observed in this preparation for a population of elements. The difference of numerical values in Fig. 1-1 and 1-2 also indicates the background activity increase after the first heat test.

<u>Adrenocortical steroid action</u>: The mechanism of action of adrenocortical steroids upon inflammatory reactions remains a matter of uncertainty and controversy, yet their clinical effect in suppressing both the tissue reaction and the pain associated with several forms of acute inflammation is well-established (see Goodman and Gilman, 1975). For this reason, we examined the effects of a synthetic steroid (dexamethasone), in clinical use as an anti-inflammatory agent, on the response and sensitization of C polymodal nociceptors. The graphs of Fig. 2B present observations on units from ears perfused with solutions containing dexamethasone (8 mgm/L) for 30 min or more prior to the first heat test. For comparison, Fig. 2A shows equivalent tests on elements studied in preparations perfused with the standard solution. The degree of sensitization, judged by the difference in frequency response between the first and second heat tests, was smaller for the units

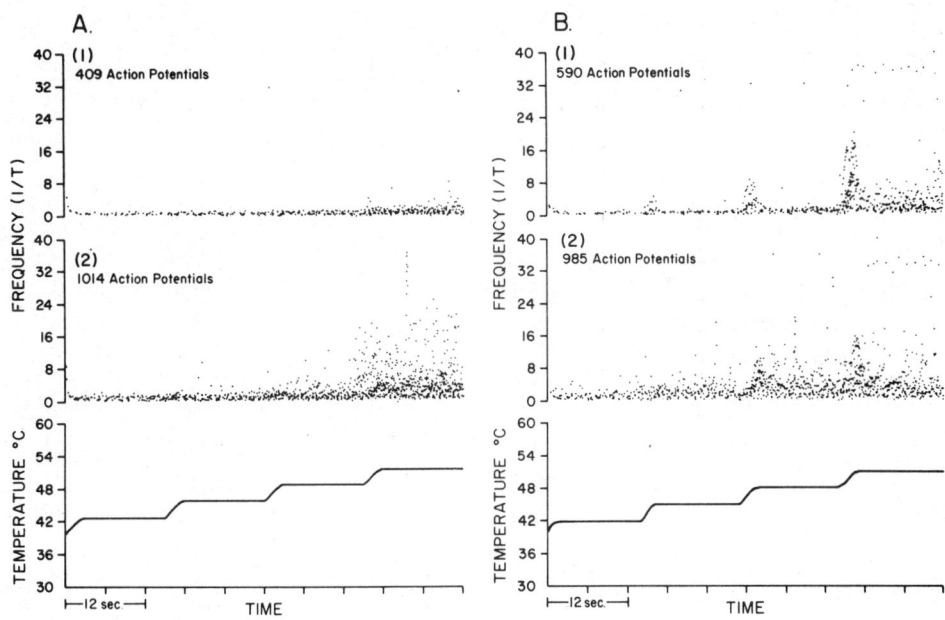

Fig. 2. Effects of dexamethasone on responses evoked by contact heat from C-fiber polymodal nociceptors of the isolated, perfused rabbit ear. Heating cycle of the type shown in Fig. 1; data from the later steps are illustrated in this figure. Discharge as function of time plotted as in Fig. 1. Total impulses (action potentials) for each display given in inset for that graph. A: All discharges recorded from ten randomly selected units in ears perfused by standard Kreb's solution for the illustrated fraction of first (1) and second (2) heating cycles. B: As for A except that perfusion at 2-4 ml/min with fluid containing 8 mgm/L dexamethasone had been underway for a minimum of 30 minutes prior to the first exposure to heat.

from ears treated with the steroid than for the control group. On the other hand, the initial heat exposure evoked a larger response from units in ears perfused with the dexamethasone solution (Fig. 2B-1) than those of the control group (Fig. 2A-1). The difference was statistically significant at the 0.05 level with respect to all tests considered: intercept, linear and quadratic trends. Moreover, a prominent dynamic component was noted during each incremental heating above 42°C for the units treated with dexamethasone. However, in contrast to the augmented evoked response, the resultant background activity of the steroid-treated elements was less than expected from control units (Fig. 3). The initial background discharge was somewhat less (20%) and persisting background discharge after the heating sequences was approximately one-half for the receptors exposed to steroids (Fig. 3B) than for controls (Fig. 3A).

Agents acting on candidate chemical mediators: Skin damage leads to an inflammatory reaction beginning in minutes and lasting for days. The processes leading to the development of inflammation responses are complex; several, possibly synergistic, chemical mediators have been implicated, including histamine, serotonin, bradykinin and prostaglandins of the E type. Evidence suggesting one or another of these compounds has come (a) from experiments in which agents presumed to interfere specifically with one or another substance have modified a test for inflammation and (b) from the collection and identification of substances in perfusates from damaged skin. Following the first-mentioned approach, we have evaluated the effects of agents, presumably acting on a candidate mediator, upon the sensitization of polymodal units. In an attempt to demonstrate the feasibility of the approach, a global experiment was tried in which a substance antagonizing with each of the four presumed chemical mediators of inflammation was added to the perfusion fluid. Fig. 4D shows that the combination of antagonists to histamine (mepyramine maleate), to serotonin (methysergide), to bradykinin (carboxypeptidase B) and to prostaglandin synthesis (indomethacin), produced a dramatic decrease in sensitization compared to the control population of Fig. 4A. (Note that the results in Fig. 4 are plotted as the mean response at each temperature in the first (1) and in the second (2) heating cycle.) Therefore, further attempts to explore specific importance of one or more intermediaries were undertaken.

The strong arguments advanced in favor of bradykinin as a chemical mediator in the production of skin pain (Keele and Armstrong, 1964) were an impetus to study the effects of agents capable of deactivation of polypeptides similar to bradykinin (Wilhelm, 1973). Fig. 4B shows data from units studied in which the perfusion fluid contained carboxypeptidase B. The difference between the mean discharge frequency between the first and second heating for the carboxypeptidase B-treated units (Fig. 4B-1, Fig. 4B-2) is slightly less

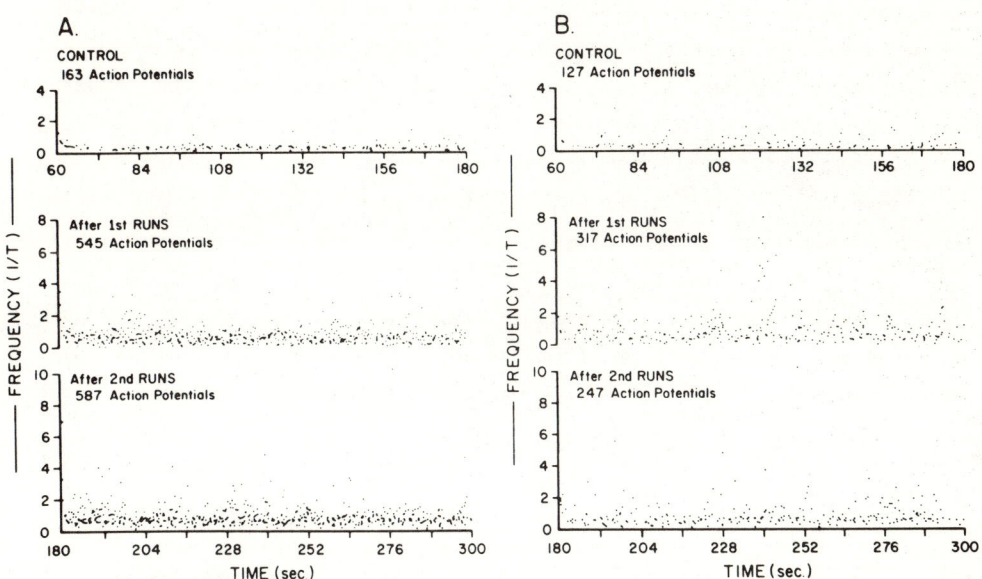

Fig. 3. Effects of dexamethasone on background discharge of C-fiber polymodal nociceptors. Plots constructed as in Fig. 1. <u>A</u>: Units from rabbit ears perfused with standard Kreb's solution. <u>B</u>: Units from rabbit ears perfused with solution containing 8 mgm/L dexamethasone. Time in seconds. Heat stimulation cycles were as illustrated in Fig. 1. <u>Control</u>: all discharges from ten units for the 120 seconds before first heating cycle. <u>After first RUNS</u> -- all discharges from the same ten units between 180 and 300 seconds after the first heat stimulation cycle. <u>After second RUNS</u> -- all discharges from the same ten units between 180 and 300 seconds after second heat stimulation cycle.

than the control population (Fig. 4A-1, Fig. 4A-2), but the variability (unit to unit) makes this difference of doubtful significance.

The literature on inflammation is suggestive of a synergism between prostaglandins of the E type and bradykinin (Wilhelm, 1973). Eight units were therefore studied in which the perfusion fluid contained both carboxypeptidase B and indomethacin. Fig. 4C indicates that while a decrease in the amount of sensitization as indicated by the difference in initial and second heating values may have resulted, it also appears on such a variable base as to be of uncertain significance. The questionable magnitude of the effects on responsiveness and sensitization obtained with the use of a proteolytic enzyme need cautious interpretation. Even though the eventual edema of the ear suggested considerable capillary permeability for solution and solutes, we had no measure of the ease with which the large carboxypeptidase B molecule passed into the interstitial space. Until there is better evidence on this point, one explanation which must be considered is that too little peptidase reached the nerve terminals to be effective. The same explanation will not account for the lack of effect of indomethacin. Within the time frame of experiments as illustrated in Fig. 4C, or in equivalent tests as a single agent, indomethacin, in concentrations which should have depressed prostaglandin synthesis, had little or no effect on polymodal responsiveness and sensitization.

Our most recent attempts to look further at the decreased sensitization illustrated in Fig. 4D have focused on serotonin. Methysergide in concentrations of 20 mgm/L of perfusion fluid has substantially depressed responses of the rabbit polymodal units to noxious heat and greatly reduced the sensitization it produces. These results are suggestive of an important part for serotonin but elimination of a possible nonspecific toxic effect by the methysergide and proof that it was acting on serotonin is necessary.

Added putative agents: An obvious approach in a search for a possible chemical intermediary is the addition of various agents to arterial blood or fluid perfusing the tissue. Experience with preparations of sensory receptors subject to such manipulation has underscored the pitfalls inherent in this avenue. A great variety of agents or circumstances can modify or initiate the response of many cutaneous sense organ types (Fjällbrant and Iggo, 1961). In our hands, synthetic bradykinin (BRS-640, Sandoz) injected as a concentrated slug (40 to 90 mgm in 1 cc) into the perfusion flow regularly has excited the polymodal units of the isolated rabbit ear, although the response has varied from a few impulses to a vigorous, short-lived discharge. Brisk responses also are routinely evoked by acetylcholine and increased K^+ concentration or, in fact, practically any agent capable of depolarizing nerve. Similar findings have been reported by Juan and Lembeck (1974). It is interesting to note that serotonin and epinephrine added to the perfusion fluid in concentrations sufficient to cause substantial vasoconstriction did not produce great changes in background activity (Perl, Kumazawa, Lynn and Kenins, 1976).

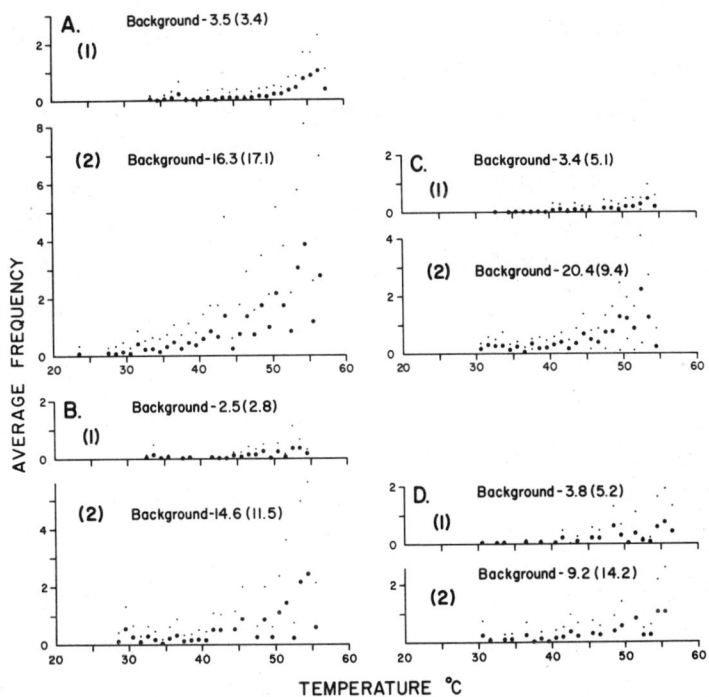

Fig. 4. Effect of chemical agents on the response of C-fiber polymodal nociceptors of the isolated, perfused rabbit ear. Mean discharge frequency, calculated from 1 second samples, (large dots) and standard error (small dots above and below each large dot) are plotted as a function of temperature during a heat stimulation cycle described in Fig. 1. (1) First heat stimulation cycle; (2) second heat stimulation cycle. Background: average discharge (standard deviation) for the last two minutes prior to the heat stimulation cycle. A: Ten units from ears perfused with the standard Kreb's solution -- same group and data used for Fig. 1. B: Eight elements from ears perfused with Kreb's solution containing carboxypeptidase B (2000 units/L) for at least 30 minutes prior to first test. C: Nine elements from ears perfused with Kreb's solution containing carboxypeptidase B (2000 units/L) + indomethacin (10 mgm/L) for at least 30 minutes prior to first test. D: Five elements from ears perfused with carboxypeptidase B (2000 units/L) + indomethacin (10 mgm/L) + methysergide (40 mgm/L) + mepyramine maleate (40 mgm/L) for at least 30 minutes prior to first test.

DISCUSSION

While these results are far from conclusive, they do point out that the development of enhanced responsiveness and background activity does not require blood-borne agents or precursors. It was surprising to find that an anti-inflammatory synthetic cortical steroid produced an apparent enhancement of the nociceptor response to first heating. On the other hand, the decrease in background activity of units exposed to dexamethasone was interesting in the light of the relief of pain often associated with the use of steroids in some inflammatory conditions. It must be recognized that the experimental design used differs from the usual clinical situation in which the adrenocortical steroids have been found to have anti-inflammatory action. Firstly, in our arrangement the cortical steroid was used prior to the noxious stimulus, while in the clinical situation, it is normally employed after tissue injury and pain have resulted. Secondly, the time scale of the present experiment just approaches those in which the corticosteroids are effective clinically; relief of pain or decrease of skin inflammation usually takes two or three hours after a steroid has been administered. Nevertheless, the very fact that a corticosteroid analogue modified the polymodal nociceptor activity under certain conditions is consistent with some link between the processes associated with inflammation and the behavior of polymodal sensory units.

The clearcut suppression of the sensitization by the use of a combination of agents which interfere with the action of several suspected chemical intermediaries for the inflammatory process is similarly consistent with some common ground for inflammation and polymodal nociceptor excitation. It must be emphasized that the experiments themselves and the nature of the results do not pinpoint a chemical intermediary. They only suggest that the action of a potent, naturally-occurring biological substance, possibly serotonin, may have a relation to nociceptor sensitization and the latter's development of spontaneous activity. To be sure, one interpretation of observations of the type shown in Fig. 4 is that a substance is released by cutaneous cells upon noxious stimulation which then produces the observed sensitization by directly causing partial depolarization of polymodal terminals. However, at this point one must still consider alternate possibilities such as (1) synergistic action between several agents acting on the sensory terminals, (2) a process in which one chemical agent is a critical link in a sequence eventually acting on the nociceptor terminals, and (3) the agent suppressing sensitization acted in a toxic and/or non-specific fashion. Obviously additional study is needed to provide clarification.

SUMMARY

1) Unmyelinated (C) fiber polymodal nociceptors in the isolated artificially-perfused rabbit ear were found to behave in a fashion comparable to such receptors in vivo. As is found for these receptors in the normally-perfused skin, repeated noxious heat produces a short latency (1-3 min), enhanced responsiveness and persisting background activity. Systematic testing of C-fiber polymodal units in the perfused preparation by identical cycles of noxious heat provided a measure of sensitization and background activity against which the effects of anti-inflammatory agents were evaluated.

2) Addition of a synthetic adrenocortical steroid to the fluid perfusing the ear led to a more marked phasic response in the initial heat test and a consistent decrease in the amount of poststimulation background activity.

3) A combination of agents presumed to interfere specifically with four putative chemical intermediaries in inflammatory reactions (histamine, serotonin, bradykinin, prostaglandin E) greatly reduced the sensitization of polymodal nociceptors when added to the perfusion fluid prior to testing by noxious heat. Carboxypeptidase B (a deactivator of bradykinin) and indomethacin (an inhibitor of prostaglandin synthesis) together were equivocally effective in modifying sensitization. Methysergide, a potent anti-serotonin agent, added alone, was highly effective in decreasing polymodal responsiveness and sensitization; however, the specificity of this action needs additional study.

ACKNOWLEDGEMENT: We gratefully acknowledge the help of Mr. Joseph Capowski in programming the digital computer for analyses of receptor discharges and Dr. James Grizzle of the Department of Biostatistics for assistance in statistical procedures. This work was supported by grants NS-11132 and NS-10321 from the NINCDS of the U.S. Public Health Service. JSK is the recipient of a special postdoctoral fellowship from the NINCDS of the USPHS and support from an A.P. Sloan Foundation Grant to the Neurobiology Program of UNC-CH. PG and VM hold predoctoral fellowships from a training grant (MH-14277) provided by the National Institute of Mental Health of the U.S. Alcohol, Drug Abuse and Mental Health Administration.

REFERENCES

Bessou, P. and E. R. Perl. (1969). Response of cutaneous sensory units with unmyelinated fibers to noxious stimuli. J. Neurophysiol. 32: 1025-1043.

Brown, A. G. and A. Iggo. (1967). A quantitative study of cutaneous receptors and afferent fibres in the cat and rabbit. J. Physiol. (Lond.) 193: 707-733.

Burgess, P. R. and E. R. Perl. (1973). Cutaneous mechanoreceptors and nociceptors. In Handbook of Sensory Physiology, Vol. II, A. Iggo, Ed., pp. 29-78, Berlin: Springer-Verlag.

Fjällbrant, N. and A. Iggo. (1961). The effect of histamine, 5-hydroxytryptamine and acetylcholine on cutaneous afferent fibres. J. Physiol. (Lond.) 156: 578-590.

Goodman, L. S. and A. Gilman. (1975). The Pharmacological Basis of Therapeutics. 5th Edition, New York: MacMillan.

Hensel, H. H. (1973). Cutaneous thermoreceptors. In Handbook of Sensory Physiology, Vol. II, A. Iggo, Ed., pp. 79-110, Berlin: Springer-Verlag.

Juan, H. and F. Lembeck. (1974). Action of peptides and other algesic agents on paravascular pain receptors of the isolated perfused rabbit. Naunyn-Schmiedeberg's Arch. Pharmacol. 283: 151-164.

Keele, C. A. and D. Armstrong. (1964). Substances Producing Pain and Itch. London: Arnold.

Kumazawa, T., J. J. G. Boivie and E. R. Perl. (1974). Cutaneous sensory units with C (unmyelinated) fibres in primate. Proc. Intl. Union Physiol. Sci. XI:

Perl, E. R., T. Kumazawa, B. Lynn and P. Kenins. (1976). Sensitization of high threshold receptors with unmyelinated (C) afferent fibers. In "Somatosensory and Visceral Receptor Mechanisms", Progress in Brain Research, Vol. 43, A. Iggo and O. B. Ilyinsky, Eds., Amsterdam: Elsevier Scientific Pub. Co., pp. 236-277.

Rischbeiter, W. (1913). Das isolierte Kaninchenohr als überlebendes Gefässpräparat (nach Krawkow-Bissemki), zur Prüfung von Gefässmitteln, speziel Adrenalin und Hypophysin. Z. ges. exp. Med. 1: 355-368.

Törebjork, H. E. (1974). Afferent C units responding to mechanical, thermal and chemical stimuli in human non-glabrous skin. Acta physiol. scand. 92: 374-390.

Wilhelm, D. L. (1973). Chemical mediators. In The Inflammatory Process. Vol. II, B. W. Zweifach, L. Grant and R. T. McCluskey, Eds., pp. 251-301, New York: Academic Press.

Discussion:

Hensel: Dr Perl, do you have any data about the natural process of desensitization after having sensitized the polymodal receptors? If so, what is the time course of desensitization?

Perl: It is very difficult to study the temporal features because each test itself may add an effect. Kumazawa and I tried the following: a unit was sensitized by several cycles of noxious heat stimulation and then tested episodically. After several tests at 3 to 5 minute intervals, the response decreased to the level observed with first stimulation. After an hour's rest, the response returned to the maximal sensitized level. Testing again after a short interval caused the response again to decrease to the first stimulation level but upon another rest the response was back up to the maximal sensitized level. We interpreted these observations as interaction between the impulse generating process and the process that produces sensitization (using up material, for example). Bessou and I also noted that if you sensitize a polymodal unit with two or three stimulation cycles and then wait for an hour or so before testing again, there was a tendency for the response to be smaller than the sensitized maximum. Then after a long wait, the response was still less. On the other hand, if we stimulated a number of times in rapid succession, the decrease with time was not so obvious. About one third of our cat polymodal units showed a parallel between changes in heat responsiveness and mechanical responsiveness. In those elements mechanical stimulation in itself produced no obvious enhancement of response, therefore it could be used as a test of sensitization. Over a period of several hours, the enhanced mechanical responsiveness also tended to go back toward the presensitized level.

Zotterman: In 1926 I worked for eight months with Sir Thomas Lewis on the "triple response" of the skin. We worked every day from nine to six on our own skins. We produced all kinds of damages and stimulus responses in the skin. We found that whatever means we used to produce "triple response" in the skin it was always associated with the liberation of some substance or substances - Lewis called it Substance H - which was taken up and transported via the lymphatic vessels. The "triple response" is also accompanied by sensations of stinging or pricking pain. That part I took up in my dissertation in 1933. Later on in 1938 I recorded the impulse traffic in fine strands of the saphenous nerve of the cat during and after a heavy stroke over the skin. I found that the afterresponse consisted entirely of slow A delta and C-spikes exactly like the response to radiating heat, where every mechanical stimulation was avoided. Further I demonstrated in 1936 that heat stimulation of the tongue surface inhibited temporarily all responses from the large mechanoceptive fibers leaving the signalling duty entirely to C-fibers. Thus noxious stimuli produce a liberation of active substances in the tissues which most likely have their influence upon the endings of the nociceptive fibers at the same time as the injurious stimuli exert a negative effect on the endings of large mechanoceptive fibers. Warming of the skin of the palm of the hand to just above 45° C will temporarily (for about 15 minutes) abolish specific tickle sensations. You get the same effect if you scratch the skin.

Iggo: Do you have any explanation for the dissociation of responses to mechanical and thermal stimuli on your nociceptors? For example, do the stimuli act on different elements in the nerve terminals? I would also like to comment on the latency of response to close arterial injections - potassium ions caused a very prompt response within a few seconds and probably by direct action on the afferent nerve terminals. In contrast other chemicals, such as histamine and 5-HT (Fjällbrant and Iggo, 1961) may excite after a latency of twenty seconds. Perhaps they are acting through an intermediary of the kind that is acting in your sensitization experiments.

Perl: We have no experimental evidence concerning the part of the neuron acted on by different stimuli. I have speculated, as you might have, on the meaning of the dissociation between the background discharge and responsiveness. Dissociation has been so regular a phenomenon that we use it to indicate when our preparations are starting to deteriorate. Late in an experiment we often find units conducting at C-fiber velocity with background discharge but cannot find a receptive field for natural stimuli. When the skin is examined at this time, edema is usually marked but we do not have a clue as to the connection between it and the process of dissociation. Capsaicin produces dissociation in a dramatic fashion. We had expected the effect of capsaicin, an extract of red pepper, to block the heat response but it did not. In the few units Lynn (unpublished) tested, the heat response remained after capsaicin was applied while mechanical responsiveness disappeared. We have noted a parallel in mechanical and thermal responsiveness during sensitization of some units but there was greater scatter in this relationship.

Handwerker: I would like to comment on a remark of Professor Perl that you can excite receptors by i.v. injections with virtually every kind of substance. As Professor Perl knows this is an oversimplification. As a rule you can say that only those substances are effective to excite nociceptors which have been shown in the old blister base experiments of Keele and others to evoke pain in low concentrations.

A second comment to the long latency of the onset of action of bradykinin: it is a pity that we cannot perform in vitro experiments with the receptors of interest. Look at the bradykinin action on smooth muscle preparations: there we have the same long latency. It was shown recently that this is not due to diffusion time, nor is it dependent on ions such as calcium. A pH effect exists but seems to be unspecific (Pagelow et al, Acta Biol. Med. Gerol., 34, 451, 1975). Thus this long latency seems to be a characteristic of bradykinic effects on membranes.

Perl: I did not mean to suggest that the effects you have described are secondary to pH changes or some artifactual alteration; however, the number of agents, some not naturally occurring, which evoke discharge or produce enhancement of response did impress us. There is an interesting difference between your results with muscle receptors and observations Bessou and I made on C-fiber receptors of muscle perfused with an artificial solution. We did not find bradykinin in concentrations of 10^{-5} gm/L to be effective in exciting most of our units while acetylcholine routinely excited every nociceptor tested. If one were to argue on the basis of this, then acetylcholine would be a good candidate for an intermediary substance. I am not aware of serious evidence pointing in that direction.

Hellekant: I have one comment and two questions dealing with the problem of increasing the background noise or decreasing the signal to noise ratio seen for example in the taste receptor when it is starting to deteriorate. How long after you cut off the blood supply are you able to record what you think is a normal response?

Perl: We have switched rapidly from blood to a solution saturated with oxygen. Normally there are some ten seconds from the time the blood supply is completely disconnected to the beginning of perfusion with artificial solutions. From this point on, in most preparations, it is possible to record normal-appearing evoked activity for four to six hours. That is, the afferent activity appears normal with the possible exception of the appearance of background discharge in some elements. Even the latter may result from stimulation because the process of moving the ear from the animal to the supporting plate could in itself cause damage. C-fiber elements in some ear preparations qualitatively seemed to respond as if they were normal for up to nine or ten hours (which is as long as we have kept such a preparation going); however, the quantitative data suggests that control elements after four hours no longer behave as they do in the intact animal. A more sensitive test may come soon. One of Dr Hensel's colleagues is looking at thermal receptors in the isolated rabbit ear. I suspect that the thermal receptors may be a better test of normal receptor behavior than nociceptors because of the thermoreceptors' inherent background discharge and their excitation by innocuous stimuli.

Hellekant: If you are not perfusing at all, how long will it respond then? Ten or fifteen minutes?

Perl: The polymodal nociceptors will respond to noxious heat and to strong mechanical stimulus for at least an hour after the circulation has been stopped. A few elements were studied after an animal's heart had stopped; up to about one hour afterwards C polymodal units responded without qualitative difference from responses in the living animal. There may have been a quantitative change which was not noted. Other receptors quit responding much sooner.

Hellekant: The solutions which you injected here apparently affected your patient. Do you think they had any effect on the receptors?

Perl: You are asking very difficult questions. We can only compare populations. It is my feeling that the artificial solutions may produce some modification of the initial responsiveness, but this is hard to establish. C polymodal nociceptors, while responding vigorously only to strong stimuli, vary a good deal in threshold. We do not have large enough populations to know whether our thresholds in the perfused preparation are equivalent to those in vivo since it takes a minimum of an hour to an hour and a half to study a unit, including 30 minutes or more to isolate the discharge by dissection. By the time two units are studied, deterioration has often set in. Even if there are some threshold changes the responsiveness which distinguishes polymodal units certainly still exists in the artificially perfused skin.

Mense: I have a question concerning your results obtained with muscle afferents. You reported that you did not get responses to chemical stimulants in the artificially perfused preparation. I would like to ask whether you have applied intra-muscular injections. I have done these injections in the muscle of the cat and I have obtained responses very regularly to these substances. I have to add that in vitro preparation of an isolated rat diafragm, we have also obtained responses of single C-fibers to substances such as bradykinin and histamine.

Perl: Let me clarify my statement in that regard. First, I did not mean to say that there were no responses by C-fiber muscle receptors to various agents added to perfusion fluid, but that in general when responses appeared they were initiated by high concentrations of substances. In the case of acetylcholine, it was 10^{-5} to 10^{-4} gm/L for most units, although a few were excited by 10^{-7} gm/L. Every unit that responded to bradykinin also responded to acetylcholine. Our injections were done differently than you reported. We injected at a constant rate and a constant concentration, using a perfusion pump. That may have influenced the effect because when rapid injections were done so that a very high concentration, relatively speaking, of the substance would reach the muscle, a somewhat larger fraction of units were excited. But still, only about fifteen elements out of one hundred elements gave a response to drug concentrations below that causing tetanic contraction. We were interested not only in testing the effect of injected agents but also the effects of pH changes. The pH of the perfusion solutions was modified by varying the buffers to levels of pH 6 and below without excitation of the units under study. Increasing lactic acid concentrations in the perfusion did not modify activity. Direct injections into the muscles were not tried. Our muscle C-fiber receptors all responded to intense mechanical squeezing or probing of the muscle. When the muscle was opened along fascial planes between the insertion and origin (usually the gastrocnemius or sartorius) the threshold for direct mechanical stimulation dropped. After exposure of the muscle, our units consistently and repeatedly were excited by localized fairly gentle mechanical stimulation.

Lindahl: Being especially interested in the connection between H-ion concentration and pain I should like to ask about skin preparation from the rabbit's ear. Did you continuously control the pH of the perfusion fluid coming back from the tissue and did you measure the pH in the tissue?

Perl: The pH of the tissue was not measured. We did measure pH of the solution after perfusing the ear. The efflux pH was slightly more acid than the starting solution, dropping from about 7.4 to 7.3. We did not find large changes in pH with fairly extensive heating of the ear by a large radiant source. But remember that we used a buffered perfusion solution. It would have taken a marked change in local hydrogen ion concentrations to significantly effect the pH of our solutions. We were aware of your work, Dr Lindahl, and were interested in the pH change not only because of it but also because pH changes have been implicated in muscle pain for many years. We could not demonstrate a pH effect on the muscle C-fiber receptors judged to be nociceptors on the basis of mechanical responsiveness.

Lindahl: Did you try lactic acid?

Perl: Yes, we tried lactic acid in concentrations high enough to produce major changes in the consistency of the muscle and to make it no longer contract on direct or nerve electrical stimulation. The receptors showed no response to the lactic acid perfusion but still responded to strong mechanical stimuli.

Gordon: This is a wild and perhaps ignorant speculation but you were talking about the dissociation that you get sometimes between mechanical and thermal responses. I suppose that the mechanical response may be attributed to some coupling between your stimulus and the receptor terminal though nobody probably knows its structure. Are any of the substances that produced this effect known to have any disorganizing effect on, for example, glabrious tissue?

Perl: The immediate answer to your question is that destructive effects are not known to occur straight off. But since the substances we used, such as capsaicin, do initiate an inflammatory response, in time one would expect some effect on supporting tissue. However, the time scale would be much longer than our observation period. Effects were looked for within thirty seconds or so after an agent was injected or within thirty minutes to an hour after perfusion was started. There is a facet of your question on which we may have evidence. At one point we tried to determine whether swelling of the tissue of the stimulated area was related to sensitization for cat polymodal nociceptors. Probes capable of detecting movements of twenty micrometers in contact with the skin while it was heated by the thermode, gave no indication of swelling. The cat skin does not seem to swell as promptly as the primate skin following insults of the type used. The rabbit ear skin does become edematous in the absence of albumen or protein substitutes in the perfusion fluid. Whether the frequent dissociation of mechanical and heat stimuli in the rabbit ear is related to actual physical distortion of the tissue I cannot say other than it seems a reasonable possibility.

Zotterman: I have some experience with this phenomenon. After fourty minutes of blocking the circulation of the arm there are no sensations at all in the fingers. When you let the blood supply come back to the hand, after about thirty or fourty seconds, you get tingling and pricking sensations. That tingling can be suppressed entirely as I have shown and described in a paper (1944) with Gernandt by breathing 10 per cent carbon dioxide in oxygen. In local inflammation of the skin I wonder if one would be able to prove that there is a break in insulation between the different fibers so the non-noxious fibers excite nociceptor fibers within the region affected.

Perl: Inflammatory changes, of course, take place over days. In our circumstance, only the first few minutes and up to the first hours were examined. In these early stages the histological changes which involve substantial alteration in the contacts between different cells are yet to take place or at least many have not taken place.

Paintal: The three papers on nociception today have all been on sensitization and its possible mechanisms. Although there are many questions unanswered, one is much more impressed by the bulk of evidence which is coming forth at a rapid speed and which has enabled us to understand the phenomena in physical parameters with the recording from the C-fibers. These phenomena have a high degree of relevance not only for physiological nociception, if I might say so, but also for various clinical conditions with pain. We will come back to that tomorrow. I would also emphasize the possibility that these studies have opened the way to re-evaluation of the old observations like the one Professor Zotterman just mentioned. These observations which were made on humans can now have their explanations in terms of neurophysiological recordings. I think that it is very important that one differentiates between various phenomena. This will be possible by the methods that are now available between substances and physical impacts which rarely mediate nociception and those which may be called paranatural. I would like to raise one question, at last. Would it be possible to save time in these studies by using mechanical stimuli, which are not noxious, to test the cause of sensitization? I can see that you must use several units to get a group to make comparisons. I would suspect that this gross modality sensitization must hold since in clinical conditions the lowered mechanical threshold giving tenderness is the regular phenomenon. One would expect that to occur also in these studies, for example in the work of Professor Perl. So my question was whether you could find a mechanical stimulus which is non-noxious to follow these stages of sensitization.

Perl: I mentioned our attempt to use that technique earlier. It seemed logical to use mechanical stimuli to test sensitization since they were less likely to cause further changes of the sense organ response; however, we spent two years in trying this approach without success. There were two problems. Firstly, the threshold of the elements is sometimes so high that they cannot be excited with any precisely controllable device, such as an electromechanically-driven probe. Secondly, we have found that there is some difference in alteration of responses to heat and to mechanical stimuli, at least in the effects occurring in the time frame we have dealt with. It may be that in the sensitization seen clinically, when inflammation is well-developed, mechanical and heat responsiveness more closely parallel one another.

Handwerker: I think that perhaps another problem is involved. Static pressure might not be the right stimulus. Perhaps you need a slow moving stimulus or something to be adequate. This makes things technically much more difficult.

Lindahl: Dr Iggo said that in injecting lactic acid preparation he did not get any increased impulses in the C-fibers. Then I think he has proved that C-fibers do not conduct pain because it is very obvious that in any human that will produce pain.

Iggo: We were looking at C-fibers supplying muscle tendons. These, like the ones Dr Perl was describing, could be excited by mechanical stimulation. This was work done ten to fifteen years ago. At that time I was very keen to explain everything with one or two experiments. I have learned better. But we did try a variety of chemicals like lactic acid and so on because these were thought to accumulate in muscles and be the cause of pain if you work the muscle. For a start we arranged the preparations so that we could occlude the blood supply to the muscle and have it occluded for perhaps an hour with C-fibers still conducting. Then we stimulated the muscle directly to cause the muscle to contract in anaerobic conditions and we hoped thereby to generate presumptive lactic acid. This certainly did not excite the C-fiber receptors we were recording from. This may have been because the receptors were in the tendon of the muscle but on other occasions we had C-endings in the belly of the muscle and these were certainly not excited by that stimulus. I was very puzzled by it. You may be right that these have nothing to do with nociception. That is one thing that I think I have learned that you have to ask the central nervous system about things and not base everything on the behaviour of the peripheral fibers.

Zotterman: Everyone who has worked electrophysiologically on peripheral nerves knows that it is a very easy way to stop spontaneous activity which you do not want to have in experiments, by just breathing carbon dioxide on them. That was the reason that I started to try to breathe carbon dioxide in order to see what the effect would be on the tingling which was suppressed entirely just by increasing the carbon dioxide. Why does it work? My theory was at that time (that was thirty years ago) that the increase in carbon dioxide tension increased the free calcium ions. That was the effect of it. I do not know whether that is proven or not. It should have been proven, of course. But that was my idea at the time. You know also that you can stop a hiccup by breathing carbon dioxide.

MECHANISMS OF MUSCLE PAIN: A COMPARISON WITH CUTANEOUS NOCICEPTION

K.-D. KNIFFKI, S. MENSE and R. F. SCHMIDT

Physiologisches Institut der Universität Kiel, Olshausenstraße 40-60, 23 Kiel, Germany

In contrast to the great amount of experimental data that have been obtained in studies on cutaneous nociception only few information is at hand concerning pain arising from skeletal muscle. In the early investigations of Lewis et al. (11) it had been demonstrated that muscular pain can be elicited in man in a well reproducible manner by ischemic contractions, the accumulation of a "physico-chemical factor" being supposed to play a role in the induction of this type of muscle pain. Later, the existence of chemo-nociceptors in skeletal muscle has been proven by Guzman et al. (8) who were able to show that the injection of small amounts of pain-producing substances into a muscle artery induces pseudaffective reactions in animals comparable to those recorded during pain in man.

As to the types of afferent fibres involved in the mediation of muscular pain, Bessou and Laporte (2) reported that during ischemic contractions the unmyelinated muscle afferents exhibited an increased impulse activity. For the pain induced by injection of algesic agents into the splenic artery in dogs this was confirmed by Lim et al. (12) who found that unmyelinated (group IV) and thin myelinated (group III) fibres were activated by pain-producing substances. The above results were obtained from multifibre recordings from undissected nerves, therefore nothing could be said about the properties of individual chemo-nociceptors. The response characteristics of single muscle receptors with nociceptive properties have been described by Paintal (17) and Bessou and Laporte (3) in their studies on muscular group III afferent fibres. At about the same time Iggo (10) succeded in recording from single unmyelinated muscle afferents; his results demonstrated that group IV units from skeletal muscle can be activated by various types of painful stimuli. Thus it appears that, similar to the nociception from cutaneous areas, pain from skeletal muscle is mediated by afferent fibres belonging to the groups III and IV. As in the skin most or all of these fibres terminate as free nerve endings (18). The thin muscle afferents differ from the corresponding cutaneous units in that they probably fulfil an additional function, namely the induction of circulatory and respiratory reflexes during muscular work (13).

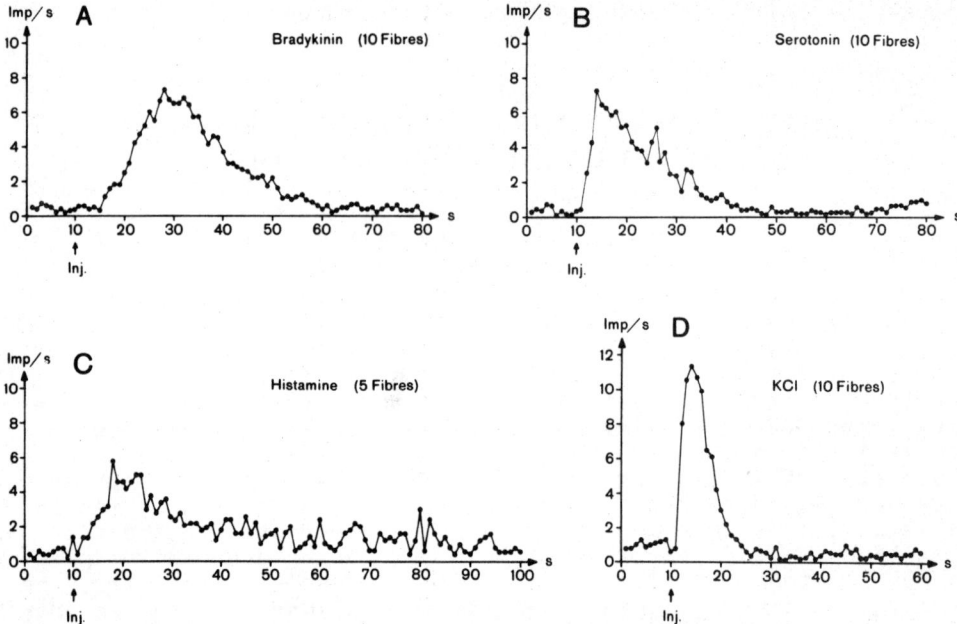

Fig. 1. Averaged responses of single group IV fibres to various pain-producing substances, injected intra-arterially. The doses administered were: bradykinin, 2.6 - 26 µg; 5-HT (serotonin), 67.5 - 135 µg; histamine, 180 µg; K^+, 1.9 - 5.9 mg (from Fock and Mense (6)).

In our studies we have tried to determine the properties of single muscle receptors with group IV afferent fibres in response to mechanical and chemical stimulation in the innocuous as well as in the noxious range. The experiments were performed on cats anaesthetized with chloralose, the muscle studied was the gastrocnemius-soleus (GS) muscle. The single fibre recordings were made from microdissected strands of the sciatic nerve or the corresponding dorsal rootlets.

Properties of group IV units. On mechanical stimulation of the muscle by locally applied innocuous and noxious pressure, most of the units (64 %) had high thresholds presumably in the painful range. Their responses were slowly adapting and showed fatigue when the high pressure stimulus was repeated at intervals of a few minutes (7). On chemical stimulation with intra-arterial injections of pain-producing substances (bradykinin, 5-hydroxytryptamine (5-HT), histamine and potassium ions) about half of the group IV units tested could be activated by quantities of the agents that are likely to be released from damaged tissues (6, 16). Bradykinin proved to be the most and potassium the least effective stimulant, the molar ratio of equi-effective doses being about 1 : 4000. Bradykinin differed from 5-HT and histamine in that its excitatory action showed no tachyphylaxis during repeated administrations.

In Fig. 1 the averaged responses of group IV afferent units from muscle to the above pain-producing substances are shown. Although equi-effective doses were administered (the number of impulses elicited by each chemical stimulus was about the same) certain differences between the effects of the substances existed. For instance the time course of the excitation induced by histamine differed remarkably from that of KCl. The former had a slowly rising and falling time course together with a long duration, whereas the latter was characterised by a shortlasting activation of relatively high frequency, followed by a phase of reduced activity. The differences in the excitatory action of the algesic agents used can only partly be explained by their differring molecular weights; evidence has been presented that separate pharmacological receptors for the substances might exist at the free nerve ending of group IV muscle afferents (9, 16). Similar suggestions have been made for cutaneous chemonociceptors (1).

TABLE I. MECHANICAL EXCITABILITY AND SENSITIVITY TO BRADYKININ OF GROUP IV AND GROUP III MUSCLE AFFERENTS

Excitability by mechanical stimulation	Number of units tested with bradykinin	Number of units excited by bradykinin
A) group IV muscle afferents		
HTP	114	51 (45 %)
LTP	6	4 (67 %)
Not excited	48	21 (44 %)
B) group III muscle afferents		
HTP	22	11 (50 %)
LTP	15	11 (73 %)
Not excited	4	1 (25 %)

Part A of this table is taken from Franz and Mense (7), part B from Mense (15).

Many of the units with a high threshold on mechanical stimulation could also be activated by the injection of bradykinin (table I A), i.e. these units had response characteristics of polymodal nociceptors and thus behaved in a way similar to certain cutaneous afferents (4). In some units, however, a sensitivity to bradykinin was associated with a low mechanical threshold lying clearly in the innocuous range (LTP units in table I).

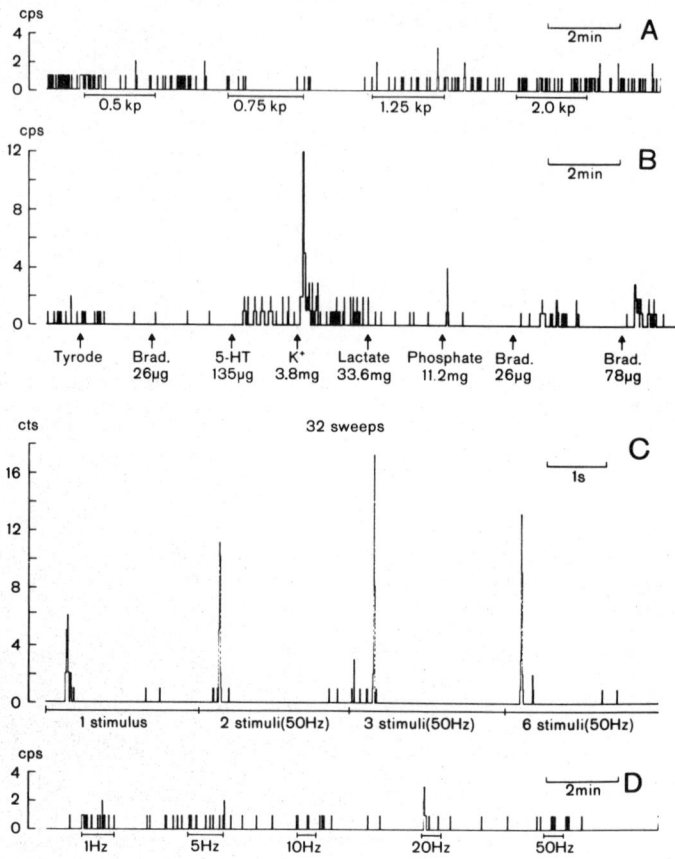

Fig. 2. Responses of a single group IV afferent unit from the GS muscle to different forms of stimulation. A: passive stretch. During the periods marked by horizontal bars, static stretch of the indicated strength was applied to the calcaneal tendon. B: intra-arterial injections of algesic agents and metabolic products. The doses indicated were administered by single injections, the volume injected was 0.3 ml for all substances. C: single contractions. At the beginning of each quarter of the histogram a single electrical stimulus or trains of stimuli with a strength of two times motor threshold were applied to the GS muscle nerve at a repetition rate of 1/2 s. The impulses evoked during 32 sweeps were summed up by a special purpose computer operated with a dwell time of 10 ms. D: tetanic contractions. During the periods marked by bars electrical stimulation of the GS muscle nerve with two times motor threshold and at the indicated frequency was performed (Kniffki, Mense, and Schmidt, unpublished).

In order to determine whether nociception as well as the circulatory and respiratory reflexes during muscle work are mediated by different populations of group IV muscle afferents, a study has been carried out in which both painful chemical and innocuous metabolic stimuli have been applied. The painful stimulation consisted in intra-arterial injections of pain-producing substances, as metabolic stimuli active contractions, passive stretch and the injection of metabolic products (lactate, phosphate) have been used. By these forms of stimulation it was possible to differentiate between three groups of GS muscle receptors with group IV afferent fibres: one responding exclusively to pain-producing substances, one responding exclusively to muscle contractions and/or stretch and a third one being activated by both chemical noxious stimulation and muscle contractions and/or stretch. While the units of the first group could serve as nociceptors, the second group could fulfil the function of metaboceptors. It has to be pointed out, however, that the magnitude of activation that could be induced in single group IV units by contractions or stretch was rather small so that the question arises whether these stimuli can be considered as adequate ones.

An example of a group IV unit belonging to the third group is given in Fig. 2. The unit could not be excited by passive stretch of up to 2 kp (A), but responded to intra-arterial injections of 5-HT, K^+ and bradykinin (B) as well as to active contractions of the gastrocnemius-soleus muscle (C, D). Fig. 2 C illustrates the result of four successive trials in which electrical stimuli in trains of different length have been delivered to the GS muscle nerve in order to induce single contractions of different force. After a latency period of 300 - 400 ms, measured from the beginning of the stimulation of the muscle nerve, afferent impulses arrived at the recording site (dorsal root L7).

By single injections of phosphate and lactate as shown in Fig. 2 B only a few group IV units could be activated. These units required a rather high dosage of the above ions to be excited, usually the concentration of the test solution had to be hypertonic to blood plasma. Therefore it is possible that the excitation was due to the hyperosmolarity of the phosphate and lactate solution irrespective of the type of ion injected.

Properties of group III units. The responsiveness of muscle receptors with group III afferent fibres to chemical noxious stimulation is quite similar to that of muscular group IV afferents (cf. Table I B). In addition, the qualitative features in the time course of excitation, some of which have been described above for group IV units, reappear in their responses (Fig. 3). Furthermore, the chemically induced excitation of group III afferents resembled that of group IV units in that their responses to bradykinin were not tachyphylactic (Fig. 3 D). Concerning their mechanical excitability a difference between group IV and group III muscle afferents exists, though. In both

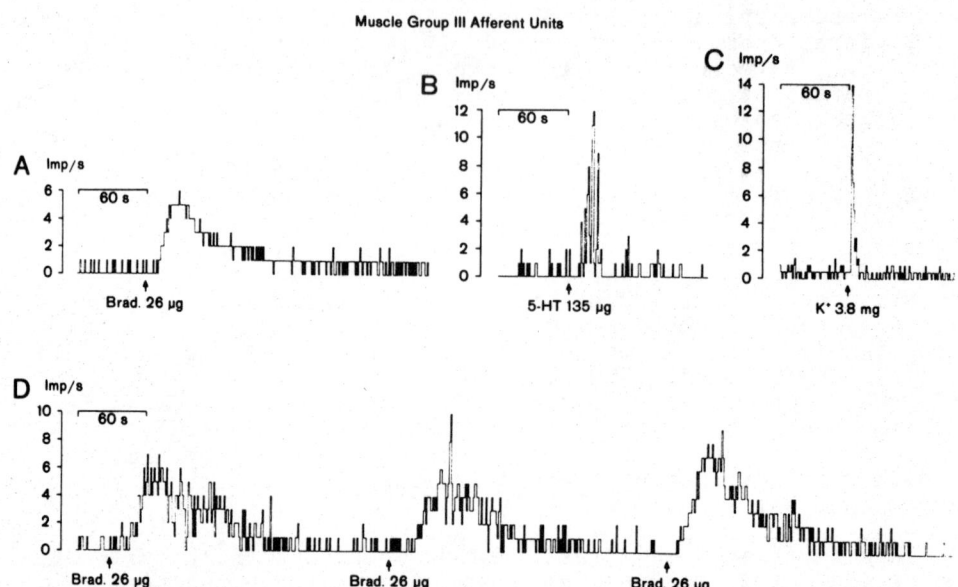

Fig. 3. Activation of four different (A-D) muscle group III afferent units by pain-producing substances. In A, B and C single intra-arterial injections of the respective agents were administered; in D the injection of bradykinin was repeated at intervals of 4 min in order to show that no tachyphylaxis is present in the responses to this substance. From Mense (15).

fibre types the units with high mechanical thresholds form the greatest group, yet among group III muscle afferents the proportion of units with low thresholds on mechanical stimulation (pressure or stretch) is much greater (35 % against 4 % in group IV units).

Total nervous outflow. As to the afferent activity elicited in a receptive region by noxious chemical stimulation, a difference exists between skeletal muscle and skin. From the studies of Fjällbrant and Iggo (5) and Beck and Handwerker (1) it is known that the injection of pain-producing substances into a skin artery activates not only unmyelinated and thin myelinated cutaneous afferents but also thick myelinated ones (group II units) that are connected to slowly adapting mechanoreceptors. Our results which were obtained with a similar technique and with similar doses of algesic agents indicate that in skeletal muscle only group IV and group III afferent units respond to intra-arterial injection of pain-producing substances, whereas group II and group I afferents are not excited (15).

Concluding remarks. From the above data it appears that, similar to cutaneous pain, the pain arising from skeletal muscle is mediated by group IV and group III afferent units. This view is supported by the recent finding (14) that the bradykinin-induced activation of group IV muscle afferents can be reduced by administration of the analgesic drug acetylsalicylic acid.

Since the application of pain-producing substances elicits an input to the central nervous system that is restricted to the group III and IV muscle afferents, this form of stimulation constitutes a useful tool for the study of the transmission and processing of nociceptive information in the nervous system. In this respect it is relevant that the algesic substances also evoke pain in man (for references see 6, 7). Thus the results obtained in mammals may give decisive clues to a more complete understanding of human pain and of its therapy.

This work has been supported by the Deutsche Forschungsgemeinschaft.

REFERENCES

1. Beck, P.W. and Handwerker, H.O.: Bradykinin and serotonin effects on various types of cutaneous nerve fibres. Pflügers Arch. 347, 209-222 (1974).
2. Bessou, P. et Laporte, Y.: Activation des fibres afférentes amyéliniques d'origine musculaire. C.R.Soc.Biol.(Paris) 152, 1587-1590 (1958).
3. Bessou, P. et Laporte, Y.: Étude des récepteurs musculaires innervés par les fibres afférentes du groupe III (fibres myelinisées fines) chez le chat. Arch.ital.Biol. 99, 293-321 (1961).
4. Bessou, P. and Perl, E.R.: Response of cutaneous sensory units with unmyelinated fibers to noxious stimuli. J. Neurophysiol. 32, 1025-1043 (1969).
5. Fjällbrant, N. and Iggo, A.: The effect of histamine, 5-hydroxytryptamine and acetylcholine on cutaneous afferent fibres. J. Physiol. (Lond.) 156, 578-590 (1961).
6. Fock, S. and Mense, S.: Excitatory effects of 5-hydroxytryptamine, histamine and potassium ions on muscular group IV afferent units: a comparison with bradykinin. Brain Res. (1976), in press.
7. Franz, M. and Mense, S.: Muscle receptors with group IV afferent fibres responding to application of bradykinin. Brain Res. 92, 369-383 (1975).
8. Guzman, F., Braun, C. and Lim, R.K.S.: Visceral pain and the pseudaffective response to intra-arterial injection of bradykinin and other algesic agents. Arch. int. Pharmacodyn. 136, 353-384 (1962).
9. Hiss, E. and Mense, S.: Evidence for the existence of different receptor sites for algesic agents at the endings of muscular group IV afferent units. Pflügers Arch. (1976), in press.

10. Iggo, A.: Non-myelinated afferent fibres from mammalian skeletal muscle. J. Physiol. (Lond.) 155, 52-53 P (1961).
11. Lewis, T., Pickering, G.W. and Rothschild, P.: Observations upon muscular pain in intermittent claudication. Heart 15, 359-383 (1931).
12. Lim, R.K.S., Guzman, F., Rodgers, D.W., Goto, K., Braun, C., Dickerson, G.D. and Engle, R.J.: Site of action of narcotic and non-narcotic analgesics determined by blocking bradykinin-evoked visceral pain. Arch. int. Pharmacodyn. 152, 25-58 (1964).
13. McCloskey, D.I. and Mitchell, J.H.: Reflex cardiovascular and respiratory responses originating in exercising muscle. J. Physiol. (Lond.) 224, 173-186 (1972).
14. Mense, S.: Pain-producing substances as stimulants for group IV afferent units from skeletal muscle. Proceedings of the First World Congress on Pain, Florence, 1975, Raven Press, New York, 1976 (submitted).
15. Mense, S.: Nervous outflow from skeletal muscle following chemical stimulation with pain-producing substances. (1976), in preparation.
16. Mense, S. and Schmidt, R.F.: Activation of group IV afferent units from muscle by algesic agents. Brain Res. 72, 305-310 (1974).
17. Paintal, A.S.: Functional analysis of group III afferent fibres of mammalian muscle. J. Physiol. (Lond.) 152, 250-270 (1960).
18. Stacey, M.J.: Free nerve endings in skeletal muscle of the cat. J. Anat. 105, 231-254 (1969).

Discussion:

Ingvar: Did you systematically explore the anoxia factor? It is well known that anoxia gives muscle pain in man. Also, stimulation (in man) with frequencies above 8 - 10/second gives rise to an increase of the intramuscular pressure which rises above the arterial pressure so that the blood flow is turned off (Nilsson and Ingvar, 1968). My second question concerns pH. Have you systematically altered the pH of the blood going to the muscle you are studying? And, furthermore, could it be that some of the solutions you have used exerted their action by their change of pH?

Schmidt: When we started this work, of course, in a kind of screening way, we did all kinds of stimulation you could think of. One in particular was that we cut off the blood supply to the muscle for a long time with and without contraction of the muscle. We got very, very few responses from these receptors. This was very discouraging. It was one of the many "downs" we had in this research. I have no definite answer to that. You have to go into that again. This was three years ago and our experience was, of course, much less. But from the first approach we did not get much and I think other people have had the same bad experience. Stopping the blood flow by itself and letting the muscle contract under these conditions which in man, of course, makes pain does not do much to these afferents, at least under the conditions we tried. This is an open question. I clearly have to admit this. Your other question is quite correct. The solution which we use here is quite acid. In the extreme you see the muscle shrink under the acid and then it might not excite the muscle. The pH question is also an unsettled one. We have not made precise measurements. But our philosophy in this is first in a screening way to find out where we get results and then to narrow down the conditions. Otherwise we would end up with quite a lot of hopeless testing.

Paintal: I would like to ask Dr Schmidt and others here whether it has been established that shutting off the arterial supply alone causes muscular pain. Of course checking both venous and arterial flows causes swelling and that leads to pain.

Schmidt: I have no answer for that.

Ingvar: This is just an extension to my previous comment. We did measure the blood flow of the muscle during various contractions. The pain appears when the blood flow is turned off by the contraction itself because the pressure inside the facia of that muscle in man increases so much that it goes above the arterial pressure.

Lindahl: I would like to put forth a very silly question. The language and the thoughts nociception, does that mean painful sensation or does that mean something that hurts? Then there is pain that does not hurt the tissue. I think we are talking about these things without any definite definitions.

Schmidt: Yes, I think you are quite right that we do not pay too much attention to these things. I think our point is purely pragmatic. We just take from the literature those substances which have been shown in man to evoke pain and which have been shown in animals by many peoples' very good work to evoke pseudo-affective responses.

Lindblom: As an answer to the question by Professor Paintal, I would remind you that nature has made that experiment many times. When you get an arterial thrombosis you certainly get immense pain.

Zotterman: I should recommend that you rupture a muscle and then stimulate the motor nerve and see what you get. Contracting a ruptured muscle causes a very awful pain and it takes 6 weeks to recover. You must make chronic experiments because most pain develops chronically.

Iggo: Algesic chemicals may not be specifically or exclusively nociceptive, so it is not sufficient simply to accept excitation by, say, bradykinin as proof of a nociceptive role. Second, you report the usual very short latency for a response to injection of potassium ions and longer latency to the algesic chemicals. Do you know whether your BK receptors etc. are in the terminals or the afferent fibers, or whether the algesic chemicals are acting indirectly? Third, we have not heard so far at this meeting of the ventral root C-afferent fibers reported by Willis and his colleagues. Do you think your muscle C-afferents may also enter via the ventral roots?

Schmidt: Thank you for the last question. Now I understand that there are three questions. The one is, do we stimulate afferents, do we stimulate the endings or do we stimulate anywhere in the course of the fibers. We have tried to test it in all possible ways you can think of by applying these substances directly on to the nerve or on the very end in the muscle. By applying the substances on the filaments which we dissected, where we have only a single active fiber and so on. In none of these conditions could we get any response from the substances.

Iggo: Did you act even further away than the end of the fibers so that you had something released by the chemical?

Schmidt: Yes, that is your second question. We have no answer to that. There is nothing in the literature which can help you except that these games which we play with the interaction of these desensitizations and tachiphylactic experiments. They still cannot all be explained. You can still work on the assumption that they work directly. We have no proof for or against this. But unless somebody comes up with an experiment which disproves this hypothesis, I think we can still stick to the simple hypothesis. In regard to the ventral root fibers I had, of course, long discussions with Bill Willis, the last time in Florence in September 1975, about these ventral root fibers and particularly whether he has any idea where they come from. All this evidence points at the moment to the idea that all these fibers are not coming from muscles and are not coming from skin but are coming from visceral structures. So we still might be on the safe side in this respect.

Perl: Dr Schmidt, I apologize but your description of background activity in unmyelinated afferent fibers from muscle prompted a comment and a question. As you know Bessou and I (unpublished) recorded from C-fibers of muscle. In contrast to your description, in one hundred C-fiber elements, we rarely (at most a few per cent) saw background discharge until damage to the muscle was produced. On another point, we did see responses to intraarterial injection of substances such as bradykinin in some elements but only at concentrations much greater than reported as effective in blister base experiments. In our experiments intraarterial injections were given when the blood supply to the muscle was blocked. The concentration of substances was specified as weight per colume; we found that bradykinin and acetylcholine were effective only at concentrations much higher than had been described as effective in blister base experiments: 10^{-4} or 10^{-5} grams per liter of bradykinin were necessary. Consequently, the question is on the actual concentration of the material you injected in the blood. Can you give an estimate?

Schmidt: With these injection experiments it is very difficult if not impossible to make any estimation of the actual concentration. We have some experience from methanol blue injections. After the methanol blue has gone further then the fiber starts to fire with 8.8 seconds delay as I mentioned. But when you look at the literature at the effective concentrations which are given in pathological states you come in the same order of magnitude of bradykinin for instance and also for serotonin values. I do not think we are too far off in the effective concentration at the endings from what might be possible concentration in pathologic tissue. But, as a matter of fact, I do not know whether the bradykinin has anything to do with muscle pain. Nobody knows.

Handwerker: It is very interesting that you found thermosensitive receptors in some of your fibers. Do you think the thermosensitivity is high enough to play a role in everyday life? Further, do you think these muscle thermoreceptors could play a role in thermoregulation?

Schmidt: Again the answer is that we do not know.

Handwerker: A definitely determined sensitivity is within the range of a few degrees Celcius. The peripheral muscles in the cat change their temperature over quite a considerable range in the times of life. The unfortunate thing is that the same effect with the same cooling and warming methods we also change or excite the background discharge of A- and C-fibers, particularly A-fibers. So again, this has to be worked out very carefully whether this has anything to do with the phenomenon. Now we have the common denominator for the metabolic steps. It is all temperature. But I think once again that it is not too sensitive.

SKIN RECEPTORS SUPPLIED BY UNMYELINATED (C) FIBRES IN MAN

H. E. TOREBJÖRK and R. G. HALLIN
Department of Clinical Neurophysiology, University Hospital, Uppsala, Sweden

Introduction.
It was recently shown that single C unit activity can be recorded with microelectrodes from intact cutaneous nerves in man (13). Afferent C units were identified, as were efferent C units of sympathetic origin (3). However, the identification of single unit potentials by means of shape and amplitude is hazardous, in part due to the low amplitudes of the C fibre signals which are often obscured by concomitant activity in myelinated (A) fibres. Therefore the human C unit samples so far presented are relatively small (4, 7, 11, 14, 16).

This paper deals with a new technique, which facilitates the identification and classification of single afferent and sympathetic C units in microelectrode recordings from intact human skin nerves (5). The technique was used to study the receptive properties of different types of afferent C units that responded to mechanical, chemical or thermal skin stimuli. Since the recordings were performed in alert subjects, the afferent C fibre activity could be correlated with perception.

Material.
Recordings were made from the radial, peroneal or saphenous nerves in 16 healthy males, aged 25-40 years. 112 afferent C units with conduction velocities ranging 0.4-1.8 m/s were studied. The receptive fields were situated in skin areas sparsely covered with hairs on the dorsum of the hand, on the lateral aspect of the calf and on the dorsum of the foot. 45 units could be identified by amplitude and shape in the original neurogram, as shown in Fig. 3, whereas the rest of the units were classified by a combination of electrical test shocks and physiological stimuli, as shown in Figs. 2 and 4.

The tests were performed in alert subject who volunteered for
these experiments, and deliberate damage of the skin was therefore avoided. This implies that the unit material is probably
biassed in favour of units of relatively low and medium thresholds compared with reported C unit samples from animal studies.

Methods.
The tungsten microelectrodes and the recording and display
systems have been described in detail elsewhere (2, 17), as have
the criteria for identification of afferent C units (14). The
stimulation procedures were similar to those reported previously
(16).

Classification of afferent and sympathetic C units in responses
to electrical stimulation in the skin.
Electrical stimulation was used to separate short latency A
fibre responses from late C fibre deflections. The electrical
shocks were delivered through needle electrodes inserted intra-
dermally close to each other in order to excite only a limited
number of nerve fibres at stimulus intensities that were well
tolerated by the subjects. Provided that the conduction distance was relatively long, the C fibre responses appeared as
separate unitary spikes due to temporal dispersion of impulses
in C fibres of slightly different conduction velocities. The
C unit potentials were converted into dots by Z-axis modulation,
and successive responses were displayed under each other in a
compact form, as illustrated in Fig. 1 (c.f. 15).

When the stimulation frequency was raised, an increase in latency of the C unit responses was observed (Fig. 1), probably due
to a frequency dependent slowing of impulse generation and transmission. When the stimulation frequency was lowered, a slow recovery occurred. With constant electrical stimulation of low
frequency (usually 0.3 Hz), only minor changes in latency of the
C unit responses were observed. If a C unit was then also activated by physiological stimuli, a slowing of conduction served

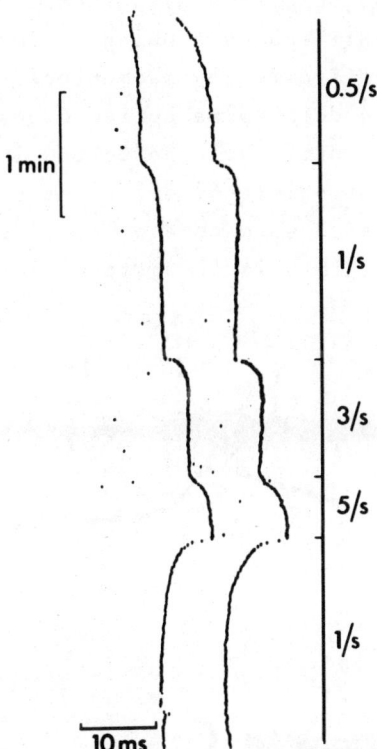

Fig. 1. Influence of electrical stimulation at constant intensity and varying frequency (indicated to the right) on the responses of two C units. The C unit potentials are represented as dots, and successive responses are displayed under each other. The recording was obtained from the radial nerve at the wrist. Conduction distance 14 cm. First 130 ms after stimulus artefacts omitted.
Note that each increase in stimulus frequency was followed by an increase in latency, and a decrease in stimulus frequency was accompanied by a decrease in latency (5).

as a sensitive index of increased firing in that particular unit.

Electrical stimulation in the skin excited not only afferent C fibres, but also induced antidromically conducted impulses in sympathetic postganglionic C fibres. Sympathetic units in the C response could be identified by the slowing of antidromic impulse conduction which resulted from repetitive firing during spontaneous or induced bursts of sympathetic discharges. Afferent C units were identified by slowing of impulse conduction as a consequence of activation by mechanical, chemical or thermal stimuli within defined receptive areas in the skin (5). In this way several C units could be tested in one recording site, even when the potentials of different units had similar amplitudes and interfered with each other in responses to physiological stimuli. This is illustrated in Fig. 2.

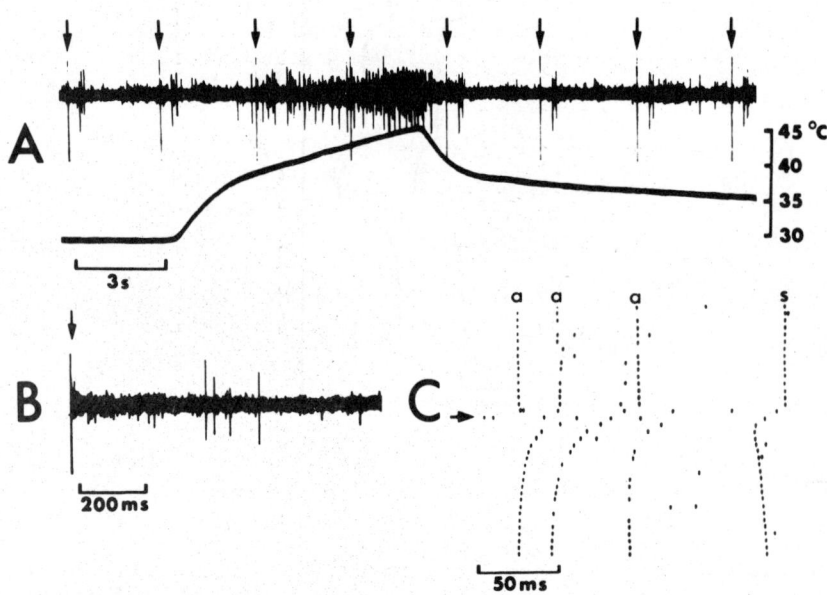

Fig. 2. Identification of physiologically activated C units in a multi-fibre recording from the peroneal nerve.
A: Upper trace shows neural responses to intradermal electrical stimulation every 3:rd s (vertical arrows indicate stimulus artefacts) and to an increase in skin temperature (indicated in lower trace).
B: Each electrical shock (vertical arrow) induced responses in four C units.
C: Compact dot display of successive C unit responses at an expanded time scale with the first 375 ms after stimulus artefacts omitted. The skin heating in A (indicated by horizontal arrow) caused a transient increase in latency of the responses in three units "a" and the reverse effect for one unit "s" (16).

It is difficult to judge from the original neurogram whether the skin heating in Fig. 2 A induced activity in A or C fibres, or if the neural activity could represent a sympathetic reflex response. An analysis of the responses to the electrical test shocks revealed that at least three C units were activated, since their conduction velocities decreased during heating (Fig. 3 C). A fourth C unit was probably not activated, the decrease in latency being due to a temperature-dependent increase in conduction velocity. The outcome of further tests established that the first three C units were afferent, with polymodal receptive properties, whereas the fourth C unit was of efferent sympathetic origin (16).

A slight influence of the electrical test shocks on the excitability of the C units could not be excluded even at stimulation frequencies as low as 0.3 Hz. The combination of electrical and physiological stimuli was therefore used only for identification and classification of different types of C units, and for a rough estimation of thresholds for different types of stimuli. For exact measurements of mechanical and thermal thresholds and for detailed studies of firing patterns, concomitant electrical stimulation was avoided.

Polymodal receptors.
Numerous afferent C units in human skin responded to a variety of mechanical, chemical and thermal stimuli. An example of this type of C unit is shown in Fig. 3. These units were not spontaneously active at normal skin temperatures and they were not activated by light touch stimuli. The thresholds for activation with von Frey hairs ranged 0.7-8.5 g. The receptive fields either were point-shaped or consisted of several spot-like receptive maxima separated by areas of relative insensitivity. A constant pressure with a nylon hair typically evoked a slowly adapting discharge (Fig. 3 B), sometimes followed by an afterdischarge. Stimuli of this type, which induced discharges at low frequency, were perceived at a latency of 1-2 s

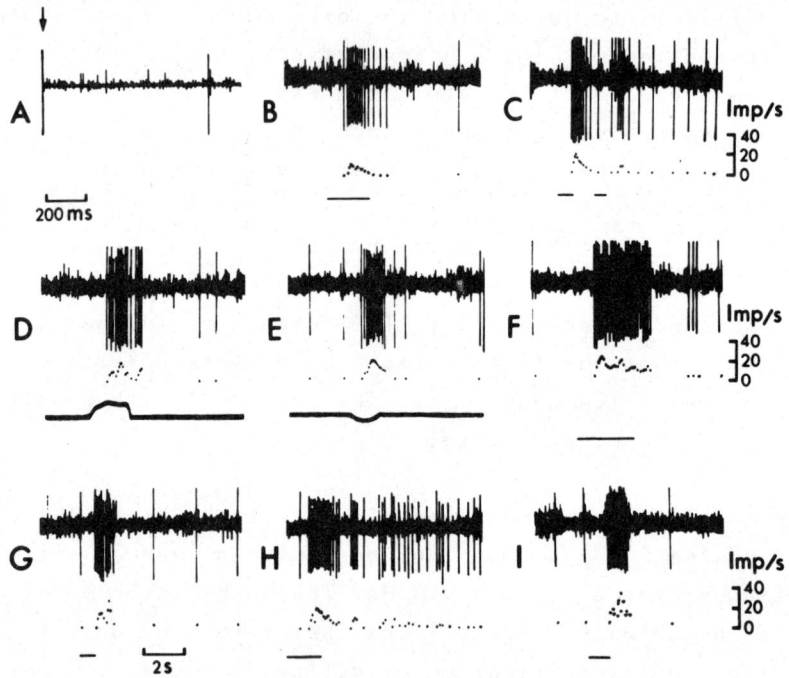

Fig. 3. Responses of an afferent C unit recorded in the peroneal nerve at knee level. Receptive area (3 x 3 mm) on the dorsum of the big toe. Conduction distance 51 cm. Conduction velocity 0.64 m/s. Various stimuli indicated by bars or deflections in a strain gauge signal under the records. "Instantaneous" discharge frequency indicated to the right.
A: Unit response to a single electrical shock in the receptive field.
B: Sustained pressure with von Frey hair, 2 g.
C: Repeated firm strokings with a small wooden stick.
D: Blunt pressure with a probe (contact area with skin 1 mm), 15 g.
E: Pointed pressure (contact area with skin 0.1 mm), 5 g.
F: Needle penetration through skin.
G: Burst induced after application of itch powder.
H: Activity induced after touching the skin with a nettle leaf.
I: Intense burst induced by touching skin with a hot match (16).

as a smarting pain sensation. Skin heating above 40–47°C was an efficient stimulus for most of the units. Cooling to about 20°C was generally an ineffective stimulus, whereas further cooling could induce sparse activity in some units. Irritant

skin stimuli, such as itch powder (Fig. 3 G) or nettle leaves
(Fig. 3 H) induced irregular bursts of impulses, accompanied
by sensations of itching pain. The C units were best activated
by intense stimuli, threatening to damage the skin, such as
skin pinches with a pair of forceps, needle pricks (Fig. 3 F),
and applications of a hot match to the skin (Fig. 3 I). Intense
responses were also induced by intradermal injections of potassium chloride, which were very painful.

Thus, these C units have similar receptive properties to the
"polymodal nociceptors" described in the cat and monkey (1, 12).
They respond rather nonspecifically to a variety of stimuli,
and the sensations aroused by the various impulse patterns of
these units are probably related not to the type of stimulus
but rather to the intensity of stimulation. Data supporting
this idea also emerged from controlled nerve compression block
experiments. When impulse transmission in A fibres was blocked,
and only C fibres were conducting (6), mechanical stimuli and
chemical irritants inducing moderate or high frequency activity
in the polymodal receptors were perceived as various intensities
of itching, smarting, stinging or burning pain. The perception
of pain when deprived of "normal" awareness of other stimulus
characteristics, such as exact location, size of skin area
involved, depth of stimulus in the skin and type of stimulus,
was rather uncomfortable.

Specific "warm" receptors.
Specific "warm" receptors supplied by C fibres have been described in the cat by Hensel, Iggo and Witt (8) and by Iriuchijima and Zotterman (10). Only a few receptors of a similar type
have so far been identified in man, indicating that they are
less numerous than the polymodal receptors. Fig. 4 illustrates
some differences in receptive properties between polymodal receptors and a specific "warm" receptor. In this radial nerve
recording several C units responded to the electrical skin
stimulation. The part of the C fibre response to be considered
(Fig. 4 A, bar) consisted of a group of C units with relatively

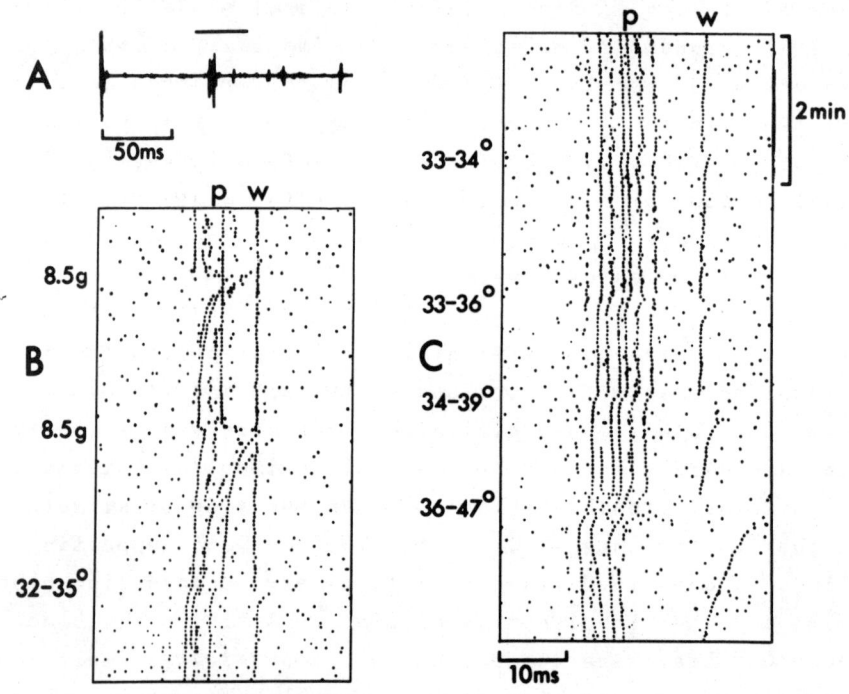

Fig. 4. Differentiation between polymodal receptors and a specific "warm" receptor supplied by C fibres. Recording from the radial nerve. Conduction distance 7.5 cm.
A: Electrical intradermal stimulation induced an extended C fibre response at a latency exceeding 75 ms. Successive dot-converted responses in the first part of the C response (bar) are shown at an expanded time scale in B and C.
B: Pressure with von Frey hair, 8.5 g, induced responses in the units marked "p" but not in the unit "w".
C: Moderate increases in skin temperature (indicated to the left) perceived as warmth excited the unit "w", and when the temperature was increased up to 47°C (perceived as heat), the units "p" were also activated.

large amplitudes, indicated by "p" in Fig. 4 B and C, followed by a unit of low amplitude, indicated by "w" in Fig. 4 B and C.

The first group of C units had polymodal receptive characteristics. They were not activated by mild cooling or slight touching of the skin. The thresholds for mechanical stimulation ranged 0.7-3.6 g. Responses were also elicited by application of itch powder to the skin. Moderate warming of the skin induced only temperature-dependent increases in the conduction velocities of these units (Fig. 4 C), but when the skin was heated up to 47°C, these temperature-dependent decreases in latencies were partly counteracted by increases in latencies indicating activation of the polymodal receptors (Fig. 4 C, bottom).

The unit "w" was not activated by mild cooling or application of itch powder to the skin. It could not be activated by relatively intense mechanical stimuli up to 8.5 g (Fig. 4 B), whereas small increases in temperature from 33 to 34° or more were sufficient to excite the unit (Fig. 4 C). From these observations it was concluded that this particular unit was a specific "warm" receptor. The conduction velocity was estimated to be 0.8 m/s.

A detailed analysis of the events occurring on raising the skin temperature from 36°C to 47°C revealed that the "warm" receptor was activated at the beginning of the temperature increase when the subject reported a sensation of warmth. The discharge frequency of the "warm" receptor increased with increase in temperature, and at about 45°C some polymodal receptors were also activated. The subject then reported a heat sensation, with a component of pain. In this experiment, similar neural events and reports of sensations were obtained on skin heating after compression block of A fibres.

It seems reasonable to assume that the sensation of warmth was induced by signals from specific "warm" receptors supplied by C fibres, and that the additional activation of polymodal receptors added to the painful heat sensation. The polymodal receptors have some characteristics in common with C "heat" receptors in the cat (9), and the distinction between these receptor groups may be only a matter of definition. We have as yet not been able to identify in man any specific receptors that are exclusively excited by high temperature. However, if there should exist such specific "heat" receptors in human skin, they might also contribute to the heat sensation.

Summary

The repeated activation of C fibres induces a frequency-dependent slowing of impulse conduction. This phenomenon has been used in a new method to identify physiologically activated C units in multifibre responses to electrical skin stimulation. Sympathetic C units can be differentiated from afferent C units, and different types of afferent C units can be classified, if appropriate manoeuvres and tests are performed concomitant with the electrical stimulation.

A large number of polymodal receptors supplied by C fibres have been identified in human non-glabrous skin. They respond to moderately intense mechanical stimuli, heat and chemical irritants. Stimuli, that efficiently activate these units, induce sensations related to pain. Specific "warm" receptors supplied by C fibres have also been identified. They respond to small and moderate increases in temperature, perceived as warmth.

Acknowledgements:

This investigation was supported by the Swedish Medical Research Council, Grant No B76-14X-02881-07B, Jörgen Schaumanns fond för dermatologisk forskning, Finsenstiftelsen, Tore Nilssons fond för medicinsk forskning and AB Förenade Liv, Stockholm.

References.

1. Bessou, P., and Perl, E.R. J. Neurophysiol., 32, 1025-1043, (1969).
2. Hagbarth, K.-E., Hongell, A., Hallin, R.G., and Torebjörk, H.E. Brain Res., 24, 423-442, (1970).
3. Hallin, R.G., and Torebjörk, H.E. Acta Soc. Med. Upsal., 75, 277-281, (1970).
4. Hallin, R.G., and Torebjörk, H.E. Acta physiol. scand., 92, 303-317, (1974 a).
5. Hallin, R.G., and Torebjörk, H.E. Acta physiol. scand., 92, 318-331, (1974 b).
6. Hallin, R.G., and Torebjörk, H.E. This volume.
7. van Hees, J., and Gybels, J.M. Brain Res., 48, 397-400, (1972).
8. Hensel, H., Iggo, A., and Witt, I. J. Physiol. (Lond.), 153, 113-126, (1960).
9. Iggo, A. Quart. J. exp. Physiol., 44, 362-370, (1959).
10. Iriuchijima, J., and Zotterman, Y. Acta physiol. scand., 49, 267-278, (1960).
11. Konietzny, F., and Hensel, H. Pflügers Arch., 359, 265-267, (1975).
12. Kumazawa, T., and Perl, E.R. Personal comunication.
13. Torebjörk, H.E., and Hallin, R.G. Acta Soc. Med. Upsal., 75, 81-84, (1970).
14. Torebjörk, H.E., and Hallin, R.G. Brain Res., 67, 387-403, (1974 a).
15. Torebjörk, H.E., and Hallin, R.G. J. Neurol. Neurosurg. Psychiat., 37, 653-664, (1974 b).
16. Torebjörk, H.E. Acta physiol. scand., 92, 374-390, (1974).
17. Vallbo, Å.B., and Hagbarth, K.-E. Exp. Neurol., 21, 270-289, (1968).

Discussion:

Paintal: I do not think reduction in conduction velocity has been seen following repeated stimulation at a slow rate. Your observations remind me of some rebound type of responses, that Dr L.C. Hunt showed me in 1956, somewhat like the late discharge in motorneurons. I wonder if you could block the rebound component with a peripheral anaesthetic block?

Torebjörk: A transient reduction in conduction velocity in nerve fibers following repeated activation has been described for instance by Gasser 1935, Tasaki 1953 and Franz and Iggo 1968. The increase in latency of the C unit responses to the repeated skin stimulation could be explained by a slowing of impulse conduction along the thin nerve fibers and perhaps also by a delay in action potential generation at the periphery. I do not think that the frequency dependent increases in latencies shown here could be explained by some rebound phenomenon.

Iggo: I think this is extremely exciting information that you are providing. Its particular value may be that you are now able to have the subject say, "well, it feels like this" and "it feels like that" while you are actually recording, because this has been the difficulty in all the animal studies.

You made a suggestion that one type of afferent fiber that responded to a variety of different stimuli may on some occasions lead to one sensation and on other occasions to a different sensation. I am not sure whether you really think this is the case or not. But it certainly seemed to be a conclusion that I could draw from what you were saying.

This kind of C fiber was first described with the responses to high temperatures and mechanical stimulation. At about the same time we were also looking at the sensitivity of the warm fibers. The warm fibers came in showing quite prominent activity at about 40°C. What we called at that time the "C-heat receptors" showed a much more striking activity when the temperature went up to about 45°. In your subjects there was a change in sensation between say the level of 40° and 45°. I wonder whether, in fact, these receptors which are responding to the high temperatures and may be excited by severe mechanical stimulation and by chemicals may not in some cases actually lead to a modification of the sensation of warmth without necessarily causing pain?

Torebjörk: The first question was whether different types of sensations could be induced by the activation of the polymodal receptors. Different subjects report their sensations in various ways when the polymodal receptors are excited by mechanical or chemical stimuli. Some speak of itching pain, others talk of stinging pain, others report burning pain. The common sensation seems to be some sort of pain, when these receptors are sufficiently activated. However, single impulses need not induce any sensation at all, and discharges at low frequency, for instance afterdischarges following a mechanical stimulus, merely induce poorly described aftersensations.

We do not know to what extent these receptors contribute to the sensation of increasing warmth, but it seems likely that they contribute to the painful component of the heat sensation. We have not been able to identify any receptors that are exclusively activated by high temperature. If such specific "heat" receptors should exist in man, they could possibly also contribute to the heat sensation, but at the present stage that question must be left open.

Iggo: If I could just come back on that. I think there certainly is varying confusion in the literature about these C receptors that can be excited by high temperatures. When I was recording in 1959 and earlier, the prominant feature of the response was that they could be excited by the high temperatures but they could also be excited by severe mechanical stimulation. I called them the C heat receptors because of this particular effect of the higher temperatures. Subsequently there have been many other recordings of, I think, almost certainly the same fibers. And there does seem now to be a bit of confusion to suggest that the ones described in 1959 are in effect different from those Perl has called "polymodal". I think that they are actually the same afferent fibers. Now, If we turn back again to this question of the response of the subject where you warmed the skin and then the temperature went higher and the subject reported pain or heat. Are you suggesting that at the low levels of intensity of activity in the warm fibers the subject has the sensation of warmth and then as you continue heating up, the higher frequency of firing in those fibers causes the heat? Or do you think, perhaps, that the change in the sensation to heat is associated with the additional input from these high temperature pain C fibers? I think that's really what I am getting at, whether you can relate the change in the quality of the sensation to the fact that you have now added in another fiber which may in other circumstances only cause pain.

Torebjörk: We have speculated a lot on that problem. The assumption that heat is induced by high frequency firing in specific "warm" receptors and an additional input from polymodal receptors is an attractive hypothesis, that fits with our experimental data, but until further experience is gained, we refrain from drawing any firm conclusions.

Landgren: My question concerns the interesting bundling of C fiber axons, which appears on the cross section of a nerve. 1) Do the different axons in one bundle take their origin from a common peripheral receptive area? 2) When you record a multiunit response do you believe that the units in this response are from one C fiber bundle? 3) Do you think there may be any "crosstalk" between C fiber axons in a bundle?

Torebjörk: We have no evidence of "crosstalk" between individual C units as they appear in our recordings. If "the single unit impulses" actually represent activity in single unmyelinated fibers or an extreme co-activation of a number of C fibers enclosed within a Schwann cell we cannot decide because we have not actually made recordings from dissected nerves to respond to that question. Other workers including Dr Iggo have also speculated on this problem. Most people agree that it would be unlikely that different unmyelinated fibers within a Schwann cell should act in such a synchrony. Several workers believe that they act as individual lines to the central nervous system.

Landgren: What about a common origin?

Torebjörk: This is also very difficult to decide because we do not see where the intraneural electrode tip is located with regard to the Schwann cells containing the unmyelinated fibers. Several C units in one recording site may have similar receptive characteristics, and their receptive fields may be clustered within a small area in the skin. This might perhaps indicate recording from several fibers within one Schwann cell. In other recording sites activity may be obtained from different types of afferent C units or from afferent and sympathetic C units, possibly indicating that the signals originate from several Schwann cell systems. The number of C units identified in one recording site is sometimes so high, that the C unit activity must derive from fibers in several Schwann cell systems.

Hagbarth: You have emphasized the desensitization of the C fibers especially when you excite them electrically. You see the increase in latency until they finally block. Yesterday we heard about the sensitization of the C fiber afferents by Perl when he excites them by heat. Have you also noticed any sensitization of the type described yesterday?

Torebjörk: We have never seen any sensitization of C receptors, possibly because we do not use such strong stimuli which are necessary to produce the sensitization.

PRELIMINARY OBSERVATIONS ON THE PATHO-PHYSIOLOGY OF HYPERALGESIA IN THE CAUSALGIC PAIN SYNDROME

G. WALLIN, E. TOREBJORK and R. HALLIN

Department of Clinical Neurophysiology, University Hospital, Uppsala, Sweden

Introduction.
Causalgia is a chronic pain syndrome which sometimes develops after damage to peripheral nerves and which is characterized always by: a) spontaneous burning pain, b) hyperalgesia and commonly by c) autonomic symptoms such as vasomotor changes or increased sweating within the causalgic region. Both the pain and the hyperalgesia often extend far beyond the area of the original lesion. Since the thirties it has been known that sympathectomy relieves the pain of causalgia and Bonica (1) includes, in addition to the main symptoms, temporary pain relief by a sympathetic block as a necessary criterion for the diagnosis. Several theories have been advanced to explain the aetiology of the syndrome but none has been widely accepted (for reviews see Trostdorf (15) and Noordenbos (12)).

During the last year we have studied hyperalgesia in a small group of causalgic patients with special emphasis on the following questions: 1) What is the link between the sympathetic nervous system and the hyperalgesia? 2) Which peripheral afferent nerve fibres contribute to the sensation of hyperalgesia?

Material and methods.
There were 4 patients, 2 males and 2 females, 25-50 years of age. At the time of investigation they had suffered from causalgia for 3-10 years. In the males the causalgia developed after crush injuries to the right foot in one case and the right hand in the other. In one female causalgia occurred in the left half of the chest after mastectomy with axillary dissection. The other female developed causalgia twice, the first time in the left hand and forearm after surgical damage to the lateral cutaneous nerve of the forearm, and the second time in the left shoulder following the sympathectomy that relieved the pain in

her hand and forearm. All had spontaneous burning pain and pronounced hyperalgesia but only minor autonomic symptoms. Sympathetic blocks relieved the pain and the hyperalgesia temporarily in all 4 patients. Control subjects were 15 healthy hospital employees, 22-40 years of age, and one patient who had undergone sympathectomy for hyperhidrosis but who had never had causalgic pain.

<u>Nerve recordings</u>. Nerve action potentials were recorded with tungsten micro-electrodes in the radial nerve at the wrist in one subject and in the peroneal nerve at the fibular head in another. Details of the micro-electrodes, the recording technique and storage and display systems have been described earlier (5). In short the micro-electrodes were inserted manually through the intact skin into the underlying nerve in which a skin fascicle innervating the desired skin area was located. Minute electrode adjustments were made until C fibre activity was found. The procedure of identifying sympathetic or afferent C fibre activity has been described in detail previously (6, 7). In suitable recording sites the C fibre activity was then monitored while hyperalgesia was either induced by intracutaneous application of noradrenaline or relieved by transcutaneous nerve stimulation.

<u>Application of noradrenaline and adrenaline</u>. Noradrenaline was applied to the skin of all patients and normal subjects either by iontophoresis of noradrenaline 0.2 mg/ml in a circular area of 2 cm^2 with a DC-current of 1-2 mA for 2 minutes (10) or by intracutaneous injection of noradrenaline 3-5 µg. Following the application the sensitivity to touch was tested qualitatively for at least one hour. In three experiments adrenaline was substituted for noradrenaline. Doses and modes of application of adrenaline were the same as for noradrenaline.

<u>Transcutaneous nerve stimulation</u> (TNS) was performed with 0.1 msec electrical pulses at frequencies between 15-100 c/sec using surface electrodes placed over the nerve supplying the hyperalgesic area. The stimulation voltage was adjusted individually until the patient felt moderate pain during the initial part of the stimulation. TNS effectively relieved the causalgic

pain and hyperalgesia for one to several days in three of the patients whereas the effect lasted only a few minutes in the fourth.

Nerve blocks. In one patient, in whom hyperalgesia could be induced by the application of noradrenaline to the dorsum of the hand, the superficial branch of the radial nerve supplying this area was blocked on several occasions by prolonged pressure. The pressure block was produced by a 2 cm wide inelastic band which was put across the wrist proximal to the hyperalgesic zone and loaded by approximately 6 kg. The sensitivity to touch, temperature and pain was continuously monitored in a qualitative way.

Results.
1) What is the link between the sympathetic nervous system and the hyperalgesia?
One possible reason for the beneficial effect of sympathectomy in causalgia is that the causalgic pain and hyperalgesia are in some way caused by abnormal sympathetic activity which is removed by the operation. Another possibility is that the sympathetic outflow is normal but that some skin receptors react abnormally to the presence of the sympathetic transmitter substance in the skin. To clarify this issue two pilot experiments were made in a patient with causalgia in whom a lumbar sympathectomy was planned because of the pain. The first experiment was made before the operation and was a micro-electrode recording of the sympathetic outflow to the causalgic skin in the right foot. The second experiment was made 11 days after the sympathectomy (which relieved the pain and hyperalgesia) and involved iontophoretic application of noradrenaline to the same skin area.

a) Recording of sympathetic activity. The result of the nerve recording is illustrated in figure 1. In short, the multiunit sympathetic activity had qualitatively normal characteristics, both at rest and in response to arousal stimuli and mental stress which are known to increase cutaneous sympathetic activity in normal subjects (3). Furhtermore, no apparent change

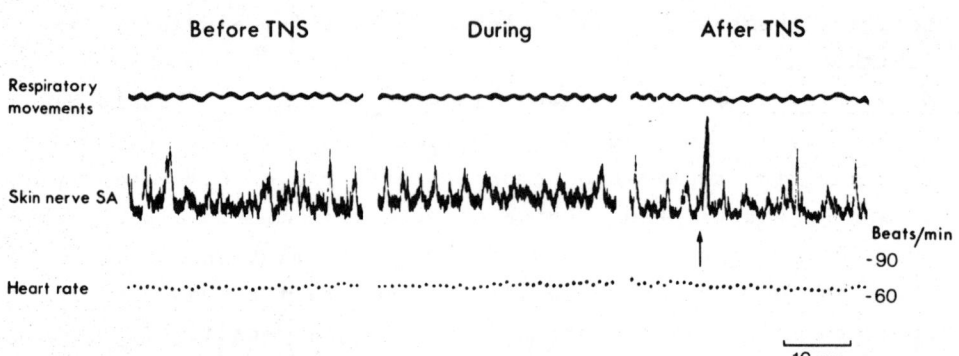

Fig. 1. Spontaneous multiunit sympathetic activity recorded in peroneal skin nerve fascicle of patient with causalgia involving the innervation zone of the impaled fascicle. Left records obtained when patient had spontaneous pain and hyperalgesia, middle records during TNS at 15/sec applied to the peroneal nerve above the ankle and right records after TNS when pain and hyperalgesia were eliminated. Arrow in the right part of the figure indicates application of tactile stimulus to the causalgic skin perceived as normal touch. Nerve record displayed as integrated activity (time constant 0.1 sec).

in the strength of the sympathetic activity occurred during or after TNS at 15 c/s which temporarily relieved both the spontaneous pain and the hyperalgesia. Although this type of multiunit recording does not provide conclusive evidence, it certainly did not suggest a direct relationship between the strength of the sympathetic outflow and the causalgic symptoms.

b) <u>Application of noradrenaline to the skin</u>. In contrast to this negative result the outcome of the second experiment was positive. Immediately after the application of noradrenaline to the previously causalgic skin area, the skin became pale and skin temperature dropped by 3-4°C. The temperature soon increased again and approached control values within 5-7 minutes whereas the pallor persisted longer. During this period light touch stimuli were perceived as normal but about 30 minutes after noradrenaline application did signs of hyperalgesia develop. The intensity of the hyperalgesia increased rapidly, and, as illustrated in figure 2, the size of the hyperalgesic zone also increased until it comprised an area approximately

10 times as large as the area originally infiltrated with noradrenaline.

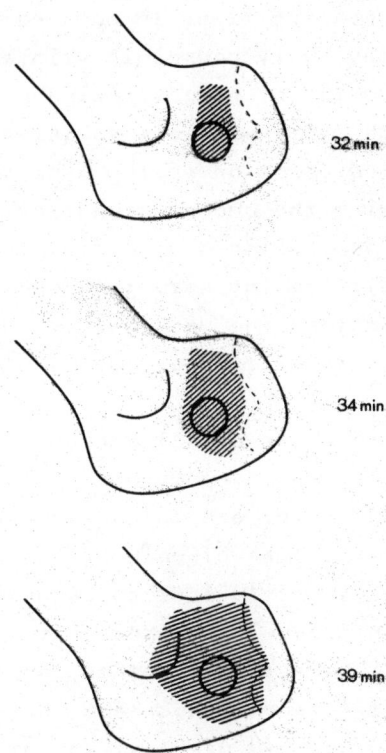

Fig. 2. Development of hyperalgesic zone (indicated by hatched area) after iontophoretic application of noradrenaline, 0.2 mg/ml to a 2 cm² area (indicated by solid circle) in a cuasalgic patient who underwent sympathectomy 11 days prior to the experiment. Hyperalgesia was first noted 30 minutes after application of noradrenaline. Same patient as in figure 1.

When the hyperalgesia was maximal the patient also felt some spontaneous pain and he reported that the symptoms were of exactly the same character as before the sympathectomy. After about 1 hour the hyperalgesia started to decrease and the sensation of touch returned to normal after 1 hour 45 minutes. Iontophoretic application of noradrenaline outside the previously causalgic skin had no hyperalgesic effect.

c) <u>Noradrenaline application in other causalgic patients</u>. Similiar experiments with similiar outcome were performed 30 times in another patient whose causalgic pain in the left hand and forearm had been relieved by cervical sympathectomy 2 years before the present investigation. In this case the hyperalgesia also developed in previously causalgic skin areas about 30 minutes after the application of noradrenaline and disappeared after $1\frac{1}{2}$-$2\frac{1}{2}$ hours. Although there was some variation from time to time the intensity and duration of the hyperalgesic reaction seemed to increase with the amount of noradrenaline applied and it could always be abolished by a few minutes of TNS. If adrenaline was substituted for noradrenaline hyperalgesia did not occur and if noradrenaline was applied to skin outside the previously causalgic area hyperalgesia did not develop.

Noradrenaline was also applied in two causalgic patients who had not been subjected to sympathectomy but who were able to relieve their hyperalgesia for one to many days by TNS. In a situation when they were free of pain and hyperalgesia noradrenaline, 3 µg, was injected intracutaneously into the causalgic skin. Both patients developed transient hyperalgesia in large skin areas in a manner similiar to the sympathectomized patients, the only difference being that the latency before the onset of hyperalgesia was 2-3 minutes. In both cases the intensity of the hyperalgesia was pronounced. Interestingly, both of them also developed transient hyperalgesia when noradrenaline, 3 µg, was injected in some other skin areas in which they had never had causalgic symptoms.

d) <u>Control injections</u> of noradrenaline, 3-5 µg, were made intracutaneously in 15 normal subjects and one patient who had undergone sympathectomy for hyperhidrosis but who had nerver suffered causalgia. Following the injections, some of these control subjects had slightly impaired perception of touch within the pale area that developed after the injection. In none did hyperalgesia occur.

2) **Which afferent nerve fibre groups contribute to the hyperalgesia?**

a) **Differential pressure blocks.** To elucidate which type of afferent nerve fibres contribute to the sensation of hyperalgesia the sympathectomized patient who had suffered causalgia in her left hand and forearm was used as experimental subject. Hyperalgesia was induced by intracutaneous injections of noradrenaline, 3 μg, into a skin area on the dorsum of the hand innervated by the superficial cutaneous branch of the radial nerve. When the first signs of hyperalgesia were perceived, firm pressure was applied over the nerve at the wrist proximal to the hyperalgesic area. After about 30 minutes the hyperalgesia started to diminish, first distally and then more proximally. Skin sensitivity was tested continuously and when the hyperalgesia was totally abolished the sensations of touch and cold were no longer perceived, whereas the patient still felt warmth and delayed pain. When the pressure was removed the hyperalgesia returned within 1-2 minutes, at about the same time as the perception of touch and cold. The same experiment was repeated seven times with similiar results.

b) **Nerve recordings.** To try to identify the fibres relaying the sensation of hyperalgesia microelectrode recordings were made in the same patient on four occasions in the superficial radial nerve at the wrist before and during noradrenaline-induced hyperalgesia. Multiunit responses evoked by tactile stimuli or by intracutaneous electrical stimulation of receptors supplied by myelinated fibres were not significantly different whether hyperalgesia was present or not. One afferent C unit with a conduction velocity of 0.8 m/s was identified. It responded to pressure stimulation with von Frey hairs from 0.7 g and greater. Some examples of the responses of the C-unit to pressure with illustrated in figure 3. The statistical analysis of the responses of this unit before, during and after hyperalgesia showed no significant differences.

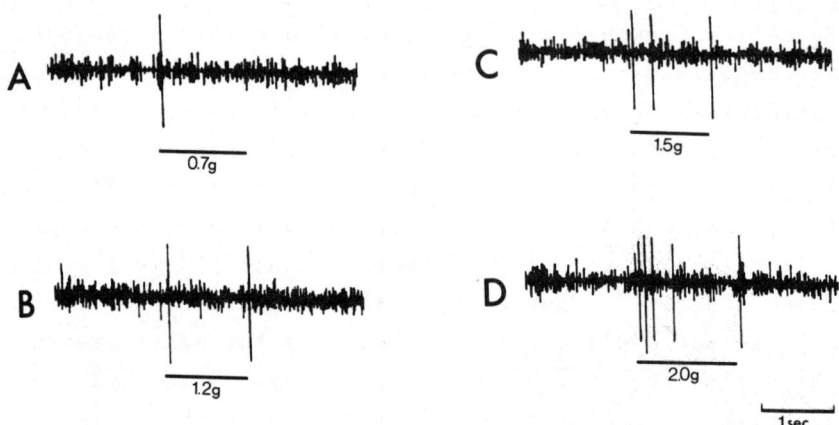

Fig. 3. Examples of single afferent C unit responses to pressure with different von Frey hairs in asymptomatic causalgic patient described in text. Horizontal bars indicate periods of mechanical stimulation with von Frey hairs at the indicated intensities. Responses were unchanged after induction of hyperalgesia by noradrenaline. Nerve recording from superficial branch of the left radial nerve.

Discussion.

Since our present material comprises only four patients, some of whom have been incompletely investigated, firm conclusions cannot be drawn. However, the fact that local application of noradrenaline to the skin of all patients, when temporarily asymptomatic, caused a transient reappearance of hyperalgesia is probably of pathophysiological significance. A possible explanation for the finding is that the presence of sufficient concentrations of noradrenaline in the skin of these patients alters the excitability of certain cutaneous receptors so that light touch stimuli are perceived as painful. Such a peripheral mechanism would explain the beneficial effect of sympathectomy in causalgia since after the operation the liberation of noradrenaline in the skin is greatly reduced. However, it does not exclude the possibility that in addition central mechanisms are involved in the production of the causalgic symptoms. It should be mentioned that causalgic skin may also be hypersensitive to more traditional "algogenic" substances. Störring and Schorre (13) reported this for histamine and in two of three patients tested we found prostaglandine E_1 to give greater hyperalgesia in previously causalgic skin than in "non-causalgic" control areas (unpublished results).

Even if an abnormal skin receptor sensitivity to noradrenaline can be verified in a larger material of causalgic patients the strength of the sympathetic outflow to the skin may still play a major role in eliciting and maintaining the symptoms. Since causalgic patients are in a more or less constant stress situation because of the pain, and since mental stress is known to increase skin nerve sympathetic activity (3) their sympathetic outflow to the skin may well be stronger than it would be in a painfree state. In addition it cannot be excluded that during the course of the disease segmental sympathetic reflexes are brought into action thus aggravating the pain. Such a localized increase of the sympathetic outflow would not have been detected in the sympathetic recording made in one of our causalgic patients but possibly would have been revealed by a simultaneous recording from the non-causalgic extremity.

In the pressure blocks the noradrenaline induced hyperalgesia was abolished when the subject had lost the perception of touch and cold but still felt warmth and delayed pain. Since prolonged pressure preferentially blocks myelinated A-fibres conveying sensations of touch and cold well before C-fibres transmitting warmth and delayed pain (4, 8, 11) these experiments suggest that the sensation of hyperalgesia was dependent upon impulse transmission in myelinated A-fibres. This conclusion is supported by the unchanged firing characteristics of the single C-unit studied in one experiment. From the present data it could not be decided which fibre type within the A-spectrum supplies the noradrenaline sensitive endings. To judge from the similiarity between afferent multiunit responses to tactile stimuli with and without the presence of hyperalgesia there does not appear to be a generalized change in receptor sensitivity. According to the literature fibres within the A δ range are known to mediate painful sensations (2, 9, 14) and it is possible that activity in these fibres contribute to the noradrenaline induced hyperalgesia.

Supported by Swedish Medical Research Council Grant No. B76-14X-03546-05, Grant No. B76-14X-02881-07B, Jörgen Schaumanns fond för dermatologisk forskning, Finsenstiftelsen, Tore Nilssons fond för medicinsk forskning and AB Förenade Liv, Stockholm.

References.

1. Bonica, J.J. The Management of Pain. Lea and Febiger, Philadelphia (1954).
2. Collins, W.F., Nulsen, F.E. and Randt, C.T. Arch. Neurol. 3, 381-385, (1960).
3. Delius, W., Hagbarth, K-E., Hongell, A. and Wallin, B.G. Acta physiol. scand. 84, 177-186, (1972).
4. Gasser, H.S. and Erlanger, J. Am. J. Physiol. 88, 581-591, (1929).
5. Hagbarth, K-E., Hongell, A., Hallin. R.G. and Torebjörk, H.E. Brain Res. 24, 423-442, (1970).
6. Hagbarth, K-E., Hallin, R.G., Hongell, A., Torebjörk, H.E. and Wallin, B.G. Acta physiol. scand. 84, 164-176, (1972).
7. Hallin, R.G. and Torebjörk, H.E. Acta soc. Med. Upsal. 75, 277-281, (1970).
8. Hallin, R.G. and Torebjörk, H.E. This volume.
9. Heinbecker, P., Bishop, G.H. and O'Leary, J.L. Arch. Neurol. Psychiat. 29, 771-789, (1933).
10. Juhlin, L. J. Invest. Derm. 37, 201-205, (1961).
11. Mackenzie, R.A., Burke, D., Skuse, N.F. and Lethlean, A.K. J. Neurol. Neurosurg. Psychiat. 38, 865-873, (1975).
12. Nordenboos, W. Pain, Elsevier Publ. Co. Amsterdam, (1959).
13. Störring, E. and Schorre, E. Dtsch. Zschr. Nervenheilk, 155, 99-126, (1943).
14. Torebjörk, H.E. and Hallin, R.G. Exp. Brain Res. 16, 321-332, (1973).
15. Trostdorf, E. Die Kausalgie. Georg Thieme Verlag, Stuttgart (1956).

Discussion:

Zimmermann: Normally the origin of causalgia is thought to be at the site of the nerve lesion, for example, in the gunshot wound or something similar. You test hyperalgesia peripheral to the nerve lesion where causalgia probably does not originate. Therefore, my question is whether you have tested other substances than noradrenaline. I would expect that other substances: chemical algogenics and subalgenic concentrations of algogenic substances could also produce hyperalgesia. I would, therefore, suggest that your hyperalgesia results from some central summation or facilitation of impulses originating at the site of the nerve lesion and from impulses coming from the peripheral territory in other nerve fibers. Perhaps you tested that?

Wallin: The causalgic pain syndrome is of course initiated by a defined nerve lesion but it is a common experience that both the pain and the hyperalgesia often occur in much larger areas than can be explained on the basis of the lesion. With regard to the question of algogenic substances Störring and Schorre found histamine to increase causalgic pain. In three of our four patients we tested the effect of intracutaneous injections of prostaglandine E_1, which causes hyperalgesia in normal subjects. Two patients got more pronounced hyperalgesia from prostaglandine in causalgic skin than on the contralateral normal side whereas there was no difference between the two sides in the third. The interpretation of these results is not clear but since causalgic skin is very sensitive to mechanical irritation it is perhaps not surprising that it may overreact to chemical irritants too. The significance of our results is that local application of noradrenaline (which is not an algogenic substance in normals) to a skin area deprived of its "physiological noradrenaline supply" by sympathectomy led to a transient return of hyperalgesia. We suggest that the effect is due to a change in the afferent inflow from certain skin receptors provoked by noradrenaline but we do of course not exclude the possibility that in addition central mechanisms operate in causalgia.

Hagbarth: I think it is very important that we make a very clear distinction between the pain as such, the spontaneous pain of these patients and the hyperalgesia that they have. This study only involves the hyperalgesia, the hypersensitivity to light touch. As you said, the pain, for instance, might originate from the nerve lesion, perhaps, to a certain extent. But I find it rather difficult to think that the hyperalgesia studied here could be initiated from the nerve stump, if that is what you meant.

Zimmermann: Yes, because it is known that in the spinal cord there is some spacial summation. If you have a site of chronic input, for example a nerve lesion, of chronic input of ongoing impulses and then you have another afferent line coming from the skin ending on the same neuron which was sensitized by your neuron, that could be a mechanism. Therefore, I would expect that noradrenaline plays a role in the production of causalgia. I would assume or suspect that it would be most effective at the site of the nerve lesion and not at the periphery.

Lindblom: You mentioned that large fiber stimulation is not known to cause pain. It is, however, in pathological conditions at least one such situation in which it is proven to exist and that is in trigeminal neuralgia. Kugelberg and I were able to show a few years ago that limited low threshold stimulation of the mechano-receptors in the skin around the face in the triggerzones was possible to precipitate the effects and in fact, nociceptive stimulation which we know activates the C-fibers was ineffective in eliciting the pain attacks. Of course, the lesion in the patient with causalgia is at the peripheral side. But it is possible that an ephaptic mechanism or what it might be could be responsible for the hyperalgesia produced by tactile stimulation. It probably was in these cases. What do you think about that?

Wallin: With regard to trigeminal neuralgia I suppose you triggered pain attacks by skin stimulation. I do not think that means that the sensation of pain was conveyed in mechanoreceptive fibers.

Hensel: You mentioned that mechanical sensations, cold sensation and hyperalgesia were abolished after pressure block. Do you have any quantitative data concerning the differential behaviour of mechanical, cold and warm sensation following pressure block?

Wallin: The test procedures used during the pressure blocks were not quantitative enough to perimit definite conclusions but we have the impression that it was not until the cold sensation was blocked that the hyperalgesia disappeared.

Zotterman: My own experience about pressure block that I did on myself is that conduction of the large fibers, the touch and pressure disappear after, say, twenty minutes. Then there is a period when you have the first pain reactions before the delta fibers are blocked. Then comes the blocking of them and you have only the C-fiber delayed pain. That delayed pain has a more nasty irradiating character.

Santini: I wonder whether you could trigger a causalgia with the Valsalva. Secondly, I wonder if you have thought of the possibility of the reverse of the chemosensitivity of the receptors which presumably trigger the causalgic syndrome.

Wallin: It is well known that causalgic pain tends to be aggravated by manoeuvres which increase the sympathetic outflow to the skin. We have not tested the effect of Valvalva´s manoeuvre since this manoeuvre increases sympathetic outflow to the muscles but not to the skin. With regard to the second part of the question the only thing we have done along those lines was to pretreat the skin with an alfa-receptor blocking drug before applying noradrenaline. In those cases hyperalgesia did not develop.

Hallin: I would like to add something to Dr Hensel´s comments concerning these pressure blocks. As I told you the other day that perceptual events progressed from the periphery centrally. And It was quite striking when we tested this particular patient that she could have her cold sensation and hyperalgesia abolished in an area peripherially but still have it in a proximal area.

Lindahl: I want to point out another possible explanation for these experiments. If you inject noradrenaline into the skin you will produce an acidosis. It is well known that acidosis in other clinical situations will produce hyperalgesia and tenderness.

Wallin: We have thought about this. However, an acidosis would occur both in normal subjects and patients, whereas hyperalgesia was induced by noradrenaline only in the patients.

Lindahl: But this patient had bad circulation from the beginning.

Wallin: This did not apply to the two patients in whom hyperalgesia was produced in skin areas in which they had never suffered nerve damage or causalgic pain.

Zimmermann: Your last comment is in favour of some central summation phenomenon of hyperalgesia. My question is, how did you measure hyperalgesia? I did not understand whether you made some comments on that. Was it quantitative psychophysical measurements or was it mere suggestive verbal communication with the patients.

Wallin: It was not quantitative. However, I would not characterize it a suggestive verbal communication with the patient. These patients had all been relieved from rather severe causalgia and when similar symptoms came back they had no difficulty in recognizing them. The noradrenaline induced hyperalgesia was usually strong enough to cause withdrawal reactions and the experience was in fact quite frightening to the patients.

Gordon: Could I try to clear my mind on one simple point? In the patients you have investigated could you attribute the symptoms to damage to one single nerve? And if so, was it possible to abolish all symptoms as Professor Zimmermann suggested, by anaesthetizing the site of injury?

Wallin: Yes, in all the patients nerve blocks were performed prior to the noradrenaline application: When the nerve (s) innervating the causalgic region was anaesthethized the pain disappeared.

Handwerker: I would like to comment not so much to the interesting contribution of Dr Wallin, but to the question of Dr Lindahl. When I applied noradrenaline close arterially in experiments very similar to those which I reported yesterday, I always found a decrease in the responsiveness of C-heat receptors to controlled radiant heat stimuli. This effect might be due to circulatory changes. I think this finding speaks against the unifying hypothesis of Dr Lindahl.

Wallin: This agrees with our findings on normal subjects in whom we tested the receptive threshold after noradrenaline application. As a rule the threshold to touch with von Frey's hairs showed a slight increase in the area treated with noradrenaline.

SINGLE AFFERENT C FIBER ACTIVITY IN THE HUMAN NERVE DURING PAINFUL AND NON PAINFUL SKIN STIMULATION WITH RADIANT HEAT

J. VAN HEES

Department of Neurology and Neurosurgery, University of Leuven, B-3000 Leuven, Belgium

The great majority of unmyelinated afferent fibers in the human cutaneous nerve belongs to the polymodal nociceptor type (3) (4). Only recently human C warm fibers are described (2). So far the studies of human nociceptive C fibers are limited to a rather qualitative description of their response to various stimuli, a consequence of technical difficulties. In the cat it is clearly demonstrated that the discharges in 'C heat receptors' are linearly related to the level of skin temperature and their thresholds were brought into relation with the human pain threshold for radiant heat (1).

Up to now we were able to make a quantitative analysis of single fiber activity in 5 polymodal nociceptive C fibers in relation to skin temperature, using radiant heat stimulation, in awake human subjects. The recordings are made with tungsten microelectrodes in the superficial branch of the radial nerve. Most of these results will be published elsewhere (5), so we will briefly resume our findings.

1) The figure represents the results of 173 stimulations in 5 different C units (in 5 different subjects). The fiber activity is expressed as the mean firing frequency during the stimulus application (about 15 seconds if tolerated). Different skin temperatures between 40°C and 55°C are administered in repeated series. Between each stimulus the skin is allowed to cool down to 35°C.

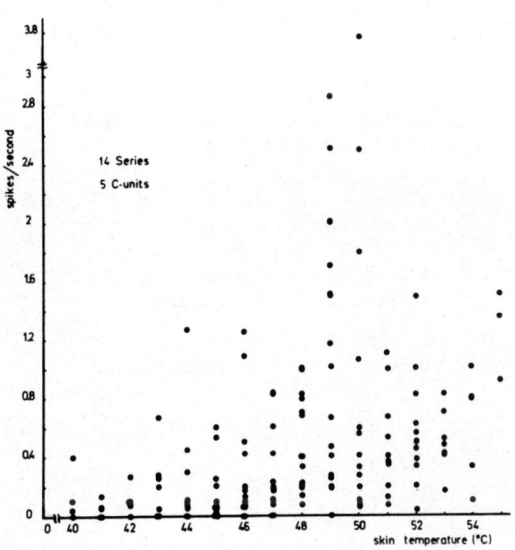

2) The afferent activity is of rather low frequency and does not as a rule exceed 2 spikes/sec even for stimuli reported as strongly painful. Thus clear pain sensations do not require a massive C fiber discharge.

3) C fiber activity of very low frequency (below 0.3 spikes/sec) does not necessarily elicit pain sensation. Almost all stimulations evoking discharge frequencies exceeding 0.4 spikes/sec are reported as painful and discharges exceeding 1.5 spikes/sec are invariably accompanied by a report of strong pain.

ACKNOWLEDGEMENTS

The author is grateful to Mrs. M. Feytons-Heeren and Mr. P. De Sutter for their skillful technical assistance.
The investigation is supported by the F.G.W.O. (grant 20.492)

REFERENCES

1. Beck, P.W., Handwerker, H.U. and Zimmerman, M., Brain Res. 67, 373 (1974).
2. Konietzny, F. and Hensel, H. Pflügers Arch. 359, 265 (1975).
3. Torebjörk, H.E. and Hallin, R.G. Exp. Brain Res. 16, 321 (1973).
4. Van Hees, J. and Gybels, J.M. Brain Res. 48, 397 (1972).
5. Van Hees, J. First World Congress on Pain, Florence 1975; to be published by Raven Press New York.

Discussion:

Zotterman: I am very happy to see my old findings made on the cat repeated on man. It is what I did on the lingual nerve of the cat in 1936. I wanted to have the heat pain spikes and the mechanoceptive spikes on the same record in order to compare the spike heights. So I asked my fellow worker to brush the tongue while another fellow was squirting hot water on it. I said "Why don't you brush the tongue?", because there were no large spikes coming. He said that he did. I was very angry with him until the other fellow said, "He did brush the tongue". But there was no response. Then I understood that heating brought the mechanoceptive myelinated fibers out of action. I would also like to tell you what happened when I told this story in a lecture in Worcester, Mass. 1940.
In the middle of the presentation a grey haired gentleman in the audience rose up and said, "Excuse me for interrupting you in the middle of your lecture but isn't this what you mean that you can't tickle a hot one?"

Hensel: I was puzzled by the extreme low frequencies you found in your units below the painful range. Our warm fibers had frequencies up to ten or fifteen per second. I would ask whether you have any comment on this?

van Hees: These are polymodal nociceptive fibers. That is my simple explanation.

Zimmermann: Concerning this question, response rates (discharge rates) of van Hees and Gybels polymodal nociceptors, what we call heat nociceptors correspond very well with the impulse rates in cats. They are so low - between one and five per second. Five impulses per second is already very high at a stimulus intensity of 50°. The average is near two impulses per second.

Torebjörk: I think that even if the impulse frequency is low, the message conveyed by a large number of C-fibers could be very important for the central nervous system. I think that the number of C-fibers that you activate by these stimuli may be considerable.

van Hees: That is true. But on the other side, people believe that there is no spatial summation at the threshold values for heat pain. So at the beginning of pain I am not sure that the number of activated C-fibers plays an important role.

Zimmermann: Concerning Dr Hensel's question on the low impulse rate of the nociceptors of man reported by Dr van Hees they correspond to our results on heat nociceptors with C-fibers in the cat. The average impulse rate at a temperature of 50° is 1 or 2 Hz. From our work on dorsal horn neurons (Handwerker, Iggo and Zimmermann, Pain 1, 1975), we realized that considerable spatial and, in part of the neurons, also temporal summation or facilitation occurs: the impulse rate may reach 150 or 200 Hz in a dorsal horn neuron during a 50° C skin stimulus. Some neurons start their discharge only some seconds after the C-afferents have started their firing, which is indicative of temporal summation and of facilitation. These units may require repetitive C volleys during electrical nerve stimulation to be excited by the C input, rather than a single volley.

Hagbarth: May I ask, how often did you see this spontaneous activity? Did you see this effect later on as described by Perl yesterday?

van Hees: I never have seen spontaneous activity in the C-fibers, not even after repeated heating.

Perl: The response of some spinal neurons to C-fiber input can be of short latency. The units described yesterday (Kumazawa and Perl) recorded from the substantia gelatinosa and excited by the polymodal nociceptors (C-fiber) respond promtly to localized noxious heat. These spinal units show phasic as well as a static response. The phasic response occurs during the rising phase of the temperature change. The polymodal nociceptors do show a burst of impulses during the phasic part of noxious heating in which impulse frequency is relatively high (10 - 50 per second) to be followed by the type of low frequency discharge described by Dr van Hees.

Hensel: Have you any idea or comment about the significance of the activity of these polymodal receptors in the non-noxious range of heating? Do they contribute to some kind of sensation? Could they be below the central threshold? What do you think about that?

van Hees: I think in normal conditions they do not evoke sensations at low frequencies. But it could be possible that the central threshold is lowered for instance by blocking input in other fibers. This is one explanation for the kind of sensation you get in partially blocked nerves when myelinated fibers are no longer conducting.

TEMPERATURE SENSITIVITY AND PAIN THRESHOLDS IN PATIENTS WITH PERIPHERAL NEUROPATHY

H. FRUHSTORFER, J. M. GOLDBERG, U. LINDBLOM and W. G. SCHMIDT

Department of Neurology, Huddinge Sjukhus, S-141 86 Huddinge (Sweden) and Institute of Physiology, University of Marburg, D-355 Marburg (GFR)

In clinical neurology quantitative methods for the estimation of nerve function are of great importance. They enable the assessment of nerve lesions which are doubtful on conventional clinical examination, and they can be used repeatedly in the same patient to follow up the course of a particular disease. A quantitative test for clinical routine work should be easy and quick in its use and it should be adapted to the patient's abilities and to the variety of deviations from the normal condition which may occur. For motor disorders several tests are available today but for sensory disturbances which are on the whole not less frequent, adequate methods have been lacking for a long time. During recent years quantitative sensory tests which can be applied clinically, have been developed for touch, vibration, and mechanical pain (Lindblom 1974; Lindblom and Meyerson 1975; Goldberg and Lindblom in preparation). Now also for thermal sensibility a test has been designed (called "Marstock" test as a fusion of MARburg and STOCKholm) by which warm, cold, and thermal pain thresholds can be quickly estimated in patients (Fruhstorfer et al. in press).

The present paper describes the results of the application of the Marstock method in a series of patients with chronic renal failure, a condition in which peripheral neuropathy is known to occur at a high percentage (Callaghan 1966; Tyler 1968; Nielsen 1971; Bergström et al. 1975). Any new method which would help to quantify the neuropathy would be a valuable therapeutic guide for the care of these patients (Nielsen 1972; Bergström et al. 1975; Dyck et al. 1975).

Uremic neuropathy usually stands for a polyneuropathy which typically starts distally in the feet with an impairment of sensation which progresses proximally. During the early days of dialysis treatment, fulminating cases with widespread pareses and muscular waisting were seen, but with modern regimens the condition, if not being totally prevented, can be kept in a restricted form with mild sensory symptoms or, which is most common, as a purely subclinical affection without obvious symptoms on routine clinical screening. According to patho-anatomical evidence the coarse myelinated afferent fibres are affected, primarily by axonal degeneration (Jennekens et al. 1969; Dyck et al. 1971; Thomas et al. 1971). In consistency, the earliest signs are impaired vibratory and discriminative sensibility or reduced conduction velocity of the peripheral nerves. Diminished deep reflexes and slight paresis of the toe extensors are also common findings. None of these signs are observed by the patients themselves. Restless legs and muscle cramps may occur early but are unspecific symptoms.

A closer study of thermal sensibility seemed to be useful in these cases as some patients had reported diminished cold sensation on the feet and lower legs on conventional screening for temperature sensibility. A differential impairment of the temperature sense could be expected in a lesion which primarily affects myelinated fibres, as cold and warm sensation are evidently mediated by myelinated and unmyelinated axons, respectively (Fruhstorfer 1976).

MATERIAL AND METHOD

The group of patients consisted of 15 persons with chronic uremia, which were admitted for neurological screening with regard to the occurrence and course of peripheral neuropathy. They were under treatment with a dietary regimen and/or hemodialysis. Most of them were ambulatory and they were all in a generally good condition and well cooperative. Most of the patients had subclinical signs of neuropathy in the form of increased vibration thresholds as measured with the standardized technique of Goldberg and Lindblom (in preparation), impaired discriminative sensibility when tested with figure writing on the feet, and/or reduced conduction velocity of the peroneal nerve. The control material consisted of 26 students and laboratory workers without known neurological disease.

The thermostimulator (area 2,5 x 5,0 cm) was composed of Peltier elements which allow a continuous stimulation of the skin. A thermocouple was attached to the stimulating surface in order to record the temperature during the test. The stimulator could either be warmed or cooled depending on the direction of the current applied. This was controlled by the patient himself who reversed a switch as soon as he felt the stimulator becoming warm or cold. For the study of thermal pain thresholds the patient was instructed to activate the switch when he perceived the stimulus as painful. As soon as the stimulator reached again an indifferent temperature of $30^{\circ}C$, the current was reversed on the operator's demand to deliver the next pain stimulus. A detailed methodological description of the Marstock test will appear separately (Fruhstorfer et al. in press).

RESULTS

The temperature record of a Marstock test reminds of the record from a Békésy audiometer. It showes a zigzag curve which initially shifts towards the warm side due to adaptation. The peak amplitude of the curve and its position on the temperature scale was taken as a measure of the temperature sensitivity of the stimulated area. The amplitude was found to be relatively small in sensitive areas like the lip or the hand, where it was normally of the order of $1-3^{\circ}C$, and it was greater in less sensitive areas such as the trunk and the feet.

Fig. 1 shows the Marstock record from a patient who on neurological examination appeared normal in all respects but for the temperature sense. Thus, the sensation of touch and pin-prick,

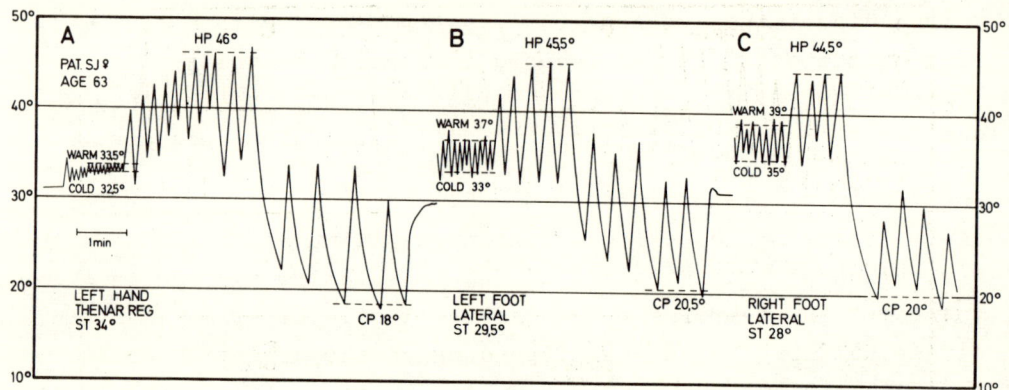

FIG. 1: Marstock recordings from a patient with chronic uremia, in A from the left thenar, in B and C from the left and right foot (lateral side). Normal warm-cold difference limens and normal heat and cold pain thresholds in all three locations. During the measurement of thermal pain thresholds the current was reversed on the operator's request whenever the stimulator reached indifferent temperatures.

muscle power and deep reflexes were normal as were the conduction velocities of the median and peroneal nerves and the vibration thresholds of the hand and feet. But both cold and warm sensation were reported to be weaker distally in the legs which suggested a neuropathic involvement of the corresponding afferent fibres. From the records in Fig. 1, it appears that the warm-cold difference limen was $1^\circ C$ ($33.5^\circ - 32.5^\circ$) in the thenar region (A), and $4^\circ C$ on the lateral side of the feet (B, C). The heat and cold pain thresholds (HP and CP) on the hand were $46^\circ C$ and $18^\circ C$, respectively. The corresponding values for the feet were of the same order (About $45^\circ C$ and $20^\circ C$). All these values are normal. Thus, in this patient, thermal sensibility proved to be normal and the suspicion of a neuropathy could be rejected.

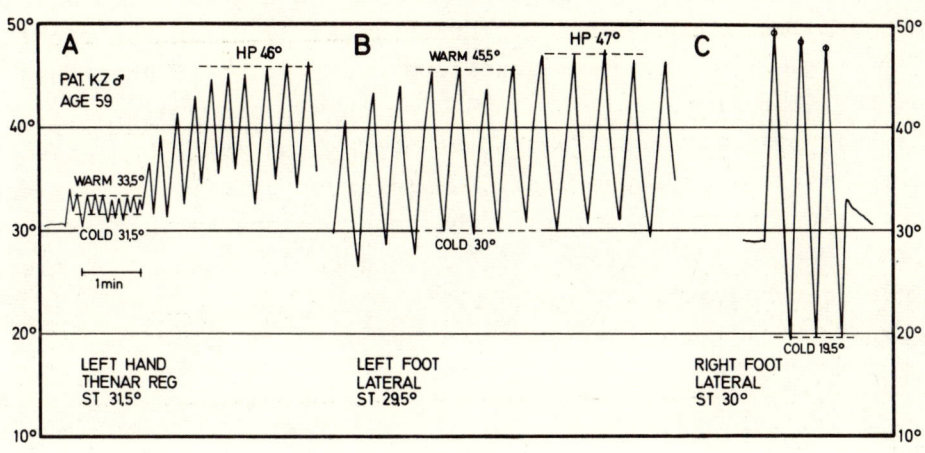

FIG. 2: Marstock recordings from a patient with chronic uremia and subclinical neuropathy: A, from left thenar region, normal; B and C, from left and right foot (lateral side), abnormal records. Note increase of warm-cold difference limen mainly towards warmth in B. In C there was no warm sensation when the temperature approached the 50°C line and switching was requested by the investigator to avoid burning (indicated by circles). Record C also illustrates a raised cold threshold.

The Marstock recording of a patient with a somewhat asymmetric but otherwise typical subclinical neuropathy is illustrated in Fig. 2. The diagnosis was based on the increased vibration thresholds in both feet, in the right lower leg and the right hand, of a defect discriminative sensibility on the feet and of reduced conduction velocities of the median and peroneal nerves. Both the warm-cold difference limen and the heat pain threshold were normal in the thenar region (Fig. 2 A). The left foot, which was the least affected one, as judged from the height of the vibration thresholds, displayed a significant increase of the difference limen which was 15.5°C (Fig. 2 B; for normal values see Fig. 3). The increase was clearly greater towards the warm side, which was contrary to what had been expected, the warm threshold being as high as 45.5°C which was just below the heat pain threshold at 47°C. On the right foot (Fig. 2 C), the warm sensation was completely abolished and the cold threshold was 19.5°C which was abnormally low. The heat pain threshold was above 50°C which was the highest stimulation temperature used. The recorded defects in warm and heat pain sensations indicate that the neuropathy in this case also affected the C-fibres. The raised cold threshold on the right foot suggests an involvement of the A-delta fibres as well.

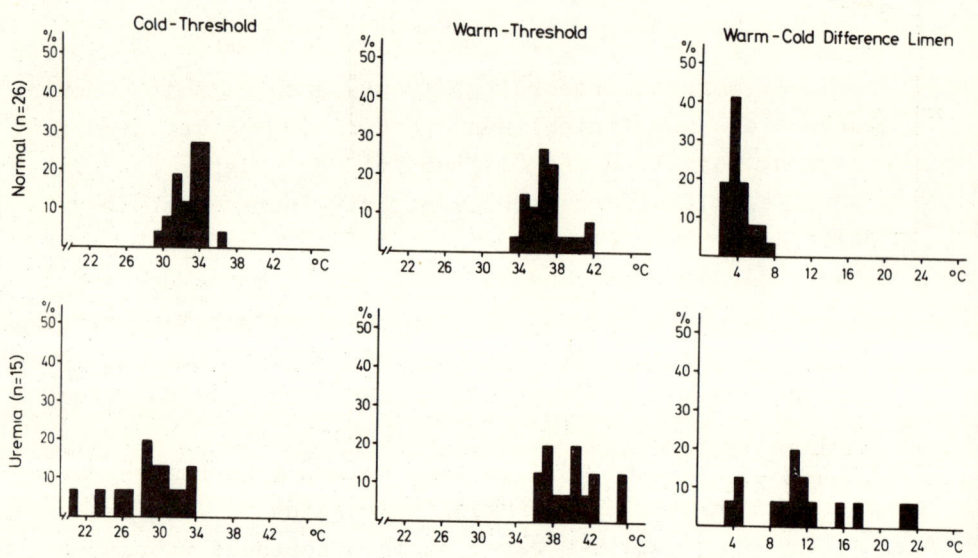

FIG. 3: Distribution of warm and cold thresholds and of the warm-cold difference limen measured on the feet in 15 uremic patients and 26 controls.

Fig. 3 shows the distributions of warm and cold thresholds measured on the feet of the uremic patients and of the controls. In the group of uremic patients both cold and warm thresholds were significantly elevated compared to the thresholds of the control group (Man-Whitney Test, P<0.01). For the verification of an impaired thermal sensibility in single cases, however, the warm-cold difference limen seemed to be the most sensitive parameter. It deviated from normal in 13 of the 15 uremic patients.

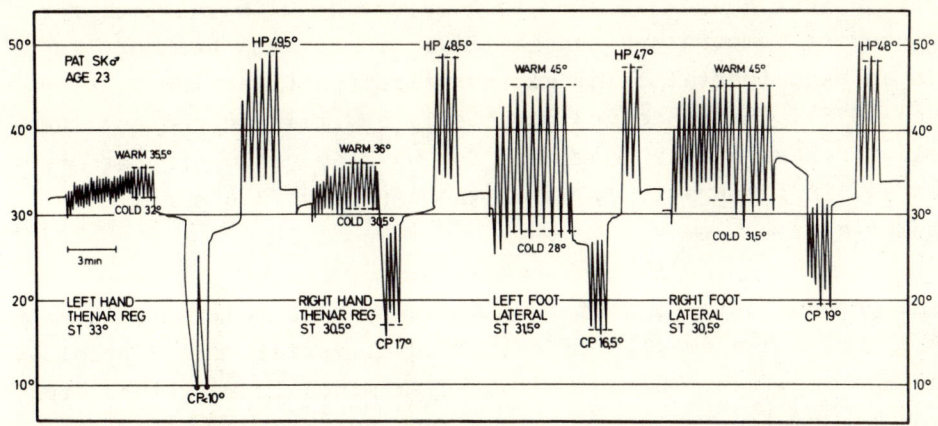

FIG. 4: Marstock records from patient with chronic uremia without other signs of neuropathy. Note increased warm-cold difference limen on both feet and on right thenar. High heat pain thresholds in both hands and no cold pain sensation in left hand above 10°C (switching was requested by the operator at 10°C as indicated by the circles).

Fig. 4 shows the Marstock recording from a patient with uremia, which displayed an increased warm-cold difference limen on both feet (left 17°C, right 13.5°C), and on the right hand where it was 5.5°C (normal ≤ 4.0°C). On the left hand no cold pain threshold could be obtained in the range above 10°C which probably is abnormal as cold pain thresholds were recorded of the other test points. The heat pain thresholds were generally high and the thenar values are probably pathological. In this patient all other neurological tests including vibration thresholds and conduction velocities were normal.

DISCUSSION

The Marstock method has been in clinical use for a little more than a year and has proved to be a useful clinical tool for measuring temperature sensibility. It has also been applied in an experimental clinical investigation (Lindblom & Meyerson 1975). The procedure gives only an estimate and not the exact values of the thresholds for warm and cold (Fruhstorfer et al. in preparation), or of the capacity to discriminate temperatures.

The present data suggest that there is a considerable interindividual and a smaller intraindividual variation and possibly an age relation. These have to be examined in a further study for the various skin areas. The existing control material, however, leaves no doubt that clearly abnormal records may be found in patients with chronic uremia. There is no reason to believe that the recorded threshold changes were due to psychological factors such as inattention or drowsiness as these patients had threshold values within normal limits on other body sites and did not show any signs of encephalopathy or myelopathy. Thus it is reasonable to interpret the results in terms of peripheral neuropathy.

The threshold increase recorded was in some cases greater toward the warm side. This finding indicates that uremic neuropathy affects besides the coarse myelinated fibres, also the unmyelinated ones, as has been demonstrated for thalidomid neuropathy (Krücke et al. 1971), which is another 'dying-back disease', for amyloidosis (Dyck and Lambert 1969), and for hereditary sensory neuropathy (Dyck et al. 1971). The observation that abnormal temperature sensibility was the only pathological sign in some patients, would imply that the unmyelinated fibres may be affected first and that the recording of temperature and pain sensibility may be important for the early detection of uremic neuropathy. To prove the correctness of these interpretations, a correlation with histological data from nerve biopsies is required and such a study is in preparation. It may be mentioned here that Schaumburg et al. (1974) in ultrastructural studies of the dying-back process, found that acrylamid intoxication produces axonal degeneration in the primary terminals of muscle spindles and in the nerve endings within the Pacinian corpuscles. These authors point out that their own results and those of others suggest a differential nerve terminal susceptibility in dying-back neuropathies. It may be speculated that some of the neurotoxic factors in uremia affect primarily the C-fibre endings.

SUMMARY

Warm, cold, and thermal pain thresholds were studied in 15 patients with chronic renal failure and in 26 normal controls. Some of the patients demonstrated a manifest neuropathy. Thermal stimulation was performed by a patient-controlled continuous stimulation technique using the Peltier effect. In the patients warm threshold, cold threshold, and the difference between them (i.e. warm-cold difference limen) deviated significantly from the control values. In some patients, only the warm-cold difference limen but not the absolute threshold values were abnormal. An increase in the warm-cold difference limen was sometimes accompanied by a raised heat pain threshold. Abnormal records were most often combined with other signs of neuropathy but could also appear in isolation. The findings indicate that besides coarse myelinated fibres, nerve fibres of fine calibre, especially C-fibres, are involved in uremic neuropathy, and that this may occur already in the early subclinical stage of the disease.

REFERENCES

Bergström, J., Lindblom, U., Norée, L.-O.: Preservation of peripheral nerve function in severe uremia during treatment with low protein high calorie diet and surplus of essential amino acids. Acta neurol. scand. 51, 99-109 (1975)

Callaghan, N.: A study of peripheral nerve function in chronic renal failure. Irish J. med. Sci. 6, 325-331 (1966)

Dyck, P.J., Lambert, E.H.: Dissociated sensation in amyloidosis: compound action potential, quantitative histologic and teased-fiber, and electron microscopic studies of sural nerve biopsies. Arch. Neurol. (Chic.) 20, 490-507 (1969)

Dyck, P.J., Lambert, E.H., Nichols, P.C.: Quantitative measurement of sensation related to compound action potential and number and sizes of myelinated and unmyelinated fibers of sural nerve in health, Friedreich's ataxia, hereditary sensory neuropathy, and tabes dorsalis. In: Handbook of Electroencephalography and Clinical Neurophysiology, Vol. 9, Amsterdam: Elsevier 1971

Dyck, P.J., Johnson, W.J., Lambert, E.H., Bushek, W., Pollock, M.: Detection and evaluation of uremic peripheral neuropathy in patients on hemodialysis. Kidney Int. 7, 201-205 (1975)

Fruhstorfer, H.: Conduction in the afferent thermal pathways of man studied by cortical evoked responses, reaction time and regional anaesthesia. This volume.

Fruhstorfer, H., Lindblom, U., Schmidt, W.G.: A method for quantitative estimation of thermal thresholds in patients. J.Neurol. Neurosurg. Psychiat. (in press)

Goldberg, J.M., Lindblom, U.: The vibration threshold in terms of displacement amplitude. (in preparation)

Jennekens, F.G.I., van der Most van Spijk, D., Dorhout Mees, E.J.: Nerve fibre degeneration in uremic polyneuropathy. Proc. Eur. Dial. Trans. Ass. 6, 191-197 (1969)

Krücke, W., von Hartrott, H.-H., Schröder, J.M. Thomas, E., Gibbels, E., Scheid, W.: Licht- und elektronenmikroskopische Untersuchungen zum Spätstadium der Thalidomid-Polyneuropathie. Fortschr. Neurol. Psychiat. 39, 15-50 (1971)

Lindblom, U.: Touch perception threshold in human glabrous skin in terms of displacement amplitude on stimulation with single mechanical pulses. Brain Res. 82, 205-210 (1974)

Lindblom, U., Meyerson, B.A.: Influence on touch, vibration and cutaneous pain of dorsal column stimulation in man. Pain 1, 257-270 (1975)

Lindblom, U., Meyerson, B.A.: Mechanoceptive and nociceptive thresholds during dorsal column stimulation in man. Proc. First World Congr. on Pain, Florence 1975

Nielsen, V.K.: The peripheral nerve function in chronic renal failure. I. Clinical symptoms and signs. Acta med. scand. 190, 105-111 (1971)

Nielsen, V.K.: The peripheral nerve function in chronic renal failure. IV. An analysis of the vibratory perception threshold. Acta med. scand. 191, 287-296 (1972)

Schaumburg, H.H., Wisniewski, H.M., Spencer, P.S.: Ultrastructural studies of the dying-back process. 1. Peripheral nerve terminal and axon degeneration in systemic acrylamide intoxication. J. Neuropath. exp. Neurol. 33, 260 (1974)

Thomas, P.K., Hollinrake, K., Lascelles, R.G., O'Sullivan, D.J. Baillod, R.A., Moorhead, J.F., Mackenzie, J.C.: The polyneuropathy of chronic renal failure. Brain 94, 761-780 (1971)

Tyler, H.R.: Neurologic disorders in renal failure. Amer. J. Med. 44, 734-748 (1968)

This work was supported by Karolinska Institutets Fonder and by the Deutsche Forschungsgemeinschaft (Fr 265/2)

Discussion:

Iggo: Is it possible that the dissociation of heat and cold pain that you reported may be due to the excitation of different sets of afferent fibers? Although the C-thermal nociceptors (C-heat receptors, C-polymodal nociceptors) may be excited by low skin temperatures, there are other C-afferent units (reported by Iggo in 1959) which are excited at skin temperatures (greater than 45° C). These latter afferent units, if present in man, may be the active peripheral elements which mediate the cold pain which survived in your patients, when the "heat pain" response was lost. However, the afferent fibers are non-myelinated, at least in the cat.

Lindblom: Yes, I think the fact that we get a dissociation in different patients may indicate what you say that there are different fiber populations, at least to a certain extent.

Franzén: I just want to remind Lindblom that we ran experiments on patients who had vascular traumatic parietal lobe lesions. They showed an increased difference limen in the way Lindblom described contralateral to the side of the brain lesion. But it was interesting to note that although they did not report any sensation of cold or warm they could say that there was a change in temperature.

Zotterman: There is a question about cold pain. When you have cold feet you get quite numb in the toes, for instance. There is no sensation of cold but you feel it very uncomfortable. The question is whether the cold fibers in the toes are still reacting at low temperatures or whether the cold sensation has its origin from the border between the cold and the warmer skin higher up.

Zotterman: As concerns ducks and other birds standing on the ice I do not believe that myelinated fibers in their toes can conduct at these low temperatures of the toes.

Lindblom: When we put thermodes on the skin and lower the temperature you feel it first as a superficial cold pain which is not at all as intense as the heat pain. If you lower the temperature further this superficial sensation disappears and is replaced by a dull, deeper aching. A very natural explanation would be that a transient cold sensation is evoked from the skin endings and then they are blocked by the cold. Then other endings are responding to the cold stimulus coming in. That may be an answer to your question. There is a zone where the temperature gradient is adequate for discharge in cold-sensitive neurons.

Zotterman: That is exactly my opinion.

Iggo: In reply to Dr Zotterman's question, the myelinated mechano-receptors and their afferent fibers are blocked at low temperatures of the skin, and the numbness of cold feet is probably due to this inactivity of the mechano-receptors. Non-myelinated fibers on the other hand, continue to conduct impulses at skin and nerve temperatures as low as +3° C. In 1959 I reported that non-myelinated afferent units could be excited at these very low temperatures in cat skin, and that the excitation was via the receptors. A nociceptive function was suggested for these C-units. They are different from the sensitive "cold" receptors.

Lindahl: I think this is of interest not only from a basic physiological point of view but also from a clinical point of view. May I ask you one question? Have you noticed this early involvement of the pain and heat sensations also in other neuropathies? And have you also noted basal-motor abnormalities in these patients indicating that sympathetic C-fibers are also not functioning?

Lindblom: Yes, we selected to study the uremic patients because we had a large number of them. We have studied other neuropathies too, for instance diabetic or toxic of various types. But so far we have only a few cases of each so I cannot communicate a systemic observation. It is well known, for example, that the diabetic neuropathy effects the sympathetic fibers as well. We often see that the skin temperature is affected indicating such a lesion.

Hensel: I would like to comment on Iggo's and Zotterman's remarks. Arctic animals standing on the ice have particular local adaptation to cold and the nerve fibers conduct at much lower temperatures than they do in the normal homeothermic animals.

MODULATION OF CLINICAL AND EXPERIMENTAL PAIN IN MAN BY ELECTRICAL STIMULATION OF THALAMIC PERIVENTRICULAR GRAY

J. GYBELS and P. COSYNS

Department of Neurology and Neurosurgery, and Department of Psychiatry, University of Leuven, B-3000 Leuven, Belgium

1. Introduction

To test the modulating effects of CNS stimulation on painsensation, we have in the course of the last ten years, used a strategy in which the subject has to make comparisons of the subjective intensity of two equally noxious electrical stimuli St 1 and St 2, a CNS structure being stimulated during the second noxious stimulus. Three categories of judgment $S_1 = S_2$, $S_2 < S_1$ and $S_2 > S_1$ are permitted. The structures of the CNS stimulated are identified by the use of scatterograms, constructed from computer data (for stimulation details, see Gybels et al. (1), and for details of plotting stimulated CNS structures, see Peluso and Gybels (2). The results have been published elsewhere (3, in press) and can be summarized as follows :
1) In the absence of paraesthesiae, as was the case when frontal (area 9 ?) and parietal (area 19 ? - 39 ?) cortex, n. C.M., n. Pf., n. V.L. and n. caudatus were stimulated, no modulation of painsensation was observed.
2) When the subject experienced paraesthesiae, as was the case with n. V.P.L. - V.P.M. and n. V.c.pc. stimulation, there was a decrease in the experimentally evoked painsensation when the noxious stimulus was near the pain threshold. With more intense pain provoking stimuli, no such effect was seen. We have extended this work now to the periacqueductal gray of the mesencephalon and periventricular gray of the posterior and caudal part of the third ventricle.
We wish to emphasize at the onset that the data are very preliminary. They are obtained from one patient, who has however been studied intensively. In view of the great current interest in analgesia from stimulation of peri-acqueductal gray in the animal, and the extreme paucity of data in the human (4), particularly when evaluated under experimentally controlled

conditions, we believe there is reason to report the results we have obtained to date.

2. Material and methods

2.1. Patient D.F. a student, now 22 years old, was operated in July 1974 via a right frontal craniotomy for a hormone producing pituitary adenocarcinoma. In December 1974, he complained of severe facial pain in the distribution of the left trigeminal nerve, due to an invasion of the neoformation in the base of the skull. He was treated successfully with telecobalt radiotherapy till December 1975, when he complained again of continuous, dull and throbbing pain particularly in and behind the left eye. Usual analgesics became insufficient and morphine-like analgesics had to be administered. General health remained good.

The patient had an IQ >120, and was particularly cooperative. Intensive psychiatric ans psychological assessment was performed using e.g. tape recorded and standardized clinical interviews, personality questionnaires, projective techniques, mood rating scales and body image and distorsion questionnaire. No psychopathological data were found in his personal, familial and social history before the illness started at age 13 with pubertas praecox and growth arrest. The last two years he mainly developed psychological features in reaction to his severe somatic condition.

As treatment for the facial pain, intracerebral self-stimulation via chronic implanted electrodes was fully explained and proposed and accepted by the patient, his family and the hospital staff.

2.2. An electrode assembly, consisting of 4 Teflon isolated stainless steel wires, each with a diameter of 110μ, and a central guide, with a diameter of 75μ, was so constructed that four points for stimulation were available. Each wire had a bare tip of 1 mm long, two successive tips were separated by a distance of 3 mm. The deepest tip to which is assigned the number 1, was stereotactically implanted at a target lying 2 mm below the commissura posterior and 2 mm at the left side from the midline. According to the Atlas of Schaltenbrand and Bailey (5) this brings electrode 1 in the vicinity of the rostral part of the periacqueductal gray matter, electrode 2 in the medial, caudal and posterior part of the thalamus, in or around the periventricular gray of the third ventricle, and electrodes 3 and 4 in or in the vicinity of the dorsomedial nucleus of the thalamus (fig. 1).

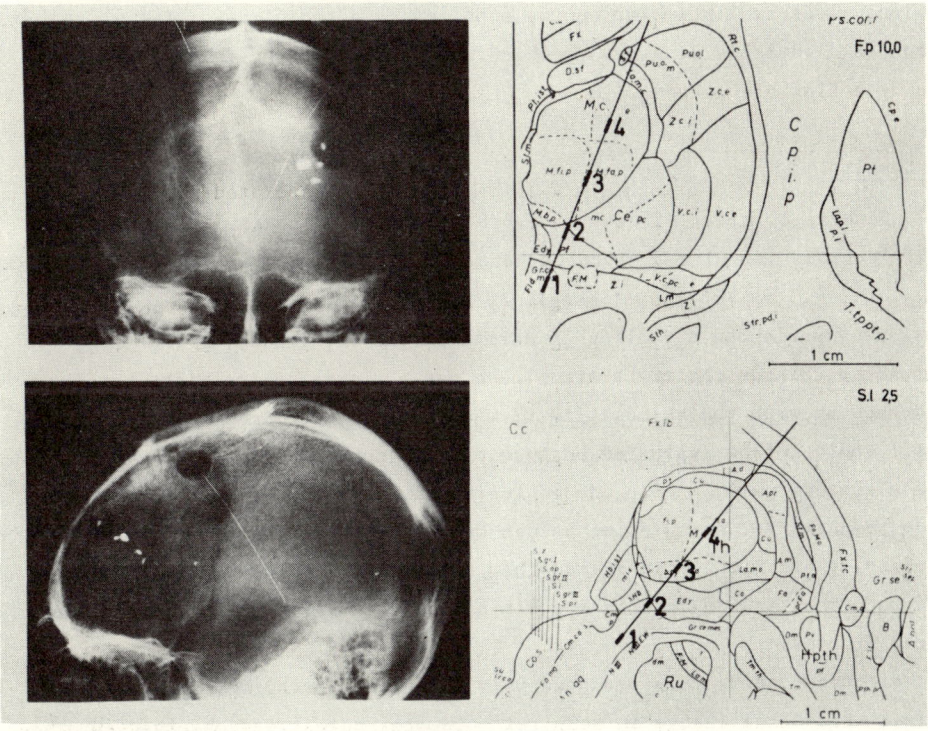

Fig. 1. A.P. and lateral X-ray. Observe the position of the implanted electrode assembly. Its position and the bare tips of the 4 electrodes are projected, respectively on frontal plane F.p 10 and sagital plane S.1 2,5 (5).

The target was choosen for the following considerations : for reasons of safety we were reluctant of placing an electrode deep in the mesencephalon; on the other hand, stimulation produced analgesia has been obtained from sites in the caudal diencephalon in animals (6), (7) and in man (Richardson, personal communication, 4). In a first stage, lasting 10 days, the four wires connected to each electrode were left outside the skin, so that the effect of stimulation of each electrode pair could be tested. Motor activity, subjective feelings, attention and mood were observed, EEG was recorded, and the analgesic action on three tests of experimentally induced and on the clinical pain were evaluated. In a second stage, the most active electrode pair (2 - 3), as far as its analgesic producing effect on the clinical pain when stimulated is concerned, was connected to a miniature radiofrequency receiver, which was implanted under the skin of the thoracic region; electrical stimulation was supplied by a radiotransmitter which produced a variable square wave which was coupled to the receiver by the use of a flexible antenna.

3. Results

3.1. General clinical effects of E.B.S. (electrical brain stimulation).
The electrode pair 1 - 2 produced paraesthesiae in the right half of the face (0.5 - 1 mA, 33 cps, 1 msec). At higher stimulus intensities the patient experienced a feeling of warmth in the right side of the face, spreading towards the right arm. These was a miosis of the right pupil, synchronous with the stimulating (2 mA, 3 cps, 1 msec) current (the left pupil could not be evaluated because of left ophthalmoplegia).
The electrode pair 2 - 3 produced the same feeling of warmth in the right face and arm. For stimulation values below the threshold for the warmth feeling, the patient volunteered that he felt "something" in the left eye, and that the tension in this eye diminished when stimulation was continued for 2 minutes.
The electrode pair 3 - 4 produced only an answer for higher stimulation values. Besides a change in respiration, motor unrest was observed in arms and legs. The patient, who otherwise was calm and cooperative felt himself become "nervous" and "restless". The pain in the face was not influenced.

3.2. Influence of E.B.S.S. (electrical brain self-stimulation).
The 3 electrode pairs (1 - 2, 2 - 3, 3 - 4) were tested during 9 days while the patient could stimulate himself (33 csec, intensity below threshold of sensation). The clinical pain was recorded five times a day by the patient himself who was instructed to rate the intensity of his pain along a 10 cm line extending from "no pain" to "unbearable maximal pain". The results of this "visual analog scale" (8) are represented in fig. 2.

It can be seen that the facial pain decreased when the electrode pair 2 - 3 was stimulated while severe pain persisted with stimulation of the other electrode pairs.
The evolution in time of the influence of E.B.S.S. with the electrode pair 2 -3 on the facial pain is represented in fig. 3.
During the first seven days of this observation, no E.B.S.S. was permitted. Analgesics had to be given to keep the patient sufficiently comfortable.

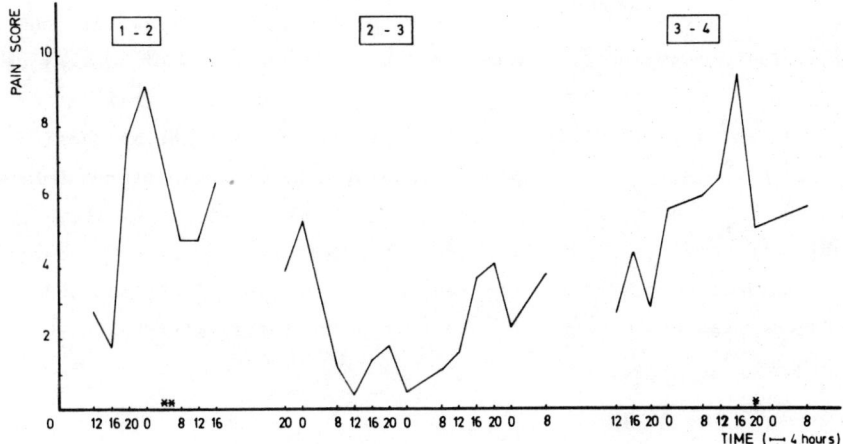

Fig. 2. See text. No analgesics were administered during the reported observation period, except in * for obvious ethical reasons.

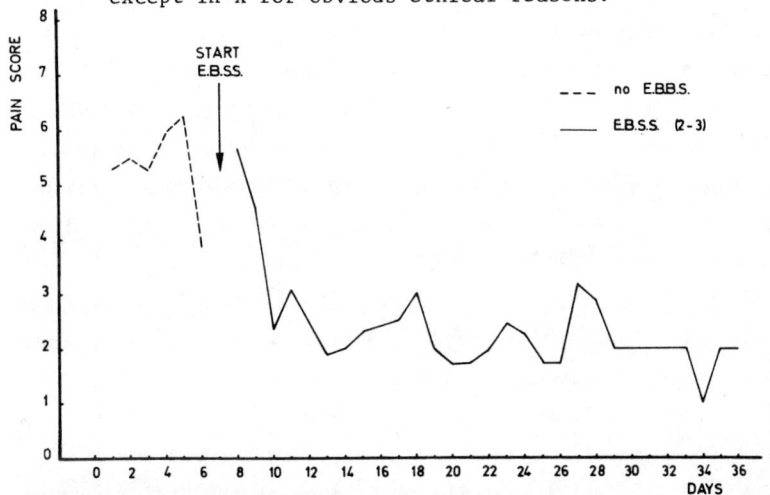

Fig. 3. See text.

When E.B.S.S. started on day 8 no analgesics were given any more. After 48 hours, one can observe a decrease in the facial pain which maintains itself during the next weeks, without however a complete disappearance of the facial pain. The patient continued to feel something uncomfortable in his left face, but this no longer interfered seriously with his daily life. From the 13th day of the above mentionned observation period, the patient developed a new pain in the left knee, left hip and left lumbal region. This new pain increased progressively without being apparently influenced by the

E.B.S.S., while the E.B.S.S. remained effective for the relief of the facial pain. On day 20, the patient needed moderate doses of analgesics to control the pain in the leg and lumbar region. What causes this latter pain is as yet not clear. In order to possibly increase the analgesic effect of stimulation of the periventricular gray we administered L-Dopa (9) at the 37th day. 1 week later the patient volunteered that the E.B.S.S. probably had some effect on the pain in the left leg as well. The patient thought this to be due to the combined effect of the stimulation and the analgesics. Possibly it might be due to a potentiating effect of L-Dopa on E.B.S.

3.3. E.B.S.S. behaviour.

Spontaneously the patient stimulated himself (electrode pair 2 - 3) during 15 to 20 minutes continuously with an intensity which was below the threshold for sensation. After 5 to 10 minutes of stimulation he felt a clear influence of the stimulation on the pain in his face. The throbbing and tension around the eye disappeared and the patient felt himself generally better. Immediately after stimulation the pain increased somewhat, but remained at a low level. During stimulation he preferred to occupy himself, such as walking or playing cards. He could not remain seated and waiting till the pain disappeared, because he felt restless and nervous. In the beginning he stimulated every time when the pain in his face became worse. After a few days, when the periorbital pain had almost disappeared, he continued to stimulate himself 5 - 8 times a day during 20 minutes. When he stimulated less often (3 - 4 times a day) the pain usually came back after a few hours. At one time he was ordered a stimulation program, consisting of 10 minutes stimulation every hour between 8 a.m. and 8 p.m. He had to give this up because the recurrence of the facial pain and he returned on his own initiative to stimulation sessions of 15 -20 minutes 5 to 8 times a day.

3.4. Influence of E.B.S. on experimental pain.

We have studied the influence of stimulation of the electrode pair 2 - 3 on three different tests for experimentally evoked pain.

3.4.1. In a first test, we have applied a noxious electrical stimulation to the skin, using a strategy as described in the introduction. From a total of 55 pairs of equally noxious stimuli, the following results were obtained : $S_2 < S_1$ 39 times; $S_2 = S_1$ 14 times; and $S_2 > S_1$ 2 times. Stimulation of the periventricular gray decreased the pain, elicited by electrical stimulation of the skin. According to the patient, in the cases where S_2 was $< S_1$, the decrease of painsensation (S_2) was small.

3.4.2. In order to use a natural noxious stimulus which can be reasonably quantified, we used radiating heat. The blackened skin was irradiated by a focussed bulb, the heating current being controlled by the output voltage of a small thermistor fixed on the surface of the irradiated skin. The subject was asked to say "yes" at the first moment of pain and to say "stop" when the pain became strong. Table I represents the results, expressed in degrees Celsius.

Table I. Influence of stimulation of thalamic periventricular gray (left side) on cutaneous pain, evoked by heating the skin.

	YES		STOP	
	M.	S.D.	M.	S.D.
Without E.B.S. stim. heat on right hand	47.2	(.78)	48.5	(.55)
With E.B.S. stim. (2 - 3) heat on right hand	48.55	(.42)	49.55	(.35)
With E.B.S. stim. (2 - 3) heat on left hand	47.35	(.63)	48.35	(.55)

Each number is the mean of 10 successive measurements. Measurements with E.B.S. were taken when electrode pair 2 - 3 had already been stimulated during 15 minutes. A statistically significant increase for the "yes" and "stop" responses is observed while electrode pair 2 - 3 were being continuously stimulated, and the focussed bulb irradiated the right hand (Wilcoscon test, T significant at .01 level).

3.4.3. In order to test an experimental pain which mimics the duration and severity of clinical pain and which is sensitive to morphine (10) we used the submaximum effort Tourniquet technique. In this test, the subject must do a fixed amount of muscle contraction with an ischaemic arm and the basic unit of measurement is the amount of time from the cessation of excercise until the pain reaches an unbearable level. In fig. 4 are represented the results for the right arm without E.B.S. and after 15 minutes stimulation of the electrode pair 2 - 3. There is no difference in the pain scores before and after E.B.S.

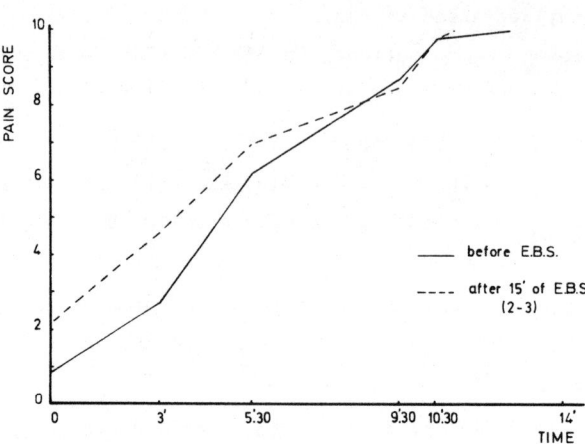

Fig. 4. See text. The ischaemic pain, measured with the visual analog scale is plotted in function of time.

4. Conclusion

No general conclusions can be drawn from the preliminary data. They suggest strongly that in man stimulation of thalamic periventricular gray can greatly reduce clinical pain without at the same time reducing to a comparable extent experimentally produced painsensation. This is puzzling in view of the results obtained in animals (6), (7), where tests for analgesia are based on experimentally provoked pain. This influence of thalamic periventricular gray stimulation on pathological pain outlasts the stimulation period, it possibly may occur only in a restricted peripheral field and it is perhaps potentiated by the administration of L-Dopa.

Aknowledgements
The authors are grateful to Mrs. Feytons-Heeren and Mr. P. De Sutter for their skillful technical assistance. The investigation was supported by the F.G.W.O. (grant 20.492) of Belgium.

REFERENCES

1. Gybels, J., Carton, H., Cosyns, P. and Peluso, F. In "Pain : Basic Principles-Pharmacology-Therapy" edited by R. Janzen, W.D. Keidel, A. Herz and C. Steichele. Georg Thieme Publishers, Stuttgart, 128-131 (1972).
2. Peluso, F. and Gybels, J. Confin. neurol. 32, 213 (1970).
3. Gybels, J., Van Hees, J. and Peluso, F. First Congress on Pain, Florence, 1975. To be published by Raven Press, New York.
4. Richardson, D.E. and Akil, H. Abstr. 7th Ann. Meeting Neuro-electric Soc. (1974).

5. Schaltenbrand, G. and Bailey, P. Introduction to stereotaxis with an atlas of the human brain. Georg Thieme Verlag, Vol. II (1959).
6. Willis, W.D., Trevino, D.L., Coulter, J.D. and Maunz, R.A. J. Neurophysiol. 37, 358 (1974).
7. Balagura, S. and Ralph, T. Brain Res. 60, 369 (1973).
8. Aitken, R.C.B. and Zeally, A.K. Brit. J. Hosp. Med. 4, 215 (1970).
9. Akil, H. and Liebeskind, J.C. Brain Res. 94, 279 (1975).
10. Smith, G.M., Egbert, L.D., Markowitz, R.A., Mosteller, F. and Beecher, H.K. J. Pharmacol. & Exp. Therap. 154, 324 (1966).

Request reprints from : J. GYBELS, Md, Agr., Department of Neurology and Neurosurgery, Akademisch Ziekenhuis Sint-Rafaël, Kapucijnenvoer 35, B-3000 Leuven (Belgium).

Discussion:

Ingvar: When you stimulate patients in this region I would like to know whether you observed any changes in level of wakefullness and also the mood.

Gybels: We have very carefully measured the following things: motor activity, subjective feeling, EEG recording, attention, mood swings and so forth. With this very intensive testing we have not seen any influence of stimulation of this leg. Not in the project mentioned.

Hagbarth: Did you try different stimulation parameters?

Gybels: No, to have an answer in this type of experiment it is better to have one bird in one's hand than to have ten in the air. So playing around with parameters of stimulus would, of course, be very interesting. But there is only a certain amount a patient can do to present reliable results from its subjective response. So we did not do this. We have changed only the stimulus frequency. They were three per second to one hundred per second and we have not seen any difference. What we did one time was to impose a stiff program of stimulation. The patient had to stimulate himself every hour during five minutes. This he did not like. He wanted to do it when he wanted a relief. While he was stimulating himself he felt what he called nervous. He wanted to be occupied; he liked walking around or playing cards.

Liebeskind: One would hope that with increasing the parameters of stimulation either in intensity or duration that one could perhaps obtain even with this particular patient an alteration in the experimental pain threshold in addition to the obtained pain relief that you found for his pathological condition. However, I entirely agree with the caution that you have used and obviously are going to continue to use. Because as you well know in the animal work it has been reported that tolerance can develop to the analgesic effect of electrical stimulation of the brain. And one would certainly want to hold on to the bird in the hand of the effective pathological pain relief and not play too seriously with attempting to get experimental analgesia with stronger levels of stimulation for fear of obtaining habituation. I should say tolerance.

Handwerker: You reported myosis among the effects of stimulation of the periventricular gray. Did you control the blood flow through the skin as well? (No) I wonder whether the feeling of warm reported by your patient might be due to an increased blood flow?

Gybels: You'll remember that the electrode is on the left side. The myosis you could control on the right side but not on the left side because of the hemiplegia. But he "felt" something on his left side. I cannot understand how he can feel something in the left side except by a vascular wave. This is a parasympathetic system. Probably something must have happened in the tension in the left eye.

EFFECTS OF MULTIFOCAL BRAIN STIMULATION ON PAIN AND SOMATOSENSORY FUNCTIONS

J. BOËTHIUS, U. LINDBLOM, B. A. MEYERSON and L. WIDÉN

Departments of Neurosurgery and Clinical Neurophysiology, Karolinska sjukhuset and Department of Neurology, Huddinge sjukhus, Stockholm, Sweden

INTRODUCTION

It is well known from animal experiments that stimulation of various brain areas will decrease or abolish responses to noxious stimulation (Cox and Valenstein 1965, Reynolds 1969, Schmidek et al. 1971, Black et al. 1972, Yunger et al. 1973). In particular, extensive studies have been devoted to the remarkable effects on pain of stimulation in the periaqueductal grey matter (Mayer et al. 1971, Liebeskind et al. 1973, Mayer and Liebeskind 1974, Liebeskind, this volume). Similar effects on pain as a result of focal brain stimulation have also been observed in man (Erwin et al. 1968, Gol 1967, Heath and Mickel 1960, Richardson and Akil 1974, Gybels et al., this volume). These results were mainly obtained by acute stimulation of various brain areas during stereotactic operations. In view of the promising results which were obtained during such experiments, methods have now been developed which makes it possible to apply this non-destructive approach to the treatment of chronic pain.

In 1973 Mazars and co-workers published a preliminary report on some patients with chronic pain who already in 1962 had had stimulatory electrodes chronically implanted in the sensory thalamic nuclei. The material now consists of 17 patients (Mazars et al. 1973) out of which 13 obtained satisfactory pain relief. Good results were achieved in phantom limb and atypical facial pain. The authors concluded that, in general, the best results were obtained with pain associated with a supposedly insufficient inflow from large caliber fibres as can be the case in lesions of periferal nerves.

Hosobuchi et al. (1973, 1974) reported on the results of stimulation through indwelling electrodes in the sensory thalamic nuclei and in the internal capsule. Some of their patients who had pain of central origin responded favourably to stimulation in the sensory limb of the internal capsule.

Richardson and Akil (1974) observed a reduction of both acute and chronic pain by stimulation in the periventricular and periaqueductal grey matter during operations in man. They, therefore, implanted electrodes in the

periventricular grey (medial to the CM-Pf complex) in 8 patients with
intractable pain. Results of up to 18 months of stimulation revealed good to
excellent control of pain. Undesirable side effects were minimal. The
decreased pain sensibility did not depend on induced paresthesias. Minutes
of stimulation could produce hours of relief.

A survey of the current literature thus shows that it is sometimes possible
to achieve complete control of chornic pain by stimulation through
indwelling electrodes in subcortical structures. At present, it is not clear
what stimulatory sites should be selected for the different types of chronic
pain. While routinely performing stimulation during the course of
stereotactic operations we have found it very difficult to evaluate
spontaneous pain effects. For these reasons we have chosen the strategy
of trying stimulation in several regions of the brain with the aid of
implanted, semi-chronic electrodes before a definite implantation is
performed. Since several electrodes are introduced into the brain it may
be argued that this procedure will increase the risk of bleeding or other
complications. However, this method has been practiced since many years in
patients with epilepsy and it has been demonstrated that serious
complications are rare. Therefore, we consider this approch justified also
in patients with severe chronic pain.

The areas selected for stimulation were the internal capsule and the sensory
thalamic nuclei. A third electrode was implanted in the medial thalamus with
its most distal tip extending into the periaqueductal grey of the
mesencephalon. Finally, a fourth electrode was implanted in the pulvinar.

METHODS AND CLINICAL METERIAL

The stimulating electrodes for temporary implantation were designed similarly
to those used by others both in experimental animal work and in patients. The
electrode material was originally steel, later exchanged for gold or platinum
in order to minimize the possible deposition of toxic metal ions during
stimulation (White and Gross, 1974). The diameter of the electrode wires was
0.1 mm and four or six wires were twisted together so that the overall
dimension of the composite electrode amounted to 0.4 mm. The distance
between the stimulating points was about 4 mm. For permanent implantation a
commercially available electrode stimulator set was used. (Medtronic).

The electrodes were implanted with conventional stereotactic technique using a Leksell instrument. The operations were performed in local anesthesia. In general, the identification of the various target areas was based on the atlas by van Buren and Borke (1972). Stimulation during the operation was only performed in the VPM-VPL nucleus in order to make certain that paresthesias could be produced within the area of pain.

Stimuli were applied between adjacent electrode points, i.e. with an inter electrode distance of about 4 mm. As a rule, the locus and polarity of stimulation were changed daily until all combinations of interconnected stimulating points had been tested. The thresholds for the production of sensory or other effects were monitored in terms of current for each electrode pair. The stimulating electrodes were left in place for about six weeks before a final decision was taken whether or not to perform a permanent implantation. In all, temporary stimulating electrodes have been implanted in five patients (Table I)

TABLE I

INTRACEREBRAL STIMULATION FOR PAIN

CAUSE OF PAIN	DURATION OF PAIN (years)	PREVIOUS TREATMENT	IMPLANTED REGIONS	PAIN RELIEF
BRACH. PLEX. INJURY THALAMIC	7	THALAMOTOMIES TNS	CAPS. INT. PULV. CM. Pf.	DYSESTHESIA REDUCED
POSTENCEPHAL. CENTRAL	3	SYMP. BLOCK. TNS	CAPS. INT. PULV. VPM. CM. Pf.	DYSESTHESIA REDUCED
PHANTOM LIMB	5	SCIAT. NERVE STRANGUL. TNS. DCS.	CAPS. INT. PULV. VPL. CM. Pf. PERIAQUEDUCT GREY	NONE
ATYP. FACIAL ANESTH. DOLOR	3	GANGL. GASS. BLOCK	CAPS. INT. PULV. VPM. CM. Pf.	COMPLETE (VPM. CAPS. INT.)
ATYP. FACIAL ANESTH. DOLOR	5	GANGL. GASS. BLOCK TNS	CAPS. INT. PULV. VPM. CM. Pf. PERIAQUEDUCT GREY	COMPLETE (VPM)

Two patients had pain of central origin. One developed this condition after having undergone thalamotomy for pain caused by a brachial plexus injury. In the other patient the pain was presumably of sequel encephalitis. Their pains were primarily located in the upper half of the body, including the face. The third patient had a phantom limb pain following the amputation of a foot. This patient also suffered from sciatic pain in the same leg, and therefore percutaneous dorsal column stimulation had been tried, but neither of the two pain components were influenced. Finally, there were two patients with atypical facial pain of the anesthesia dolorosa type. In both, the pain was located in the area of the second trigiminal branch and had originally started in connection with operations performed on the maxillar sinus. They had both been treated with several gasserian blockades resulting in a marked facial hypesthesia.

Subjective responses to stimulation.

Stimulation within the sensory nuclei of the thalamus (VPM, VPL) and within the posterior limb of the internal capsule regurlarly produced paresthesias. The thresholds were found to vary considerably in different locations of one and the same structure. The lowest thresholds amounted to 0.15 - 0.30 mA and the highest to 5 - 7 mA. In one of the patients with pain of central origin there was a tendency to a spontaneous decrease of the thresholds for paresthesias during the course of stimulation.

The distribution of the paresthesias varied with the stimulus parameters as well as with the locus stimulated. In particular, pulse duration was found to be critical. Thus, for instance on one occasion increasing the duration from 0.1 ms up to 0.3 ms caused the paresthesias to spread from the hand and the face to the entire half of the body.

Two of the stimulating points of the electrode in the internal capsule were located closer to the anterior limb and stimulating through these produced motor responses in the contralateral face and arm. As appears from fig. 1 the tip pole of the electrode in the internal capsule was located very close to the lateral geniculate body (CGL in the figure). Stimulation applied to this region often caused visual phenomena and one patient reported the apperance of a light spot of bluish-pink-colour.

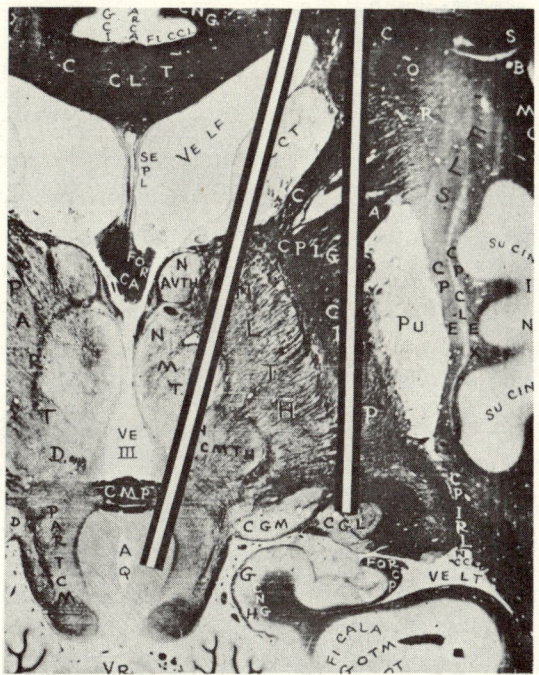

FIG. 1 Reconstruction of electrode tracks in the internal capsule (right) and in the medial part of the thalamus and the periaqueductal grey.(Atlas by Riley, 1960).

Stimulation of the pulvinar and the medial part of the thalamus (CM, Pf) inconsistently produced paresthesias at a higher threshold than when stimulating in VPM or the internal capsule. In two of the patients stimulation of what was supposed to correspond to the upper part of the periaqueductal grey matter was accompanied by diplopia and vertigo, presumably due to activation of the oculomotor nuclei. In one of the patients with facial pain stimulation at low frequencies, around 10 Hz, in the periaqueductal or paraventricular grey matter resulted in a pleasant feeling of warmth in the contralateral half of the face. Increasing the frequency, without changing the current strength, evoked sharp paresthesias in the hand.

Clinical results

Both patients with facial pain have experienced complete alleviation of pain with stimulation in VPM and in the internal capsule. In one of them stimulation in the pulvinar was also effective. The apperance of paresthesias was a prerequisite for obtaining pain relief. One of these patients has had a permanently implanted electrode in VPM since six months. The other one is still under examination with temporary electrodes but is scheduled for permanent implantation in the near future. During the first week of stimulation both patients had to stimulate themselves at least four times a day to obtain pain relief. Later the post-stimulatory pain free period increased in length and the patients can now do with stimulation only twice a day. The pain is felt to subside within about 20 minutes of stimulation and it disappears completely after a further 20 - 30 minutes. The optimal stimulation frequency is between 50 and 100 Hz. In the patient who is still under observation it has been possible to obtain partial relief of facial pain during low frequency stimulation within the periaqueductal grey matter. However, it seems that there is no poststimulatory effect comparable to that obtained with stimulation within the sensory thalamic nucleus.

The two patients with pain of central origin experienced a marked reduction of their dysesthetic, superficial pain component as a result of stimulation in the VPM and the internal capsule. The pain was influenced only in areas which were invaded by the paresthesias. Although the partial relief of the dysesthetic pain was of same benefit to the patient enabling them to use more freely their dysesthetic hand and arm, the overall suffering was not reduced to the extent as to justify permanent electrode implantation. Stimulation at other sites, including the internal capsule, was ineffective. The patient with phantom foot pain did not experience any considerable pain relief apart from short periods of time when there was a feeling of warmth occurring as an off-effect following stimulation in VPL.

Electrophysiological observations

Recording of the electrical activity from the different structures into which the electrodes were inserted was performed in all patients examined. Fig. 2 shows the activity in leads from different depths of CAPS INT, VPM, PULV and CM. The patient was in states of quiet and aroused waking. This pattern of activity in the depth recordings was characteristic for all patients examined. Particularly noteworthy is the high amplitude slow activity from the deepest recording point in the CAPS INT and the spindles of rhythmic 8 c/s activity, most pronounced in the deep parts of PULV and CAPS Int. VPM, on the other hand showed an inconspicuous, low voltage, mixed frequency activity. The arousal reaction in response to eye opening was characterized by desynchronization of the activity and disappearance of the spindles. During the course of the recordings some of the patients had attacks of spontaneous pain. This did not influence the basic patterns of activity.

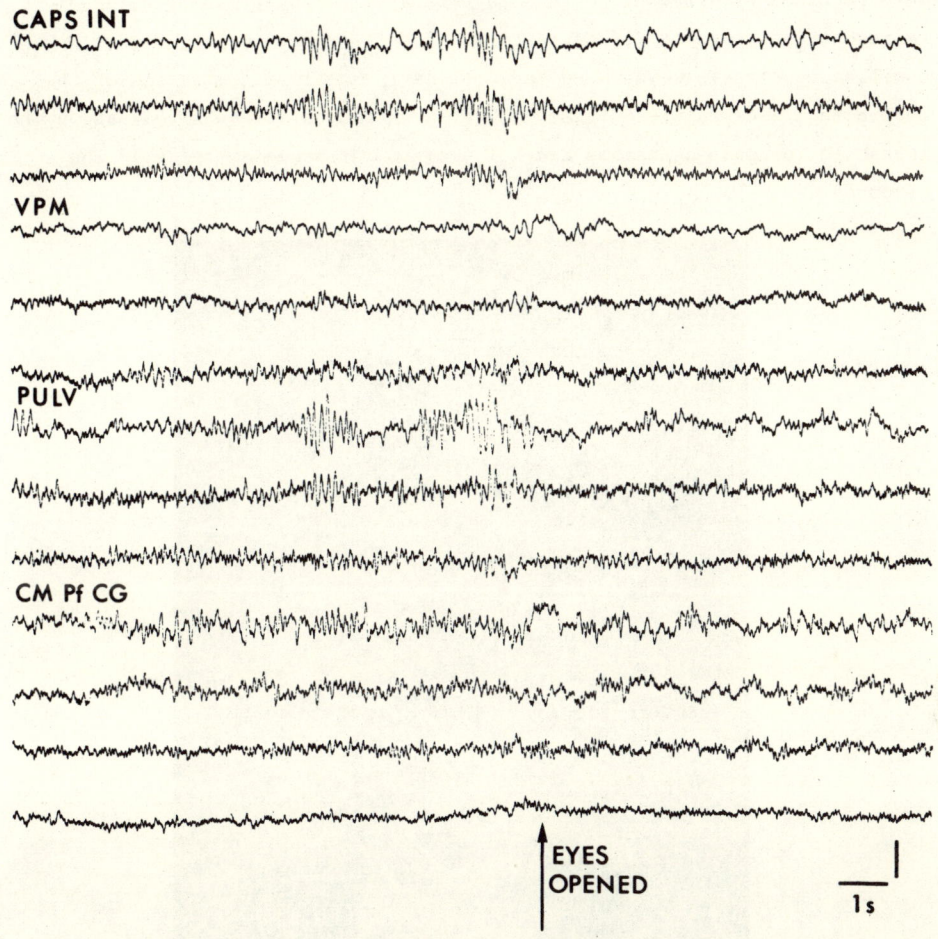

FIG. 2 Spontaneous electrical activity in different subcortical structures (CAPS INT, internal capsule; CM Pf CG, centre median-parafascicularis-central grey complex). Vertical bar denotes 200 μV for the uppermost channel and otherwise 50 μV.

As a means of further checking of the functional localization of the electrode points peripheral stimuli of different modalities (visual, auditory, somatosensory) were delivered and the evoked potentials recorded from the different intracerebral electrodes. In fig. 3 the responses in CI, VPM, Pulv and CG to electrical stimulation of the 3:rd finger on the left hand were recorded with the aid of a data retrieval computer. The records represent the averaged responses to 30 stimuli. A slow sweep of the oscilloscope tracings was used and both early and late components of the responses are demonstrated. Increasing the stimulus strength well above the threshold for pain sensation did not seem to influence appreciably the responses.

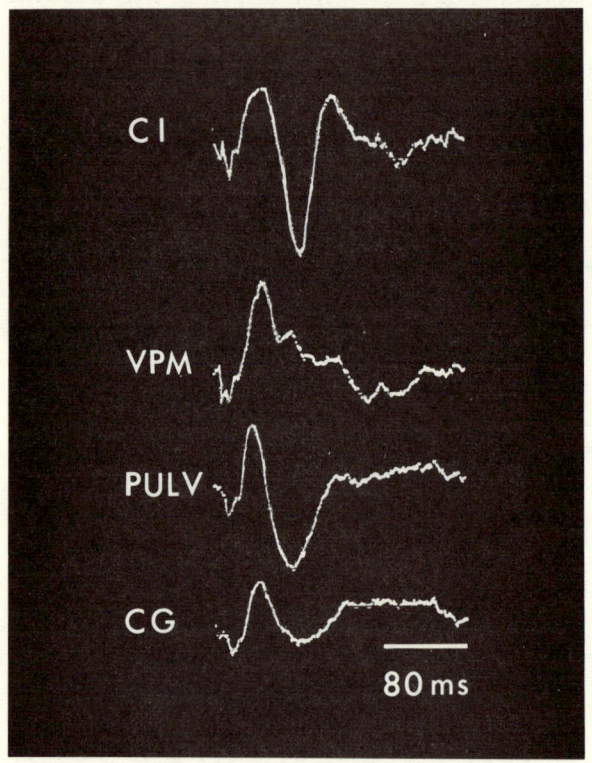

FIG. 3
Somesthetic evoked responses in the internal capsule (CI), VPM, pulvinar (PULV) and centre median (CM). Averaged responses to 30 consecutive stimuli delivered at one per second.

Effects of dorsal column stimulation (DCS) and supraspinal stimulation on somatosensory functions.

In previous studies it was reported that dorsal column stimulation influenced the perception of sensory stimuli applied to the skin (Lindblom and Meyerson 1975 a, 1976). Tactile, vibratory as well as mechanical and thermal pain stimuli were used. During DCS there was, concomitantly with a relief of pain, a considerable increase of the tactile and vibratory thresholds when measured in segments below the implanted spinal electrode. A similar effect on the perceptual magnitude of supraliminal stimuli could also be observed (Lindblom and Meyerson 1975 b). The changes of sensory perception persisted for some time after cessation of the DCS but these effects were short lasting in comparison with the effect on spontaneous pain. A typical example of the changes of vibratory thresholds caused by DCS is showed in fig. 4. There are several reasons to assume that DCS exerts its influence on mechanoceptive functions primarily by producing a central, possibly supraspinal, inhibitory state. It is not probable that blocking of the primary afferents is of prime importance.

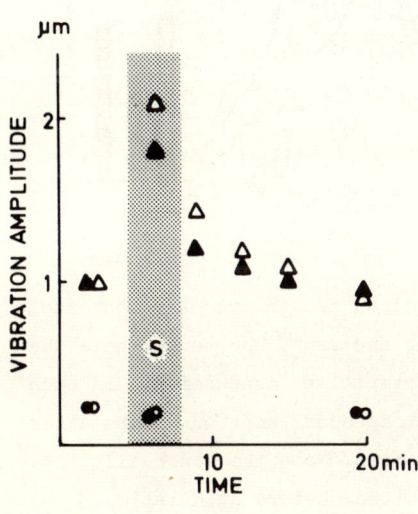

FIG. 4. Effect of dorsal column stimulation at a thoracic site (S) on vibratory thresholds in metatarsal (triangles) and carpal (circles) regions. Filled and open symbols represent right and left side respectively. Note post-stimulatory elevation of the thresholds in the feet. (From Lindblom and Meyerson, 1975 a).

In contrast to the effective suppression of spontaneous pain by DCS, experimental pain induced by mechanical stimuli or heat was uninfluenced when tested within areas of normal skin sensitivity. (Lindblom and Meyerson 1975 a. For methods, see also Frushtorfer et al., this volume). Some of the patients suffered from localized hyperpathia as part of their chronic pain condition and within these skin regions the thresholds for induced pain were abnormally low. As a result of DCS these thresholds increased to a level comparable to that obtained in normal skin areas (fig. 5).

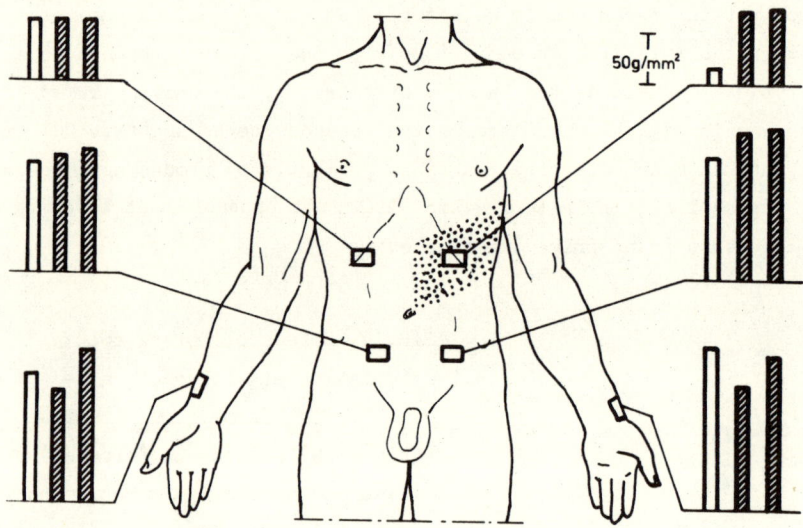

FIG. 5. Effect of dorsal column stimulation on mechanical pain thresholds measured in different regions on the trunc and arms. The bars denote the threshold values obtained during three consecutive measurements in each region, before (open), during (second bar, hatched) and four hours after (third bar, hatched) dorsal column stimulation. Note the abnormally low pain threshold in the area of hyperesthesia (dotted) before stimulation.

This rise in threshold occurred in parallel to the relief of the spontaneous pain. The effect persisted as long as the pain relief, i.e. for about three hours after the stimulator had been shut off. Mechanical and heat pain thresholds were similarly influenced. Thus, it appears that DCS, albeit capable of relieving spontaneous pain, does not influence the experimental skin pain except in areas where there is a disturbance of nociception of a causalgia type.

Some preliminary experiments have now also been performed on patients with intracerebral, stimulating electrodes in order to test whether or not stimulation of higher order neurons in the lemniscal system i.e. the VPM and the internal capsule, has the same effect on somatosensory perception as DCS. So far we have not been able to demonstrate with certainty any such effects. Despite the fact that sensory skin function were tested in areas in which paresthesias were felt during stimulation of the VPM or the internal capsule, the skin thresholds for tactile and vibratory as well as for thermal and mechanical pain stimulation - both inside and outside the area of spontaneous pain - remained unchanged. This was also the case when the intensity of the cerebral stimulation was increased to a level that was just tolerable to the patient. The results were furthermore independent of whether or not the stimulation was effective to relieve the spontaneous pain.

On the other hand, preliminary observations indicate that low frequency stimulation in the periaqueductal grey matter may significantly influence the pain thresholds. Such an experiment is illustrated in figs. 6-8. The mechanical pain threshold was found to increase, sometimes with more than 50% (fig. 6).

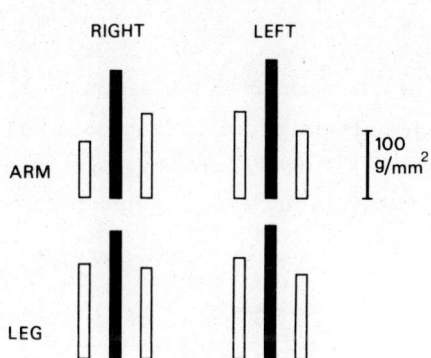

FIG. 6. Threshold values obtained before (first open bars in each group of three), during (second filled bars) and two hours after (third open bar) low frequency stimulation of the periaqueductal grey.

These effects could occur in legs or arms on both sides and persist for many hours. It should be emphasized that the thresholds for vibratory stimuli applied to areas adjacent to those in which pain was tested were not influenced by the stimulation in this experiment.

Periaqueductal stimulation seemed to have an effect also upon thermal nociception both with regard to heat and cold, (for methods, see Fruhstorfer et al., this volume). This effect occurred bilaterally in both arms and legs. The records in fig. 7 illustrate that during right-sided periaqueductal stimulation the patient failed to perceive the "burning" sensation of cold pain whithin the applied temperature range.

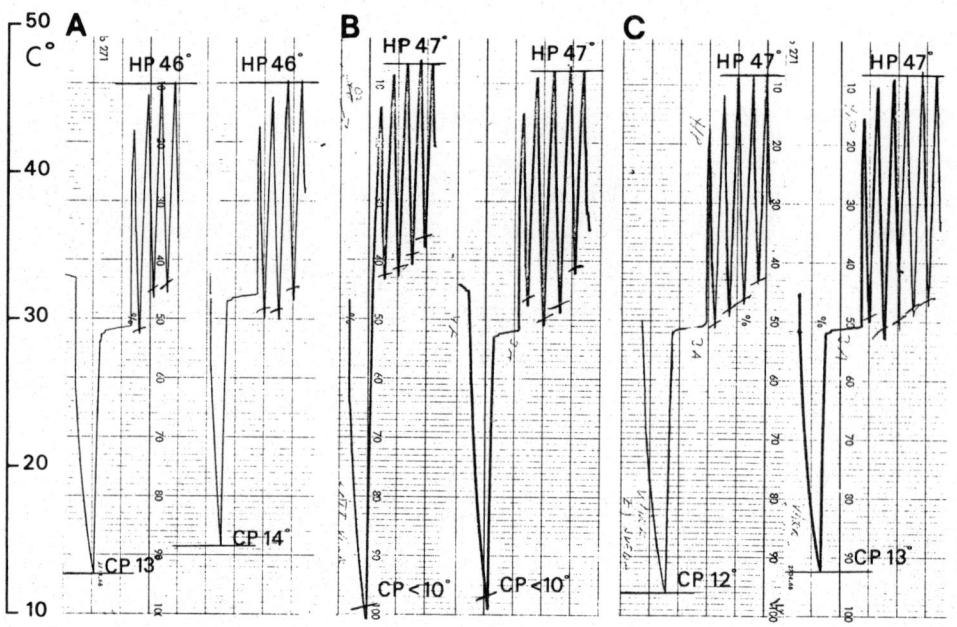

FIG. 7. Effect on cold (CP) and heat pain (HP) thresholds in the hands of right-sided periaqueductal stimulation (low frequency, moderate intensity). A. Control. The first record from the right and the second from the left hand. B. During stimulation. CP was not possible to elicit until well below 10°C. Marginal effect on HP. C. Control after stimulation.

In fig. 8 is shown that when the intensity of stimulation was increased also
the heat pain thresholds were affected. The magnitude of heat pain threshold
increase generally amounted to not more than 2 - 3° but these changes were
highly reproducable and could be demonstrated when measured both on the trunk,
the arms or the legs.

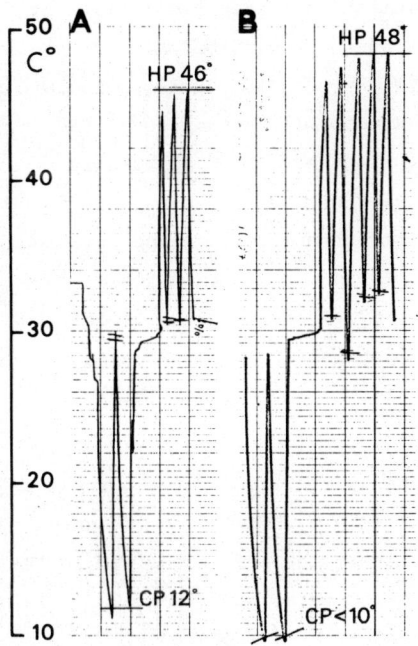

FIG. 8. Effect on cold and heat pain
thresholds (CP, HP) in the hands of
high intensity periaqueductal
stimulation. A, before, and B, during
stimulation with effect on both CP
and HP.

COMMENTS

The finding in the present study that stimulation of the thalamic sensory
nucleus (VPM) can alleviate facial pain (anesthesia dolorosa) confirms earlier
observations by Mazars et al. (1973) and Hosobuchi et al. (1973). In addition,
it seems that such pain may be suppressed by stimulation of the sensory
portion of the internal capsule (Hosobuchi et al. 1974). A prerequisite for
pain relief as a result of stimulation in these structures is the simultaneous
provocation of paresthesias. Also during dorsal column stimulation the
presence of paresthesias is generally necessary to obtain pain relief and it
might be that the same pain inhibitory mechanisms can be activated during
stimulation anywhere along the lemniscal system: the dorsal columns, the
sensory thalamic nucleus and the sensory portion of the internal capsule. This
assumption is further supported by the observation that the time course of
pain relief during and following stimulation is similar in any of these

structures. The intimate association between the sensation of paresthesias and relief of pain seems to indicate that activation of pain suppression mechanisms requires a stimulation intensive enough to evoke cortical excitation (cf. Nashold et al. 1972).

In one of the two patients with facial pain it was possible to obtain pain relief associated with paresthesias by stimulation in the pulvinar. In view of the fact that this thalamic nucleus is not considered to be part of the afferent, somesthetic system the occurrence of paresthesias during stimulation was an unexpected finding. However, there is a possibility that such effects may be evoked by spread of current to neighbouring structures containing somatic, afferent fibres en passage. Very little is known about the functions of the pulvinar but apparently it is of some importance for the appreciation of pain as evidenced by the well-known fact that lesions in this region may alleviate pathological pain similarly to what may be achieved by lesioning parts of the medio-basal thalamic nuclei. To the best of our knowledge, however, it has so far not been reported that also stimulation within the pulvinar may be accompanied by a relief of pain.

It has earlier been reported that DCS can cause an increase of the thresholds for vibration and touch (Lindblom and Meyerson 1975 a). Such effects could not be reproduced during stimulation in the sensory thalamic nuclei or in the internal capsule. This difference may be explained by assuming that DCS activates a larger number of neurons than stimulation of supraspinal structures. On the other hand, intracerebral stimulation of high intensity was tried in an attempt to enlarge the stimulus field but even this stimulation proved ineffective. An alternative explanation would be that the inhibitory effect induced by DCS on sensory threshold function occurs at a subthalamic level and there are experimental indications that such events may take place in the dorsal column nuclei (Brown and Martin 1973).

In one patient stimulation of the periaqueductal grey caused a reduction of the pathological pain. This effect was achieved without any concomitant paresthesias. This observation is in accordance with those made by Richardson and Akil (1974) and Gybels et al. (this volume). Stimulation of the periaqueductal grey also induced an increase of the threshold for experimental pain induced by mechanical or thermal stimuli. The effects of stimulation were not at all of the same magnitude as the very marked hypalgesia found in animals during the same type of stimulation (e.g.

Liebeskind et al. 1973). Also Gybels et al. (this volume) have found that periaqueductal stimulation may influence the appreciation of experimental pain (see also Richardson and Akil 1973). The fact that we found this effect in only one of the two patients who had electrodes implanted in the central grey matter seems to indicate that minor differences in electrode positions may account for considerable differences in the pain blocking effect of stimulation as described in animal experiments (Liebeskind et al. 1973). The periaqueductal grey stimulation had to be kept at a fairly low intensity in order not to provoke nausea and vertigo and it is possible that this low level of stimulation is not sufficient to induce a level of hypalgesia comparable to that obtained in animals.

The study was supported by grants from Karolinska Institutet and from the Swedish Medical Research Council (B75-14X-4505-01 and B75-14X-4256-02).

REFERENCES

Black, P., Cianci, S.N.,and Markowitz, R.F. Alleviation of pain by hypothalamic stimulation in the monkey, Confin Neurol., 34 (1972) 374-381.
Brown, A.G. and Martin, H.F. Activation of descending control of the spinocervical tract by impulses ascending the dorsal columns and relaying through the dorsal column nuclei, J. Physiol. (Lond.) 235 (1973) 535-550.
Cox, V.C.,and Valenstein, E.S. Attenuation of aversive properties of peripheral shock by hypothalamic stimulation, Scince, 149 (1965) 323-325.
Erwin, F.R., Mark, V.H.,and Stevens, J., Behavioral and affective responses to brain stimulation in man, Proc. Amer. psychopath. Ass., 58 (1968) 54-65.
Fruhstorfer, H., Goldberg, M.R., Lindblom, U.,and Schmidt, W., Temperature sensitivity and pain thresholds in patients with peripheral neuropathy. (1976) This volume.
Gol, A., Relief of pain by electrical stimulation of the septal area, J. Neurol. Sci., 5 (1967) 115-120.
Gybels, J., van Hees, J., and Peluso, F., Modulation of experimentally produced pain in man by electrical stimulation of some cortical, thalamic and basal ganglic structures. This volume.
Heath, R.G., and Mickle, W.A., Evaluation of seven years' experience with depth electrode studies in human patients. In E.R.Ramey and D.S. O'Doherty (eds) Electrical Studies of the Unanesthetized Brain, Hoeber New York, 1960, pp. 214-247.
Hosobuchi, Y., Adams, J.E., and Fields, H,L,. Chronic Thalamic and Internal capsular stimulation for the Control of Facial Anesthesia Dolorosa and Dysesthesia of Thalamic Syndrome, Adv. Neurol. 4 (1974) 783-87

Hosobuchi, Y., Adams, J.E., and Rutkin, B., Chronic thalamic stimulation for the control of facial anesthesia dolorosa. Arch. Neurol. 29 (1973) 158-161.

Liebeskind, J., Modulation of pain by central nervous system stimulation. (1976) This volume.

Liebeskind, J. M., Guilbaud, G., Besson, J.-M., and Oliveras, J.-L., Analgesia from electrical stimulation of the periaqueductal grey matter in the cat: behavioral observations and inhibitory effects on spinal cord interneurons, Brain Research, 50 (1973) 441-446.

Lindblom, U., and Meyerson, B.A., Influence on touch, vibration and cutaneous pain of dorsal column stimulation in man, Pain,1 (1975) 257-270.

Lindblom, U., and Meyerson, B.A., Mechanoceptive and nociceptive thresholds during dorsal column stimulation in man. Abstract, First World Congress on Pain, Florence 1975 b p. 201.

Lindblom, U., and Meyerson, B.A. On the Effect of Electrical Stimulation of the Dorsal Column System on Sensory Thresholds in Patients with Chronic Pain. In A. Iggo and O. B. Ilyinsky. (eds.) Progr. Brain Res. 43 (1976) 237-241.

Mayer, D. J., and Liebeskind, J.C., Pain reduction by focal electrical stimulation of the brain: an anatomical and behavioral analysis, Brain Research, 68 (1974) 73-93.

Mayer, D. J., Wolfe, T.L., Akil, H., Carder, B., and Liebeskind, J. C., Analgesia from electrical stimulation in the brainstem of the rat, Science, 174 (1971) 1351-1354.

Mazars, G., Merienne, L. and, Ciolocca, C., Stimulations thalamiques intermittentes antalgiques. Rev. Neurol., 128 (1973) 273-279.

Nashold, B., Somjen, G. and, Friedman, H., Paresthesias and EEG Potentials Evoked by Stimulation of the Dorsal Funiculi in Man. Exper. Neurol. 36 (1972) 273-287.

Reynolds, D. V., Surgery in the rat during electrical analgesia induced by focal brain stimulation, Science 164 (1969) 444-445.

Richardson, D. E. and, Akil, H., Chronic self-administrated brain stimulation for the relief of intractable pain. Abstr. 7th Ann. Meeting Neuro electric. Soc., 1974.

Riley, H. A. An atlas of the basal ganglia, brain stem and spinal cord. Hafner Publ. Comp. N. Y. 1960.

Schmidek, H. H., Fohanno, D., Erwin, F.R., and Sweet, W. H., Pain threshold alterations by brain stimulation in the monkey. J. Neurosurg. 35 (1971) 715-722.

van Buren, J. M., and Borke, R. C., Variations and connections of the Human Thalamus, Springer-Verlag, Berlin Heidelberg New York 1972.

White, R. L., and Gross, T. J., An Evaluation of the Resistance to Electrolysis of Metals for Use in Biostimulation Microprobes, IEEE Trans. Biomed. Engin., 211 (1974) 487-490.

Yunger, L. M., Harvey, J. A., and Lorens, S. A., Dissociation of the analgesic and rewarding effects of brain stimulation in the rat. Physiol. Behav., 10 (1973) 909-913.

Discussion:

Zotterman: I have some recent personal experience about the effect of vibratory stimulation of the skin on chronic pain. After fracturing my left radial bone I had for several weeks chronic pain in my left hand. This pain disappeared when I tapped with my right long finger on the plaster bandage for half a minute or so. The most remarkable phenomenon, however, was that the relief of pain outlasted the tapping for several minutes. This is most interesting because it raises the question of what is really happening after the stimulation comes to an end. What causes the relief of pain for such a long time after stimulation? Does the mechanical stimulation set up a long lasting state of an inhibitory potential or a circuit or is the inhibition of the pain due to an accumulation of an inhibitory transmitter which will outlast the mechanical stimulation for long periods?

Meyerson: May I add that this long lasting stimulus effect has been observed for a long time. There is also a tendency that its duration increases. It is also apparent in these experimental situations where we have tested thresholds within areas of hyperalgesia when we managed to abolish the hyperalgesic state during several hours after dorsal cord stimulation.

Franzén: Do you have an idea how large the field is that you cover with your electrode? It is quite an area that you are stimulating, maybe.

Meyerson: It is very difficult to say anything about this. Since it is a bipolar stimulation between these two adjacent stimulating points, I think it is fairly restriced but I cannot state it in terms of quantitative measurements.

Gybels: I have two very short questions. One, what was the sensation when you stimulated VPL in the patient with anaesthesia dolorosa during the stimulation of CPM? Two, the threshold measurements you made with the periaqueductal stimulation were they made while the patient was having a heat sensation?

Meyerson: Stimulation within the essential thalamic nuclei in the two anaesthesia dolorosa patients produced paraesthesias involving primarily the aching face sometimes extending out into the arm. That very much depended upon an interplay between the intensity of stimulation and the duration. The threshold for inducing warmth was about **1 or 1.5 milliamp.**

Gybels: That was not my question. The threshold measurements you showed were made three days ago. Were they made while the stimulating electrode in the periductal gray produced a heat sensation or not?

Meyerson: Yes, it did. There was a subjective feeling.

Zimmermann: You reported the long term effect of the dorsal column stimulation on the mechanical pain threshold in the algesic skin. Did you also make similar observations on the vibratactile threshold?

Meyerson: Yes, we did. The poststimulatory effect after electrical and tactile stimulation, I mean the increase of threshold did not last more than a maximum of fifteen minutes. It was usually five, ten, or fifteen minutes. It was not at all of the same order of magnitude that could be observed with the abolishment of hyperalgesia.

Zimmermann: Was the column stimulation different in effectiveness as regard to vibratactile and pain threshold?

Meyerson: With regard to the time course, yes.

Landgren: My point is relevant to the possible explanations of the long lasting effects of these stimuli. I would suggest that tetanic stimulations will make synchronervous factors more effective in a way similar to that which Bliss et alia have shown for hippocampus where you can show certain synapses being passivitated for hours by repeated stimulation. One can make hypothesis that central synchronervous activation could evoke long lasting phenomena that could explain this.

Zotterman: The question is what is happening in the neurons in the spinal cord when the response lasts for hours after the cessation of the stimulation. Can it be metabolic changes of any kind or accumulation of any special inhibitory substances? There cannot be any lesion so it must be either accumulation of inhibitory substance or some oscillating or reverberating circuit. Could such a circuit go on as long as two hours?

Landgren: Posttetanic potentiation of synaptic activity can last that long.

Hagbarth: Either it is chemical substances accumulating somewhere or post-tetanic potentiation or reverberating circuits operating somewhere it is hard to explain the very sudden return of pain that sometimes occurs following a long period of pain relief. Following TNS-stimulation or sympathectomy you can have a long period of pain relief for perhaps weeks and then suddenly one day at a certain moment the pain comes back again. It is not always a gradual return. That's rather difficult to explain both in terms of chemical substances and reverberating circuits.

Zotterman: Yes, this is a great problem which we must attack.

Sjölund: I would like to ask about the induction time for algesia. Was there a difference when you induced an algesia because on dorsal column stimulation the onset is rather sudden? You get it very soon after you start stimulating. How long did it take?

Meyerson: I cannot say precisely but it very much followed in parallel with the relief of the spontaneous pain. That differs from case to case. In some cases the effect is rather instantaneous and just takes five minutes or something like that. In other cases we had to wait for ten or fifteen minutes before the patient could experience any considerable relief of pain. They had to wait still longer to get complete relief. It has been very difficult to follow the time course precisely because you miss it many times while testing and so on.

Sjölund: I meant the increase in pain threshold when you stimulate periaqueductal gray.

Meyerson: In the periaqueductal gray it happened rather soon, about ten minutes or so.

ACTIVATION PATTERNS INDUCED IN THE DOMINANT HEMISPHERE BY SKIN STIMULATION

D. H. INGVAR, I. ROSÉN, M. ERIKSSON, and D. ELMQVIST

Department of Clinical Neurophysiology, University Hospital, Lund, Sweden

INTRODUCTION

The cerebral events which accompany perception of cutaneous and other sensory stimuli still remain by and large unknown. Studies of evoked potentials, the CNV response, as well as various EEG reactions, have shown that specific and unspecific components of afferent volleys have different distribution on the scalp, and furthermore, that certain electrical events correlate not only to the intensity of the stimulation but also to the level of wakefulness and to psychological factors like expectation or preparedness.

Findings made with electrophysiological techniques are, however, often difficult to interpret, and they cannot be translated into mass activity terms or into psychophysiological concepts. It is for example not possible to say with certainty that an increase of a potential amplitude signals involvement of more neurons, i.e. demonstrate an increase of the metabolic "work" of the brain - or an increase of the perceptual qualities of the stimulus. One further major drawback of the electrophysiological techniques is their limited capacity for studies of the distribution of function in the brain.

In the present paper we summarize measurements of the regional cerebral blood flow in man during skin stimulation. We have used ^{133}Xenon technique to measure the blood flow in 32 regions simultaneously in order to study the distribution of cerebral function. This is possible since, normally, the blood flow of the brain is controlled directly by the metabolic activity$_1$of the active neurons themselves (cf. Ingvar and Lassen 1975) .

In the measurements to be summarized below we have studied the effects of electrical stimulation of the right thumb region upon the blood flow in the left hemisphere. Two intensities were used corresponding to touch and slight pain.

MATERIAL AND METHODS

Details of the investigations will be given elsewhere[2, 3, 4]. The clinical material included three groups, 1/ neurologically normal patients (studied for suspicion of organic dementia or other psychiatric disorders), 2/ patients with diffuse or focal brain lesions, and 3/ patients with chronic schizophrenia. The rCBF measurements were made as a part of routine clinical investigations. The ^{133}Xenon technique implies the injection into the internal carotid artery of a small saline bolus in which 3-5 mCi of the isotope is physically dissolved. The uptake and clearance of the gamma-emitting isotope is recorded with a 32 detector device placed at the lateral side of the patient's head. By means of a computer, flow parameters are calculated for each detector field (central distance about 25 mm). In the present context, the main emphasis will be given to the f_{init} parameter which is calculated from the initial part of the clearance curve and which is mainly determined by the flow of the grey matter of the lateral surface of the hemisphere. Controls of the arterial pCO_2 and the blood pressure was made at each measurement.

The rCBF distributions were plotted as topographical charts in which the hemisphere mean flow was used as reference. The detector fields were localized with small lead markers upon a lateral skull X-ray of the patient's head from which a hemisphere outline was drawn.

In the present studies, three rCBF measurements were made in each patient: A/ at rest with closed eyes and with silence in the laboratory, B/ during weak electrical stimulation of the right thumb region with an intensity just above threshold, C/ during intense stimulation, about 4 times the threshold, at which the patient experienced definite discomfort or slight pain. Finally, D/ another rest study was made in most cases.

As will be shown in a forthcoming publication[3] the present technique enables quantitative analysis of cerebral events related to perception (and to consciousness) in patients with severe brain lesions.

In patients unable to communicate perceptual and discomfort thresholds, electroneurography and cortical evoked potential studies were made with identical stimulation parameters as those during the rCBF study in order to acertain a normal afferent conduction.

In the following, the results from the neurologically and psychiatrically normal patients will be emphasized. In the discussion, some pertinent findings in patients with focal brain lesions and with chronic schizophrenia will also be taken up.

RESULTS

In Table 1, the mean hemisphere blood flow values are given for the 8 neurologically and mentally normal patients.

It is seen that there was no change of the respiration (as reflected in the mean arterial pCO_2) during resting, and the two stimulation conditions (sens I and sens II). During high intensity stimulation there was a slight increase (ns) of the blood pressure.

The mean hemisphere blood flow values increased slightly during touch and significantly during pain. This increase was mainly confined to the parameters pertaining to the grey matter (f_{init}, f_{10} and f_g). The flow of the white matter, f_w, and g % remained essentially uninfluenced.

In Figure 1, the distribution of the flow values at rest and during touch and pain are shown. It is seen that at rest the normal "hyperfrontal" distribution was found with a high flow (function) anterior to the rolandic and sylvian fissure and low

Table 1.

n = 8, Age: 57 (42-68), Sex: 4 m /4 f

	BP	pCO_2	f_{init}	f_{10}	f_g	f_w	g %	$CMRO_2$
REST I	141 12	35.7 2	48.5 13	43.2 9	68.8 15	20.0 4	46.1 3	2.47 0.4 n = 5
SENS I	142 12 n = 7	36.3 4	50.8 12	45.1 8	70.6 15	18.4 4	44.9 3	2.52 0.3 n = 5
SENS II	149 17 n = 7	36.3 2 n = 7	54.7 15 n = 7	46.3 10 n = 7	76.6 20 n = 7	18.3 5 n = 7	42.1 5 n = 7	2.99 0.4 n = 5
REST II	152 9 n = 7	36.8 4 n = 6	54.9 11 n = 7	48.3 4 n = 3	81.0 9 n = 3	21.0 4 n = 3	44.3 3 n = 3	2.54 0.7 n = 2
Test of significance								
REST I/ SENS I	p<ns	ns	ns	ns	ns	ns	ns	ns
REST I/ SENS II	p<ns	ns	0.02	0.02	0.05	ns	ns	p 0.02
REST I/ REST II	p<ns	ns	ns					

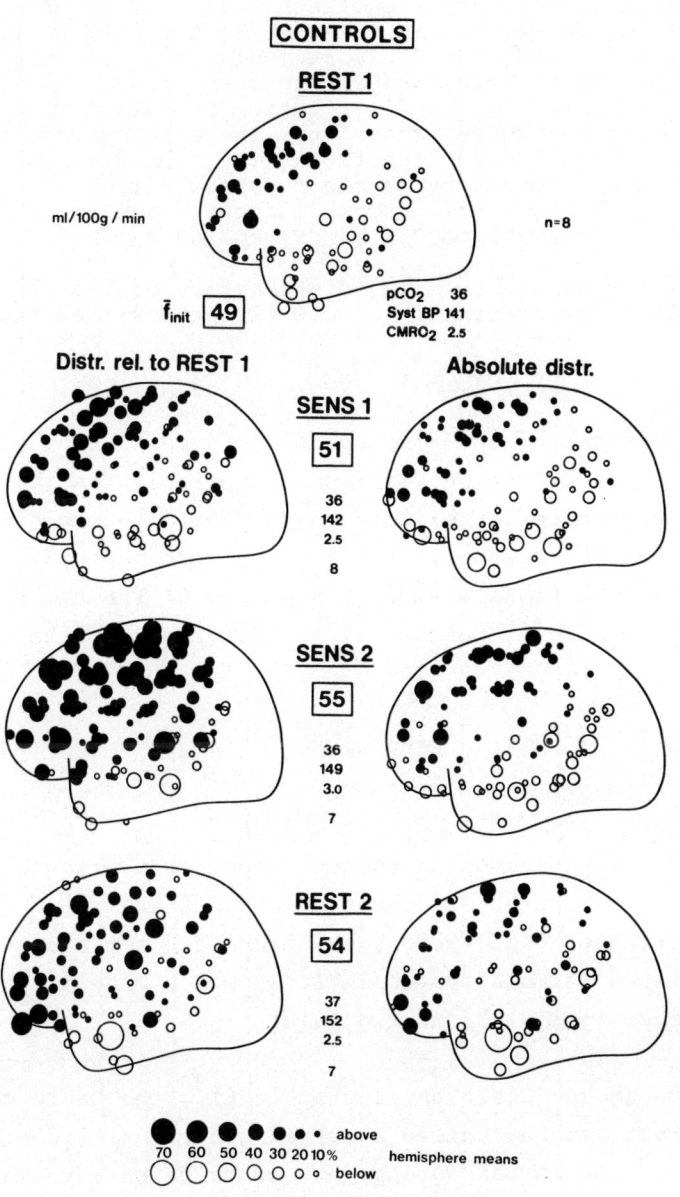

Figure 1. <u>Effects of skin stimulation of the right hand upon
the blood flow and its distribution in the left hemisphere.</u>
Eight neurologically normal patients were studied. The flow
distributions are plotted in relation to the hemisphere means
according to the scale at the bottom of the figure. In the right
row the absolute distribution at the respective levels are
shown. In the left row the distribution in relation to the
rest I conditions. There is a slight increase during touch
stimulation (sens I) and significant increase during pain
(sens II). The cerebral hyperemia remained during a second resting study (rest II). During sens II there was also an increase
of the $CMRO_2$ (from 2.5 to 3.0 ml oxygen/100 g/min.).

Note finally that the relative distribution of the flow (right
row) remained "hyperfrontal" in all situations. See text.

flows in postcentral and temporal structures. During both touch
and pain the distribution remained essentially the same if the
plottings were made in relation to the absolute new hemisphere
mean flow values. However, if the plots were made relative to
the resting conditions a general increase of the hemisphere
flow was seen also in postcentral structures, especially during
pain.

During the final resting rCBF study, a remaining moderate cerebral hyperemia was usually found.

Measurement of the cerebral oxygen uptake from arterial blood
samples and from cerebral venous samples taken from the jugular
bulb demonstrated that the oxygen uptake did not change between
rest and touch stimulation while it showed a moderate significant increase ($p < 0.02$) during pain.

In the coma group (Rosén and Ingvar 1976)[3], the basic conditions at rest usually showed a marked general flow decrease.
Skin stimulation in this group gave no reactions in the cases
with very deep coma caused by massive diffuse cortical lesions,
and various deviating patterns, including cerebral vasoconstric-
tions in the remainder of the patients.

In chronic schizophrenia the rCBF effects of skin stimulation were less pronounced than in the mentally normal patients. The difference between the normals and the schizophrenics were in many respects significant[4] (cf. Franzén and Ingvar 1975).

DISCUSSION

Other types of cerebral activation such as voluntary motor activity, speech, reading and psychological testing give rise to activity patterns which differ from those evoked by skin stimulation. Thus, voluntary motor activity causes a localized increase of function in the rolandic region, often with an emphasis of postcentral regions, speech and reading involves large parts of the rolandic regions, as well as premotor and posterior sylvian ones[1].

In the present context it should be emphasized that touch did not essentially change the resting pattern of the normal (conscious) dominant hemisphere. The flow distribution remained "hyperfrontal" and the cerebral oxygen uptake was not altered.

In contrast, higher intensity stimulation augmented the blood flow significantly in the grey matter. This increase was widespread, but, when plotted relative to the new high hemisphere mean, a "hyperfrontal" distribution was definitely retained. The oxygen consumption of the hemisphere showed a slight increase in this situation.

It is of interest that in the rest study following intense stimulation, the cerebral blood flow remained high, while the oxygen consumption again showed lower values. This indicates that even slight pain may induced long standing effects upon the cerebral blood flow, possibly caused by tissue lactacidosis.

The touch-pain rCBF pattern thus highly ressembled the resting blood flow pattern. It was also very similar to the one recorded during problem solving[6,7]. One gets the impression that the brain may attain various "levels" of consciousness,

the lowest represented by the resting condition awake without
any form of induced problem solving or increase of the sensory
input. The next level can be represented by low intensity skin
stimulation (touch). Finally, there are the two higher levels
of problem solving and pain which both, like the two first
mentioned, show a "hyperfrontal" distribution of the blood
flow.

We have previously interpreted the hyperfrontal flow distribution as signalling a relatively high degree of activity in
efferent structures located in the prerolandic and frontal
parts of the brain. Apparently, these regions are continuously
active with synthetizing an adequate behavior for the organism.
This synthesis becomes even more marked when the sensory input
is augmented, when mental problems are presented to the brain
and, especially, when the individual is perceiving pain. The
common denominator of all these four stages would thus seem to
be a "problem solving" mode of cerebral activity which, as it
seems, is mainly located to precentral and frontal structures.

It should be added that occasionally we observed a diminution
of the flow during high intensity skin stimulation. This could
have been due to cerebral vasoconstriction since the flow
diminution was general and there was no respiratory changes
which could have explained it. Findings of this type indicate
that the cerebral blood flow reaction to pain may contain two
or more components of which, under normal conditions, the increase due to cerebral vasodilatation appears to dominate.

Finally, the sensory rCBF patterns described above may be compared with the one induced by voluntary motor activity. As
mentioned, the motor pattern is characterized by a marked peak
of activity in the rolandic region with a diminution of the
flow in frontal parts. The sensory patterns, on the other hand,
all showed a "hyperfrontal" distribution. This difference
appears at first to be paradoxical, viz. the voluntary motor
activity activates brain regions posterior to those activated

by an augmented sensory input. Elsewhere the phenomenon has been termed "the sensory-motor paradox" [7]. This finding which requires closer study with techniques permitting better localization, indicates, in general, that the "brain work" carried out during motor activity is to a large extent confined to postcentral structures activated by the feed back control of the movement in question. Contrarywise, the brain work caused by cutaneous sensory perception, especially by perception of pain, is to a major extent carried out by premotor and frontal brain structures in which the behavioral responses to the perceived stimulation are synthetized.

Acknowledgements: Aided by grants from the Swedish Medical Research Council (project nr B75-14X-84-11C), from the Wallenberg and the Thuring Foundations, Stockholm.

REFERENCES

1. Ingvar, D.H. and Lassen, N.A., (eds.), Brain Work, Munksgaard, Copenhagen, 1975.
2. Ingvar, D.H., Rosén, I. and Elmqvist, D., To be published, 1976.
3. Rosén, I. and Ingvar, D.H., To be published, 1976.
4. Ingvar, D.H., Franzén, G. and Rosén, I., To be published, 1976.
5. Franzén, G. and Ingvar, D.H., J. Neurol. Neurosurg. Psychiat. 38, 1027-1032, 1975.
6. Risberg, J. and Ingvar, D.H., Brain, 96, 737-756, 1973.
7. Ingvar, D.H., In: Brain Work, Ingvar, D.H. and Lassen, N.A. (eds.), Munksgaard, Copenhagen, 1975, pp. 397-413.

Discussion:

Hyvärinen: I was very happy to see the confirmation of the sensory-motor paradox with studies of circulation in cortical regions in man. In electrophysiological experiments in moving, non-anaesthetized monkeys we have observed a similar phenomenon that has puzzled us and caused doubts among some sensory physiologists to whom we have presented it. We performed experiments on monkey subjects in which the correct detection of a cutaneous vibratory stimulus was alternately made relevant and irrelevant for obtaining juice reward. A separate light signal turned on before the trials signalled whether the detection of the stimulus was going to be rewarded or not. Under the relevant condition the monkeys appeared attentive to the stimuli but they were quite inattentive during the irrelevant trials. During the performance of this task we recorded cellular activity in the sensory and motor cortices.

We found little effect of attention in the postcentral cortex but a considerable enhancement of the sensory responses during the relevant situation in the motor cortex. (Compare figure 3 from S I with figure 6 from motor cortex in Hyvärinen et al "The Neurosciences. Third Study Program", Eds F. O. Schmitt and F.G. Worden, MIT Press, Cambridge, Mass. 1974, pp. 311-317). Later work in our laboratory has confirmed this finding (Poranen, A., In preparation) in the type of task mentioned above.

Ingvar: Yes there are many things that we would like to do but there are certain very great limitations here.

Granit: What do you mean by a simple movement? Opening and closing the hand, according to Duchenne, who describes this in great detail, are exceedingly complex sequences of action and inhibition of individual muscles. A really simple movement should be used.

Ingvar: We will try to do this but we have not had access to the machine with the high resolution yet. But I agree with you that even this is a very complex thing. When I mean simple it is not involving a problem as such because when I do this I can even talk to Professor Granit. I do not have to play a little melody. There is no problem.

Franzén: You mentioned that schizophrenic patients showed a lowering of activity following the tactile stimulation or electrical stimulation. How is it if you record a primary cortical potential?

Ingvar: We do not know. There is some work done on evoked potentials done on schizophrenics which is in line with these findings but we have not done it yet.

Franzén: What happened with the right hemisphere?

Ingvar: It is okay I can assure you.

von Euler: What about the lateralisation?

Ingvar: I can answer that. They have done bilateral studies in Israel with this technique and it turns out that you can activate the right hemisphere with music. Non-verbal stimulation activates the right hemisphere more than verbal. This has also been done with an inhalation technique by Risberg in Lund.

Perl: I want to ask Dr Ingvar two questions. One is: you injected all of your substances, as I understood it, into the carotid artery. And it is known that there is a differential distribution of blood flow not only to the brain stem but in part to the cerebrum according to some sort of laminar flow within the basilar and the internal carotid artery distribution. And I wondered what effect that might have upon the relative distribution of effects you described. The second is: you seemed to have rather consistent results but I wondered what kinds of control you had on the flow patterns after the effect.

Ingvar: The first question about the carotid distribution is indeed as you say that the distribution of an isotope is different in different patients depending upon the development of their cerebral-vascular tree. However, we are only measuring the tissue which receives isotopes and the method is independent of how much isotope comes in. It is the rate change once the isotope has gotten there that counts. And that is why we are so fortunate that we do not have to pay attention to the exact distribution of the bolus pools. But I agree that we measure only tissue that gets isotope of course.

It is another fortunate anatomical fact that the carotid system does perfuse the cortical mantle of the hemisphere. And this is the part that we see best with our method. So what we are looking at in this chart is in fact the distribution of activity in the cortex. The deepest tracks are not seen so well due to the internal absorption of this type of isotope so it is the cortical mantle. The controls proved to present a difficulty. But as I thought I showed to you the resulting distributions which you get under controlled conditions, silence, pads over the eyes, etc. is very consistent in relative terms. People may be at slightly different levels but neurologically normal, mentally normal. Really they give very consistent results.

If, Mr Chairman, I may make a comment myself on the implications of our findings for the type of studies that I have been listening to here for three days I would put in a word of caution. I think we have not quite realized how much we do change the cerebral activity in our subjects simply by talking to them. Simply by inducing an idea or a concept. So I think that you - the circulatory people and the more neurophysiologically oriented people - have to be extremely careful about what we tell the patients because the whole landscape might be changing by telling the patient something which will lead to the formation of new concepts.

Zotterman: It would be very interesting to see what happens when you have lost all sensations in your right arm for instance. You try to move it but you cannot. Normally an enormous afferent inflow occurs from the active arm. The questions are, will the "intention" of moving that arm be enough to induce an increased bloodflow in the actual parts of the cortex or is it afferent inflow induced by moving the limb which is responsible for the local cerebral vascular reaction? And finally I want to remind you that Pavlov conceived the cortical motor area as a sensory proprioceptive area.

EVIDENCE PERTAINING TO AN ENDOGENOUS MECHANISM OF PAIN INHIBITION IN THE CENTRAL NERVOUS SYSTEM

J. C. LIEBESKIND, G. J. GIESLER, Jr., and G. URCA

Department of Psychology, UCLA, Los Angeles, California 90024, U.S.A.

Since Reynolds (1) first reported that abdominal surgery could be performed without apparent discomfort during electrical stimulation of the midbrain central or periaqueductal gray matter (PAG) in the unanesthetized rat, a considerable literature has rapidly developed reinforcing and extending his original observation. The efficacy of stimulation-produced analgesia (SPA) has been demonstrated in the cat (2 - 5) and monkey (6) as well as the rat (e.g., 7), and information is now available from Richardson and Akil (8) and more recently from J. E. Adams (personal communication) that chronic, clinical pain states in addition to normal pain appreciation can be blocked with electrical stimulation in homologous medial brain stem regions in man. Evidence for SPA has been obtained employing a wide variety of nociceptive stimuli including pinprick, noxious heat or cold, strong pinch, electric shock applied to the skin, peripheral nerves, and the dental pulp, and the injection of chemical irritants into cutaneous or visceral tissues (for references, c.f., 9). In the rat, SPA has been found equi-analgesic to morphine in doses ranging from 10 - 50 mg/kg depending on the analgesic test employed and the intensity and duration of the central stimulating current (10). Using pinches of the limbs or tail, for example, complete inhibition of all nociceptive manifestations can be shown with PAG stimulation no matter what force of pinch is applied (7, 10). To obtain a comparable degree of pain inhibition with morphine, a dose sufficient to produce considerable ataxia and rigidity of the limbs (50 mg/kg) is required (10). Additional evidence for the exceptional potency of SPA is the fact that it readily yields suppression of even spinally mediated nociceptive reflexes (e.g., rat tail-flick test), reflexes known to be resistant to all but narcotic analgesic drugs (11).

SPA may manifest itself after only a few seconds of intermittent stimulation and then may endure for many minutes or even hours after stimulation is terminated (7, 10). In the rat, considerable variation in the time course of SPA is seen; and although the problem has yet to be systematically investigated, no obvious correlation between SPA duration and exact locus of the stimulating electrode has been noted. In the cat and monkey (2 - 6), the post-stimulation duration of analgesia is generally shorter than in the rat. Fortunately, relief from chronic pain in man has been seen to outlast the period of central stimulation by up to 24 hours (8 and Adams, personal communication). Although extensive clinical tests are still needed, this feature of SPA encourages the belief that brain stem stimulation may soon become a major weapon in the neurosurgeon's armamentarium of techniques for the treatment of intractable pain states in man.

An important consideration is the specificity of the analgesic effect of brain stimulation. For example, SPA might be regarded as merely a side effect of intense activation of central motivational or motor systems. In the rat, however, reliable and potent SPA has been found at electrode sites yielding reward (self-stimulation) and aversion (escape) as well as at sites of apparently neutral motivational sign (7, 10). At the same time we have failed to find SPA in other rewarding or aversive brain regions, for example, lateral hypothalamus and septal area (7, 10), locus coeruleus (J. M. Liebman, personal communication), ventrobasal thalamus and midbrain reticular formation (7, 10). Even at sites yielding both SPA and self-stimulation (for example, the ventral, caudal PAG), the two phenomena can be pharmacologically dissociated (c.f., 12 - 14). Moreover, in a recent report Basbaum et al. (15) showed that restricted spinal cord lesions can eliminate SPA without affecting the rewarding properties of brain stimulation.

In some rats and cats SPA is seen in association with various motor manifestations, but in others there is no indication from merely observing the animal that the stimulating current is on. Even when stimulation-elicited behaviors are apparent, they invariably terminate with the offset of stimulation, whereas analgesia typically persists (7). In a careful study in the monkey recently reported by Goodman and Holcombe (6), a "therapeutic index" was calculated for each stimulation site as a function of the ratio of the current thresholds for motor side effects to the thresholds for analgesia. An index greater than 1.0 reflected the attainment of significant analgesia at current levels below those producing motor signs. Fifteen of 40 electrode placements in this study yielded a therapeutic index greater than 1.0, one placement giving an index of 12.0. The best placements were found in PAG and neighboring medial brain stem loci. The value of this approach for ultimate clinical applications should be evident.

SPA has been most frequently observed with electrodes placed in the PAG. This structure is known to receive an important contribution of fibers from the anterolateral quadrant of the cord (16, 17). In fact, it has been recently shown with the horseradish peroxidase technique that PAG receives afferents from laminae in the dorsal horn known to contain cells uniquely or differentially responsive to noxious stimuli (D. L. Trevino, personal communication). The role of the PAG in nociception has also been suggested by electrophysiological recording and stimulation studies (18 - 20). It might reasonably be suggested, therefore, that SPA results from a functional lesion of this area or the temporary disruption of the pain message at this level. This interpretation is not supported, however, by other findings. For example, we failed to show any evident reduction in the response to noxious footshock following electrolytic destruction of even wide portions of the PAG in the rat (21), a finding also recently reported by Bevan and Pert (22). Reversible lesions of this area by microinjections of a local anesthetic have also been found not to increase pain threshold (23); and, in fact, both Huprich (24) and Rhodes (25) in our laboratory have found that rats with caudal PAG lesions are actually hyperreactive to noxious stimuli. Rather than SPA being attributable to disruption of nociceptive transmission locally in the PAG, it has since our first work with the phenomenon (7) seemed more likely to us that it works by <u>activating</u> a natural or endogenous pain inhibitory mechanism in the PAG which serves to block pain transmission elsewhere in the nervous system. More evidence related to this important matter will be detailed below.

SPA from some sites is accompanied by a certain amount of cortical spiking (25), but this is not true for sites in the caudal PAG (25); and in general, there is a negative correlation between the elicitation of electrographic or motor seizure activity and the occurrence of SPA (10, 25). SPA is not specifically associated with either evident drowsiness or arousal, nor is it accompanied by obvious deficits in other sense modalities (7). In fact, in both the rat and the cat, SPA is sometimes seen at the same time that the animal manifests hyper-responsiveness to light touch (2, 7). Moreover, in the cat SPA has been shown to block selectively the jaw opening reflex to noxious dental pulp stimulation without affecting a similar response elicited by innocuous tooth tap (26). One of SPA's most striking features is the fact that its peripheral distribution is frequently limited to one or two limbs or the tail or head (7, 10, 27). This finding has been more reliably made in the rat than in the cat or monkey (3, 6), and it is more evident with stimulation sites in caudal PAG (10) than with more rostral placements (25). Seeing analgesia on one limb but at the same time not on another makes it difficult to believe that SPA will ever be found attributable to a non-specific mechanism.

Electrophysiological evidence of SPA's selective effect on nociceptive mechanisms is gradually being accumulated. Stimulation in the vicinity of the dorsal raphe nucleus in the ventral, caudal PAG of the cat, shown to elicit behavioral analgesia in the awake animal, was also found to suppress the responding of wide dynamic range (lamina 5-type) interneurons in the dorsal horn of the spinal cord evoked by noxious peripheral stimuli without similarly affecting the responses of some of these cells to innocuous inputs and without affecting the responses of lamina 4-type cells to light tactile stimuli (2, 3). A similar specificity has been recently reported by Morrow and Casey (28) who found that PAG stimulation in the rat preferentially blocked bulboreticular neurons responding to noxious inputs. Oleson and Liebeskind (29), studying evoked potentials and multiple unit activity in various mesencephalic and diencephalic areas, found that responses evoked in the PAG and in the medial and ventrobasal thalamus by noxious footshock were markedly attenuated by SPA, whereas responses in these same areas evoked by innocuous air puffs were either unaffected or actually enhanced. Findings such as these not only indicate the selectivity of SPA's action on nociceptive mechanisms but also suggest that SPA's suppressive effects, whether occurring primarily in the spinal cord or simulataneously at higher levels as well, do in any case involve sensory neural elements participating in central processes of pain perception.

The initial work with SPA concentrated on the effects of stimulation within the caudal PAG. However, the phenomenon of SPA is by no means limited to stimulation sites in this area. Scattered placements in the medial diencephalon were found to produce good analgesia in our earliest studies (7, 10). A more detailed mapping of this region was recently completed by Rhodes (25) who found the most consistent and powerful effects throughout a medial system extending from rostral PAG and the pretectal region just ahead of it into the periventricular regions of the caudal thalamus and the posterior hypothalamic area. The pretectal area and the gray matter surrounding the third ventricle also yield excellent analgesia in the monkey (6) and in man (8, Adams, personal communication). High therapeutic index scores were obtained at this level in the monkey, and stimulation here in man is said to be without the annoying side effects that are sometimes found with stimulation in the PAG (8). In the cat, midbrain stimulation sites other than those in the immediate vicinity of the dorsal raphe nucleus in ventral, caudal PAG give powerful aversive and motor reactions (2, 3, 5). This fact coupled with the short post-stimulation duration of SPA in this species has precluded adequate testing of much of this region. On the other hand, still more caudal placements in the area of the nucleus raphe magnus of the cat (30) and the rat (31, 32) have been found very effective in eliciting SPA. It thus appears that a large portion of the medial brain stem, extending from at least the level of the rostral medulla to the level of the caudal diencephalon, participates in this pain inhibitory function. However, the ultimate boundaries of this system have, no doubt, yet to be disclosed.

The medial brain stem analgesia system just described has been found to contain both ascending and descending monoamine-containing axons and cell bodies, including principally serotonin (33, 34) and the catecholamines, dopamine and noradrenaline (35, 36). Immunohistochemical evidence for the existence of adrenaline-containing axons (37) as well as axons containing substance P (38) has also recently been discovered. The serotonin-containing midbrain raphe nuclei are known to project primarily in a rostral direction, whereas the hindbrain raphe nuclei are known to send their serotonin-containing axons into the spinal cord (33, 34). In fact, according to these authors (33), many descending serotonin fibers terminate in the intermediate zone of the spinal gray matter, a region thought to play a key role in the production of primary afferent depolarization (39, 40). The medial brain stem analgesia system, therefore, seems on anatomical grounds well suited for both the gating of in-coming sensory information in the cord and for additional modulation of this information once it has been relayed to supraspinal structures.

A great deal of recent information suggests there are some remarkable parallels between the sites and mechanisms of morphine's analgesic action and the sites and mechanisms of action of SPA. Stereospecific receptor binding of opiate agonists and antagonists has been found within the rodent and primate brain (41 - 43). Opiate receptor sites are distributed widely but unevenly in brain tissue, with a heavy concentration found in the periaqueductal and periventricular gray (42, 43). These sites are of particular interest not only because of their considerable overlap with the SPA system but also because of a series of studies showing that these same regions, and especially the PAG, are most sensitive to morphine when directly applied via microinjection cannulas (44 - 47). Most recently, Yaksh et al. (23) have extended this observation in the rat by showing that analgesia can be obtained with microinjected morphine into PAG according to a crude somatotopic map, analgesia on the body deriving from microinjections into caudal PAG and analgesia on the head deriving from more rostral injection sites. This rough somatotopy corresponds well with the preferential, rostro-caudal distribution of somatic and visceral afferents to the PAG of the rat seen in evoked potential mapping studies (19, 24). Moreover, microinjection of somewhat higher doses of morphine into the PAG results in hyper-reactivity to innocuous stimuli in the rat (44, 46) as has also been observed in some rats and cats during SPA (2, 7).

Similarities between SPA and morphine have also been noted in studies of tolerance. That tolerance develops to repeated systemic injections of morphine is well known. Of interest here are two very recent reports of the role of PAG in mechanisms of tolerance development. Jacquet and Lajtha (48) have shown that tolerance develops to microinjections of morphine in the PAG and that cross-tolerance is found between locally and systemically administered morphine. Similarly, Mayer and Hayes (49) report the development of tolerance to repeated exposures of SPA with PAG electrodes, the effects of which slowly disappear over several weeks of non-exposure. They also observed that following the development of tolerance to systemically administered morphine, cross-tolerance to SPA was present. Again, the return of normal SPA levels was seen several weeks after discontinuation of morphine.

Evidence also exists that SPA and morphine analgesia share an at least partly common neurochemical basis. Interactions between morphine analgesia and drugs affecting transmission in central monoamine systems have been demonstrated in many studies. It has been frequently observed, for example, that drugs interfering with tryptaminergic or catecholaminergic mechanisms reduce morphine's analgesic action. More specifically, although some controversies in this literature exist, good evidence is available that drugs blocking serotonin and dopamine also block morphine analgesia, whereas drugs blocking noradrenaline in fact potentiate it (50 - 53). Similarly, Price and Fibiger (54) have recently shown that biochemical lesions of the dorsal noradrenergic bundle originating in locus coeruleus (but not equivalent lesions in the ventral noradrenergic bundle) enhance morphine analgesia, whereas when such lesions were placed in the dopamine-rich substantia nigra, morphine analgesia was reduced.

A quite parallel involvement of monoamine systems in SPA has been recently reported by Akil and Liebeskind (14). It was shown that SPA from PAG stimulation in the rat, as measured by the tail-flick test, is greatly reduced by either a dopamine receptor blocker (pimozide) or a serotonin synthesis inhibitor (PCPA) but is enhanced by a dopamine receptor stimulator (apomorphine) or the monoamine precursors (L-DOPA and 5-HTP). On the other hand, depletion of noradrenaline (disulfiram) led to an increase in SPA, and when a combination of drugs (AMPT + L-DOPA) was given such that dopamine levels were high and noradrenaline levels were low, a particularly potent degree of SPA was seen. From such evidence that SPA and morphine analgesia have comparable pharmacological susceptibilities, we have suggested (14) that they must both depend, at least in part, upon a common neural substrate.

Morphine and SPA are now known to have similar, lamina-specific suppressive effects on spinal cord activity. Both powerfully inhibit responses to noxious stimuli of lamina 5-type cells without affecting responses to innocuous stimuli of lamina 4-type cells (3, 55).

Evidence is also accumulating that the descending serotonin system originating in nucleus raphe magnus and terminating in the dorsal horn of the spinal cord plays a role of special significance in mechanisms of SPA and morphine analgesia. Interference with this pathway by pharmacological means (56) or by electrolytic destruction of the raphe magnus (32) reduces morphine's analgesic effectiveness. Similarly, Basbaum et al. (15) have now shown that selective unilateral transection of the rat's dorsolateral funiculus, in which run the descending serotonin fibers destined for the dorsal horn, results in a complete block of SPA measured with foot pinch on the side ipsilateral to the lesion. SPA to pinch of the contralateral foot remains unaffected. Preliminary evidence from Basbaum (personal communication), from D. D. Price (personal communication), and from our own laboratory (in work by G. Olson) is also showing that the analgesic effect of systemically administered morphine depends in part on the integrity of this same pathway. It will be recalled that electrical stimulation of the raphe magnus induces analgesia in the rat and cat (30 - 32). In the context of such findings, other preliminary work from our laboratory (31) showing that both morphine and SPA from PAG stimulation significantly augments spontaneous multiple unit firing in the raphe magnus becomes especially interesting. Several very recent anatomical studies appear to shed additional light on these descending paths. With injections of tritiated amino acid into selected areas of the cat PAG, Ruda (57) has disclosed a heretofore unrecognized neural connection between the ventral PAG and the nucleus raphe magnus. Moreover, with the horseradish peroxidase technique, direct connections from the PAG of the cat to the lumbar segments of the cord have now been established by Kuypers and Maisky (58). Finally, Randic and Yu (59) have shown that microiontophoretic application of serotonin within the spinal cord of the cat has a direct inhibitory effect on neurons located in laminae 1 and 2 which respond to noxious stimuli. The functional significance of these findings, of course, remains to be determined. However, the importance of the pathway involving the PAG, nucleus raphe magnus, and the descending serotonin fibers in mechanisms of morphine analgesia and SPA seems apparent. Furthermore, the results of the experiment by Randic and Yu (59) suggest the possibility that the release of serotonin in the dorsal horn by these descending fibers represents at least one final step in the process of pain inhibition. In fact, recent work by Repkin, Proudfit and Anderson (60) is entirely consistent with this view. These authors report finding antidromic spike conduction in dorsal roots of cats and an enhancement of such spiking following systemic morphine administration. The morphine-induced enhancement, in turn, is blocked by anti-serotonin drugs. The authors conclude that serotonin-mediated primary afferent depolarization (presynaptic inhibition) may be the mechanism underlying morphine analgesia.

The final point to be discussed relevant to the apparent communality between mechanisms of SPA and morphine analgesia is, perhaps, the most significant of all. SPA in the rat (61, 62), in the cat (30, 63), and even in man (Richardson & Akil, and Adams, personal communication) can be blocked by naloxone, a specific morphine antagonist. The effect is, however, highly variable from animal to animal; and in our most systematic study to date (62), an average reduction in degree of analgesia of only 38% was obtained. It may well be that several different underlying mechanisms of SPA exist, not all of which are morphine-like and hence naloxone-sensitive. So far, careful histological examination of electrode sites from which naloxone-sensitive and naloxone-insensitive SPA was obtained has failed to reveal any clear anatomical basis for these different systems. The possibility remains that such systems, if they do in fact exist, are sufficiently intermingled to escape dissection with such gross instruments as our stimulating electrodes.

Much of the data reviewed above, and especially the fact that SPA may be even partially antagonized by naloxone, supports our earlier contention (7) that an endogenous mechanism of pain inhibition functions within the medial brain stem. The demonstration of opiate receptor binding sites in the PAG (42) lends still more credence to this view. Recent discoveries by Hughes (64 - 66) and others (67 - 70) and several preliminary reports following up on Hughes' work now make this hypothesis most tenable indeed. Hughes first extracted and purified an endogenous substance from the brains of guinea pigs, pigs, rabbits, and rats which exerted a specific, naloxone-reversible, morphine-like effect, the inhibition of neurally evoked contractions in the mouse vas deferens and guinea pig myenteric plexus bioassays. This discovery of a morphine-like factor in the brain was confirmed using somewhat different techniques by Pasternak et al. (67), and it has been reported by Terenius and Wahlström (68, 69) to exist as well in human cerebrospinal fluid. Interestingly, the level of this factor appeared to be lower in the cerebrospinal fluid of trigeminal neuralgia patients (69). A functionally related, but structurally somewhat different substance has also been isolated by Teschemacher et al. (70) from pituitary extracts. It has been suggested by all of these investigators that the morphine-like substance is the endogenous ligand for opiate receptors. Supporting this view, the substance is unevenly distributed in the brain and in gross dissection appears to be most heavily concentrated in regions where opiate binding sites are most plentiful (64, 67). Preliminary work with the fraction prepared by Snyder's group (67) has shown that microinjections of this substance into the PAG of rats yield significant analgesia in the tail-flick test, an effect reversed by naloxone (A. Pert, R. Simantov, and S. H. Snyder, in preparation).

Hughes and co-workers (66) have now identified the biochemical structure of and synthesized this morphine-like substance, termed by them "enkephalin". It appears to be composed of at least two structurally similar pentapeptides, differing from each other only by the presence of methionine or leucine in the fifth amino acid position. The methionine form was shown to be roughly four times more active than the leucine form in bioassay. Studies are certainly now in progress in several laboratories which will map the brain regions most sensitive to microinjections of the synthesized product and which will attempt to relate the resulting regional specificity to that already established by morphine microinjection. Preliminary work by J. Belluzzi, N. Grant and L. Stein (personal communication) with methionine-enkephalin (synthesized according to Hughes' description by V. Garsky at Wyeth Laboratories) indicates that 40 - 100 µg of the material injected into the lateral or third ventricles yield significant tail-flick analgesia in all rats tested. The peak analgesic effect occurred after approximately 6 min, and the duration of the effect varied between 5 and 10 min. Vehicle injections were inactive.

Obviously, many important questions still need to be answered before the functional significance of these fascinating discoveries can be fully understood. One interesting question is whether or not the endogenous substance is liberated in the brain tonically in some degree, or only phasically under a special set of circumstances. Jacob et al. (71) have recently reported for the first time that systemic administration of naloxone in the rat and mouse decreased jump latency in the hot-plate test, a finding which supports the existence of some level of tonic activity in the endogenous analgesia system. We have been attempting to replicate and extend this important observation in the rat hot-plate and tail-flick tests, so far, however, without success. On the other hand, preliminary evidence again from Stein's group (L. Stein, C. D. Wise and J. Belluzzi, personal communication) shows that electrical stimulation of the dorsal raphe nucleus in the rat, confirmed by these workers to yield potent analgesia in the tail-flick test, releases an enkephalin-like substance which is collected via a push/pull cannula (placed 3 mm caudal to the stimulating electrode below the fourth ventricle) in a perfusate of Krebs' solution. Pooled samples of perfusate collected for 10 min prior to stimulation were compared with pooled samples collected during the 10 min stimulation period. Samples were run through a Biogel, and a single bump of peptidic material was found. The material collected during stimulation, but not that collected before stimulation, was shown to have positive activity in an opiate receptor binding assay. It thus appears that, whether or not some perhaps low level of enkephalin is released tonically in the untreated animal, under conditions of analgesic brain stem stimulation, a compound very much like it is released in substantial quantity. These findings especially, then, begin to lend the weight of hard evidence to our contention (7, 9, 10, 14, 62) that an endogenous, pain inhibitory substrate exists within the medial brain stem which is activated by electrical stimulation and by morphine. In particular, they support the hypothesis (14) that electrical stimulation releases enkephalin or in some other way makes it available for binding at opiate receptor sites, whereas morphine, by resembling the natural substance, interacts with these receptors directly.

These proposed mechanisms do not preclude the existence of other possible modes and sites of action of SPA and morphine analgesia. The fact that SPA is differentially sensitive to naloxone in different animals and is, most frequently, only partially antagonized by this drug suggests that other medial brain stem systems of pain modulation do in fact exist which are not dependent upon the release or availability of enkephalin. Moreover, considerable evidence has been accumulated to indicate that morphine's suppressive action on spinal cord nociceptive processes is exerted not only by the reinforcement of descending control mechanisms of brain stem origin, but also by direct action on the spinal cord itself (c.f., for example, 72). In fact, very recent information shows opiate receptor sites to be distributed throughout the spinal cord dorsal horn but most densely in the superficial layers where, following dorsal root section, an approximately 50% reduction in binding occurs (C. LaMotte, C. D. Pert and S. H. Snyder, personal communication). It seems, then, that at least some portion of the analgesic mechanism of opiate drugs may involve structures as early in the pain path as primary afferent terminals. By what pathways and mechanisms SPA affects dorsal horn cells (2, 3) has yet to be determined, but an action on primary afferent terminals has in no way been precluded by the results so far obtained.

Finally, if pain inhibition is, as we suggest, a normal property of the medial brain stem, then it must be the case that other systems have access to this function and serve normally to turn it on and off. Speculations concerning the role played by the endogenous analgesia system in biologically adaptive mechanisms are interesting to make and may prove heuristic. Obviously, the system is not often or easily accessed since noxious stimuli are almost invariably perceived as such. It would not, under most circumstances, be adaptive to inhibit the useful warning signs which normal pain messages provide. On the other hand, it would be biologically adaptive to inhibit pain during certain, very strong drive states such as sexual arousal, aggression and fear, and especially during the goal-directed behaviors associated with these drives (copulation, fighting and flight) where feeling pain might be disruptive to effective performance of these behaviors of still greater survival value to the organism and species than nociception itself. The situational determinants of the system's operation are surely complex, however, since one can also imagine that in a state of fear or apprehension, where options for flight or self-defense are either not available or not chosen, pain inhibition might usefully be reduced to allow the organism heightened awareness of danger signs in his environment. The fact that the PAG and other portions of the medial brain stem appear to be critically involved in the expression of fear (21), in mechanisms of affective attack (73, 74), shock-elicited defensive behavior (75) and interspecific aggression (76), in the processing of somatic and visceral nociceptive information (18, 19, 24), and in the regulation of sympathetic and parasympathetic tone (24) suggests that speculations such as these are not gratuitous and can be subjected to empirical test. For example, Komisaruk (77) has recently reported that vaginal cervix probing in the rat selectively blocks both unit firing in the thalamus and various behavioral responses evoked by noxious but not innocuous stimuli.

The existence and operation of a pain inhibitory system has long been inferred from the occurrence of certain pain states in man thought to result from lesions in the rostral brain stem. Hyperpathia and spontaneous pain characterize this so-called "thalamic pain" syndrome, suggesting, of course, that the damaged or functionally impaired brain stem structures serve normally to block pain perception. It is also interesting to speculate that endogenous anti-nociceptive mechanisms are shut off in pain patients addicted to narcotic analgesic drugs. It is known that cross-tolerance to SPA occurs in morphine-dependent rats (49). This finding might serve to explain the recent observation by Erickson et al. (78) that in their experience with pain patients, detoxification from narcotic drugs rarely increases and usually decreases complaints of pain.

We are surely provided with powerful, endogenous mechanisms of pain inhibition even though most of us are almost totally incapable of voluntarily bringing them into play. In view of the remarkable rate of progress made during the past few years in identifying and understanding the neuroanatomical, neurophysiological and neurohumoral bases of anti-nociception, it begins to seem hopeful that a non-invasive, non-addictive means to control pain will soon be found.

REFERENCES

1. Reynolds, D.V., Science 164, 444 (1969).
2. Liebeskind, J.C., Guilbaud, G., Besson, J.-M. and Oliveras, J.-L., Brain Res. 50, 441 (1973).
3. Oliveras, J.-L., Besson, J.-M., Guilbaud, G. and Liebeskind, J.C., Exp. Brain Res. 20, 32 (1974).
4. Melzack, R. and Melinkoff, D.F., Exp. Neurol. 43, 369 (1974).
5. Gebhart, G.F. and Toleikis, J.R., Fed. Proc. 34, 439 (1975).
6. Goodman, S.J. and Holcombe, V., Proc. First World Congress on Pain, Florence, Italy (1975).

7. Mayer, D.J., Wolfle, T.L., Akil, H., Carder, B. and Liebeskind, J.C., Science 174, 1351 (1971).
8. Richardson, D.E. and Akil, H., Abstr. 7th Ann. Meeting Neuroelectric Soc. (1974).
9. Liebeskind, J.C., Proc. First World Congress on Pain, Florence, Italy (1975).
10. Mayer, D.J. and Liebeskind, J.C., Brain Res. 68, 73 (1974).
11. Grumbach, L., In Pain (Knighton, R.S. and Dumke, P.R., Eds.) Little, Brown, Boston, 163 (1966).
12. Liebman, J.M., Mayer, D.J. and Liebeskind, J.C., Behav. Biol. 9, 299 (1973).
13. Liebman, J.M. and Butcher, L.L., Naunyn-Schmiedeberg's Arch. Pharmacol. 277, 305 (1973).
14. Akil, H. and Liebeskind, J.C., Brain Res. 94, 279 (1975).
15. Basbaum, A.I., Marley, N. and O'Keefe, J., Proc. First World Congress on Pain, Florence, Italy (1975).
16. Bowsher, D., Brain 80, 606 (1957).
17. Mehler, W.R., Ann. N.Y. Acad. Sci. 167, 424 (1969).
18. Becker, D.P., Gluck, H., Nulsen, F.E. and Jane, J.A., J. Neurosurg. 30, 1 (1969).
19. Liebeskind, J.C. and Mayer, D.J., Brain Res. 27, 133 (1971).
20. Wolfle, T.L., Mayer, D.J., Carder, B. and Liebeskind, J.C., Physiol. & Behav. 7, 569 (1971).
21. Liebman, J.M., Mayer, D.J. and Liebeskind, J.C., Brain Res. 23, 353 (1970).
22. Bevan, T. and Pert, A., Fed. Proc. 34, 713 (1975).
23. Yaksh, T.L., Rudy, T.A. and Yeung, J.C., Proc. Soc. Neurosci. 5, 283 (1975).
24. Huprich, S.T., Doct. Diss., UCLA (1975).
25. Rhodes, D.L., Doct. Diss., UCLA (1975).
26. Oliveras, J.-L., Woda, A., Guilbaud, G. and Besson, J.-M., Brain Res. 72, 328 (1974).
27. Balagura, S. and Ralph, T., Brain Res. 60, 369 (1973).
28. Morrow, T.J. and Casey, K.L., Proc. First World Congress on Pain, Florence, Italy (1975).
29. Oleson, T.D. and Liebeskind, J.C., Proc. First World Congress on Pain, Florence, Italy (1975).
30. Oliveras, J.-L., Redjemi, F., Guilbaud, G. and Besson, J.-M., Pain 1, 139 (1975).
31. Oleson, T.D. and Liebeskind, J.C., Physiologist 18, 338 (1975).
32. Proudfit, H.K. and Anderson, E.G., Brain Res. 98, 612 (1975).
33. Dahlström, A. and Fuxe, K., Acta physiol. scand., suppl. 247, 64, 5 (1965).
34. Fuxe, K., Acta physiol. scand., suppl. 247, 64, 1 (1965).
35. Lindvall, O. and Björklund, A., Acta physiol. scand., suppl. 412, 1 (1974).
36. Lindvall, O., Björklund, A., Nobin, A. and Stenevi, U., J. Comp. Neurol. 154, 317 (1974).
37. Hökfelt, T., Fuxe, K., Goldstein, M. and Johansson, O., Brain Res. 66, 235 (1974).
38. Hökfelt, T., Kellerth, J.O., Nilsson, G. and Pernow, B., Science 190, 889 (1975).

39. Eccles, J.C., Kostyuk, P.G. and Schmidt, R.F., J. Physiol., Lond. 161, 237 (1962).
40. Besson, J.-M. and Rivot, J.P., J. Physiol., Lond. 230, 235 (1973).
41. Pert, C.B. and Snyder, S.H., Science 179, 1011 (1973).
42. Kuhar, M.J., Pert, C.B. and Snyder, S.H., Nature (Lond.) 245, 447 (1973).
43. Lowney, L.I., Schulz, K., Lowery, P.J. and Goldstein, A., Science 183, 749 (1974).
44. Jacquet, Y.F. and Lajtha, A., Science 185, 1055 (1974).
45. Pert, A. and Yaksh, T., Brain Res. 80, 135 (1974).
46. Sharpe, L.G., Garnett, J.E. and Cicero, T.J., Behav. Biol. 11, 303 (1974).
47. Wei, E., Sigel, S. and Way, E.L., J. Pharmacol. exp. Ther. 193, 56 (1975).
48. Jacquet, Y.F. and Lajtha, A., Brain Res. in press (1976).
49. Mayer, D.J. and Hayes, R.L., Science 188, 941 (1975).
50. Cicero, T.J., Meyer, E.R. and Smithloff, B.R., J. Pharmacol. exp. Ther. 189, 72 (1974).
51. Nakamura, K., Kuntzman, R., Maggio, A.C., Augulis, V. and Conney, A.H., Psychopharmacologia (Berl.) 31, 177 (1973).
52. Saarnivara, L., Ann. Med. Exp. Fenn. 47, 103 (1969).
53. Tenen, S.S., Psychopharmacologia (Berl.) 12, 278 (1968).
54. Price, M.T.C. and Fibiger, H.C., Brain Res. 99, 189 (1975).
55. Kitahata, L.M., Kosaka, Y., Taub, A., Bonikos, K. and Hoffert, M., Anesthesiology 41, 39 (1974).
56. Vogt, M., J. Physiol., Lond. 236, 483 (1974).
57. Ruda, M.A., Doct. Diss., Univ. Pennsylvania (1976).
58. Kuypers, H.G.J.M. and Maisky, V.A., Neurosci. Letters 1, 9 (1975).
59. Randic, M. and Yu, H., Proc. Soc. Neurosci. 5, 151 (1975).
60. Repkin, A. H., Proudfit, H. K. and Anderson, E.G., The Pharmacologist 16, 203 (1974).
61. Akil, H., Mayer, D.J. and Liebeskind, J.C., C.R. Acad. Sci. (Paris) 274, 3603 (1972).
62. Akil, H., Mayer, D.J. and Liebeskind, J.C., Science in press (1976).
63. Akil, H. and Richardson, D.E., Soc. Neurosci., 4th Ann. Meeting (1974).
64. Hughes, J., Brain Res. 88, 295 (1975).
65. Hughes, J., Smith, T. Morgan, B. and Fothergill, L., Life Sci. 16, 1753 (1975).
66. Hughes, J., Smith, T.W., Kosterlitz, H.W., Fothergill, L.A., Morgan, B.A. and Morris, H.R., Nature in press (1975).
67. Pasternak, G.W., Goodman, R. and Snyder, S.H., Life Sci. 16, 1765 (1975).
68. Terenius, L. and Wahlström, A., Acta pharmac. tox., suppl. I, 35, 55 (1974).
69. Terenius, L. and Wahlström, A., Life Sci. 16, 1759 (1975).
70. Teschemacher, H., Opheim, K.E., Cox, B.M. and Goldstein, A., Life Sci. 16, 1771 (1975).
71. Jacob, J.J., Tremblay, E.C. and Colombel, M.-C., Psychopharmacologia (Berl.) 37, 217 (1974).
72. Le Bars, D., Menetrey, D., Conseiller, C. and Besson, J.-M., Brain Res. 98, 261 (1975).

73. Hunsperger, R.W., Helv. Physiol. Pharmacol. Acta 14, 70 (1956).
74. Chi, C.C. and Flynn, J.P., Science 171, 703 (1971).
75. Edwards, M.A. and Adams, D.B., Physiol. & Behav. 13, 113 (1974).
76. Chaurand, J.P., Vergnes, M. and Karli, P., Physiol. & Behav. 9, 475 (1972).
77. Komisaruk, B.R., Proc. First World Congress on Pain, Florence, Italy (1975).
78. Erickson, D.L., Michaelson, M.A. and Acharya, A., Proc. First World Congress on Pain, Florence, Italy (1975).

Discussion:

Perl: Thank you, Dr Liebeskind for a very provocative paper. It is good that we have some evidence that the nervous system does have the mechanism in some way to fit with common experience, namely that sometimes pain reactions do not occur.

Zimmermann: PCPA has been established to interfere with serotonin synthesis, I think. Has anybody used the substance to check whether the effects are compatible with your story?

Liebeskind: Yes, we have. An article on that came out recently. PCPA blocks stimulation produced analgesia as does morphine analgesia. A note was published on that in the London Journal about a year ago.

ACUPUNCTURELIKE ELECTROANALGESIA IN TNS-RESISTANT CHRONIC PAIN

M. ERIKSSON and B. SJÖLUND

Department of Clinical Neurophysiology and Institute of Physiology, University of Lund, Lund, Sweden

In conventional Transcutaneous Nerve Stimulation (TNS) for pain relief, based on the Melzack-Wall gate theory[11], stimulation frequencies of 20-200 Hz with intensities of up to three times perception threshold are used. This probably means that mainly coarse myelinated fibers of mixed nerves are stimulated, and as recently shown by Handwerker, Iggo and Zimmermann[4], dorsal horn neurones activated by noxious C-fiber input and possibly mediating pain centrally, are inhibited by electrical stimulation of group II myelinated nerve fibers, supporting the notion of a segmental interaction. According to several clinical reports, e.g. by Shealy and Maurer[13] and by Long[7], the results of high frequency TNS in patients with chronic pain conditions indicate that 25-40 % of the patients find the induced analgesia sufficient for long term treatment.

To improve the results of TNS we have used experiences from the Chinese electro-acupuncture, where inserted needles are stimulated electrically, often with a very low frequency[6]. Chiang and coworkers[3] claim that afferent impulses from muscle nerves are necessary to produce acupuncture analgesia. Similarily, in a Swedish investigation, Andersson and associates[2] have shown that an increase in tooth pain threshold of healthy adults during electro-acupuncture occurs only when strong muscle contractions are elicited in adjacent regions. It was necessary to use stimulation strengths of 5-8 times perception threshold[5], and moreover, surface electrodes were found to be more effective than needles, probably because the amount of current passed could be larger. These findings might indicate that deep high threshold receptors or nerve fibers were involved. The effect began and passed off gradually with a time course much resembling that found for the raphe descending control system of the cat by Melzack and Melinkoff[10].

Activation of this system can suppress behavioural responses as well as lamina V cell activity evoked by noxious stimulation as established by Mayer, Liebeskind, Oliveras and others[8, 12].

For the present study, 50 consecutive patients with chronic pain conditions, referred to a Neurosurgical Clinic for pain alleviation, were used. Conventional high frequency TNS was carefully tried out on every patient in one to several 2-4 hour sessions with variation of electrode positions and stimulation parameters. As evident from Table I, 20/50 (40 %) experienced a satisfactory analgesia with daily stimulation during more than one month of observation.

Table 1

TNS IN CHRONIC PAIN

	Analgesia	No effect
HIGH FREQUENCY STIMULATION	20/50	30/50
LOW FREQUENCY STIMULATION	10/30	20/30
TOTAL	30/50	20/50

The remaining 30 patients were subjected to acupuncturelike, low frequency stimulation via standard TNS surface electrodes. Care was taken to stimulate nerves to myotomes segmentally related to the painful area. To ensure strong muscle contractions and thereby hopefully an effective impulse flow from deep receptors, a new portable stimulator was developed by a Swedish manufacturer according to our specifications. This device gives 0.2 msec constant current square pulses of up to 80 mA at loads of maximally 2500 Ohms. Since the current needed to get strong contractions and possibly analgesia is 5-8 times the sensory threshold, i.e. up to 80 mA on single shock stimulation, we decided to use short trains of stimuli with an internal frequency of 100 Hz and 70 ms duration with a repetition rate of 2 Hz.

This tetanic stimulation reduced the current needed for muscle contractions to half or two thirds of the single shock values. The stimulator was also used for the conventional TNS of this study.

Out of the 30 patients not responding to conventional TNS, 10 experienced significant pain alleviation from acupuncturelike TNS during more than one month of observation. As shown in Table I, this means that another 20 % of the patients benefitted from TNS, giving a total value of 60 % (30/50) success with a combination of high and low frequency stimulation. To evaluate the pain relief, patients were asked to score their pain intensity before and during stimulation on a 1-5 intensity scale in a questionnaire, sent to their homes after 1 month of stimulation treatment. In Fig. 1 the histograms illustrate that about 1/3 of the patients with both high and low frequency stimulation experience total pain relief, whereas the remainder generally have a more than 50 % alleviation. However, when determining the induction time of analgesia (upper part of Fig. 2) it was found that while most patients with conventional TNS experience analgesia immediately or within 10-15 minutes, the induction times on low frequency stimulation center around half an hour and none has an immediate effect. (Difference highly significant; $p < 0.001$ in Student´s T-test.) The poststimulus duration of analgesia on the other hand (lower part of Fig. 2) did not differ for the two groups, except that the three patients with no aftereffect at all were in the high frequency group.

The long induction time found for analgesia from low frequency stimulation fits well with the earlier mentioned experimental observations on tooth pain thresholds and with the characteristics of the raphe system. In this context, it is interesting to note that naloxone, known to block the descending effects of raphe stimulation[1], has recently been shown to abolish acupuncture analgesia in normal subjects by Mayer and coworkers[9] using a double blind test, possibly implying a role for the raphe system in acupuncture analgesia.

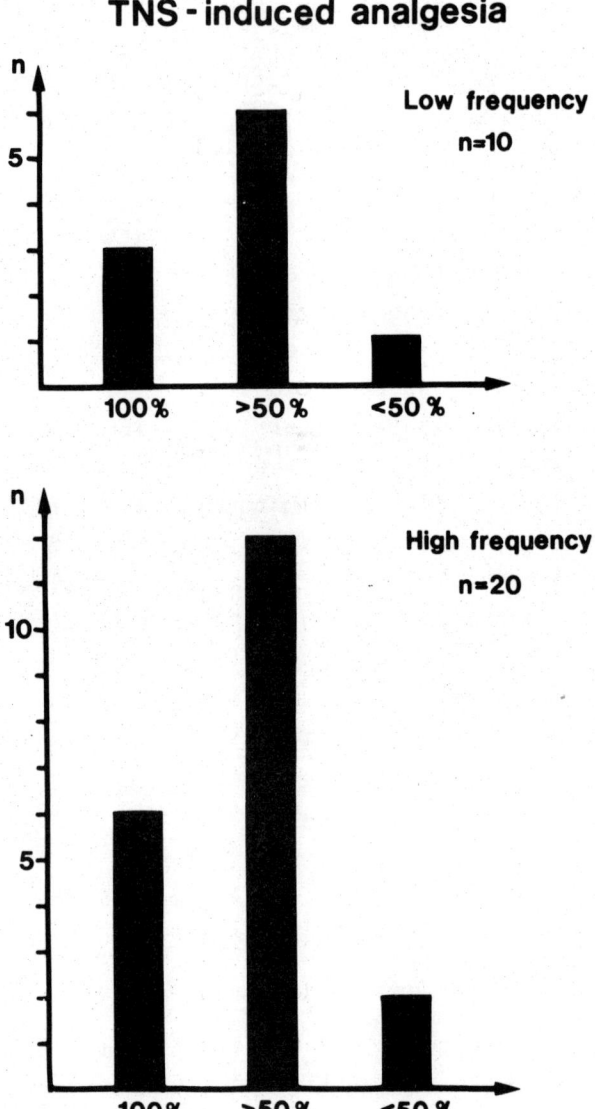

Fig. 1. Number of patients (n) experiencing different degrees of pain alleviation. Calculated from self scoring of pain intensity on a 1-5 scale before and during stimulation.

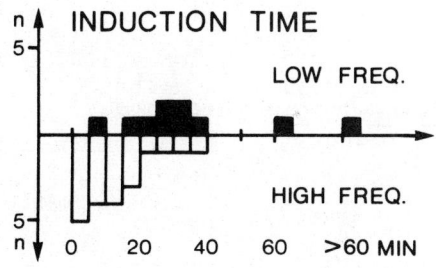

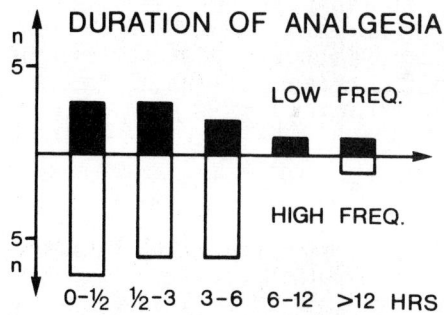

Fig. 2. Upper part: Induction time for analgesia. Lower part: poststimulus duration of analgesia. Data from patients reports. Filled blocks = low frequency stimulation; empty blocks = high frequency stimulation; n = number of patients.

REFERENCES

1. Akil, H., Mayer, D.J. and Liebeskind, J.C., C.R. Acad. Sci. (Paris) 274, 3603-3605 (1972).
2. Andersson, S.S., Ericsson, T., Holmgren, E. and Lindqvist, G., Brain Res. 63, 393-396 (1973).
3. Chiang, C-Y., Chang, C-T., Chu, H-L., and Yang, L.F., Scientia Sinica 16, 210-217 (1973).
4. Handwerker, H.D., Iggo, A., and Zimmermann, M., Pain 1, 147-165 (1975).
5. Holmgren, E., Dissertation, Göteborg, 1975.
6. Kaada, B., Hoel, E., Leseth, K., Nygaard-Østby, B., Setekleiv, J. and Stovner, J., T. norske Laegeforen. 94, 417-442 (1974).
7. Long, D.H. and Hagfors, N., Pain 1, 109-123 (1975).
8. Mayer, D.J., Wolfe, T.L., Akil, H., Carder, B., and Liebeskind, J.C., Science 174, 1351-1354 (1971).
9. Mayer, D.J., Price, D.D. and Rafii, A., Abstract, The First World Congress on Pain, Florens, 1975.

10. Melzack, R. and Melinkoff, D.F., Exp. Neurol. 43, 369-374 (1974).
11. Melzack, R. and Wall, P.D., Science 150, 971-979 (1965).
12. Oliveras, J.L., Besson, J.M., Guilbaud, G., and Liebeskind, J.C., Exp. Brain Res. 20, 32-44 (1974)
13. Shealy, C.N. and Maurer, D., Surg. Neurol. 2, 45-47 (1974).

Discussion:

Zimmermann: Could you please make some comment on the spectrum and pattern of nerve fibers which you stimulated with your either high or low frequency stimulations?

Sjölund: That is, of course, the main question. What kind of afferents are we stimulating? I think the main problem here is what kinds of afferents are stimulated in the low frequency type. We have no idea at all. You need to have heavy muscle contractions to get the effect. Also there is a clear but not complete segmental arrangement much the same finding as Anderson and Holmgren have made that you need to have rather significant stimulus myograms rather closely related to the painful area.

Zotterman: Close to the pain threshold or to the production of paresthesias?

Sjölund: Yes, that is correct.

Lindahl: I find these results very interesting. It does mean, I suppose, that if you stimulate in the real acupunctural point from a classical view you will get better results than if you irritate some other place.

Sjölund: I cannot tell. We have not followed any meridian lines. But our experience is that you must be close. From what I know of the literature some of the acupuncture points are far from the painful area. So this would not fit with the Chinese idea.

Lindahl: We have made some experiments in Linköping. We have stimulated in subjects, not patients, acupunture points and points one centimeter beside. Testing the arrousal in formatio reticularis we got significant difference in the arrousals between these two types of stimulations. From our point of view it is quite obvious that the "pure" points do something else than points around.

Perl: Could you correlate the "pure" points with something else?

Lindahl: Yes, the "pure" points are physically quite different from the surrounding skin. But no correlation with nerves. It is a close criteria. Our treatment was without electricity, just putting in the needless.

Ingvar: You refer the analgesia to the muscle contractions. Then one would have a blocking effect upon pain. Have you any comment?

Sjölund: That is something that these patients spontaneously tell you that after some exercise they feel less pain.

Granit: I was just wondering along the same lines. What does a muscle contraction mean? It merely means that now you have reached the fastest fibers. Does it mean that the muscle has to be contracting and stimulating some sensory endings? For that you would have to try some blocking techniques and some passive stretches of more to find out what amount of contraction is needed. As such it is not a clear definition.

Sjölund: No, I agree completely. The receptor problem is still there.

Perl: The chairman might make a gratuitous remark. I wonder or not we are moving around the active sites in the cortex that Dr Ingvar has suggested.

IMMUNOHISTOCHEMICAL STUDIES ON THE DISTRIBUTION OF SUBSTANCE P AND SOMATOSTATIN IN PRIMARY SENSORY NEURONS

T. HÖKFELT, J-O. KELLERTH, R. ELDE, R. LUFT, O. JOHANSSON, G. NILSSON, B. PERNOW and A. ARIMURA

Departments of Histology, Pharmacology and Anatomy, Karolinska, Institute and Departments of Endocrinology and Metabolism and of Clinical Physiology, Karolinska Hospital, Stockholm, Sweden and the Veterans Administration Hospital and Tulane University School of Medicine, New Orleans, Louisiana, U.S.A.

INTRODUCTION

Primary sensory neuron have been extensively studied from the structural point of view and the cell bodies in the spinal ganglia have been subdivided into several groups on the basis of morphological criteria (see 1). However, comparatively little is known about the chemical characteristics of these neurons, especially with reference to their transmitter substance(s). Early studies by Hellauer (11), Lembeck (20) and Pernow (25) revealed a higher concentration of Substance P (SP), a principle originally discovered by von Euler and Gaddum (10) and recently isolated and structurally characterized by Chang, Leeman and Niall (5), in the dorsal than in the ventral roots. It was, in fact, suggested that SP may act as a neurotransmitter in primary sensory neurons. On the other hand, glutamate has been a strong candidate for being released from the nerve endings in the spinal cord of the central branches of sensory neurons (see 9). More recently biochemical and electrophysiological studies by Otsuka and collaborators have strongly supported a transmitter or modulator role of SP in primary sensory neurons (19, 31, 32).

In the present article we summarize some of our immunohistochemical (14, 15, 17, 18, 21, 22) results on the distribution in primary sensory neurons of SP and of somatostatin (SOM), a tetradecapeptide recently discovered by Guillemin and collaborators (4, 33) and ascribed a role as a hypothalamic hormone inhibiting the secretion of growth hormone. Our findings indicate that on the basis of immunohistochemical criteria, primary sensory neurons in spinal ganglia can be divided in at least three subgroups: 1) SP-containing neurons, 2) SOM-containing neurons and 3) neurons that probably contain neither of these peptides.

IMMUNOHISTOCHEMICAL LOCALISATION

Methodology

Antisera to SP, coupled to bovine serum albumin (BSA), and to SOM, coupled to human α-globulin (HAG), were raised in rabbits (see 23 and 2, respectively). For immunohistochemistry the SP antiserum and SOM antiserum were pretreated with BSA and HAG, respectively. The same sera pretreated with SP and SOM, respectively, were used as control sera. It has been established that no cross-reactivity occurs between anti-SP and SOM or between anti-SOM and SP (15).

Various tissues of rat and cat and the post-mortem spinal cord of man have been studied. All tissues were fixed with 4% formalin, prepared according to Pease (24). The rats and cats were perfused via the ascending and thoracic aorta, respectively, whereas the human tissue was fixed by immersion. After fixation for 2-6 hrs the tissues were rinsed and cut on a Dittes cryostat. The indirect immunofluorescence technique of Coons and collaborators (see 7) was used. Briefly, the sections were incubated with the rabbit antiserum to SP or SOM, diluted 1:20 or 1:40, rinsed in phosphate buffered saline (PBS), incubated with sheep anti-rabbit fluoresceinisothiocyanate conjugated antibodies (Statens Bakteriologiska Laboratorium, SBL, Stockholm, Sweden), rinsed in PBS, mounted and examined in a Zeiss Junior fluore-

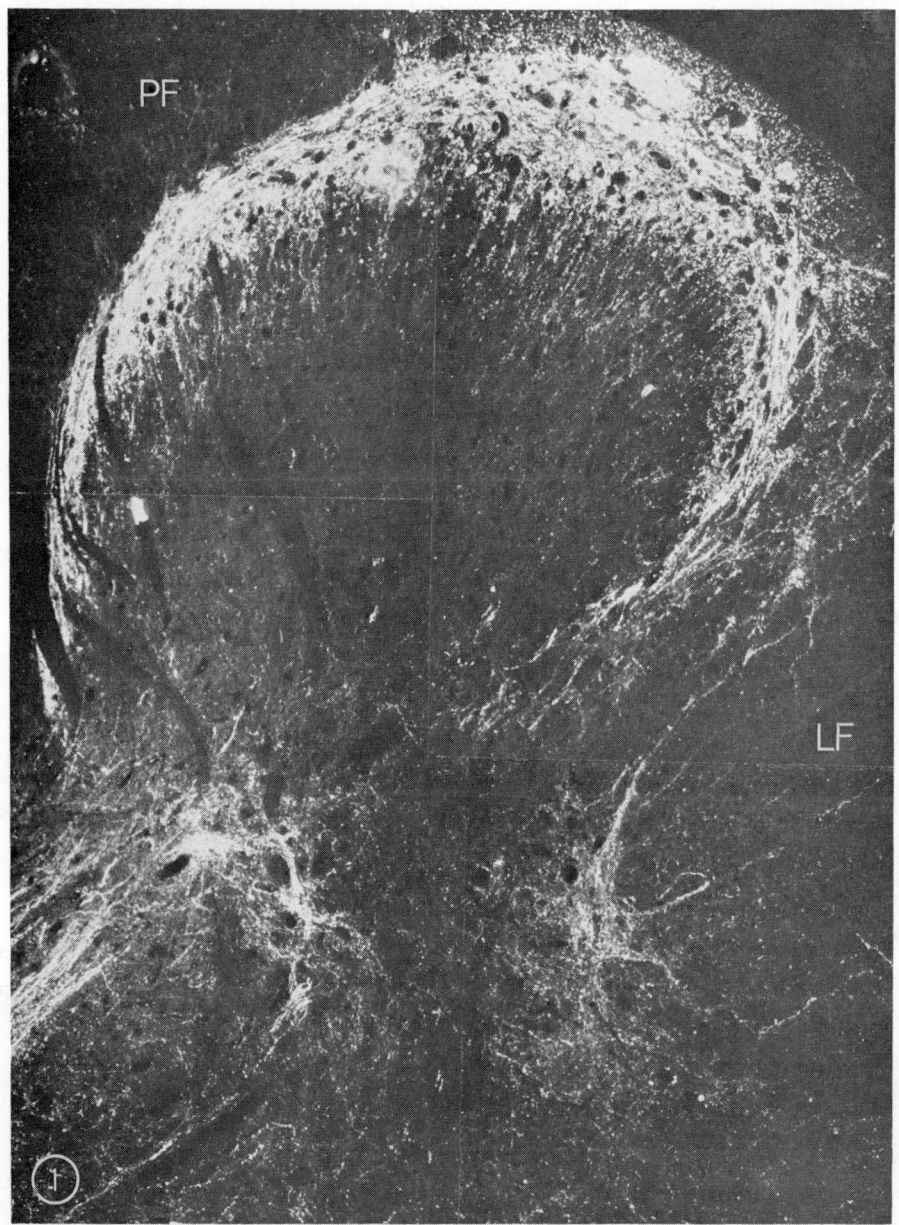

Fig. 1. Immunofluorescence micrograph of the dorsal horn of the cat spinal cord after incubation with SP antiserum. A dense plexus of fluorescent fibers is observed in Lissauer's tract and in laminae I and II extending ventrally along the periphery of the horn. PF = posterior fasciculus, LF = lateral fasciculus. From Hökfelt et al. (18). Magnification 104X.

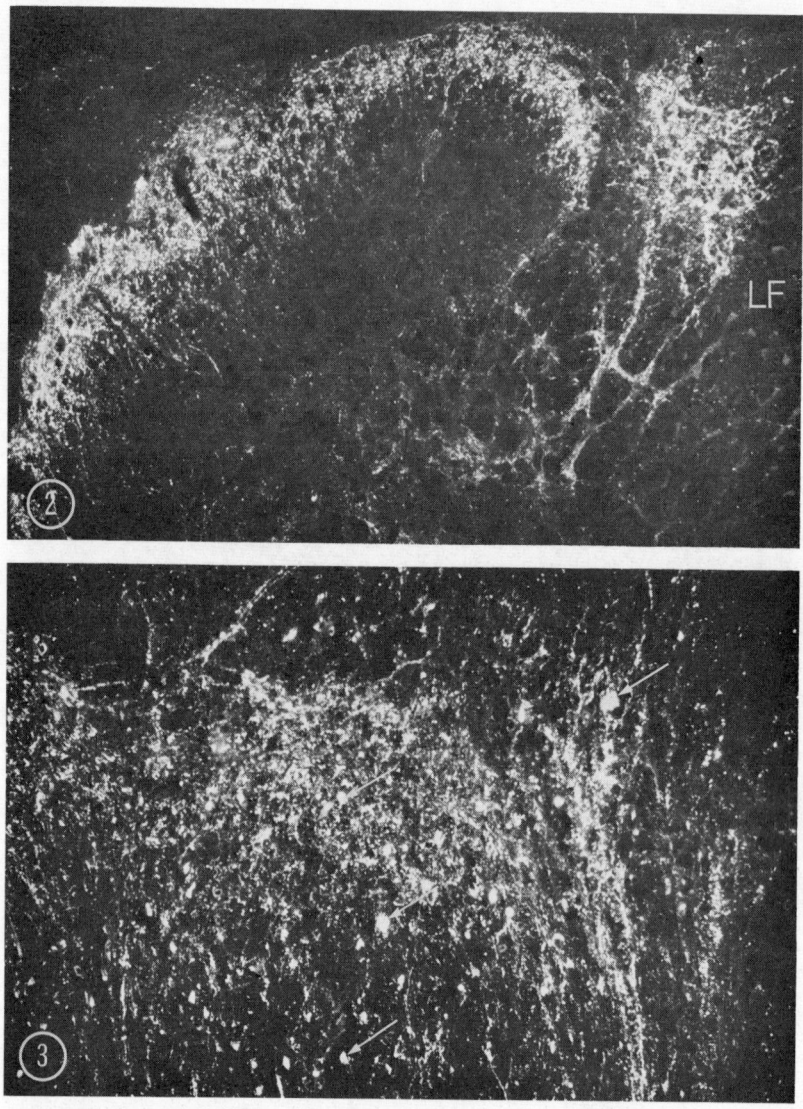

Figs. 2 and 3. Immunofluorescence micrographs of the dorsal horn of rat (Fig. 2) and man (Fig. 3) after incubation with SP antiserum. In the rat the highest concentration was found in laminae I and II and in the lateral fasciculuc (LF) immediately adjacent to the dorsal horn (Fig. 2). Also in man the SP-positive fibers are observed mainly in the two first laminae (Fig. 3). Arrows point to autofluorescent structures. Magnification 104X.

scence microscope. For further details see ref. 16.

In some cases consecutive sections of the spinal cord, intestine and spinal ganglia of the rat were incubated alternatively with antiserum to SP and SOM, respectively.

Substance P

Spinal cord. A dense network of SP positive fibers was found in the dorsal horn of the spinal cord of cat (Fig. 1), rat (Fig. 2) and man (Fig. 3). In the cat and rat the highest concentrations were observed in Lissauer's tract and in lamina I and II (29), with some fibers extending into lamina III. In the lateral and medial aspects of the rest of the dorsal horn numerous SP-positive fibers were present whereas only few fibers were observed in its central parts. The ventral horns (Figs. 4-6) and the area around the central canal (Fig. 7) contained a network of moderate density. In the rat fluorescent fibers could also be seen in the dorsal roots. In man the SP positive fibers had approximately the same distribution although autofluorescent material interfered with the specific immunofluorescence and the fluorescence was weaker than in the experimental animals. This is probably due to the differences in fixation conditions and post mortem time. After transection of the dorsal roots in the cat a marked decrease in the number of SP-positive fibers was observed in the dorsal horn (Figs. 17, 18).

Peripheral tissues. SP positive fibers were found in most peripheral tissues, sometimes in relation to blood vessels, secretory cells and ducts. A very dense network of SP-positive fibers was observed in the gut (see 22) (Fig. 8). Of special interest was the presence of fluorescent fibers in the skin of the cat hind paw (Figs. 9, 10). These axons were in most cases running in the connective tissue just beneath the epithelium and occasionally penetrating into the epithelium. Sweat glands were often surrounded by SP-positive fibers (Fig. 11).

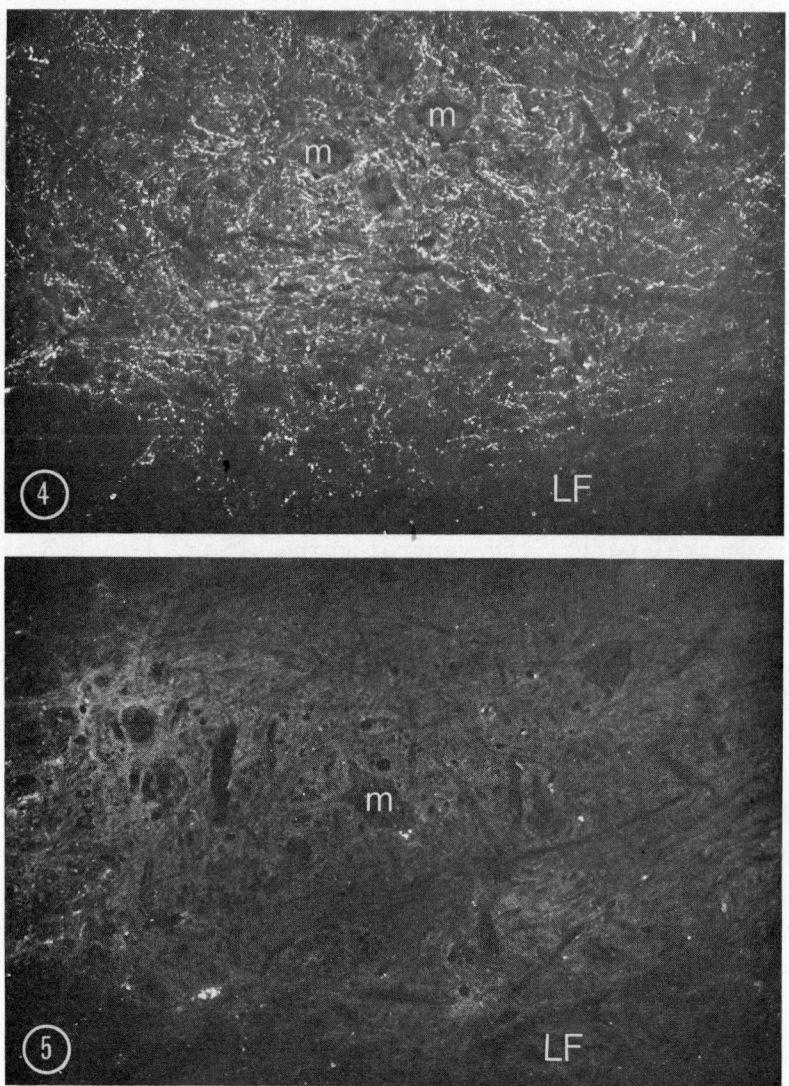

Figs. 4 and 5. Immunofluorescence micrographs of the ventral horn of the cat spinal cord after incubation with SP antiserum (Fig. 4) and control serum (Fig. 5). Numerous SP-positive fibers are found after incubation with the specific antibodies whereas almost no fluorescent structures are observed in the controls. m = motoneurons. LF = lateral fasciculus. From Hökfelt et al. (18). Magnification 104X.

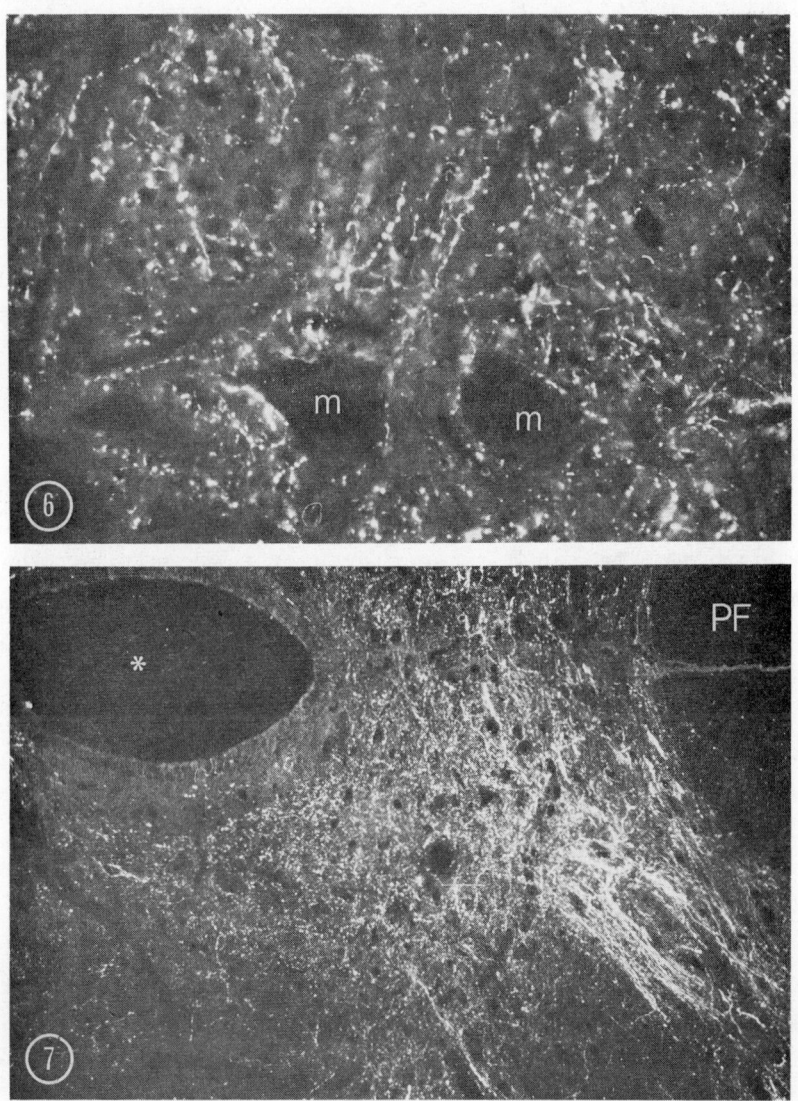

Figs. 6 and 7. Immunofluorescence micrographs of the ventral horn (Fig. 6) and area around the central canal (asterisk) (Fig. 7) of the cat spinal cord after incubation with SP antiserum. m = motoneuron. PF = posterior fasciculus. From Hökfelt et al. (18). Magnification 256X. (Fig. 6) and 104X. (Fig. 7).

Spinal ganglia. In the rat spinal and trigeminal ganglia several SP-positive cell bodies and fibers were observed (Figs. 12, 14). The fluorescent cell bodies were almost exclusively of the small type and probably did not constitute more than 20% of all neuronal cell bodies. In the cat no SP-specific immunofluorescence could be observed in cell bodies of the L6, L7 or S1 ganglia. Therefore we used experimental procedures aimed at arresting outtransport of substances produced in the cell body, such as colchicine treatment (9) or ligation of the dorsal root close to the ganglion. After both procedures SP-positive cell bodies could be observed in the cat spinal ganglia (Fig. 13) and furthermore, on the proximal side of the ligation accumulations of SP in probable axons could be observed.

Somatostatin

Spinal cord. In the rat a dense plexus of SOM-positive fibers was observed mainly in lamina II and to a lesser extent lamina I and in Lissauer's tract (Fig. 16). No fluorescent fibers could be observed with certainty in the ventral horns. In the cat a moderately dense network of weakly fluorescent fibers were present in lamina II and a sparse network in the ventral horns (unpublished findings).

Peripheral tissues. In the rat SOM-positive fibers have been observed in the lamina propria and in the submucosal and the myenteric (Auerbach's) plexus of the gut, especially of the colon and distal parts of the small intestine. So far no SOM-positive fibers have been observed in the skin, neither of the rat nor of the cat.

Spinal ganglia. Several SOM-positive neuronal cell-bodies were present in rat spinal ganglia (Fig. 15). They were exclusively of the small type and seemed to be less frequent than the SP--positive ones. No fluorescent fibers could be observed.

Other tissues. SOM has been found in nerve fibers in wide-spread

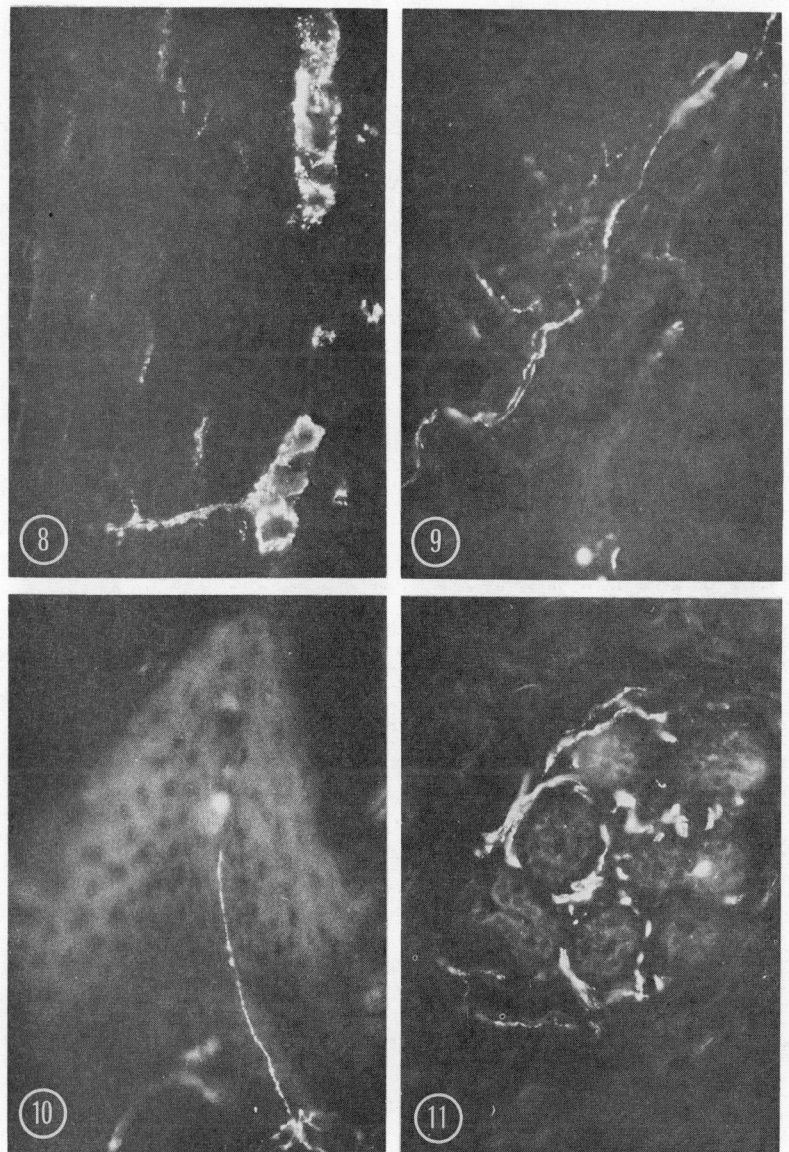

Fig. 8-11. Immunofluorescence micrographs of the rat stomach (Fig. 8) and the skin of the cat hind paw (Figs. 9-11) after incubation with SP antiserum. SP-positive fibers are seen around the Auerbach's plexus (Fig. 8), under the epithelium (Fig. 9), occasionally within the epithelium (Fig. 10) and around sweat glands (Fig. 11). From Hökfelt et al. (18). Magnification 192X.

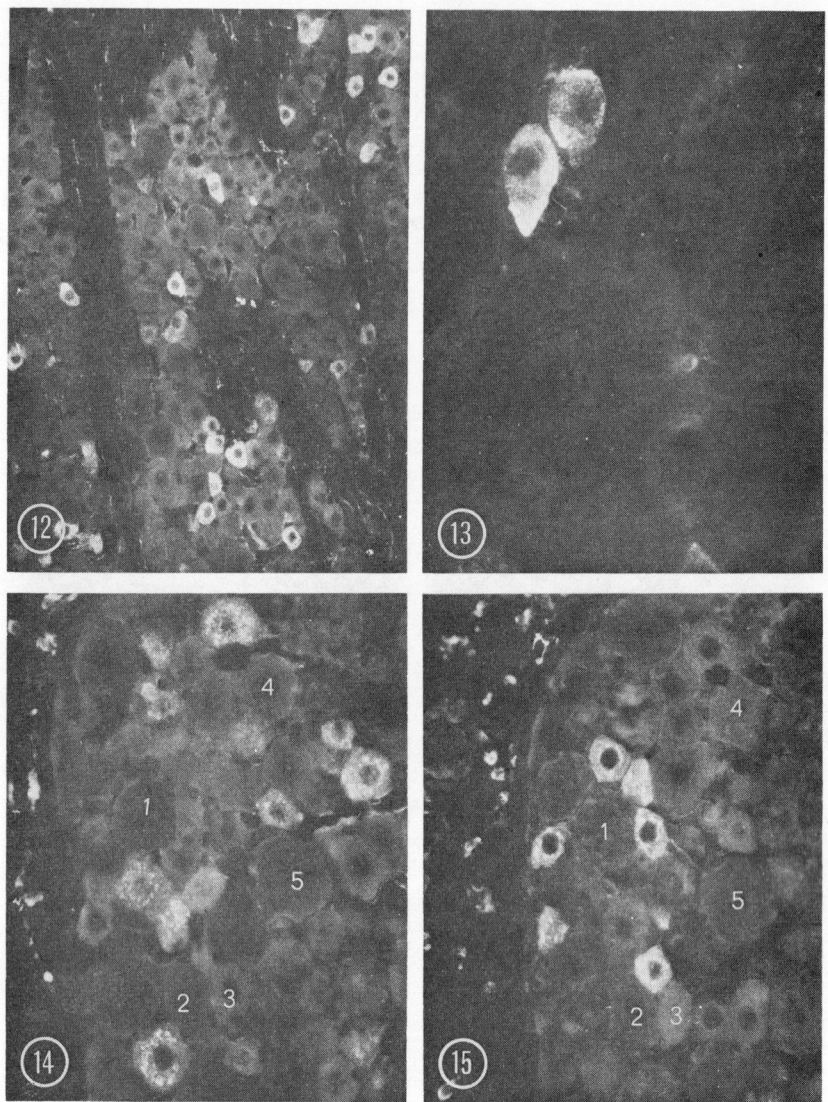

Figs. 12-15. Immunofluorescence micrographs of rat (Figs. 12, 14, 15) and cat (Fig. 13) spinal ganglia after incubation with SP antiserum (Figs. 12-14) and SOM antiserum (Fig. 15). Fig. 13 shows a ganglion after compression of the dorsal root. Note that only small cells exhibit a specific immunofluorescence. Figs. 14 and 15 represent consecutive sections and it can be established that the SP- and SOM-positive cells are not the same ones. To facilitate comparison some of the cells appearing in both sections have been labelled 1-5. From Hökfelt et al. (15 and 18). Magnifications 104X. (Fig. 12), 256X. (Fig. 13) and 192X. (Figs. 14, 15).

areas of the central nervous system, including the median eminence, many hypothalamic nuclei and nuc. accumbens and in neuronal cell bodies in the anterior hypothalamic periventricular area. However, SOM is also present in endocrine-like cells in the Langerhans' islets of the pancreas (A_1-cells), in the thyroid gland and in the stomach and gut (for ref. see 13).

Staining of consecutive sections with Substance P and somatostatin

Spinal cord. In the rat there was generally a similar distribution of SP- and SOM-positive fibers in the dorsal horn (Figs. 16, 17), whereas no SOM-positive structures were found in the ventral horn. However, there was an impression that in the dorsal horn, the SP-positive fibers were located more dorsally than the SOM-positive ones. Thus, the SP fibers seemed to be most numerous in lamina I and II, whereas the SOM fibers appeared most numerous in lamina II. This difference seems to be more pronounced in the cat (unpublished results).

Intestine. The SP-positive fibers were considerably more numerous that the SOM-positive ones whereas, qualititatively, their distribution in the colon and lower part of the small intestine was very similar. However, the SP-positive fibers were found not only in the basal parts of the lamina propria but also in its apical parts.

Spinal ganglia. It could clearly be established that SP-immunoreactivity and SOM-immunoreactivity were present in different cell populations (Figs. 14, 15).

Control experiments

After incubation with control sera none of the structures described above exhibited immunofluorescence.

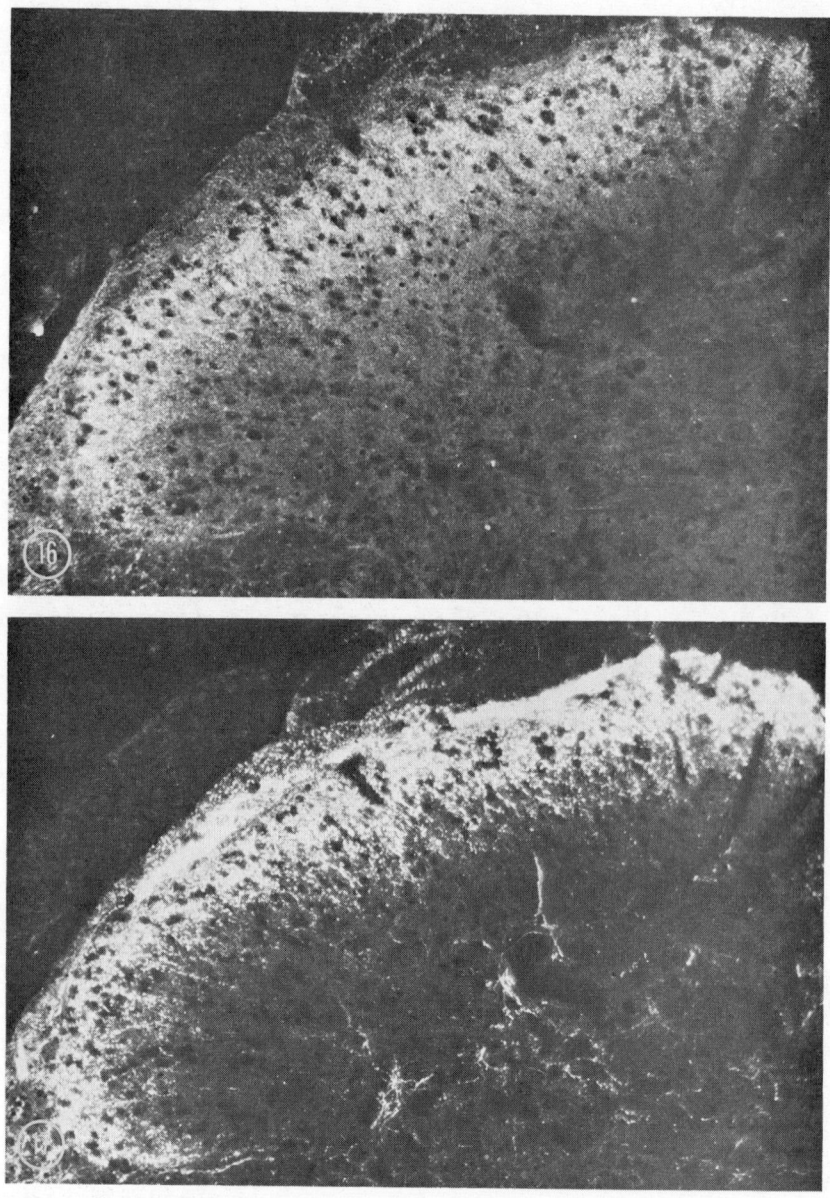

Figs. 16 and 17. Immunofluorescence micrographs of consecutive sections of the dorsal horn of the rat spinal cord after incubation with SOM antiserum and SP antiserum, respectively. The distribution of SOM- and SP-positive fibers in the dorsal horn is very similar. From Hökfelt et al. (15). Magnification 104X.

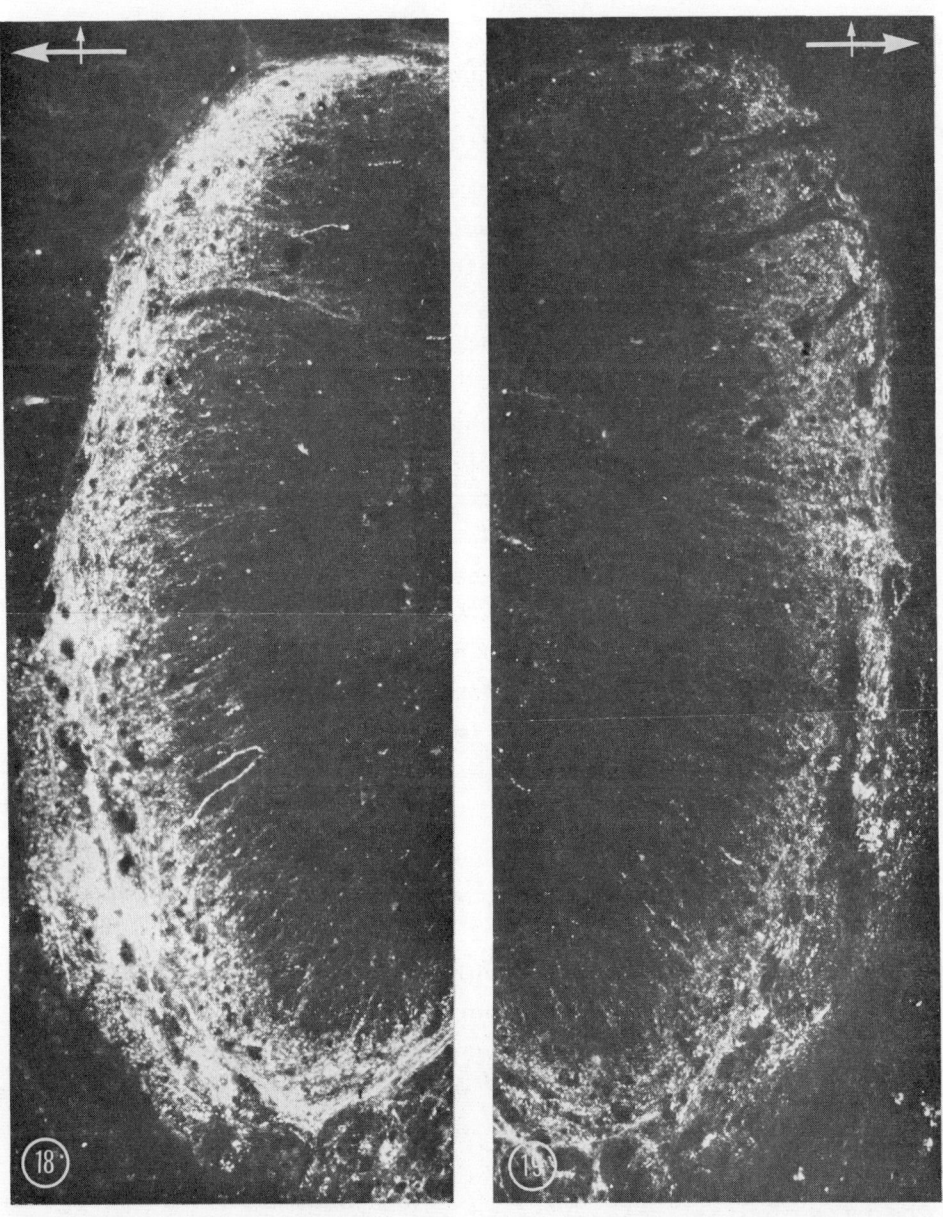

Figs. 18 and 19. Immunofluorescence micrographs of the dorsal horn of control side (Fig. 18) and lesion side (Fig. 19) ten days after dorsal rhizotomy, a marked decrease in the number of SP-positive fibers is observed on the lesion side. Big arrow points dorsally, small arrow medially. Magnification 104X.

COMMENTS

The present results give evidence for SP-positive and SOM-positive cell bodies in spinal ganglia and nerve fibers in the dorsal horns of the spinal cord and in many peripheral tissues including skin. Thus, there exist in all probability two populations of primary sensory neurons containing SP and SOM, respectively. The distribution of both SP- and SOM-positive fibers in the dorsal horn is very similar to the distribution of small--caliber primary afferents as described on the basis of classical neuroanatomical techniques by Szentágothai (30, see also 28). With regard to SP these findings are in good agreement with earlier biochemical results (31, 32), whereas, to our knowledge, SOM has so far not been demonstrated in sensory neurons. It should, however, be emphasized that although the immunoreaction observed is specific in the sense that it is abolished by pretreatment of the antisera with SP and SOM, respectively, cross--reactivity with other, unknown peptide(s) cannot be excluded. Thus, it is probably more appropriate to use the terms SP-like and SOM-like immunoreactivity (SPLl and SOMLl).

Qualititatively, both SP and SOM neurons belong to the small--sized neurons (type B of Andres (1)). The SP fibers in the ganglia and in peripheral tissues seem to be thin, unmyelinated fibers. Quantitatively, these two types of neurons do not seem to constitute more than about 25% of all neurons in spinal ganglia, although careful calculations are necessary to establish their true numbers. Furthermore, since it is difficult to visualize certain peptides in cell bodies (see above), negative results have to be interpreted with caution. Thus, it cannot be excluded that more primary sensory neurons than 25% contain SP or SOM.

The physiological role(s) of SP and SOM in sensory neurons is not clearly defined. The Japanese group has shown that SP exerts an _excitatory_ action on the membrane potential of spinal motoneurons (19, see also 12), supporting earlier hypotheses (11, 20, 25) of SP being the transmitter of primary sensory neurons. The role of SOM is at present not understood. In several brain areas SOM exerts a depressant action (27) and in several peripheral tissues SOM inhibits secretion of hormones such as insulin and glucagon (for ref. see 13). Thus, whereas SP could act as an excitatory transmitter substance in primary sensory neurons, SOM, or a cross-reacting peptide, may more likely represent an inhibitory principle. The latter idea is, however, at present without any experimental support.

If there exist subpopulations of primary sensory neurons characterized by certain peptides, the question arises whether or not these different systems have a defined function, i.e. are involved in the conduction of a specific modality. Recent electrophysiological studies by Henry (12) indicate that SP may be involved "in regulating the level of excitability of spinal neurones in nociceptive pathways". Our findings that the SP neurons are of the small type (B-group according to Andres (1)) and in all probability have unmyelinated fibers are in conformity with this view. Furthermore, the extensive networks of SP--positive terminals in lamina I agrees well with the results of Christensen and Perl (6), who found that cells responding specifically to noxious mechanical and thermal stimuli are located in this lamina.

CONCLUSIONS

With the indirect immunofluorescence technique of Coons and collaborators evidence has been obtained that substance P (SP) and somatostatin (SOM) are present in primary sensory neurons. Both peptides were found in neuronal cell bodies of the small type in spinal ganglia, in probable nerve fibers in the dorsal horn of the spinal cord and in peripheral nerves in many tissues including skin. Staining of consecutive sections of spinal ganglia, however, clearly demonstrated that SP and SOM are present in different cells. Thus, at least three populations of primary sensory neurons may exist based on immunohistochemical criteria: SP-positive and SOM-positive neurons and such containing neither of these peptides. Quantitatively the two groups may constitute approximately one quarter of all neuronal cell bodies in spinal ganglia.

ACKNOWLEDGEMENTS

This work was supported by grants from the Swedish Medical Research Council (04X-2887, 04X-2886, 19X-3412, 04X-04495), Magn. Bergwalls Stiftelse, Knut och Alice Wallenbergs Stiftelse and Harald och Greta Jeanssons Stiftelse. R.E. was supported by an NIH National Research Service Award NS 05047-01 from the NINCDS.

The skilful technical assistance of Miss A. Nygård is gratefully acknowledged.

REFERENCES

1. Andres, K.H. 1961. Untersuchungen über den Feinbau von Spinalganglien. Z. Zellforsch. 55: 1-48.
2. Arimura, A., Sato, H., Coy, D.H. and Schally, A.V. 1975. Radioimmunoassay for GH-release inhibiting factor. Proc. soc. exp. Biol. (N.Y.) 148: 784-789.
3. Barry, J., Dubois, M.P. and Poulain, P. 1973. LRF-producing cells of the mammalian hypothalamus. Z. Zellforsch. 146: 351-366.
4. Brazeau, P., Vale, W., Burgus, R., Ling, N., Butcher, M., Rivier, J. and Guillemin, R. 1973. Hypothalamic polypeptide that inhibits the secretion of immunoreactive pituitary growth hormone. Science 179: 77-79.
5. Chang, M.M., Leeman, S.E. and Niall, H.D. 1971. Amino acid sequence of substance P. Nature New Biol. 232: 86-87.
6. Christensen, B.N. and Perl, E.R. 1970. Spinal neurons specifically excited by noxious or thermal stimuli: the marginal zone of the dorsal horn. J. Neurophysiol. 33: 293-307.
7. Coons, A.H. 1958. Fluorescent antibody methods. In General Cytochemical Methods (ed. Danielli, J.F.) pp.399-422. Academic Press, New York.
8. Curtis, D.R. and Johnston, G.A.R. 1974. Amino acid transmitters in the mammalian central nervous system. Rev. Physiol. 69: 97-188.

9. Dahlström, A. 1970. The effects of drugs on axonal transport of amine storage vesicles. In New aspects of storage and release mechanisms of catecholamines.(eds. Schumann, H. J. and Kroneberg, G.) pp.20-36. Springer, Berlin, Heidelberg, New York.

10. Euler, U.S.v. and Gaddum, J.H. 1931. An unidentified depressor substance in certain tissue extracts. J. Physiol. (Lond.) 72: 74-87.

11. Hellauer, H. 1953. Zur Charakterisierung der Erregungssubstanz sensibler Nerven. Naunym-Schmiedeberg's Arch. exp. Path. Pharmak. 219: 234-241.

12. Henry, J.L. 1975. Substance P excitation of spinal nociceptive neurones. Neuroscience Abstracts I: 390.

13. Hökfelt, T., Efendić, S., Hellerström, C., Johansson, O., Luft, R. and Arimura, A. 1975a. Cellular localization of somatostatin in endocrine-like cells and neurons of the rat with special reference to the A_1-cells of the pancreatic islets and the hypothalamus. Acta endocr. 80 Suppl.200: 1-41.

14. Hökfelt, T., Elde, R., Johansson, O., Luft, R. and Arimura, A. 1975b. Immunohistochemical evidence for the presence of somatostatin, a powerful inhibitory peptide, in some primary sensory neurons. Neuroscience Letters 1: 231-235.

15. Hökfelt, T., Elde, R., Johansson, O., Luft, R., Nilsson, G. and Arimura, A. 1976. Immunohistochemical evidence for separate populations of somatostatin-containing and substance P-containing primary afferent neurons. Neuroscience, in press.

16. Hökfelt, T., Fuxe, K., Goldstein, M. and Joh, T.H. 1973. Immunohistochemical studies of 3 catecholamines synthesizing enzymes: aspects on methodology. Histochemie 33: 231-254.

17. Hökfelt, T., Kellerth, J.-O., Nilsson, G. and Pernow, B. 1975c. Substance P: Localization in the central nervous system and in some primary sensory neurons. Science 190: 889-890.

18. Hökfelt, T., Kellerth, J.-O., Nilsson, G. and Pernow, B. 1975d. Experimental immunohistochemical studies on the localization and distribution of substance P in cat primary sensory neurons. Brain Res. 100: 235-252.

19. Konishi, S. and Otsuka, M. 1974. The effects of Substance P and other peptides on spinal neurons of the frog. Brain Res. 65: 397-410.

20. Lembeck, F. 1953. Zur Frage der zentralen Übertragung afferenter Impulse. I. Mitteilung. Das Vorkommen und die Bedeutung der Substanz P in den dorsalen Wurzeln des Rückenmarks. Naunyn-Schmiedeberg's Arch. exp. Path. Pharmak. 219: 197-213.

21. Nilsson, G., Hökfelt, T. and Pernow, B. 1974. Distribution of substance P-like immunoreactivity in the rat central nervous system as revealed by immunohistochemistry. Med. Biol. 52: 424-427.

22. Nilsson, G., Larsson, L.I., Håkansson, R., Brodin, E., Sundler, F. and Pernow, B. 1975. Localization of Substance P-like immunoreactivity in mouse gut. Histochemistry 43: 97-99.

23. Nilsson, G., Pernow, B., Fischer, G.H. and Folkers, K. 1975. Presence of substance P-like immunoreactivity in plasma from man and dog. Acta physiol. scand. 94: 542-544.

24. Pease, D.C. 1962. Buffered formaldehyde as a killing agent and primary fixative for electron microscopy. Anat. Rec. 142: 342.

25. Pernow, B. 1953. Studies on substance P. Purification, occurrence and biological actions. Acta physiol. scand. 29: Suppl.105, 1-90.

26. Powell, D., Leeman, S., Tregear, G.W., Niall, H.D. and Potts, J.T.Jr. 1973. Radioimmunoassay for Substance P. Nature New Biol. 241: 252-254.

27. Renaud, L.P., Martin, J.B. and Brazeau, P. 1975. Depressant action of TRH, LH-RH and somatostatin on activity of central neurones. Nature (Lond.), 225: 233-235.

28. Réthelyi, M. and Szentágothai, J. 1973. Distribution and connections of afferent fibers in the spinal cord. In Handbook of sensory physiology, Vol. II (ed. Iggo, A.) pp. 207-252.

29. Rexed, B. 1954. A cytoarchitechtonic atlas of the spinal cord in the cat. J. comp. Neurol. 100: 297-379.

30. Szentágothai, J. 1964. Neuronal and synaptic arrangement in the substantia gelatinosa Rolandi. J. comp. Neurol. 122: 219-240.

31. Takahashi, T. and Otsuka, M. 1975. Regional distribution of Substance P in the spinal cord and nerve roots of the cat and the effect of dorsal root section. Brain Res. 87: 1-11.

32. Takahashi, T., Konishi, S., Powell, D., Leeman, S.E. and Otsuka, M. 1974. Identification of the motoneuron-depolarizing peptide in bovine dorsal root as hypothalamic Substance P. Brain Res. 73: 59-69.

33. Vale, W., Brazeau, P., Rivier, C., Brown, M., Boss, B., Rivier, J., Burgus, R., Ling, N. and Guillemin, R. 1975. Somatostatin. Rec. Progr. Horm. Res. 31: 365-392.

Discussion:

Perl: This paper is now open for discussion. May I take the chairman's prerogative and ask you to speculate about the possible correlation between the substances that Dr Liebeskind talked about, encephalin and somatostatin in particular, or Substance P. I know it is said to be different than Substance P but it was reported by Snyder's group by Pert actually, to concentrate again in the superficial lamina of the spinal cord. Is it possible that the internal morphine-like substance as tested in fact could be nothing or less than a receptor that has a common affinity for a transmitter and for some agents?

Kellerth: I will attempt to answer that question. Actually, the trouble with somatostatin is dealing with Substance P. It has been suspected for a long time that Substance P might be a transmitter substance. But there have been some difficulties with this. First, with regards to the effects of iontophoretic application on neurons. The effects have sometimes been reported to be very slow and rather long-lasting which one would not expect if it was a transmitter substance with a momentary action. Secondly, it has also been reported sometimes not to have any effect at all. This might also be explained by technical difficulties because, if, when you use these multi-barrel electrodes, you record their activity in the vicinity of the cell soma that is also where you inject the substance you are testing. Now if the receptors are located far away, on the dendritic tree, you would have several other facts to calculate, for example, diffusion, dilution and so on. So negative results would not be that crucial, I think. But so far no one has shown that Substance P is actually released during neural stimulation. And that is something that we are trying to design experiments for now, to find out if it actually is or not.

Uvnäs: I would like to ask you if your technique or the techniques of others permit one to see if these substances (Substance P or somatostatin) if they are localized in radices or in the cytoplasm. I heard somebody say that one substance was localized in the cytoplasm. Now this is of importance, of course, if you discuss how it could be stored and how it could be released since most transmitters, as I know, are localized and stored in a way so they are ready for excitosis. Can you give me a comment?

Kellerth: We cannot tell from our light microscopical pictures. What you need then, of course, is electron microscopic pictures. We intend to try to get those too. But at this point I would not like to tell whether they are in vesicles or not.

Zimmermann: I have two questions: 1) Most probably there are many other aminoacids and polypeptides transported in axonal flow, which subserve the various synaptic and trophic functions of the nerve terminals. Did you try other substances with your method, or did you try these two, and found them? 2) How do you explain the persistence of some Substance P in the laminae I to III of the dorsal horn after complete deafferentation?

Kellerth: The answer to your second question might of course be that you also have intraspinal pathways descending or ascending that pass through this region. So far we have only done hemi-sections of the spinal cord which unfortunately did not seem to influence it very much. It still persisted after rhizitomy in combination with hemi-section. But we now plan to do total section of the spinal cord to see if that would effect the persistent activity. As to the first question, we did not try other substances.

Zimmermann: You found both these substances?

Kellerth: Substance P is the only substance which has been debated for several years. Somatostatin has also been discussed for some time. People have found it in more and more places. We had antibodies against it so we tried it.

Zotterman: You know that there are children born without any perception of pain. They have been found to have an extra chromosome between 14 and

15. They have succeeded in helping them to reach adult life. Generally in the past they have met their fatal accident fairly early in life. They scald themselves in hot water etc. But they have sensations of cold and warm so you have to warn them that when they feel very warm then that may be very dangerous for them. They crack their teeth and legs and so on and have fatal accidents because they cannot feel any pain. They have examined them post mortem, of course, but they found no difference whatsoever in the central or peripheral nervous system. Therefore it would be very interesting to see how this Substance P and somatostatin appear in these cases. The next thing I would like to propose is that you looked for it in rats deficient in the essential amino acid tyrosin. They show an enormous irritability. They jump high on the slightest touch.

Ottoson: There is a recent case described where a boy was born without pain. When he was examined later on they found no fine C-fibers in the dorsal root.

Santini: As you know glycine and glutamic acid and alanine and aspartic acid are produced in dorsal root ganglia along the dorsal root fibers. I have tried to interfere with the ganglionic production of these amino acids by injecting dopa or serotonin and in other cases monaminoxidase inhibitors. I could get a significant and drastic decrease of these amino acids in the dorsal root ganglia which were transported in a minor amount to the spinal cord. So I wonder whether this could also be the case for Substance P and somatostatin.

CONCLUDING DISCUSSION

WHAT ABOUT THE FUTURE?

Perl: It is now time for the discussion in which we are supposed to look into the future. I am going to do a terrible thing. Those of you who have not run out of the room may be called on to make comments because I believe it is perhaps worthwhile to hear from some people who have sat through this meeting and might now think and give us the benefit of their ideas. Professor Paintal, do you have any view for the future? You gave us a unifying hypothesis to start off with which you wanted us to challenge. Would you like to say something about what you see or what you would like to see?

Paintal: I have really learned a lot from this. I thought that by the end of this meeting somebody would be having a sack of tomatoes to throw at me. But nobody has thrown any tomatoes so I am very unhappy at my hypothesis of course. I had wished that somebody would have challenged it and said this is what is wrong with it because it would help me to go further along these lines. But it seems to me that when one considers these stimuli we have seen a lot of work being done on the injection of drugs and here I would only use one minute in connection with what Dr Perl said with regard to infusion. The infusion was the injection. I think the injection is a very useful device. It is reproducable and it has several merits over the infusion because the infusion if you ever use drugs for stimulating sensory receptors you find that during the course of the infusion the receptor itself gets anaphylactic or into the presistent presence of the substance. Apart from that I think that as far as the muscle receptors are concerned a lot of work really needs to be done here on the muscle C-fibers because it looks to me that even though people have shown resting discharges in C-fibers nobody has told what is the possible natural stimulus of these C-fibers. That is a resting discharge but what is it being produced by? That we do not know. Some indications have been given that it might be due to the experimental procedure itself owing to the fact that during the course of the experiment you get more resting discharges. I think this is a very important thing to look at because muscle pain is an important feature of our lives. At one state I had asked somebody whether any work had been done on the pain from ligaments in cases like lumbago and slipped discs and so on where the slightest movement make you shriek with pain. These things have not been tested and I suppose animal models would be available to test these things like that tyrosine deficient rat for instance that suddenly jumps.

Perl: I think that Professor Iggo was curteous enough to come back into the room knowing that he might be called on. I am going to call on him and ask if he has any ideas he would like to share with us as to the future in particular or the past as he sees it.

Iggo: Well, I think there are one or two areas where I can see we are going to need help of the multidisciplinary kind. It was really quite interesting to have the last paper presented by people who are now using biochemical techniques because the meeting has been very strongly influenced by our honorary president Yngve Zotterman's life-long interest in electrophysiology. And I think it is fair to say that a large part of the results we have been talking about have been electrophysiological in origin. And yet the nervous system has a chemical basis. We have had people going to the shelf and taking down the bottle and putting in a slug of this or a slug of that and seeing what happened. But I think that we are going to have to spend much more time in the future actually being concerned with the chemistry of the receptor systems. Yes, but I think we are going to need a lot more of it. We now are learning more about the chemicals which have a fleeting existence in the nervous system which are going to need new techniques to detect. I have kept coming back several times in this meeting to the question of what happens between the injection and the discharge of the impulses. Often a latency of several seconds is involved. In fact these chemicals are not acting at a single site. It is quite clear from quite old recordings that histamine, for example, although it may be altering the sensitivity of the receptor in some way is also effecting transmission at some peripheral part of the fiber. So that is one area where I think we can expect to see big developments. Another point that stuck me I suppose partly from my own work but also listening to the discussions was that it is clearly insufficient to imagine that the central nervous system behaves much the same way as the peripheral afferent fibers particularly in the question of the way information is coded. With carefully controlled quantitative stimulation of the receptors and with computers to back us up we can now provide a very quantitatively exact description of the peripheral stimulus in terms of the interspike interval in the afferent fibers. But except in perhaps a rapidly adapting system the nervous system does not simply take over the peripheral input and reproduce it exactly. As the dorsal horn cold neurons show it seem to behave in a rather unfriendly way. So I think there is going to have to be some new development in our thinking about what the central nervous system does with these often very finely graded and quantitatively expressed peripheral data. I think that a third comment that I might make is that for a long time I think again because we were recording from the afferent fibers we tended to believe that impulses that followed each other at high frequency were the things that really mattered. That a brisk discharge with lots of impulses was really what was making the nervous system work. Well, the muscle afferent fibers have shown you can have very low rates of discharge in the afferent fiber and yet these might be having quite potent central actions although that is not yet properly established. And I think we are going to have to pay more attention perhaps to these rather low-frequency noisy little bits of activity occurring out in the periphery. This goes back to my previous comment that central nervous system is not just reproducing what comes in. Also the small fibers as several people have mentioned may have their actions much amplified in the central nervous system. So that is a third area where I think we are going to have to have fresh ideas.

Perl: Dr Gybels, I see you here. Since you have come from a different viewpoint than the electrophysiologist at least at first start would you like to make some comments about the future?

Gybels: Very few comments. I think electrophysiology has not helped us very much in understanding what is going on in the patient with pain. I am afraid that I will have to go on in a very painstaking way noting exactly what the patient is going to say and use some good techniques of electrophysiology to collaborate between the two. But I think it will be a long and hard way.

Ingvar: Partly in connection with Dr Gybels comment I think it is pertinent to bring up a clinical application of this knowledge on pain. We are as most of you are aware faced with an increasing number of patients who are deeply unconscious or who have very large and extensive defects of their central nervous systems. These are often chronic ward cases who are in the hospital for many, many years where the clinician stands there and asks himself how much does the patient suffer? I think it is extremely important that we apply our knowledge to this group of patients in order to find out whether they have cerebral pain reations so that we can plan the treatment. The number of such patients as you all know is increasing and the problem is rather imminent. What shall we do to these patients and how shall we handle them? Which patients suffer and which patients do not suffer? And there is where we come in with the ethical problem.

Paintal: I got the impression listening to these talks that the use of the computer has gone down. Is that a fact? I thought that a few years ago everybody used some kind of a computing system. I actually saw data in the raw this time and that was a real pleasure. Is this because people are preferring raw data to cox data? Is my impression correct that people are now giving up processing as an essential element in their experiments?

Many voices: "We're just not mentioning it." "Yes, we do." "It turns up because we have so much work to do. But we often have to go back to the records." "It saves a lot of labour. And labour is expensive."

Iggo: I think that question is rather like asking why don't we still put up illustrations of our oscilliscopes? We do use computers.

Perl: I think that may be a sampling error. We use it but do not mention it. It is a bad thing to do to a friend. But we are talking about the future. Dr Hensel you made the mistake of walking in and I know that you have some ideas about how we might do things in the future that is some possibilities where we might learn something by doing some things in the future that we do not do now. I wondered if you had come up for Professor Zotterman and give him the benefit of some of your ideas.

Hensel: I would say that after having done so much work in recording afferent traffic in the peripheral nerve and in the spinal cord and thalamus and so on I think it might be worthwhile now to return to sensation and to retry the whole story again as we have actually started to do it in Marburg. I think it would be worthwhile with such a lot of information about what is going on in the nervous system to try to put together the picture and ask what all this nervous traffic and information might be good for. I think it would be necessary now to try to get again the whole picture and to become a bit more interested in sensation again. That would be one of my suggestions for future work.

Perl: I am using up all my good will but I see George Gordon back there looking pensive. Would you like to add something to this, speculation for the future?

Gordon: I had hoped that I had been keeping what is now called a low profile but I am not, unfortunately, built that way. So I was noticed. It strikes me that there is one aspect of semiaesthetic mechanisms which has not been very much stressed here but which must very much be a feature of the future. It is of course a very well known fact that tactile discrimination to take a single sensory phenomenon is very much more effective when the finger moves over the object which it is exploring. In other words, we have perhaps been speaking of sensation in a kind of artificial isolation from movement. There have been various references the paradox for instance, and some of the comments that Dr Hyvärinen has made making it clear that there is a link between what starts in the skin and what comes out in the finger. This must be a kind of sequential circuit when you are exploring and recognizing objects. So in the future I can see that we shall have to make what may be quite a difficult and painful recap in the first place with people who have always considered themselves to be motorphysiologists. I think that is perhaps enough for me to say. I hope that will happen in the next year or two.

Perl: Thank you. I had about two hours more notice than several of you on the fact that there was going to be this sort of a summing up attempt. And since I promised not to write this down, Yngve, I am going to point out a few things. It is a little over a hundred years since our knowledge of neuroanatomy began to fall into what you might consider a modern perspective. I know that it is about seventy years since Sherrington published his lectures on the integrative action of the nervous system and fifty years since Adrian and Zotterman first recorded the discharges of single impulses. I should observe that things have changed in our knowledge. It is painfully slow but we do understand more than we did a hundred years ago. I should submit that we probably know a good deal more about many things including pain than we did a hundred years ago. Also, we might be able to deal with people somewhat more intelligently than what we would have then. I think that Professor Iggo has already commented on some of the things that struck me. I noticed a few others too. One, it is perfectly obvious that we still do not know how receptors are activated. We do not know the intimate processes of receptor activation. That still lies before us. We know a little bit about what receptors say to the central nervous system. I do not have any great hopes for seeing answers to how all receptors are activated in the future that I can participate in but I think there might be some changes. The last paper that we heard brought home the fact that we still have a lot to learn about central transmitters in fact we have just scratched the surface; we hardly know anything. I do suspect that we are going to learn more about central transmitters and that we are going to learn using the combination of techniques that involve electrophysiology, anatomy and biochemical approaches. As Dr Hyvärinen pointed out to us there is still a lot to learn about central processing of information. We have again only barely scratched the surface. We do not even know the circuitry for most of the projections that we are talking about. We just know the major pathways. We do not know any of the intimate details and some of those are dreadfully important. We have heard about inhibition, we have heard about lots of other things where we can modify some of the central projections. It is obvious that this is a fruitful field and that is a field that perhaps some combination of some electrical physiology and biochemical approaches might be useful as well as some of the newer anatomy. Finally, I think that Dr Ingvar has pointed out something that neurophysiologists by and large have ignored namely the relation of metabolic activity to the central nervous system action and how metabolic activity may influence central nervous system action. By and large we have not used metabolic tools to follow central nervous system action because it has not been fast enough. But perhaps the future will bring us some modifications of these tools that will allow us to follow metabolic activity. Obviously if there is a blood flow change there is some change in metabolic activity. These are important clues. And I predict that we will see some increasing knowledge about the relation between metabolic activity and the way that the brain works. If there are any other comments that anyone in the audience would wish to make, this is the moment. Professor Zotterman, do you have any thoughts?

Zotterman: I have no future as an experimenter as I have no lab any longer. It moved to Uppsala. This is in contrast to you others who can go home and start continuing your useful work. About twenty years ago I was asked by a morning paper what I thought about the future of the study of the nervous system. I can recollect at the moment that I said that we are looking forward to an era where we can, for instance, use electricity instead of some drugs which have too complicated effects. You press a button and you go to sleep when you put an electrode here or there.

Generally I would say that I have been delighted to see how much you now can get out of experiments on monkeys and on human subjects. All the animal experiments I did in the 1930's on pain fibers can now be made in men by more sophisticated methods. But I also worked on man in the 1930's because I always wanted to check the results of my animal experiments on myself or my assistants by psychophysical methods. After all it is the physical correlate to our experienced sensations which is the big game we are hunting. It has of course been an enormous pleasure for me to see so many of my old observations confirmed from recordings from human nerves. I look forward now to an era where more experiments can be performed on man and much more information particularly about the functions of the nervous system will be obtained on man. After all, there is a great difference even between the cat, which is a comparatively high mammal and man. For that reason I am looking forward very much to the future developments of physiological, still more sophisticated methods which can be used in experiments on man. I look forward to an era of intimate team work by neurophysiologists, psychologists, biochemists, neurobiologists, circulatory physiologists, clinical scientists and pharmacologists etc, the whole spectrum of life scientists.

Iggo: I do not know if there is any formal end to this meeting. But just in case everybody goes away before we discuss this matter of pain I would like, I think, on behalf of all to thank, if nobody else is going to do it, the organizers, Zotterman, Lindblom, Vallbo and Hagbarth who put together this meeting. It has been, I think, we all agree, an exhausting but exhilerating event. For Yngve in particular I can imagine that he can now look back on half a century of contributions to sensory physiology. And although other people have without a doubt done their bit to make this meeting a success I think it is to him that we really ought to now be saying thank you for a very splendid occasion.

Zotterman: As a matter of fact mutual contributions have made it. I know that this was the exact time to have this meeting because there has been such an advance of knowledge in the last five years particularly as the experiments have focused on primates and humans. Thank you very much for coming and for taking all the trouble in preparing your papers. I know what it means and I feel extremely grateful that so many, who are so busy in actual research, as all of you are, have taken the time and the trouble to come to this place here up in the high north during such a winter as we are having now. Thank you from all my heart.